The Family Guide to Homeopathy

Dr Andrew Lockie was born in Glasgow and was brought up in the countryside in the Central Lowlands of Scotland. He graduated in Medicine from Aberdeen University, then moved to London and gained his membership of the Faculty of Homeopathy after studying at the Royal London Homeopathic Hospital. After a short spell in practice he gained his membership of the Royal College of General Practitioners, his diploma in Obstetrics and Gynaecology, and the Family Planning Certificate, working in the Oxford region and the New Forest. In 1978 he returned to London and opened his first homeopathic practice in Ealing, supplementing his income at first by working for the local GP deputizing service. Later he opened two branch surgeries in Surrey and became Medical Director of the Enton Hall Health Hydro before consolidating his practices in Guildford, where he is now based.

Dr Lockie is a homeopathic consultant to the *Journal of Alternative & Complementary Medicine* and has written numerous articles for both the medical and the lay press. He has been the guest homeopathic doctor on the Peter Murray Show on LBC, and has made other radio and TV appearances.

Dr Lockie is married to an acupuncturist. They have four children and live in Surrey.

THE FAMILY GUIDE TO HOMEOPATHY

The Safe Form of Medicine for the Future

Dr Andrew Lockie

TO GMJ, who showed me the thing I most needed to know

HAMISH HAMILTON LTD

Published by the Penguin Group
Penguin Books Ltd, 27 Wrights Lane, London W8 5TZ, England
Penguin Books USA Inc., 375 Hudson Street, New York, New York 10014, USA
Penguin Books Australia Ltd, Ringwood, Victoria, Australia
Penguin Books Canada Ltd, 10 Alcorn Avenue, Toronto, Ontario, Canada M4V 3B2
Penguin Books (NZ) Ltd, 182–190 Wairau Road, Auckland 10, New Zealand

Penguin Books Ltd, Registered Offices: Harmondsworth, Middlesex, England

First published in Great Britain by Elm Tree Books 1989
Published in paperback by Hamish Hamilton Ltd 1990
7 9 10 8 6

Copyright © Dr Andrew Lockie, 1989

The moral right of the author has been asserted

Typeset by Cambridge Photosetting Services
Reproduced, printed and bound in Great Britain by
BPCC Hazell Books
Aylesbury, Bucks, England
Member of BPCC Ltd.

Contents

ACKNOWLEDGEMENTS

To Babs, for her love, support, understanding, and wisdom

To David, Kirsty, Alastair and Sandy, for their love and tolerance of their fazed father

To Anne Cope, for her editorial skill and stamina

The author would like to thank the following people and organizations:

Ainsworths, Nelsons, and Weleda (product information)
Nim Barnes (preconceptual care)
Sally Bundy (hyperactivity)
John Davidson (electromagnetic phenomena)
Chris Donne (for typing a mountain)
Light Research Council
Hahnemann Society
British Homoeopathic Association
Faculty of Homoeopathy
Jeanette Marshall (nutrition)
Simon Martin (for pointing me in the right directions)
Tony Pinkus (interesting conversations of a political nature)
David Reynolds (at whose instigation the book was written)
Vicky Rippers (clinical ecology)
Caroline Taggart, for her faith and encouragement
Richard Solway and Geoffrey Taylor Institute (water filters)
Margaret Williams (for keeping my practice ticking over)
Helmut Ziehe (building ecology)

For information about alternative therapies the author would like to thank:

Hazel Bentley, Sandra Billings, Pat Chittananda, Farida Davidson, Stephen Davis, Jesper Dokkedal, Philip and Carol Grealy, Nida Ingham, Sue Makin, Rosemary Nott, Robert Tisserand, Richard Thomas, Michael Van Straten, Jeff Wictome, Arvid Willen, David Wood, even though much of the excellent material had to be edited out.

The publishers would also like to thank:

Philip Boys and Steve Parker (editorial assistance), Shona Grant (illustrations), Norman Reynolds (text design)

The author would also like to express his appreciation and gratitude for the expert scrutiny of the proofs of the book and the constructive criticism afforded him by his colleagues:

Dr Nuria Booth
Dr Michael Callander
Dr 'Jace' Clarke
Dr David Curtin
Dr Charles Forsyth
Dr Mike Hart
Dr Roger Lichy
Dr John Nicholls
Dr David Owen

INTRODUCTION

'The Physician's highest calling, his only *calling is to make sick people healthy – to heal, as it is termed.'*

Hahnemann, Organon VIth Edition.

Thank you for acquiring this book. Whilst it is loosely based on *Ruddock's Domestic Physician,* an early twentieth century family guide to Homeopathy, I have tried to make it completely relevant to the needs of the end of the 20th century and those of the 21st.

I felt it had to be written because orthodox medicine is quite clearly failing to meet the medical needs of the population. Contrary to what politicians claim, more and more patients being treated by the National Health Service does not represent a success. On the contrary it means that it has failed to cure people. I believe there are several reasons for this. The single most important one is the deliberate move away from looking at people *as a whole.* This is in spite of impressive evidence that what takes place in the intellect, emotions and, perhaps, soul of a human being directly affects their body, and vice versa.

This has led to an increasingly mechanistic view of disease and consequent reliance on physical methods of treatment such as drugs, surgery, radiation and other 'high tech' methods. Whilst there can be no denying that these have been successful in some disorders, they are not appropriate for the majority of diseases seen in general practice. They are also responsible for at least 14% of hospital admissions, which represents the tip of an iceberg. People have lost confidence as a result: in fact some 50% of drugs prescribed are never taken.

It has also been shown that the very foundations of scientific medicine in theoretical physics are 20 years out of date. Even so it is from this standpoint of observational objectivity, which has proved to be untrue, that critics of alternative or complementary medicine launch their attacks.

Thanks mainly to public opinion, however, times are changing. The last twenty years have seen a dramatic rise in interest in alternative or complementary medicine amongst doctors and other health care professionals. The importance of treating disease gently by nurturing and stimulating the body's own immune system and other healing mechanisms is being increasingly acknowledged.

It is now recognised by most health care profes-sionals that no *one* system of medicine has all the answers for all the ills that afflict mankind, any more than any one doctor can hope to cure every problem in every patient every time. We all need to work together. The main problem is to know which is the most appropriate treatment for any particular patient. Obviously, the less life-threatening and more chronic the condition, the more sense it makes to use non-toxic and immune-system-boosting therapies first, and only to progress to potentially harmful methods if these fail or the situation becomes more critical. In the case of acute, serious illness we still have to rely heavily on proven orthodox methods, at least until we have had more experience of using alternative or complementary therapies in these situations.

This is the spirit in which this book has been written. It is offered to assist you in helping yourself in minor accidents and ailments and to tell you when to stop. It is also to support you when facing more serious situations. It tells you who to call and how quickly to act, and also what you can do whilst waiting for assistance.

Please read the opening chapters carefully, espe-cially Parts 1 and 3 and the opening remarks to Part 5, before attempting to use the book, so that you are familiar with the philosophy of homeopathy, and with the way the book is constructed. Please pay particular attention to the meaning of the symbols used for determining how to get assistance. Please note that throughout this book, when you are referred to a 'homeopath' this means a medically qualified homeo-pathic physician. If a medically qualified homeopathic physician is not available in your area and you wish to consult a non-medically qualified homeopath, the author advises that you do this under the continuing observation of your own GP.

I hope that when you have done all this and used the remedies for yourself, you will agree with me that Homeopathy goes a long way towards meeting Lord Colwyn's criteria for an ideal medical system. These are that it should be effective, have minimal or no risk for the patient, strengthen the constitution (increase well being and the ability to live life to the full) and not palliate, not be expensive, be accessible and under-stood by all members of the public and be linked to the general ecological good.

Finally, please remember that no book can be a

substitute for a good and caring physician and so, if you are in doubt, CALL YOUR DOCTOR!

Introduction for Health Care Practitioners

It is my sincere hope that all my fellow practitioners, especially homeopaths, will find this book of use in their practices. It represents a synthesis of what one man has experienced in his vocation over the years. Inevitably this is bound to be more concentrated in some fields than others and so, where I have felt my knowledge to be inadequate I have borrowed from the experience of others. My main sources are listed in the bibliography at the end of the book. I would welcome any suggestions and constructive criticism, sent to me c/o my publisher.

My intention has been to keep the indications for each remedy short as I feel people become over-powered otherwise and lose interest. It was for that reason that I included the mini repertory or General Remedy Finder. I hope this will encourage people to look for the other symptoms making up the Totality of the case and thus to appreciate more about how we work in practice. On the other hand I hope that by giving strict rules and duration guides, I have succeeded in getting them to ask for help when the case is not suitable for self care. This is always a difficult balance to achieve and I would, again, welcome any comments you may have on whether this has been achieved. I also hope I can be forgiven for using the American spelling of Homoeopathy, which has been done for the sake of simplicity.

I offer this book to my colleagues in General Practice and Hospital Medicine in the hope that it may inspire them to experiment with this remarkably safe addition to their therapeutic armamentarium. I hope they will be as satisfied with it as I have become over the years. If they wish to take it further, I can assure them of a warm welcome at the courses run in various parts of the country. Simply phone the Education secretary at the nearest Homeopathic hospital and ask for details of the Postgraduate curriculum. For addresses and phone numbers see 387–8.

Part 1

WHAT IS HOMEOPATHY

HOMEOPATHY is an exceptionally safe form of medicine which treats the whole individual. It is equally concerned with maintaining good health and aiding recovery from ill health, and like all forms of medicine – even those which use powerful drugs and high technology surgery – relies for its effects on the body's own powers of self-regulation and self-healing. Since its development nearly two hundred years ago homeopathy has benefited millions of people, young and old, from all walks of life, in countries all over the world.

The word 'homeopathy' (also spelt 'homoeopathy') comes from two Greek words, *omio* meaning 'same' and *pathos* meaning 'suffering'. A homeopathic remedy is one which produces the same symptoms as those the sick person complains of, and in doing so sharply provokes the body into throwing them off. 'Like may be cured by like', also expressed as *similia similibus curentur*, is the basic principle of homeopathic therapeutics. The opposite therapeutic approach is 'allopathy', which is defined as a system of therapeutics in which diseases are treated by producing a condition incompatible with or antagonistic to the condition to be cured or alleviated.

The idea that remedies and symptoms sharing certain key features might interact in such a way as to banish illness, and the implied corollary that two similar states of discomfort cannot exist in the same body, was not new even two centuries ago. The great achievement of Samuel Hahnemann, the founder of homeopathy, was that he systematically studied, for himself, all the orthodox medical remedies of his day, noted their effects on healthy people, and then used this knowledge to give very specific and safe treatment to sick people. This was revolutionary in an age when medicines were indiscriminately prescribed, often in poisonous quantities.

Homeopathy is a naturopathic form of medicine – it seeks to assist Nature rather than bludgeon her, to assist the body's own healing energies rather than override them. The 'disease' is not only the virus or the bacteria – these are merely the organisms which move in when the body's defences are low. The discovery of legions of microorganisms since Hahnemann's time has done nothing to alter this fundamental truth. The fever, the inflammation, the diarrhoea, the headache – these are not the disease either, but the body's attempt to return to normality. Such ideas may be difficult to adjust to if one has been brought up in the belief that both attack and cure come from the outside, but they are ideas which have been accepted by humanistic physicians since the time of Hippocrates.

Another tenet of naturopathic and therefore of homeopathic philosophy is that every person is different. The same remedy, the same diet, the same general advice does not necessarily help everyone with the same ailment. Indeed there is no such thing as the same ailment; the course of a particular kind of cancer in one person will not be the same as that in another. Accordingly, homeopathy has the most flexible system of remedy prescribing of any system of therapeutics, as this book demonstrates. The most effective remedy is always the one which matches three things: the physical symptoms, the mental and emotional symptoms, and the general sensitivities of the person concerned. It is also taken in the least possible dose for the least possible time.

If homeopathy is, or becomes, your first line of health care you will probably want to consult a professional homeopath from time to time. Indeed his or her skills should complement and guide your own. The purpose of this book is to enable you to give homeopathic First Aid and to help you decide on a sensible course of action for ailments and diseases already diagnosed. It will also enable you to treat homeopathically the symptoms which do not add up to any particular ailment, symptoms which general practitioners see most of and find hardest to treat.

Homeopathy is also a rational system of medicine. If the body's defence systems are handicapped by poor diet, bad habits, destructive emotions, and environmental stresses, it stands to reason that homeopathic remedies, of themselves, will be of limited benefit. If you consult a homeopath, he or she may suggest a change of diet or lifestyle before prescribing any remedy. Homeopathy is not a system for those in search of instant, easy answers, although it can act very swiftly in acute conditions. It requires careful self-monitoring and a willingness to stick to a course of action. The prize is higher vitality and greater resistance to all disease processes.

The beginnings of homeopathy

The 'father' of homeopathy was Samuel Christian Hahnemann, born in Dresden, now in East Germany, in 1755. Despite his humble background – his father worked in a porcelain factory – he acquired a good education, became fluent in eight languages, and studied chemistry and medicine. He then set up in practice as a physician. But the accepted medical customs of his day, which included excessive purging, blood-letting, and cavalier prescribing of drugs which often caused more suffering than they cured, gnawed at his conscience, and after a few years he turned to translating rather than doctoring to earn his living.

It was while he was translating a treatise on herbs by a Dr Cullen of Edinburgh that he came across the tiny seed which was to flower into a whole new system of medicine. Cullen stated that quinine, an astringent substance purified from the bark of the cinchona tree *(Cinchona calisaya)*, was a good treatment for malaria because it was an astringent. Why, Hahnemann wondered, should quinine have an effect on malaria when other, more powerful, astringents did not? He decided to investigate. For several days he dosed himself with quinine and noted down his reactions in great detail. It seemed that in a healthy person, himself, quinine produced all the symptoms of malaria – fever, sweating, shivering, weakness. Was this why it also cured malaria?

Fascinated, Hahnemann repeated the quinine tests, which he called 'provings', on his acquaintances, again noting their reactions in meticulous detail. He then went on to test other substances in widespread use, such as arsenic, belladonna, and mercury. There were strict requirements for the people involved in these provings. They had to be healthy in mind and body; they could not take anything which might confuse the results, such as alcohol, tea, coffee, or spicy foods; and they were to avoid 'all disturbing passions'.

Hahnemann found that people's responses varied. Some of his volunteers showed one or two mild symptoms in response to a particular substance, but others experienced vigorous reactions with many and varied symptoms. The symptoms most commonly found for each substance he called 'first line' or 'keynote' symptoms. 'Second line' symptoms were less common, and 'third line' symptoms rare or idiosyncratic. Together these symptoms added up to a 'drug picture' of the substance concerned.

Using the results of his provings, Hahnemann went on to test various substances on sick people. But before he did so he questioned them thoroughly about their symptoms, general health, way of life, and attitudes, and gave them a physical examination. From each interview and examination he built up what he called a 'symptom picture', then prescribed the substance whose drug picture most closely matched it. The closer the match, the more successful the treatment. What he had suspected from his early experiments with quinine was indeed proving to be the case: a remedy and a disease which produce the same symptoms cancel each other out in some way. The adage *similia similibus*

curentur, 'like may be cured by like', was true. In his first essay on the subject, *A New Principle for Ascertaining the Curative Powers of Drugs and Some Examination of the Previous Principles*, published in 1796, he stated: 'One should imitate Nature, which at times heals a chronic illness by another additional one. One should apply in the disease to be healed, particularly if it is chronic, that remedy which is able to simulate another artificially produced disease, as similar as possible, and the former will be healed. . .' The name he gave to this new principle of healing was 'homeopathy'.

This was not the end of the story, however. To Hahnemann's dismay some of his patients reported that their symptoms actually got worse before they got better. To prevent such 'aggravations', as he called them, Hahnemann started to dilute his remedies. First he made a tincture of the substance concerned, leaving it to stand in a solvent, usually pure alcohol, for one month. He then strained off the liquid, the 'mother tincture'. Then he took one drop of mother tincture and added it to 99 drops of pure alcohol, a dilution factor of 1:100. To mix the one drop with the 99 thoroughly he 'succussed' the mixture by repeatedly banging it on a hard surface for a specific length of time. The dilution process could be repeated again and again, with each successive dilution having one hundredth the strength of the preceding dilution. If the substance was insoluble, it was triturated, or ground up, before being dissolved into solution.

To Hahnemann's surprise, diluted remedies not only forestalled 'aggravations' but seemed to act much faster and more effectively. They were, paradoxically, weaker but more potent. The process of successive dilution and succussion 'potentized' the original substance in a way which is difficult to explain.

Today, in Britain, most homeopathic remedies are available in centesimal potencies, that is successively diluted by a factor of 100. It is also possible to obtain some of them in decimal potencies, successively diluted by a factor of 10, or as mother tinctures. In this book 6c is the potency recommended for most acute or self-limiting ailments, and 30c the potency recommended in chronic conditions or emergencies. 6c means that the remedy has been diluted six times by a factor of 100, and 30c that it has been diluted 30 times by a factor of 100. This means that 30c remedies are many, many times more potent in homeopathic terms, although they contain much less original substance. A small range of remedies can be bought in most ordinary chemists, mail order companies offer a wider range, and homeopathic pharmacies and hospitals the widest range of all (see addresses p. 387–8). Many of the commonest remedies are sold as lactose (milk sugar) pilules which have been impregnated with potentized solution; these are taken by dissolving them on the tongue. Others are available as solutions which can be dropped directly on the tongue (the recommended method if you are allergic to lactose) or onto lactose pilules. Some can be obtained in lactose powder form, others as creams or ointments, and a few as injections, although only medically qualified homeopaths are allowed to give such injections. Suggestions for building a home medicine chest appear on page 35.

However, before we return to Hahnemann's work, it is important to point out that there is no such thing as a 'homeopathic remedy'. This is not a perverse statement. A remedy can be prepared homeopathically, by successive dilution and succussion and in accordance with standards laid down by the Medicines Act, but it will not *act* homeopathically unless its drug picture matches the symptom picture of the person taking it. Herein lies the art of homeopathic prescribing. An over-the-counter product which commends itself to a thoroughly miserable hay fever sufferer because it says 'for hay fever', may indeed work, but only fortuitously. A remedy specially selected to match the sufferer's constitution and personality as well as his or her most distressing hay fever symptoms would be a surer route to eventual cure. A fundamental tenet of homeopathy, and of all the healing arts, is that there is no such thing as a disease purely of the mind or body. Mind and body are one. Influence one and you influence the other. Stress one and you stress the other. The beauty of homeopathy is that its prescribing system, although complex, takes full account of the physical and the mental.

It is not difficult to imagine the scorn which Hahnemann's contemporaries poured upon his claim that weaker remedies produced stronger effects. This ran, and still runs, completely counter to the principles of clinical pharmacology. At dilutions above the eleventh or twelfth centesimal potency, does even one molecule of the original substance remain in solution? Modern physics affords a glimmer of an explanation why the energies of the original substance persist through successive dilutions and succussions, but how did Hahnemann answer his critics two centuries ago? Then, as today, the cures achieved by homeopathy are real. They cannot be dismissed because the mechanism of cure is not fully understood.

Being a chemist, Hahnemann knew that whatever active principles his dilute remedies contained, they could only be present in infinitesimal quantities. And yet the merest trace of them was enough to produce a strong effect. At some level in the body, he reasoned, there must be something which responds to such tiny hints, an extremely subtle something capable of switching the body from sickness to health, and vice versa. He called that something the 'Vital Force'.

It was this force which was responsible for the orderly and therefore healthy running of the body, and for coordinating the body's defences against disease. In fact Hahnemann thought of the Vital Force as a form of electromagnetic energy or vibration. If this coherent energy became jangled and disturbed by stress, poor diet, lack of exercise, inherited constitutional prob-

lems, or climatic change, illness would result. The signs and symptoms of the illness were the body's attempts to restore order.

Most of the ailments doctors see are 'acute' – they onset quickly, run a fairly well-defined course, and then clear up of their own accord with or without treatment. Hahnemann's rationale for prescribing homeopathic remedies in such cases was that they hastened recovery. The Vital Force, temporarily depressed, was more than equal to bouncing back. He discovered that in outbreaks of acute infection – measles for example – where the basic symptoms are usually the same for most people, the same remedy could be routinely prescribed for those afflicted; he also prescribed the same remedy as a preventive.

By contrast, 'chronic' or long-standing illnesses represent a series of minor victories and capitulations on the part of the Vital Force. Though relapses may be followed by remissions, the general trend is downwards. In his writing Hahnemann likened this process to a wearying civil war, with both sides alternately losing and winning battles. In such circumstances, the Vital Force stands sorely in need of mercenaries, or rather correctly prescribed homeopathic remedies.

Perhaps a less bellicose analogy is better suited to the spirit of homeopathy today. Let's imagine, instead, that the Vital Force is a trampoline and that the stresses which beset us all from time to time are stones dropped on to it at random from a great height. If the Vital Force is flowing strongly, the trampoline will be taut; any stone falling on to it, even quite a big one, will be flung off. A homeopathic remedy will merely provoke a quicker recoil.

But if the Vital Force is weak and confused, the trampoline will sag; it will not have the recoil energy to fling off the stones, so the stones will settle and make it sag even more. The only way to provoke a recoil sufficient to throw off the stones is to bounce something much heavier on to the trampoline, in the hope that the recoil will be fierce enough to throw off the stones along with the heavy object. This, essentially, is what homeopathic remedies do in cases of chronic illness; they are the stimuli which energize the Vital Force.

Although Hahnemann did not understand the immune system or the intricacies of homeostasis (the body's ever vigilant self-steadying mechanism) as we understand them today, or appreciate that where infection is present so are viruses, bacteria and other microorganisms, his intuition that it is some quality or energy in the individual which makes for health or illness is difficult to quarrel with.

Hahnemann gradually re-established himself as a physician, using his new homeopathic methods. However it was not long before he realized that certain patients, whom he had treated for acute conditions, were returning to him complaining of new sets of symptoms. These often seemed to declare themselves after stressful events. As the years passed, it became clear to him that such patients were treading a descending spiral of health, despite intervals of feeling reasonably well. Were their episodes of acute illness a manifestation of some deeper malaise? In treating the symptoms of each acute episode, was he not repressing the fundamental, underlying problem or 'miasm'? 'Miasm', meaning 'taint', was the word Hahnemann used to describe these putative, deep-seated tendencies.

Hahnemann recognized various miasms, some of which we now know to be mediated by specific micro-organisms which can indeed provoke repeated episodes of deepening illness if treatment is inappropriate or delayed; among them were syphilis, gonorrhea, tuberculosis, and cholera. Another was 'psora', which manifested itself in skin eruptions. Modern public health measures have made such taints less frequent, but the miasm concept continues to be useful and is much discussed among homeopaths. We now know that many bacteria and viruses, including those associated with measles, chickenpox, influenza, and AIDS, seem to create, in predisposed people, a vulnerability to all sorts of seemingly unconnected ailments. Depression and anxiety seem to underlie a host of conditions, from migraine to cancer. Hereditary conditions also have a miasmatic character. The task of the homeopath is to look for and recognise such disease patterns and attempt to treat them. By diligent research, mainly with sick people, Hahnemann developed remedies which seemed to work at the deeper miasmatic level. He also gave strict advice on the sort of diet and lifestyle his patients should follow – no perfumes or scented waters, no tooth powders, no snuff, sparing use of tobacco, no woollen underwear, no excessive bathing, no card playing, only occasional visits to the theatre, only moderate studying, and no madcap riding or cab-driving.

The first edition of *An Organon of Rational Healing*, the best-known and most comprehensive of all Hahnemann's writings on the nature of health, disease, and homeopathic healing, was published in 1810. He revised the book five times before his death in 1843, each time searching for greater understanding of the potency of homeopathic remedies and the nature of the Vital Force. At the time of writing it is still in print.

The spread of homeopathy

During the nineteenth century Hahnemann's ideas spread quickly from Germany across Europe and then to the Americas, and also eastwards to Asia. Today homeopathy is well respected in some countries, notably in Britain, France, Germany, Netherlands, Greece, India (where it is recognised and supported by the state), South Africa and South America, but mistrusted in others.

Homeopathy 'arrived' in Britain in 1832 when a Dr Hervey Quin began to minister to fashionable society from premises at 19 King Street in London's West End. Quin had travelled to Germany to consult Hahnemann on his own account and learned homeopathy from the Leipzig homeopaths. Later Quin became the first President of the British Homeopathic Society, founded in 1844. Thereafter, despite opposition from orthodox physicians, homeopathy steadily grew in popularity. Quin set up the first homeopathic hospital in London in 1850. The first royal patron of homeopathy was Queen Adelaide, consort of William IV, who, from 1835 until her death in 1849, was the patient of Dr Ernst Stapf, one of Samuel Hahnemann's closest colleagues. Three very distinguished homeopathic physicians have served the present Queen in the past, Dr John Weir, Dr Margery Blackie, and Dr Charles Elliott. Currently, Dr Ronald Davey holds this position.

In the United States the fire of homeopathy was lit by Dr Constantine Hering (b.1800). As well as formulating the Laws of Cure summarized below, he pioneered the use of 'nosodes', remedies made not from plants or minerals but from diseased tissue or from bodily secretions. In 1838 he and his colleagues used a homeopathic preparation of infected sheep's spleen to cure anthrax, at one time an almost certainly fatal disease.

Materia Medicas and Repertories

Hahnemann originally published the results of his provings in the form of a book called a *Materia Medica*. This listed, under each remedy, the symptoms that the remedy produced in healthy people. Later work has increased the number of substances used as remedies to 3000, although not all of these have been tested with the same thoroughness as Hahnemann's original investigations. The *Materia Medicas* of today contain not only details of symptoms from provings, but also the effects of poisons from the science of toxicology and details of symptoms from clinical observations.

Most of the remedies found in *Materia Medicas* nowadays were discovered in the last century or in the early part of this century. Many homeopaths agree that there is an urgent need to update the information, in order to find out if the twentieth century environment has changed people's responses to remedies. Some work has been done – in England, in mainland Europe and in the USA – but there is still much to do.

Materia Medicas are used to find out which symptoms a remedy might cause. Homeopaths have also developed remedy finders or *Repertories*. In a repertory, there is a series of headings concerned with parts or systems of the body, such as mental, vertigo, head, eyes, nose and so on down to toes. Under each heading there is a list of symptoms, such as pain, redness or swelling. Alongside each symptom are printed all the remedies known to produce that symptom, together with any factors which may affect it. The symptoms are graded, the most well proven being given in bold type, the second in italic and the third in plain roman. In our repertory, or General Remedy Finder, I have stuck to a single grading system for simplicity.

Homeopathic laws

The 'Laws of Cure' were partly devised by the physician who established homeopathy in America, Dr Constantine Hering. They state that cure takes place from the top of the body downwards, from the inside outwards and from the most important organs to the least important. Cure takes place in reverse order to the onset of symptoms. Therefore, for example, an ill person will start to feel better emotionally before the physical symptoms disappear and a long-standing complaint will take longer to disappear than a recent one.

Other homeopathic laws state:
1. Small stimuli encourage living systems, medium stimuli impede them and strong stimuli tend to stop or destroy them altogether. (Arndt's law.)
2. The quantity of action necessary to effect a change in nature is the least possible, and the decisive amount is always the minimum – perhaps an infinitesimal amount.
3. Functional symptoms are produced by the Vital Force in exact proportion to the profundity of the disturbance, and functional symptoms come before structural change.

Constitutional prescribing

Most people, when they are ill, suffer not only from the basic diagnostic symptoms of the disease, but also from other symptoms which are specific to each person. In orthodox medicine, these individual symptoms are mostly unimportant. But in homeopathy, they are vital for giving the correct prescription. This is why different patients may receive different remedies for the same disease.

Many homeopaths who worked on the provings, especially the American, James Tyler Kent, noticed that different types of people reacted strongly to certain remedies and proposed that people could be placed in different categories, called "constitutional types". Homeopaths talk of, for example, "phosphoric types" (people who react strongly to phosphorus) or "arsenicum album types" (those who react strongly to arsenicum album). The belief is that people of one type share similarities in terms of body shape, character and personality, and the sorts of diseases from which they suffer. For instance, natrum mur people tend to be pear-shaped, have a dark complexion, be fastidious and rigid in personality, keep themselves to themselves, crave salt and suffer from constipation. Lycopodium types tend to be tall, gangly and of stooped appearance, with an anxious expression, a craving for sweets, and a propensity to produce intestinal gas.

Of course, constitutional types have their limitations. In reality, each person is an individual, and so there are as many constitutional types as there are human beings, and account must be taken of the sum total of the person's inherited predispositions, past illnesses, diet, general reactions to the environment, intellectual and emotional features, and general attitude to life. This is what is meant in this book by 'constitutional treatment'.

Finding a homeopathic practitioner

In Britain today there are two basic kinds of homeopathic practitioner. One is the medically qualified homeopath. There are about 600 such in Britain. They have studied at an orthodox medical school and later at one of the homeopathic hospitals (see addresses p. 387–8). They have access to conventional methods of diagnosis and treatment as well as homeopathic techniques.

The second is the lay homeopath. He or she has no orthodox qualifications and thus lacks the clinical experience of the full spectrum of disease. The situation is further complicated by the greatly varying standards of homeopathy taught in the different colleges. The Society of Homeopaths (address p. 388) is endeavouring to standardize qualifications.

If you wish to contact a homeopath, ask the advice of a National Health Service general practitioner – usually, your own family doctor. If you have any difficulties, contact the British Homeopathic Society (address p. 387).

You may be put in touch with a homeopath who uses less conventional methods. There are many concepts which go under the name of homeopathy today. The practitioner is the best guide to the one which will best suit your needs. If you discover that your homeopath's philosophy and practice do not meet your expectations, you are of course free to find another practitioner.

The homeopathic practitioner must put the care and cure of his or her patients above any particular beliefs about which branch of homeopathy is right. As Hahnemann himself said, it is not so much the theories about the causation and treatment of illness that are important, but the results.

The consultation

At your first consultation with a homeopath, there are a great many questions to answer. He or she will want to know about the symptoms of your illness and what affects them, about your medical history from your mother's pregnancy onwards, your appetite, likes and dislikes, and the regularity of your bodily functions.

Some questions are aimed at deciding which constitutional group you fit into. Your activities, occupational and recreational, are discussed, along with your emotional state.

The homeopath will prescribe a remedy, which he may dispense himself or which you can obtain from a homeopathic pharmacist; he may also give you advice on any changes you should make in your lifestyle and on the sort of diet you should follow. Hahnemann stated that nutrition was one of the principal factors which could modify the body's response to disease. He was very strict about what his patients ate, especially those with chronic illness.

In a second consultation where constitutional treatment is concerned the homeopath must interpret your response to the prescription in detail, and decide how to continue treatment.

Controversy and proof

Homeopathy is a living, evolving form of treatment. Throughout its history there have been controversies and arguments. There was a split in the homeopathic world when Hahnemann introduced his theory of the Vital Force and how it could be influenced by remedies diluted, one to 100, perhaps 30 times (30c) or more. Some homeopaths, such as Kent and now Vithoulkas supported his theory. Others believed that Hahnemann left science behind at this point. One of these was the British homeopath, Richard Hughes. He produced his own *Materia Medica* called *The Cyclopedia*, (1884–91), based on laboratory findings and low potencies, without regard for the theory of the Vital Force. Those who followed him tended to see homeopathy in more conventional scientific and medical terms. It was as a result of this split that homeopathy foundered in America some years before the introduction of antibiotics. One living homeopath who champions the middle road, using both approaches with great skill and expertise, is the Argentinian Dr Francisco Eizyaga. (For further details see *The Two Faces of Homeopathy* by Anthony Campbell (see p. 389)).

Does homeopathy stand up to scrutiny by modern medical and scientific methods? Lack of convincing scientific proof is one of the great stumbling blocks to homeopathy's acceptance by the general medical community. Many reasons are quoted for this failure, such as lack of money, lack of time and lack of interest. (Although it should be said that many homeopaths are not interested in providing proof, because they know from their own experience that it works.)

There are three main areas which must be explored in an effort to overcome this lack of evidence. First, tests called clinical trials must prove that homeopathic remedies, as prescribed, actually benefit patients. Second, there must be proof that the highly diluted remedies have a measurable effect on living organisms, to show that they do contain some of the original substance. Third, the theoretical mechanism behind the potentization effect must be explored.

Clinical trials

In conventional medicine, all new drugs must undergo clinical trials before being licensed for prescription by doctors. There have been few well-run clinical trials in homeopathy. In 1854, there was an outbreak of cholera in London. The mortality rates were compared for homeopathic and orthodox hospitals. The former had a mortality rate of 16.4 per cent, while the rate in the latter was 51.8 per cent. The Board of Health at the time attempted to suppress these damning figures. It was only after the matter was raised in Parliament that the figures were duly recorded.

During World War II there were experiments on the homeopathic treatment of mustard gas burns, for the Ministry of Defence. Controlled trials of mustard gas nosode 30c, and a remedy called *Rhus tox 30c*, showed a protective effect when these were given as a preventative measure.

A more recent study was conducted in 1980 by Gibson and colleagues, in Glasgow. It compared homeopathic treatment of rheumatoid arthritis with orthodox treatment by the drug aspirin. The results showed that the improvement rate was higher among the former group. However, a combination of aspirin and homeopathic remedies was even more effective.

Smaller trials have shown that *Arnica 30c* can significantly control pain and bleeding after dental treatment, and that *Borax 30c* and *Candida nosode 30c* are effective treatments for vaginal discharge.

In 1986 there was a double-blind study of the homeopathic treatment for hayfever, by Reilly. This showed significantly reduced symptoms in patients taking prescribed homeopathic remedies, compared with those taking a placebo. There have been other trials but their results are open to question and cannot be used as proof.

The overall conclusion is that, where results are available, they show homeopathy to be of benefit. But many people demand better clinical trials, and more of them, before they will accept that homeopathy works.

The effects of high dilutions

What about the evidence that living systems can be influenced by substances in high dilution? It is known that animals can be extraordinarily sensitive. For example, salmon in the ocean can detect the "scent" of their home river water at dilutions of one part in 1,000,000. The human nose is capable of detecting the foul-smelling substance mercaptan at concentrations of only one part in 500,000,000,000 parts of air.

In 1940, Dr W E Boyd conducted an important experiment in Edinburgh. He showed that the chemical mercuric chloride, diluted to 60c, had a measurable effect on the rate at which an enzyme, diastase, affected starch. Similar experiments have been done using animal tissues in the laboratory, including frog's heart and rat's uterus. Yeasts and plants have also been tested. All the results demonstrate that substances "in potency" (diluted to typical homeopathic concentrations) have effects on living tissues. Many other experiments are recorded, but most have not been repeated and have been criticized for their accuracy. However, recently there has been a worldwide standardization of homeopathy, which it is hoped will give future scientific experiments their due credence.

The theories behind potentization

When a substance is diluted one to a 100, for 12 times (the 12c potency) or more, then it is likely that in any one sample, nothing of the original substance remains – it is pure solvent. Naturally, it is difficult to give a chemical explanation for how such infinitesimally small doses, or even no doses at all, produce their effect.

One possibility is the "placebo effect". It has been shown that up to three-quarters of patients will feel better if given a "treatment" which is actually only a placebo. It appears that, if they think it will cure them, then this belief is enough, and they do improve. But it seems unlikely that babies or animals would respond to this effect – and respond they do, to homeopathic remedies.

It has also been proposed that minute quantities of a remedy may act as a catalyst, a substance that speeds up the chemical workings of the body and so stimulates its innate healing powers. However, the extreme dilutions seem to preclude this.

It may be that physics, rather than chemistry, holds the answer. Experiments have been conducted using Raman lasers and nuclear magnetic resonators (NMR machines, used in medical scanning) to reveal the electromagnetic or vibratory properties of remedies in high dilutions. Evidence indicates that the structure of the solvent molecules may be electrochemically changed by succussion (the violent mixing used when diluting potencies). The solvent molecules may be imprinted and "remember" the vibratory properties of the original tincture. When the remedy is given to the patient, this "memory" is communicated to the living system and stimulates the effect that we see.

A recent experiment to demonstrate potencies was carried out in France by Doctor Benveniste and its results were published in the prestigious *Nature* magazine. It provoked a flurry of comment and resulted in the rerun of the experiments under the 'scientific' eyes of a fraud detector, a journalist and a magician. The resulting furore has done little to clarify the issue of potentization and much to discredit the objectivity and reputation of the orthodox scientific community.

Homeopathy and conventional medicine

Homeopathic remedies are not exclusive to homeopathy. For example, cis platinum is used in the treatment of many types of cancer, in both homeopathic and conventional medicine. Cis platinum, in common with many other drugs used in cancer treatment, is itself a "carcinogen" (cancer-inducing drug). Similar experiments include quinine, digitalis and emetine. Orthodox medicine also employs dilutions of allergens (the allergy-causing substances) to treat the allergies themselves.

Remedies which are presented as homeopathic cures for certain conditions, such as lumbago or sleeplessness, may give results – but they are not being used homeopathically. Rather, they are being used as orthodox drugs, without regard for the individuality of symptoms.

It is important that homeopathic physicians use orthodox methods of diagnosis. This permits understanding of how an illness might progress without treatment, which in turn helps in assessing the response to the remedy. Such diagnosis also helps the practitioner to identify symptoms that are characteristic to the individual, rather than the illness – information which is vital to prescribing the correct remedy. And qualified homeopaths are aware when it is necessary to recommend that a patient sees an orthodox physician. In addition the repetories include many examples of orthodox diagnoses.

Conventional surgery is used in conjunction with homeopathy in certain cases. For example, there may be an injury or physical blockage in an internal organ, or an illness may be draining the body's ability to cure itself. Homeopathic remedies also help in the healing of the wound made by the surgeon's knife. And homeopathy interacts with toxicology, the study of the effects of poisons on the body. Although remedies are so dilute that they are not poisonous, their toxic effects must be understood.

There are many similarities between the concepts of homeopathy and the new, expanding fields of immunology and allergy study. Indeed, the homeopathic approach to preventative medicine is reflected by the immunizations of orthodox medicine.

Homeopathy and non-orthodox medicines

There are many complementary, alternative or other non-orthodox medicines which share concepts with homeopathy. In particular, common to many such therapies is the concept of a natural healing force by which the body cures itself, given the right circumstances. In its use of natural remedies, homeopathy resembles herbal medicine and aromatherapy. In its use of subtle diagnosis it resembles iridology and kirlian photography. In its emphasis on the calmness of the mind it has a close harmony with yoga, meditation and relaxation techniques. Homeopathy can be used together with hypnotherapy and psychotherapy. And if structural problems are interfering with the progression of a cure, most homeopaths will send patients for physiotherapy, osteopathy, chiropractic or massage. (See p. 391 for further reading on these subjects, and p. 386–7 for useful addresses.)

Part 2

PREVENTION IS BETTER THAN CURE

HUMAN nature is such that it is always easier – and probably always will be – to take a pill than to change a way of life. Most people want quick solutions. They want health with the minimum of fuss and effort. They don't want to worry about the food they eat, the air they breathe, the neighbourhood they live in, and so on. And while there are professionals to provide the quick solution, who is to say that such people are less healthy than those who worry interminably about saturated fats, additives, nitrates, fluoridation, toxic metals, ozone depletion, radiation, and so on? In this modern world of ours, driven by short-term profit rather than thought for the future, there is indeed a lot to worry about – a great deal of this chapter is taken up with the nutritional, environmental, and cultural hazards of living in Britain today. The trick is to strike a balance between constructive worry and neurotic worry. There are many small changes in lifestyle which are practical and affordable; try these first, feel the benefits, and then larger changes may be possible.

This is not an exhaustive list of environmental factors which may be hazardous to health nor is it intended to be. I have tried to highlight broad areas of concern and to give you, where possible, means to avoid them. If you suspect that something in your environment may be upsetting you, but are afraid that you are making a fuss about nothing, discuss it with your homeopathic physician. He will either be able to deal with it himself or will suggest further action if necessary.

The preventive role of homeopathy

At the deepest level, homeopathy is preventive in intent. Homeopathic remedies do not wade in and 'zap' offending organisms, leaving the immune system less able to cope than before. Quite the opposite. They nudge the immune system – not only the white cell populations of the body but also the mental and emotional states which keep those populations healthy – into greater responsiveness and readiness so that disease is kept away or prevented from recurring. In fact, homeopaths are trained to look for diseases *before* they happen. When a homeopath prescribes constitutionally, he or she is prescribing not only for the present ailment but for tendencies which have not yet manifested themselves as medically recognized ailments.

The foetus in the womb can be treated homeopathically to minimize imbalances inherited from the mother and father. Homeopathic treatment of childhood ailments lessens the risk of the latent weaknesses they cause being activated in later life – infants and children, with their newly minted immune systems, respond excellently to homeopathic treatment. Homeopathic immunization against the graver diseases of childhood is not usually offered unless a child is particularly at risk; most homeopaths prefer to take the route of boosting general resistance to disease, rather than exposing a child unnecessarily to the influence of powerful disease organisms. That said, homeopathic immunization has never damaged anyone, although the properly conducted trials that are needed to show that it is as effective as orthodox immunization have not been done.

In adults, prompt homeopathic treatment of minor illnesses can often prevent persistent, and sometimes serious, complaints developing in later life. At all points in the cycle of development, birth, growth and maturity, subtle symptoms of constitutional weakness can be picked up by careful homeopathic analysis and treated before they burgeon into chronic and entrenched disease.

Unfortunately, no one has yet invented a way of trying out homeopathic and orthodox remedies on the same person and comparing their effects over a lifetime, but the following hypothetical case history shows how a homeopathic physician might approach a case of late-onset asthma.

At nine months old, the future Mrs X develops eczema; the ointment used to treat it leaves her skin very dry. Apart from dry skin and constipation, she is a generally healthy child. At the age of 14, she has a bad fall from a horse. A year later she develops hay fever, which turns into allergic rhinitis (a runny nose all year round). Skin tests show that she is allergic to house dust, house dust mites, grasses and horses. Desensitizing injections clear up her runny nose but leave her feeling unwell for some time afterwards.

In the early 20s she is underweight and suffers from an almost continuous nasal drip (catarrh dripping down the back of the throat). In her late twenties she marries and has two children, both full-term, healthy babies. Apart from dry skin, constipation, occasional nosebleeds and irregular periods, she feels reasonably well throughout her 30s. In her early 40s, she loses two people very close to her, her mother and eldest son. Shortly afterwards, she develops asthma.

She consults a homeopathic physician for the first time. High potency *Natrum mur* is prescribed to help her through the grieving process, and she is advised to cut down on salt and carbohydrates. A month later, the asthma has all but disappeared, but she continues to suffer from dry skin, constipation, and catarrh at the back of the throat; if anything, she reports, her throat feels worse than before; and she also feels chilly and irritable, and has had several boils. Hepar sulph. is prescribed. This clears up the boils and the catarrh, but the runny nose remains. Allium and Arnica clear up the runny nose; Sulphur clears up the dry skin and the constipation. At this juncture the eczema she had as a very young child reappears. Since there is a family history of tuberculosis and allergies, she is given Tuberculinum; this clears up the eczema. She is then advised to follow the 'twice a week' eating rule (see p. 24). She continues in good health, visiting the homeopath at infrequent intervals, until the age of 75 when she dies of pneumonia.

The homeopathic treatment involves a peeling away of layers of illness, removing symptoms in the reverse order in which they appeared, each time reaching farther back into the chain of cause and effect.

There is little doubt that predispositions to certain groups of ailments run in families. Mrs X's Achilles heel, so to speak, was her respiratory tract. Had she been treated homeopathically from childhood onwards, this vulnerability might have been dispelled. Even from the age of 45 onwards, homeopathic health care prolonged her life and enhanced her quality of life.

Unlike many other modes of 'health care' which swing into action once health has broken down, homeopathy is based upon helping the organism to resist breakdown.

EXERCISE

Strenuous exertion is no longer a necessary part of daily life. Millions of people in the West today spend a third of their lives sitting in offices or behind steering wheels. Nevertheless, the human body is designed for muscular activity and does not function or maintain itself properly without exercise.

The most natural way to exercise, and therefore the easiest, is to build some moderately strenuous activity into your daily routine. Walk briskly to the station, get off the bus two stops earlier, cycle to work, use the stairs rather than the lift. . . If you cannot do any of these things, try to set aside a few minutes each day and work through an exercise routine.

Bear the following points in mind whenever you exercise:

1. Always warm up carefully before you start, especially if the surroundings are cold, to avoid damage to muscles and tendons.
2. Practise new movements slowly to avoid wrenching a muscle. Set yourself realistic targets.
3. Do not wear clothing which will stop the evaporation of sweat, as this may cause dehydration.
4. Wear shock-absorbing footwear.
5. Slow down gradually at the end of an exercise session and do not get chilled afterwards.

The dangers of exercise are illustrated by the following list of problems encountered by the incautious: damage to muscles and joints, bone fractures, heart attack, asthma, amenorrhoea (stopping of periods), heat stroke, weight loss and urinary tract infections such as cystitis. It is vitally important that exercise is taken seriously, and all the rules are followed, in order to avoid these problems.

The dynamic exercises described on pp. 21–22 should be done vigorously enough to make you breathe hard and sweat a bit, which is when the real benefits to the heart and vascular system occur. But to begin with, here are some gentler exercises to tune up the body.

Breathing How well do you breathe? How often do your lungs get a full change of air? When you take a deep breath do you just puff your chest out and draw your shoulders up, or do you breathe with your abdomen as well? Every cell in the body requires a constant supply of oxygen, so the ability to breathe fully and freely is very important. If posture is poor – rounded or high shoulders, poking chin, hollow chest, flabby abdomen – breathing will be shallow. In severe cases, breathing out too much carbon dioxide can cause dizziness, palpitations, tingling in the arms, and even angina like pains in the chest and arms (see HYPERVENTILATION p. 181).

You can train yourself to breath properly by a variety of techniques, but I would like to introduce you to a yoga technique called *pranayama*, in which the diaphragm is used properly and inhalation is imagined as beginning below the navel and spreading all the way up to the forehead. Sit on the floor in the lotus or half lotus position, or sit straight in a chair if you find it easier. Keep your chin level, stretch your neck up and forwards, and look straight ahead. Exhale slowly through both nostrils, and as you reach the end of the out-breath pull your stomach in. Hold your stomach in for one second. Now inhale as deeply as possible, feeling the air enter your abdomen first, then fill your chest, then fill the top of your lungs beneath your collar bones. As you breathe in, imagine a wave of energy travelling up from your abdomen to your forehead. Hold the in-breath for one second, then exhale slowly as before, pulling your stomach in at the end of the out-breath. Pause for one second before inhaling again.

To be of real benefit, this exercise should be repeated 10–15 times at one sitting, and 10–15 times a day, whenever you have a quiet moment. It is an excellent antidote to stress and anger.

Posture Most body movements involve the spine, the axis to which the rib cage, shoulder girdle, and hip girdle are attached. The ideal spine is neither straight nor over-curved, but has four gentle curves – cervical, thoracic, lumbar, sacral – which nicely balance each other so that no single group of muscles has to work overtime to keep the body erect. When posture is correct, breathing is fuller and easier, and wear and tear on all the load-bearing joints of the body is less. In the long run, this may prevent degenerative conditions such as 'slipped' discs and osteoarthritis.

Strained spinal ligaments and muscles certainly affect the way we carry ourselves, but many back problems are actually caused by faulty posture, by the positions in which we habitually stand, sit, or lie, and of course by the emotional states which make us adopt positions of strain and tension.

At a much deeper level, posture can be a mirror of suppressed emotions, and if posture and mobility can be improved, some of these tensions can be gently dissolved.

Try this simple exercise. Stand with your back to the wall, with heels, buttocks, and shoulders touching the wall. Your head does not have to touch the wall. Imagine the back of your neck lengthening – think 'up' and 'forwards' as you do this, and keep your chin level. Imagine the back of your rib cage widening. Imagine your lower back lengthening – think 'coccyx under', release the tension in your legs, and slightly flex your knees. Let your heels take about 70 per cent of your weight. Allow your hands to hang lower and lower on your thighs. Take a few quiet breaths, and feel a new sensation of balance and relaxation. Now you are ready to walk away from the wall! Your new stance will seem strange at first, but with practice it is possible to acquire a new set of posture reflexes which will discharge stress rather than store it.

When you sit, try not to imitate the proverbial sack of potatoes. Sit as erect as possible – this is the position of least strain – with a small cushion in the small of your back if necessary. Cross your ankles but not your legs. In the car, an adjustable lumbar support is a good idea. Try not to stretch or twist over your desk or work area – simultaneous stretching and twisting are responsible for many pulled backs. If you are obliged to sit for long periods, get up and stretch every hour or so – this will give your mind and your body a change. Or you could invest in a chair with a forward sloping seat, because it obliges you to sit up straight with your feet firmly on the floor. Kneeling or 'back' chairs are unsuitable for people with knee problems and should not be used for longer than two hours at a time. (For further information, consult a seating consultant such as Alternative Sitting, address p. 386.) If you have to stay in bed for any length of time, avoid half-lying.

Although this position is allowed and even encouraged in hospitals, it puts considerable strain on the lumbar spine. Half-reclining in low armchairs does the same.

If you can, sleep on your back with a single, low pillow. This is preferable to side-lying, which twists the spine and compresses the ribcage and shoulder area.

If you have posture-related problems, consult a physiotherapist, chiropractor, osteopath, or Alexander teacher. The Alexander Technique (see p. 386 for address of society of teachers) is a very good and thorough way of unlearning bad posture.

Salutations to the sun This is a body toning sequence which synchronizes stretching and bending with breathing. I thoroughly recommend it as a way of starting the day. Do not force the movements, especially if you are a bit stiff in the mornings. Work within your limits, allowing gravity and your own body weight to do the stretching and bending. The entire sequence can be done in seven in-breaths and out-breaths. Synchronizing breathing and movement will prevent over-stretching. Breathing should be relaxed, not forced.

If you have the perseverance to run through this sequence three times each morning, you will soon notice that your body feels more alive and relaxed throughout the day. If you are rather creaky to start with, the changes will be more gradual. Be patient with yourself.

Spine and neck The simplest and most effective exercises you can do to keep your back and neck supple are side-bending and head rolling.

Again, work within your existing limits. With repetition those limits will extend. To start with, lean sideways, sliding your hand slowly down the outside of your leg. Your feet should be parallel and about a shoulder-width apart, and your knees straight but not locked. Your lower hand should merely rest against your leg. Bend and straighten slowly, and be conscious of stretching up and over rather than sagging sideways! Hold the bend for 30 seconds, not forgetting to breathe, before straightening up. Repeat five times.

When side-bending is comfortable with your arms by your sides, try side-bending with your arms above your head. You'll find this puts a lot more strain on the lumbar spine, so go gently. Hold for 30 seconds, then straighten up. Repeat five times.

Head rolling simply involves rolling your head round in a full circle *very slowly*. Do not force the movement. Let gravity assist the rolling forwards and backwards. Repeat two or three times in both directions.

Slantboard exercises These have many beneficial effects. In an inclined supine position with the head lower than the feet, at an angle of 25–30° to the horizontal, many stretching and toning exercises are helped by gravity, blood flow to the heart and brain is improved, and the abdominal organs are gently repositioned and decompressed.

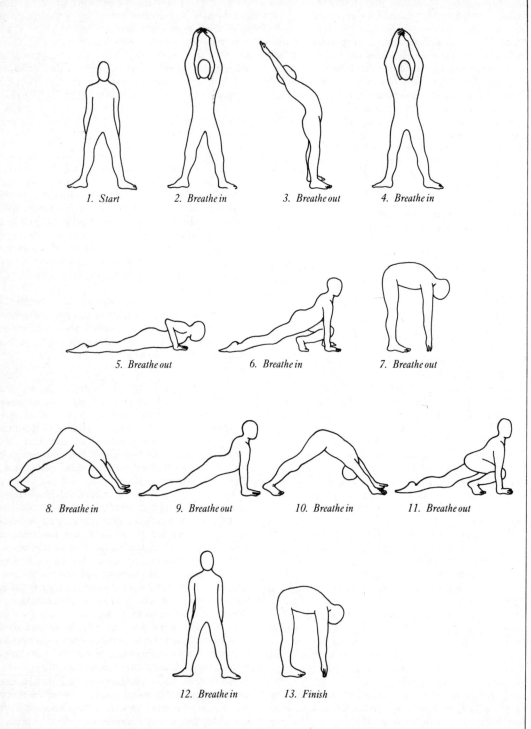

1. Start   2. Breathe in   3. Breathe out   4. Breathe in

5. Breathe out   6. Breathe in   7. Breathe out

8. Breathe in   9. Breathe out   10. Breathe in   11. Breathe out

12. Breathe in   13. Finish

Salutations to the Sun: work from left to right on the first two, then right to left, left to right and right to left, so that you finish in the 'start' position

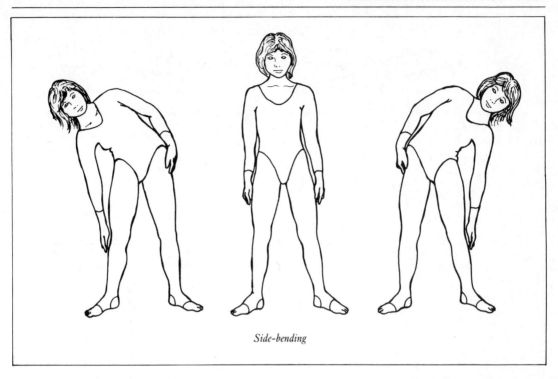

Side-bending

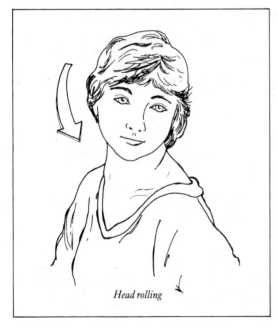

Head rolling

Dynamic exercises The purpose of dynamic (as opposed to static) exercise is to increase the capacity of the lungs and heart, strengthen muscles, increase suppleness and flexibility, and improve circulation. All of these things help to relieve stress. They also whittle away excess weight, not least because they tend to put a brake on appetite, and they improve coordination. The result is greater vitality and resistance to disease, especially heart disease.

Before starting any form of dynamic exercise, find out how fit you are, then build up gradually to a level of fitness appropriate to your age and general health. If you are over 60, or over 45 and have never done any vigorous exercise, or if you smoke heavily or are more than 15 per cent overweight, see your doctor before starting any strenuous form of exercise.

To find out how fit you are, try the following test (but stop at once if you start to gasp, or feel sick or dizzy). Step up on to a 20-cm (8-in) high step with your left foot, bring the right foot up beside the left, then step down with the left and bring the right foot down beside it. Now step up with the right foot. Repeat, at the rate of 24 step-ups a minute (this may take a bit of practice), for 3 minutes. Wait 1 minute, then take your pulse at the wrist, using the second hand of your watch. Count the number of beats in 30 seconds and double the count to give the rate per minute. Don't use your thumb to take your pulse; just place the tips of your fingers lightly along the inside of your wrist on the thumb side.

There are one or two caveats, however. Always wait 2 hours after eating before doing slantboard exercises, and do not do them at all if you have high blood pressure, heart problems, kidney problems or hiatus hernia. If you have a lower back problem, avoid exercises 5 and 6.

SLANT BOARD EXERCISES

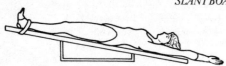

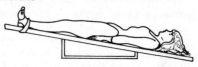

1. *Abdominal stretch: raise arms above head, then lower them to the sides. Repeat 10 to 15 times*

2. *Uplifting organs: hold your breath and bring abdominal organs towards shoulders; breathe out and let organs return to former position. Repeat 10 to 15 times*

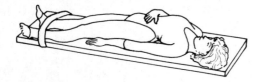

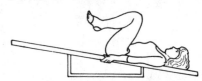

3. *Colon rejuvenation: lean to one side and stretch. Pat stretched side of abdomen vigorously with open hand 15 to 25 times. Change sides and repeat. Repeat 3 or 4 times for each side*

4. *Enforcing circulation: bend legs as shown and relax. Turn head from side to side 5 or 6 times. Lift head slightly and rotate 3 or 4 times in both directions. Repeat from beginning 2 or 3 times*

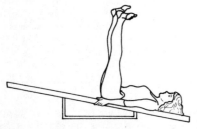

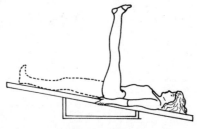

5. *Ligament stretch: rotate legs outwards in circles 8 to 10 times, then inwards 8 to 10 times. Increase gradually to 25 times*

6. *Muscle toner: raise both legs to vertical position, then lower first one leg, then the other, slowly, keeping knee straight, 15 to 25 times. Raise both legs and lower together slowly, 3 or 4 times. Increase gradually to double this number*

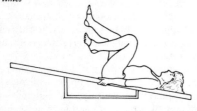

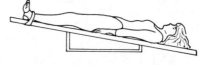

7. *All-in-one exercise: raise legs to vertical position, then bicycle 15 to 25 times. Increase speed gradually over a few weeks*

8. *The basic position: lie flat on your back with feet under straps, allowing gravity to help put abdominal organs in proper position and letting blood circulate to head. Keep this position for 5 to 15 minutes. Always do this at the end of a series of exercises*

Results	Male	Female
Excellent	less than 68	less than 76
Good	68–79	76–85
Above average	80–89	86–94
Below average	90–99	95–109
Very poor	more than 100	more than 110

A 'very poor' result tells you that you should begin exercising very gently. Do about 5 minutes a day every day for a month, not allowing your pulse rate to exceed 100. In the second month increase the exercise period to 10 minutes.

If the result of your fitness test is 'below average', exercise for 10 minutes a day, keeping the pulse below 110. Keep the rate below 120 if your result is 'above average'. After a month or so you should be fit enough to continue with the main exercises. If you can comfortably walk 8 km (5 miles) you should be fit enough to undertake any form of vigorous exercise such as dancing, squash, tennis or jogging. Swimming is undoubtedly the best type of exercise because the water takes the weight off your joints and also provides gentle, yielding resistance to movement. Cycling is also good.

It is very important to stress that any discomfort in the chest, neck, abdomen, jaw, arms or shoulders while exercising must not be ignored. Play safe and see your doctor.

When you are approaching fitness, exercise regularly. Three, or at least two, times each week is recommended, for 20 to 30 minutes each time. Some people find competition a spur to fitness; others are content to monitor their own performance and try to improve on it each time.

MORE GOOD HEALTH HABITS
Dental care In 1945 Dr Western Price recorded some of the effects of western 'civilisation' upon primitive peoples. These effects included the appearance of diseases and tooth decay not previously experienced by these people, before the introduction of western foods.

The following nine-point plan can prevent tooth decay.
1. Don't eat sweets, especially between meals.
2. Eat a balanced diet with lots of wholefoods.
3. Eat chewable (but not sweetened) foods, such as raw fruit.
4. Ensure a balanced diet during pregnancy, to strengthen the teeth of the unborn child.
5. Brush teeth at least twice a day, after meals. Ask your dentist to show you the correct way to brush, and use plaque-disclosing tablets every few weeks to highlight the areas you miss.
6. Use dental floss, following the instructions carefully to avoid gum damage.
7. Fluoride can be given to children under 12 to help strengthen teeth. But – too much fluoride can cause mottling of teeth, so consult your dentist about the use of fluoride drops or tablets, and in any case stop them two days a week.
8. Unless you live in an area of chalky soils, where caries (tooth decay) is less common, take cod liver oil capsules and eat some dairy products.
9. Neutralise acid-producing foods such as meat or sugar by eating alkaline foods, such as cheese, at the end of the meal.

Pre-conceptual care You owe your baby the best possible start in life. So when you begin to think about pregnancy, make sure you and your partner are in good health and physically fit. Pregnancy and birth are strenuous activities. Stop smoking and stop drinking alcohol at least three months before you plan to conceive, and if you are taking any medication, consult your doctor about giving it up.

Stop taking oral contraceptives or have any intra-uterine device removed three months before you intend to become pregnant, and use barrier methods

such as the sheath or cap in the meantime. Unfortunately, there is no homeopathic contraceptive. Good supplies of vitamins A, C, E and the B complex, zinc, iodine and selenium are necessary for fertility. See PART 6 for sources in the diet.

Read the section on general nutrition and diet (p. 23–27) and ensure your diet is wholesome and nutritious, with adequate vitamins and minerals. Have constitutional homeopathic treatment, particularly if you have any long-standing health problems; if you have back trouble, see a physiotherapist, osteopath or chiropractor before conceiving.

If you are worried about specific problems, e.g. if you have a history of any hereditary diseases, or have previously given birth to a baby with a congenital abnormality or had recurrent abortions, it is worth consulting Foresight (address page 384) for specialized care.

Having a healthy baby should never be put in jeopardy. Remember that relaxation, rest and exercise are vital.

NUTRITION
The subject of nutrition is vast, but I will try to answer some basic questions: How has our diet changed in recent times – and for worse or better? What should we eat? How should food be produced, stored and cooked? How is food absorbed by the body – and do you need to take supplements?

Our evolutionary past Some 40,000 years ago our ancestors were probably mainly vegetarian, eating roots and seeds and fruits, with meat only occasionally. These hunter-gatherers would have been continually on the move; they picked their food fresh, they shared it and did not store it. This situation had its advantages. Modern examples of hunter-gatherers such as the Bushmen of Botswana, are rarely obese, have few signs of malnutrition or high blood pressure, and they have low blood cholesterol levels and no tooth decay.

Gradually, hunting took over from gathering. More meat was included in the diet, and the extra protein, especially, was linked with an increase in stature (as it is today). Remember that the fat content of the meat from wild animals, at about 4 per cent, is much lower than that of today's domestic animals – which can be up to 30 per cent. But the diet at this time was still high in fibre, calcium and Vitamin C, and low in fats, sugar and salt.

By about 10,000 years ago, people were beginning to grow and store crops and rear animals in one place. The resulting development of the structured society encouraged increasingly concentrated human populations and a reduced variety of food.

The modern diet The majority of the world today is still predominantly vegetarian, for economic, ecological, philosophical, religious and even political reasons. The diseases linked with over-consumption of refined carbohydrates and animal fats are mainly confined to the 'developed' societies: obesity, degenerative diseases, dental decay, coronary artery disease, diabetes, gallstones and diverticular diseases. But there is also a high level of malnutrition among the poor of the developed world.

Although there has been a marked change in diet over the last 40,000 years, there has been little change in our bodies to cope with it. Physical and biochemical evolution simply does not work that fast. In order to avoid the diseases of over-nutrition, the World Health Organization has redefined the ideal diet to conform more closely to that of our hunter-gatherer forefathers – indeed, the very diet our bodies are designed for.

There are four main categories of diet. Vegans eat no animal protein of any kind; lacto-vegetarians include milk products and sometimes eggs in their diet; an omnivore wholefood diet includes all types of wholefoods (foods not processed, treated or refined by industry); while a western omnivore diet includes refined and processed foods.

The 'twice a week' rule This memory aid helps you to simplify diet planning and include in your diet the right proportions of the various types of food. Foods are divided into groups and you should eat foods from each group no more than twice a week.

Group 1 – meat and poultry
Group 2 – fish
Group 3 – eggs
Group 4 – cheese
Group 5 – sugar in concentrated form (sweets, cakes)

In addition, keep milk to an average of less than 250 ml (about ½ pint) per day.

The rest of your diet should be made up of wholemeal bread and flour, cereals, grains, nuts and seeds, vegetables, legumes and fruit, organically grown if possible. You will then be eating a well-balanced diet which your digestive system is designed for and which satisfies your body's nutritional needs.

Organic foods are grown in humus-rich soils without artificial fertilisers and pesticides. Demand for organically grown vegetables is increasing and some supermarkets are now promoting their organic ranges. Vegetables with split stalks, cracked skins or an unnaturally bright green or pasty yellow colour are unlikely to be organically grown. Look out for a range of organically grown vegetarian meals soon to be marketed by ARK.

If you have any bad habits, nutritional or otherwise, indulge them only twice a week – though preferably not at all. Use small amounts of salt or Ruthmol for cooking, if at all. Do not add salt to your food at the table. If you have a sweet tooth, eat muesli bars, dried fruit, carob chocolate or cakes and biscuits made with unrefined sugars.

Remember that even if you are eating a pesticide-free, organically grown, additive-free diet, you are still in danger if your diet is very restricted and you eat too much of one particular food. Variety is the spice of life!

Children's food Old habits die hard, and eating habits are moulded in childhood. Try to educate children in the ways of a good diet. Many of the factors associated with heart disease, such as poor diet, start when we are young. Use the twice-a-week rule (above), but increase the amount of protein from animal and vegetable sources. Avoid salt and too much fat. Read labels on foods and avoid additives if possible. The additives E250, E251, E310, E311, E312, E320, E321 and Ethoxyquin are not allowed in foods meant for children, but they are sometimes found in adult foods that children eat. Some children are especially susceptible to certain foods or to additives, and food allergy may lead to behavioural problems.

Children often go through 'faddy' phases of refusing to eat, or eating only certain things. There appears to be no medical basis for this, unless they are actually ill. The problem usually resolves itself if you pay it as little attention as possible. The child may well be trying to get a reaction, and if an emotional battle develops, it can be very difficult to overcome. Continue to serve food only at normal meal times, even when it is not eaten. Try serving the same food in different guises, puréed or cut into interesting shapes. Give only small amounts. Encourage the child to eat a small piece of everything on the plate, not just one item. Make sure he or she has not eaten sweets or biscuits or had a large drink before a meal. No one can eat when the stomach is already full!

To reassure yourself, try keeping a diary of everything that your child eats over a two-week period. Food intake over a day may not be adequate, but you will probably find that the diet averages out. Children will not starve themselves to death, and their metabolism is much more efficient than an adult's.

The tongue bears taste buds that are sensitive to salt and sugar. In ancient times these flavours were probably provided by fruits, wild honey and vegetables. Today there is salt or sugar in many processed foods. Children readily develop a taste for them, so try to avoid using junk food as a treat. A recent research project involved removal of sugar, food colourings and preservatives from the meals served in a residential school. Fresh, unrefined foods were substituted. The startling results included higher academic achievements, less fighting and better behaviour.

Healthy alternatives to junk food are not difficult to find. Instead of fizzy drinks and adulterated squash, give mineral water, unsweetened fruit juices or non-additive squash. Ice-cream and yogurt can be bought without additives and with a low fat content. Sweets and snacks can be replaced by muesli bars, dried or fresh fruits, and carob can be used instead of chocolate. Make your own cakes, biscuits and puddings using low-sugar recipes, wholemeal flour, fresh and dried fruits and yogurt. Burgers, sausages and fishfingers can also be made at home or bought as low fat, additive-free products. Soya products can replace meat, but beware of colouring chemicals. Choose additive-free crisps or try tortilla chips and corn chips.

Children can be raised on vegetarian diets. But great care must be taken, especially on vegan diets, that the combinations of foods give adequate amounts of nutrients. Expert planning is needed. Contact the Vegan Society (address p. 383).

The elderly and food Elderly people need less energy, and so they tend to eat less: but their food should still be of a high nutritional quality. Yet because of poverty or an unwillingness to cook when living alone, the reverse is often the case. Older people should avoid too much fat, salt, sugar and red meat, and eat plenty of wholegrain bread, cereals, vegetables, fruit and fish. It is best to eat several small meals and healthy snacks rather than one large daily meal. Elderly people who rarely get out in the fresh air may need to take Vitamin D supplements. Go easy on tea and coffee, since they contribute to insomnia. Some drugs interfere with absorption of nutrients, so consult a doctor about your diet if you are taking medication.

Fasting Eating nothing, on occasions, can be good for you, provided your general health is satisfactory. Complete abstinence from solid food rests the digestive system and allows the body to cleanse itself of toxic residues. Also, any unknown allergens in your diet will cease to bother you. If you are in any doubt about your fitness to fast, consult a homeopath or doctor. When you fast, take plenty of additive-free fruit juices, herb teas or mineral water. Do not fast for longer than three days. After a fast, gradually introduce easily-digested foods such as yogurt, fruit and vegetable stew. (For more information about fasting, see Part 6.)

Digestion Digestion is the process that changes food into a form which the cells of the body can use. The mouth, stomach and intestines, and the organs associated with them, form the digestive system. Digestive capabilities vary from person to person and deteriorate as we get older. The liver is the central organ for the breakdown of digested nutrients (catabolism) and the building, from them, of chemicals required by the cells of the body (anabolism). The processes of body chemistry are called metabolism.

In order to eat enjoyably and healthily, it is necessary to understand what is in the food we eat, and why the body needs it – or not.

WHAT IS FOOD?

Energy Food contains energy, usually measured in calories. One calorie is the amount of heat required to raise the temperature of 1 gm of water by 1°C. The 'calorie' of the nutritionist is in fact equivalent to one kilocalorie (1,000 calories) of the physicist, and is written Calorie (capital C). This is the convention we adopt here. In addition, very up-to-date energy measurements are sometimes given in joules (J). One Calorie equals about 4.2 joules.

The body needs energy for all its processes, physical, mental and chemical. The number of Calories the body requires varies according to age, sex, build, and activity level (which is closely linked to occupation).

Average daily Calorie requirements

Children	varies greatly, 1,000–3,000 at school age
Teenager	varies greatly, 2,000–3,000
Woman	sedentary, 2,000 active, 2,300–4,000
Man	sedentary, 2,500 active, 3,000–5,000
Elderly person	1,000–2,000

If the energy in food is not used by the body, by being converted into growing tissue or movement or warmth, then it is stored, generally as fat. This is what makes people overweight (see OBESITY, page 260).

Carbohydrates These are the chief source of energy for bodily functions and muscular exertions. Carbohydrates come in the form of sugar, for example in fruit and vegetables, or starch, for example cereals, potatoes and bread. It is better to take carbohydrates in their unrefined or wholefood form, when the foods rich in them also contain fibre, vitamins and minerals, and the digestive system is better able to cope with them.

Snacks containing high levels of refined carbohydrates (such as chocolate bars) lead to a sudden rise in blood sugar level. When the level begins to drop again there is often a craving for sugar, dizziness, trembling and headaches. Long-term over-indulgence in refined carbohydrates leads to obesity and caries and may be involved in such diseases as diabetes, high blood pressure, atherosclerosis, cancers of the digestive tract, gastric ulcer, anaemia and kidney disorder.

Fats Fats in food are the most concentrated forms of energy, producing twice the number of Calories per gram as carbohydrates and proteins. The substances that give fats their flavours, textures and melting points are called fatty acids and these may be 'saturated', 'unsaturated' and 'polyunsaturated'. These names derive from the nature of the chemical bonds within the molecules. Suffice to say that 'saturated' fatty acids come mainly from animal sources (lard, dripping) and are usually solid at room temperature. They are less healthy than 'unsaturated' and 'polyunsaturated' fatty acids, which come from vegetable sources and are usually liquid. They can be solidified by a process called hydrogenation to give the familiar vegetable-oil margarines.

Three fatty acids, linoleic, arachidonic and linolenic, are essential in the diet because the body cannot make them itself. They are necessary for the transport and breakdown of cholesterol and lowering the blood pressure, and they are involved in blood clotting and inflamation.

Fat deficiency is rare in the west today, but it can lead to deficiency of fat-soluble vitamins. Signs include dry skin and eczema, sterility in men, retarded growth and poor vision. Too much fat in the diet is much more likely and so animal fats, processed foods and fried foods should be kept to a minimum. Over-indulgence in fats leads to obesity and atherosclerosis which can in turn be involved in kidney failure, angina, stroke and heart attack.

Proteins These are the 'building blocks' in food, the construction materials for growth and repair of cells. The body needs proteins throughout life, but the need is greatest during infancy, pregnancy and after illness or injury.

Protein may also be used as an energy source. If carbohydrates or fats are lacking in the diet, protein is converted to fat by the liver and burned to provide energy, or burned directly. It yields the same amounts of energy, weight for weight, as carbohydrate.

During digestion, proteins are broken down into units called amino acids. The body requires 22 different amino acids, but it can make 13 itself from other amino acids. The remaining 9 are called essential amino acids because they must be present in the diet. Meat and dairy products contain all the essential amino acids, but individual vegetable foods may contain only some of them. It is important, therefore, in a vegetarian diet, to eat a variety of fruits, nuts, cereals, legumes and vegetables that provides all the essential amino acids.

While proteins are obviously essential to the healthy body, they are dangerous in excess. Obesity, kidney disorders and gout are linked to a diet too high in certain proteins. A diet rich in animal proteins leads to diseases such as kidney stones, high fat levels in the blood, high blood pressure and the formation of cancer-inducing agents in the bile.

Dietary fibre The indigestible parts of plants such as cellulose, lignin and pectin are known as 'fibre' or 'roughage'. They cannot be broken down by our digestive system and therefore pass through it. On the way, fibre aids digestion, absorbs water and makes the stools larger and softer, so preventing constipation. It takes up wastes such as toxins and bile salts and removes them in the stools.

Bowel problems such as diverticular disease, irritable bowel and some cancers of the bowel may be caused by lack of fibre. However, too much fibre can lead to blockage of the intestine, poor absorption of vitamins and minerals, and grain-sensitive bowel inflammations such as coeliac disease. About 30 gms (approximately 1 oz) per day of fibre is suitable for the average person: you should manage this easily if you eat wholefoods.

Vitamins These are organic substances which the body cannot make, but which it requires in small amounts (the exception to this is Vitamin D which can be made from sunlight). Vitamins are either fat- or water-soluble. The fat-soluble vitamins, A, D, E and K can be stored in the body, but the water-soluble B group and C are quickly excreted. Vitamins often work together or with minerals, and their absorption in the gut may be aided or prevented by certain minerals. (See Part 6 for more details of individual vitamins and minerals.)

Supplements You should not need extra vitamins or minerals if you are eating a well-balanced diet with plenty of wholegrains, raw fresh fruits and vegetables. There are conditions where supplements may be recommended, such as alcohol abuse, smoking, taking the oral contraceptive pill, pregnancy, dieting, illness and exposure to radiation. Supplements may also be required by bottle-fed babies, lactating mothers and elderly people.

If you are feeling low physically and mentally, a month's course of multi-vitamins and minerals may give you a boost. I would recommend a multi-vitamin preparation which contains less than 25 mgs of any one of the B vitamin group and is free of additives and colourings. Children's chewable vitamins and minerals are available.

Additives Food has probably always been mixed with other things – herbs, salts, spices, for example – to make it more appealing to eat. In the past 30 years, however, there has been a massive explosion in the chemical adulteration of food. It probably represents the biggest uncontrolled experiment ever performed. However, the results will be hard to analyse. We know some of the short-term effects on the body of individual chemicals added to food, but there is no way of telling what the combined long-term effects will be.

Additives in food are used to colour, flavour, preserve, sweeten, emulsify, stabilise, acidify, thicken, anti-oxidise . . . and of course increase the profits of the growers and processors and sellers. Meat carcasses are sometimes injected with polyphosphates to increase water intake, in order to make them heavier. Antibiotics and even hormones are routinely fed to animals to speed up growth rates. There are 1,200 legal additives for ice cream! Some people – especially children – are extremely allergic to many of them (see Children's food, above).

Naturally-occurring toxins As well as the additives we put in food, there may also be natural toxins (poisons). Some plants produce toxins to avoid being eaten by animals. These are often destroyed by cooking, are not dangerous to humans in small amounts, or are chemically neutralised in the whole plant. Examples include bananas, legumes (especially red beans), potatoes, mushrooms, brassicas, rhubarb, cheese, almonds, quail and certain fish. There are also foods which often seem to raise allergies in certain people. For example, wheat causes the digestive disorder known as coeliac disease. Aflatoxins are present in some nuts.

Infections and parasites are often present in foods: salmonella in chickens, listeria in certain cheeses, brucellosis in meat, tuberculosis in milk, and worms and flukes in meat and fish. Fresh vegetables may have fluke eggs or moulds on their surfaces. Infections such as dysentery and gastroenteritis may be caught from food due to bad hygiene.

Better livestock health and the introduction of pasteurised milk should have removed these risks, although it is possible they have increased the risks for other usually better adapted to parasites. The use of antibiotics and overcrowding of animals for slaughter has increased the risk of salmonella. If, however, you eat untreated products from untested animals, take care to prepare and cook the food properly. Thorough washing of food, cooking to adequate temperatures, correct storage, good hygiene and not reheating food will prevent most infections from being transferred.

Preserving food From earliest times people have preserved food by heating, drying, pickling and salting, in sugar or vinegar or alcohol. Modern methods include canning, cooling or freezing, chemical preservation, and more recently, irradiation. Food decomposes because of the enzymes in it or because bacteria or fungi contaminate it, and preservation kills or slows the contaminants.

Preservation has become essential for city living. It has also removed seasonal and regional restrictions on availability. In some cases it may not be harmful: research has shown that a diet based on modern canned foods gives no adverse effects.

Irradiation uses gamma-rays to kill bacteria in foods. It is already in use in certain countries such as South Africa, the Netherlands, Japan and the USA. Irradiation gives a longer shelf-life, it leaves no taste, and no chemicals are introduced. It destroys vitamins, however, and the long-term effects are not known. Because the word 'radiation' has negative associations, there are moves to call the process by another name, such as 'picowaving'.

Cooking food When buying and preparing food, select the best quality food possible and bear in mind its origins, production and processing.

Take care when storing, preparing and cooking food, that the nutrients are not damaged and toxic chemicals are not introduced. For instance, avoid preparing vegetables in advance, since they will lose their vitamins if allowed to soak for long in water. Microwave cooking causes a loss of nutrients, but whether this is greater than in any other form of cooking is not yet known. Toasting and browning alters the chemical composition of the surface layers and may destroy amino acids and vitamins. Frying is to be avoided if possible; not only does it increase the amount of fat in the diet, but high temperatures can produce carcinogens in fats.

Food, cooked or raw, should always be kept covered in the fridge. Frozen food should be defrosted thoroughly and as quickly as possible before cooking.

Utensils Even the implements you use when cooking can affect health. Rinse detergents thoroughly from kitchenware, since experiments have linked them with eczema and damage to the intestinal lining. Iron utensils are recommended since they distribute heat evenly for thorough cooking, and they may also be a source of iron in the diet! Earthenware pots are sometimes glazed with lead or cadmium, which can be dangerous; white porcelain or glass containers are more suitable. Copper, brass and aluminium pans should be avoided. Aluminium, especially, may be associated with digestive-system complaints ranging from mouth ulcers to piles. Non-stick teflon coatings may lead to gut trouble when they start to peel off.

HEALTH HAZARDS IN PERSPECTIVE

Many environmental hazards of recent decades are inevitable spin-offs from the great technological advances of the last century. There is no doubt that these advances have brought benefits to people across the world. Yet they are not without drawbacks. Reassessing our needs and balancing them carefully against benefits and scientific 'progress' must be an ongoing process. Scientists can predict most short-term toxicological (poisonous) effects of a new substance on animals and people. But the long-term effects of these substances are difficult to study; when more than two substances interact it is impossible to predict the way they are going to behave.

When determining the toxicity or otherwise of a substance it is necessary to study what happens to it and its breakdown products in the body. By modern scientific methods it is possible to do this even where two substances are mixed together but not if more than two are involved. One could even speculate that some are already 'potentized', having been diluted in rivers and lochs and then succussed over weirs and waterfalls and through gurgling pipes and taps! When one considers the thousands of chemical substances loose in our environment, many of them new to the planet, one can appreciate the problems involved in trying to identify potential toxins. Perhaps homeopathy can help.

Some years ago I first heard of the possible link between aluminium and Alzheimer's disease (see PRESENILE DEMENTIA page 134). I compared the symptoms of the disease given in a standard textbook with the mental symptoms of aluminium found in the records of the provings and discovered that they were virtually identical. In theory at least it should be possible, by conducting provings of everyday

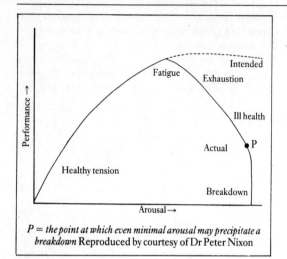

P = the point at which even minimal arousal may precipitate a breakdown Reproduced by courtesy of Dr Peter Nixon

chemicals, either alone or in combination, to discover what their most likely side effects will be, if any.

STRESS

Stress can be defined as anything which puts a load on the systems of the body. Many people are exhausted for a variety of reasons, from lack of sleep to prolonged emotional stress. Paradoxically, the more exhausted you become, the more energy you may appear to have and the less able you may be to sleep. It is like comparing your level of energy in the body to a bank account which has a current and a deposit account. When you are overtired over a long period of time, you have to supply the current account from the deposit account. The danger of this is, of course, that if you have an unexpected demand which has to be met from the deposit account, you may end up in debt or bankrupt, in other words, ill or worse! To avoid this, you have to spend less: cut down the amount of energy you put out to 75% so that 25% is constantly going into the deposit account.

Stress affects different people in different ways. Some can cope with being sent into space in a capsule, others find it hard to leave their own homes. How stress affects us can be shown on the graph above.

As stress increases, so does performance and efficiency – up to a point. That's where fatigue sets in. This breaking point does, of course, vary from person to person. Like the White Queen in *Through the Looking Glass*, 'It takes all the running you can do to stay in the same place. If you want to get somewhere else, you must run at least twice as fast as that.' Few of us can run twice as fast as our bodies will allow. If fatigue is not corrected, it leads to exhaustion ('burn out') and, inevitably, ill health.

Stress produces an increase in the hormones adrenaline, noradrenaline and cortico steroids, among others. In the short term these cause an increase in breathing and heart rates, queasy stomach and tense muscles. There is an enormous list of long-term complaints linked to high stress – just a few of them are high blood pressure, mental problems, hair loss, skin complaints, ulcers in the mouth, asthma, angina, nervous twitching, gastritis, peptic ulcer, ulcerative colitis, irritable bowel syndrome, menstrual problems in women, impotence and premature ejaculation in men, irritable bladder, heart disease, cancers, lung ailments, sclerosis of the liver, accidental injuries and even suicide. Diseases such as multiple sclerosis, diabetes and herpes genitalis may be aggravated by stress.

Some people become addicted to the 'buzz' of adrenaline caused by stress, seeking thrills and 'living in the fast lane'. They may take to dangerous sports or drugs such as cocaine, and without help they will become exhausted and burnt out.

Short-term or acute stress can usually be dealt with. Often some small incident, such as a shoe lace snapping, will cause the person under stress to do the same – snap, perhaps shout and get physical – and release the tension. The safety valve has worked.

Long-term stress The major causes of long-term or chronic stress involve feelings such as lack of purpose, alienation and helplessness. For example, stress is often seen in cases of poverty and unemployment. Stress also occurs in unhappy families and is often related to lack of communication. There may be a stereotyping of each partner's role, classically resulting in frustration for the woman and alienation of the man from his children.

Greater vulnerability to stress may also be caused by such factors as lack of closeness to parents and family, loneliness, or trying to accomplish too much in too little time. Any situation where difficulties cannot by discussed and overcome will lead to stress: sex, class and mothers-in-law being classic examples.

How to measure stress There are several questionnaires that identify stressful life events, from which you can get a rough idea of your own situation. Here is one. The total score gives an indication of the degree of stress you have been exposed to, and perhaps your likely vulnerability to stress-related illness. (This is simplified from a questionnaire devised by Lyle H. Miller and Alma Dill Smith of Boston University Medical Centre.) But remember that no such questionnaire can take into consideration individual differences in response; it is only a guide. Score your answers: 1 yes/always; 2 probably/usually; 3 I suppose/it depends; 4 rarely/not a lot; 5 no/never.

Do you:
1. Take at least one hot, balanced meal per day?
2. Have seven hours' sleep at least four nights per week?
3. Give and receive affection frequently?

4. Have a relative within 80 km (50 miles) on whom you can rely?
5. Exercise to perspiration at least twice per week?
6. Smoke less than ten cigarettes per day?
7. Take alcohol less than five times per week?
8. Keep within the appropriate weight for your height (see page 261)?
9. Have an adequate income for your needs?
10. Get strength from religious, philosophical or some other deeply-held beliefs?
11. Regularly attend a social gathering?
12. Have a network of friends and acquaintances?
13. Have a close friend to confide in?
14. Have good health?
15. Express feelings of anger or worry?
16. Have regular domestic discussions with those you live with?
17. Do something for fun at least once per week?
18. Organize your time effectively?
19. Drink less than three cups of caffeine (tea, coffee or cola) per day?
20. Have a quiet time to yourself each day?

Add up your score. If the answer is less than 50 you probably cope well with stress. Increasing scores indicate increasing vulnerability to stress.

How to cope with stress Stress can be relieved by taking control of the situation. Here are a few simple guidelines:
1. Deal only with things that you can do something about.
2. Take one problem at a time.
3. Talk problems over with other people and listen to their advice, but without complaining or burdening them.
4. Act positively, even if you make the wrong decision; remember everyone makes mistakes.
5. Don't harbour grudges.
6. Relax daily.
7. Occupy yourself rather than just sitting in solitude.
8. Have routines for mealtimes, sleep, exercise, relaxation.
9. Don't dwell on problems after 8 o'clock at night.
10. Admit to yourself if you are becoming overwhelmed by your problems and seek help from your GP, homeopathic physician, health visitor, the Samaritans, a trusted friend or relative – someone you respect and who can be objective.

Anything which gives satisfaction calms the mind and helps to dissipate stress. It varies with the individual: massage, exercise, a hot bath, holiday, music, craft, cinema, sexual intercourse – each gives satisfaction to someone. For many people this is enough to keep them balanced. For others, external sources of satisfaction are not sufficient and they need an internal technique for developing peace of mind. Such techniques include yoga, t'ai chi, biofeedback, self hypnosis, autogenic training, progressive relaxation of the muscles, deep breathing, Alexander technique, psychotherapy or meditation.

Meditation This is one group of techniques for relaxing the body and achieving peace of mind. Research has shown that meditation can stimulate the immune system and reduce inflammation, blood pressure and the likelihood of heart attacks.

The simplest form of meditation is called the relaxation response and was devised by an American cardiologist, Dr Benson. It is summarised in four simple steps:
1. Assume a comfortable position.
2. Close your eyes.
3. Concentrate on a single word, sound or phrase.
4. Cast off other thoughts.
At first you may find it difficult to concentrate on the word, but it will become easier. Do it for 15 minutes each morning and evening, getting used to sitting still.

Yoga techniques such as pranayama breathing (see page 18) and the candle technique are also ways of meditating. The candle technique should be done in the evening. Sit looking at the flame of a candle from about one metre away, for five minutes. Blow out the candle and lightly cover your closed eyes with the palms of your hands; you should see the after-image of the candle in the middle of your forehead. After a while it will tend to slip away, but if you concentrate, you can bring it back and practise holding it for as long as possible.

Deep meditation is the experience of being totally at peace, no matter what is happening outside. With practice you can withdraw your concentration totally from your external senses and focus inwards.

Meditation has been attacked as self-centred escapism. But if you become more at peace with yourself, then your attitudes to and relationships with other people may be more peaceful. Meditation is not in conflict with any religious beliefs – indeed, often it serves to enhance them.

THE AIR WE BREATHE
Without air, or more accurately the oxygen it contains, the biochemical processes which sustain life cease. Cells and tissues die. Clean air, then, is the most important factor in sustaining life.

Chemicals which pollute the air are rarely toxic to all living things. More often they affect only a few people badly, or only their long-term effects are harmful. Atmospheric pollution occurs from numerous sources. Industry accounts for much of it. Careless incineration of waste can lead to the release of dioxins, organo-arsenides and PCBs (poly-chlorinated biphenyls) into the atmosphere – all amazingly dangerous chemicals that contaminate grazing land and can be found in the milk of farm animals. Fluoride emissions from aluminium smelters have been shown to kill cattle and destroy woodlands. Fumes from such processes as dry cleaning contain chloroethylene, which may lead to nausea, headache, fatigue, confusion and poor co-ordination.

Non-industrial pollution There are also many non-industrial sources of air pollution. Carbon monoxide can be emitted from gas installations in the home and may lead to vague 'flu-like symptoms or un-explained headache, nausea, vomiting, tiredness and muscular weakness. Many household insecticides con-tain organophosphates which have been implicated in the development of aplastic anaemia and types of leukaemia in children. Fluorocarbons from aerosol cans are heavily implicated in the depletion of the protective ozone layer in the upper atmosphere, poten-tially leading to an increase in the ultraviolet radiation which triggers certain skin cancers. And of course there is acid rain, smog and the other major causes of massive air pollution, and their links with illnesses such as bronchitis.

Causes of unexplained depression and ill-health may include noxious fumes liberated slowly from rubbers and plastics found in homes, shops and offices, and from air-fresheners. Some curtain and drapery materials contain synthetic textiles or are chemically treated for fire resistance, mould resistance, moth resistance and other resistances. Any of these chemicals may upset a particularly susceptible person.

Ionizers Many people, especially those suffering from asthma, hay fever, migraine or peptic (duodenal) ulcer, often feel well when near mountains or in the country-side after rain. This may be because of the high concentration of negative ions in the atmosphere. Pollution of the air in and around buildings leads to the loss of negative ions, but they can now be replaced by machines. The use of ionizers has been shown to be beneficial for respiratory and circulatory conditions.

Humidifiers Central heating tends to dry out the air, especially when the temperature outside is low and the air's capacity to hold moisture is reduced. Dry air seems to aggravate influenza, colds, migraine and sinus problems. Humidification can be achieved simply by putting bowls of water in a room (out of reach of pets and children). Special humidifier trays can be pur-chased to hang on radiators; electric humidifiers spray fine jets of water vapour into the atmosphere.

THE WATER WE DRINK

In the western world, tap or 'drinking' water is usually safe bacteriologically – the microbes that cause major infections such as cholera and dysentery are not there. But there may be other contaminants which come from agriculture or industry. These contaminants may affect some people more than others, producing skin symptoms such as redness and itching. Nitrates, nitrites, chlorine, fluoride and sulphoxides in water may cause allergenic responses giving rise to a wide variety of symptoms in the abdomen, respiratory tract and nervous system. These include abdominal pain, ulcers of the mouth, sore throat, abdominal distension, diarrhoea, unusual vaginal discharge, fre-quent urination, headache, irritability, tiredness, dizzi-ness and confusion, and Raynaud's syndrome. Lead and copper levels may be high in water because of contamination from old piping. Allow water to run for a full minute before drinking or cooking with it, if unsure or worried.

Water testing If you think your water may be causing problems, ask the local Water Authority to test it. If levels of contaminants are within the legally acceptable range, it may be that you are very sensitive to them. You may be tempted to solve the problem in your home by treating your water. Water from water softeners should not always be used for drinking, since they remove vital trace minerals such as magnesium and calcium. There is also evidence that hard water has a protective effect against coronary artery disease. There are now water filters on the market which remove contaminants. But some of these also remove trace minerals, and they may harbour bacteria. Bottled water may be the answer.

Swimming is an excellent form of exercise, but even then there are drawbacks. Indoor swimming can lead to problems with chlorine (or bromide) sensitivity. Swimming in the sea in some parts of the world has become a hazardous business because of bacterial or chemical pollution.

TOXIC METALS

Some metals are essential as minerals for the body, in tiny amounts (see page 346–9). But most metals are extremely toxic in larger quantities. They are found everywhere – in the air around us, in food and in water, in buildings, clothes and machinery.

Aluminium High levels of aluminium affect the central nervous system, bones, liver and kidneys. Accumula-tion in the body may be involved in hyperactivity in children, joint problems, Alzheimer's disease and presenile dementia. Food and water may be contami-nated when cooked in aluminium utensils or stored in aluminium foil (see page 27, 349). The metal is also found in coffee whitener and antacids; it is released from the soil by acid rain. Its toxic effects in the body are aggravated by deficiency of magnesium and calcium.

Arsenic Arsenic can be found in shellfish, animal feed additives, insecticides, wallpapers and ceramics. It is a well-known poison and large doses are fatal.

Cadmium Zinc is an important constituent of some bodily enzymes. Cadmium replaces zinc in these enzymes, affecting the kidneys and causing high blood pressure. It is found in cigarette smoke, plumbing alloys, soil and old plaster. There are cadmium 'hot spots' near industrial works and it is found in many foods and in rubber products. It is especially dangerous to pregnant women and children.

Lead There has been a great deal of research on the toxicity of lead. High levels of lead in body tissue are known to be potentially fatal. Symptoms include anaemia, colicky abdominal pain and damage to the nerves or brain (see BRAIN DAMAGE, PERIPHERAL NEUROPATHY). Many authorities are now convinced that even low lead levels can cause 'subacute' poisoning, leading to stillbirths or congenital abnormalities, learning and behavioural problems, cancers, heart disease and high blood pressure, kidney and metabolic disease, immune system problems, and vague symptoms such as lethargy, depression, muscular aches and pains and frequent infections. Lead is found in traffic fumes, fruit and vegetables exposed to these fumes, some unlined saucepans, old paints, dust, water from lead pipes or lead-alloy-sealed copper piping, cracked lead-glazed earthenware, bone meal, old toy soldiers, dolomite stone, cigarette ash and tobacco.

Mercury High levels of mercury contamination are known to cause problems with the nervous system. Hatters used to suffer from mercury poisoning as a result of the mercury originally used in hat production – hence the saying 'mad as a hatter'. Small quantities of mercury may cause multiple sclerosis-type symptoms. Mercury is found in fish and shellfish taken from waters polluted with effluent, especially from paper-making factories, drinking water, weed killers, dental amalgam and treated wheat.

RECREATIONAL AND 'STREET' DRUGS
Drug-taking for 'fun' is not new. Evidence suggests that human cultures through history have used various drugs to relieve tension, promote sociability or for religious reasons. In war they have been used to increase aggression and remove concern about personal safety. In today's westernised societies they include caffeine, tobacco, alcohol, and 'soft' and 'hard' drugs. Addiction to certain drugs, legal or illegal, is dealt with on page 108. Yet dependence on the 'everyday' drugs – tobacco, alcohol and caffeine – affects far more people. Alcoholism is dealt with in detail on page 109.

Tobacco Smoking tobacco causes 50,000 premature deaths in the UK each year. Tobacco smoke is toxic because of the various components such as tars (which cause cancers), nicotine (a stimulant drug) and carbon monoxide (which lowers the ability of the blood to carry oxygen). Commercially prepared cigarettes also contain saltpetre to keep them alight. On average, the five minutes someone takes to smoke a cigarette shortens his or her life by the same time. It is estimated that if you smoke between 15 and 20 cigarettes a day you are 15 times more likely to die of cancer of the oesophagus, twice as likely to die of cancer of the bladder, and twice as likely to die of a heart attack, as someone who does not smoke.

A pregnant woman who smokes tobacco is more likely to have a miscarriage or premature delivery. Growth of the baby in the womb may be slow, possibly due to the effects of cadmium in the smoke (see Cadmium, above). There is also an increased risk of the baby being ill or dying in the first year of life. Other dangers include an increase in infantile colic and low intelligence. Smoking when pregnant is hardly giving your child a good start in life.

Other adverse effects from smoking include an increased incidence of kidney disease, stroke, chronic bronchitis, emphysema, heart failure, high blood pressure, and cancer of the cervix. These effects are more likely if smoking started during teenage years, and they are heightened by taking the contraceptive pill.

There is also a danger from 'passive' or 'secondary' smoking, that is, breathing other people's tobacco smoke. You may not smoke but there might be a heavy smoker at home or at work. If you live in a smoky atmosphere you are also more likely to suffer from the long catalogue of smoking-related diseases.

Nicotine in tobacco smoke paralyses the small hairs (cilia) which sweep up debris from the lungs, and stimulates the production of mucus which then cannot be removed by the cilia. A cough develops to remove this excess mucus (smoker's cough). Smoking increases the requirement for vitamins A, B_1, B_2, C, D, bioflavinoids and zinc, and therefore symptoms of deficiency in these vital nutrients may also develop.

People smoke despite strong and continual medical warnings. Why? Some groups of people seem more likely to smoke than others, such as soldiers, criminals, prostitutes, taxi drivers and sailors. One common factor may be long periods of boredom with brief periods of hazardous activity. Smoking relieves boredom because nicotine, in small quantities, stimulates the brain. In large quantities it has a sedative effect. It can also heighten the experience of well-being in an enjoyable situation. And there is also an element of ritual in manipulation of the cigarette and the lighter.

How to stop smoking It is difficult to stop smoking unless you really want to. The reason for stopping may be your own health or the health of your family, or your financial situation. It is pointless trying to stop without working out in your own mind why you smoke, and developing other ways of satisfying these needs. If you smoke because you are anxious, take some form of relaxation or try meditation (see Stress, page 27–9). If you smoke because of boredom, find other ways of amusing yourself.

There appears to be little point in changing to a low-nicotine or low-tar brand of cigarette; statistics show they are also harmful to health. This may be because people who smoke low-tar cigarettes tend to smoke more often or smoke more of the cigarette itself, or inhale more deeply.

If you want to stop smoking, follow these steps:
First, record your smoking habits in detail over a

seven-day period. Against each cigarette make a note of the situation, and rank your 'craving' from 0 to 5.

Second, cut down over four to ten weeks, by smoking the first cigarette of the day later and leaving out the cigarettes that you crave least. Eventually you should get down to the two or three cigarettes that you enjoy the most, for instance with a cup of coffee after a meal.

Third, develop some other habit that avoids both of these situations together. For instance, instead of the coffee after the meal, wash the dishes or go for a walk. Chew gum if you need something in your mouth.

Nicotine gums help some people (4 mg strength for over 20 cigarettes per day, 2 mg strength for under 20 cigarettes per day, on prescription from your doctor). Once the physical craving has gone, you can change to ordinary chewing gum – preferably a low-sugar one such as Orbit.

The habit of chewing tobacco is spreading from America to the UK. This may lead to ulceration in the mouth and also create a state of nicotine dependency . . . leading to smoking.

Caffeine Caffeine is found in tea, and coffee and drinks such as cola and chocolate. One survey found that one Australian in three was physically dependent on caffeine! They drank more than five cups of medium-strength instant coffee daily, approximately 200 mg of caffeine per day. There was also an association with smoking more cigarettes.

Caffeine has been shown to remain in the body of a pregnant woman for up to 20 hours, for up to 13 hours in a woman on the pill, for up to 7 hours in non-smokers, and for up to 3 hours in children. In non-smokers it causes irritation of the lining of the stomach, an increase in acid production, and it may aggravate peptic ulcers. Interestingly, decaffeinated coffee aggravates stomach ulcers more than normal coffee.

Caffeine can relax the lower end of the oesophagus, resulting in reflux of acid. It also causes irritability, insomnia in some people, quickening of the pulse rate and palpitations. There may be loss of the mineral potassium, deficiency of vitamin B_1, decreased absorption of iron from the intestine, nervous excitability, loss of fluids, anxiety, possibly cancer of the pancreas, genetic aberrations and hypoglycaemia. Caffeine generally increases the metabolic work load.

Tea has half the amount of caffeine as coffee. It is associated with peptic ulcer irritation, and has been shown to decrease absorption of proteins, iron and vitamin B_1. It does, however, contain high levels of the essential element manganese.

So what should you do when faced with this array of possible health hazards from coffee and tea? Restrict the drinking of ordinary coffee – one or two cups per day – but moderate use of decaffeinated coffee and tea daily (up to three cups) should do no harm. Substitutes include Maté and Rooibosch teas, herb teas, and grain coffees such as Caro Extra and Barley Cup, made from roasted grains of cereals and dandelion roots. Végétal by Triggs is a good example of a pleasant salt-free drink.

Chocolate can be replaced by carob in both drinks and sweets. Cola drinks should be avoided and replaced by, for example, fruit juice.

ENVIRONMENTAL HEALTH HAZARDS

Employment Each year one million people are off work for more than three days through injury or industrial disease, and a staggering ten million require first aid for injuries sustained at work.

To avoid becoming one of these statistics, always follow safety instructions and make sure the equipment you use is in proper working order. Use an air filter, masks, eye and ear protectors, reinforced footwear, helmets and heavy gloves as necessary. If they are not provided they should be. They are for your safety – don't be a Rambo! If you feel ill after starting a new job or using a new process, explain it to your GP and report it to the person responsible for health and safety where you work.

Unemployment Problems linked to the low incomes of the long-term unemployed include inadequate housing, which can in turn lead to illness. There may not be money for proper food or heating. Children in such families tend to be small and at greater risk of accidental death and injury. Malnutrition, coronary artery disease, peptic ulcers and certain cancers are commoner in poorer people. Those with inadequate incomes lack the resources of choice, influence and ability to shape their environment. They tend to have low self-esteem and cope less well with crisis. Hormone levels and the immune system may also be affected. Stress caused by the hopelessness of unemployment is associated with increased drug abuse.

The home Until recently, houses were built of tried and tested natural materials such as wood and bricks. Over the last few decades, some of these materials have either been treated with chemicals or replaced by synthetic products. There are new forms of heating and endless uses for electricity.

Numerous childhood ailments are connected with damp housing. Mould spores are often responsible, and reducing condensation by extractor fans or open windows can prevent their growth. Consider that a family of 5 produces two buckets-full of condensation in one day.

The bed A bed should be a psychological retreat from the world, a place of ease and relaxation, as well as giving you a comfortable and refreshing night's sleep. The ideal interior-sprung mattress is one which has individually-pocketed springs that independently support each part of the body. Turn the mattress regularly to prevent uneven wear and replace at the manufacturer's recommended time or before if it becomes too saggy. Pillows should fill in the curves between the head and the shoulders. Neck sufferers may benefit from special supporting pillows.

Clothes and cosmetics The skin absorbs substances from its surface – witness the steroid ointments used in some types of eczema and dermatitis. Many nail varnishes, deodorants, antiperspirants and shampoos contain formaldehyde, and some include aluminium. Avoid them if your skin is broken, irritated or sensitive. If you are healthy and hygienic, body odour should not be a problem. Vary brands and, where possible avoid aluminium; health food shop products are usually aluminium free.

Pets Animals have long been domesticated for food and materials – and for companionship. People sometimes find it easier to express their emotions to their pet than to another person. Pets relieve loneliness and can give security. Bear the family pet in mind, however, when dealing with unexplained allergies, and respiratory or bowel disorders. In particular don't allow young children to play unattended in parks or gardens where there may be animal excreta.

Sound The loudness of sound is measured in decibels (db). A watch ticking generates 20db, while normal speech is about 60db. Amplified rock music generates 100db and may cause pain and injury to the ears. A jet engine at close range, at 130db, will permanently damage unprotected ears very quickly. Hearing, like sight, is a very precious sense – guard it carefully (see EARS page 157*ff*).

Weather and electromagnetic phenomena The weather is blamed for many illnesses, especially by British people! Research in Germany does suggest that a wide range of illnesses are worse in certain weather conditions. These include angina, 'flu, depression and rheumatic diseases.

The weather has always been with us but we are now surrounded by man-made electromagnetic radiations, at home, at work and out of doors. Whether these are capable of causing disease is not established for certain, but two areas of concern are high voltage electricity cables and VDU screens. If you are living in close proximity to power lines and are suffering from unexplained mental or physical ill-health bear them in mind. Avoid using VDUs if you are pregnant. Otherwise only use them for an hour at a time with a ten minute break for a maximum of four hours a day. Make sure the display is sharp but not too bright, with no flickering, glare or reflection and follow the Health and Safety Executive's recommendations for seating etc.

Rock and mineral deposits also give off electromagnetic radiation. If you feel that you have become unwell, or cannot sleep since moving house or changing your bedroom you may be exposed to this, or other magnetic phenomena. Try moving your bed or sleeping in a different room.

Radioactivity High doses of radiation of a high frequency do physical damage to the cells of the body. At this time $\frac{2}{3}$ of radioactivity is still from natural sources. Most of the remaining $\frac{1}{3}$ comes from the medical use of X-rays.

In the event of another Chernobyl-type disaster, immediately adopting the following measures will help reduce your exposure until the danger is past:
1. Reduce animal products, including milk.
2. Eat food which is packed in air-tight containers.
3. Avoid foods exposed to rainwater.
4. Eat 2 or 3 apples four times daily (provided they were collected before the fallout, obviously).
5. Take a multivitamin and mineral supplement and consider giving iodine to children – but only under medical supervision.
6. Contact your homeopathic physician to see if homeopathic remedies are required.

Light Light is part of the electromagnetic spectrum, blurring into ultraviolet at one end (higher frequencies) and infra red at the other.

Ultraviolet not only tans the skin but it can also burn. The hazards of sunlight include cataracts and malignant melanoma, particularly in light-skinned people. Sunlight may also cause problems in people taking certain drugs, such as the phenothiazines – which are used in the treatment of schizophrenia.

The disadvantages of sunlight, however, are far outweighed by its advantages, provided that exposure to strong sunlight is done gradually or high factor creams are used at first. Apart from being essential for the formation of vitamin D in the skin, sunlight may also help to prevent depression. Exposure to sunlight on a daily basis is recommended, even in cloudy weather.

There are inherent dangers in the use of sunbeds. Protective measures described in the instructions, such as eye goggles and test doses, must be carefully followed.

Finally, avoid looking directly into both sun and artificial light, and use full spectrum tubes if you have to replace old fluorescent strips. Eyesight is most precious; guard it well (See EYES, page 149*ff*).

Travel For general advice, obtain a copy of *Traveller's Health* by Dr R. Dawood (see bibliography, page 390). Books are also available to help you overcome jet lag. Take out health insurance.

Homeopathic alternatives are available for all the usual immunizations. There is no proof at present that they are effective although they can certainly be used where you are unable to take the ordinary immunizations.

In addition to your usual first aid kit you may wish to take remedies for travel sickness (page 219). special remedies for possible hazards such as snake poisoning (see First Aid page 90–92), and two remedies for the bowels: Phosphoric acid 30 for mild traveller's diarrhoea and Arsenicum album 30 for gastro-enteritis!

PREVENTING ACCIDENTS AND EMERGENCIES

Although you may be more aware of an accident happening say, on holiday, the stark truth is that most occur around the home and on the roads. One accident in four involves a child under 5; elderly people are also particularly susceptible. Research has shown that poorer people, the unemployed and the socially disadvantaged are more likely to suffer serious injury. These facts reflect the high cost of safety equipment for children and old people. There are grants for people on low incomes to help make their homes safer. (See also First Aid, page 85pp).

A great deal of care and thought should be put into making your home a safe place. Pay particular attention to preventing burns and fires, cuts, scalds, falls, electrocution, drowning and suffocation. Unprotected fires and cookers, wide-opening windows, loose wiring and unsecured floor coverings should all be avoided. Have adequate lighting, and safety glass in internal glazed doors. Keep sharp implements and tools locked away. Make sure electrical equipment, wires, plugs and sockets are safe or out of reach of children. Be a good neighbour; the elderly living alone should have regular visitors.

The roads account for an alarming number of accidents each year. If you have been driving a long time, I advise taking an advanced driving test.

Checklist for children
1. Do not leave young children to play, bath or eat unattended.
2. Satisfy yourself about safety precautions in the kitchen, at school, at playmates' homes and on outings.
3. Keep medicines, domestic cleaners, disinfectants, alcohol, cigarettes, decorating materials and garden chemicals out of reach of children. Teach youngsters not to eat any berries or fungi they may find.
4. Never allow a young child on the road alone and teach children the Green Cross Code. Always use suitable seats, belts and door locks in the car. If on the road at night, wear luminous clothing and carry a torch.
5. Supervise children near water and teach them to swim as early as possible.

No checklist can be exhaustive. Preventing accidents to young children, where a few seconds damage can kill them or scar them for life, is well worth the few minutes it takes to make things in their environment as safe as possible.

FINALLY

We could spend our entire lives worrying about avoiding hazards and preventing ill-health; briefly, the most important things to remember are:
1. Stress is part of the modern world: try and find a way of coping with it.
2. Eat healthily, breathe properly, take plenty of exercise, especially in fresh air and maintain good posture.
3. Try to avoid contamination of your body and environment.
4. Treat ill-health by homeopathic means as much as possible: do not resort automatically to orthodox medicine.

Part 3

HOMEOPATHIC REMEDIES

THERE are now more than 3000 homeopathic remedies in use throughout the world, most of them derived from plants and minerals, some from animal and human tissues or secretions, a few from the micro-organisms which multiply during disease processes, and even a few from modern drugs. You will find all the remedies mentioned in this book, some 250 in all, listed on pp. 77–83, with their full Latin names and common names.

Since many of the commonly used abbreviations of remedy names are neither consistently used nor particularly meaningful to the non-homeopath, remedies in this book are generally referred to by the first part of their Latin name, with a suffix if there is any chance of confusion. For example *Allium cepa* is simply referred to as Allium, whereas *Allium sativa* is Allium sat. *Mercurius solubilis* is simply Mercurius, but *Mercurius corrosivus* is Mercurius corr. *Nux vomica* is simply Nux, but *Nux moschata* is Nux mosch. If in doubt about which remedy is meant, turn to pp. 77–83. More detailed information on 60 of the remedies can be found in the appendix, p. 355.

For everyday home use a stock of three or four dozen remedies would be more than adequate. Suggestions for building a Home Medicine Chest appear opposite. To spread the expense, buy the starter remedies, ointments, and mother tinctures first, and add the other remedies later.

Where can I buy homeopathic remedies?
Some chemists and healthfood shops stock a small range of remedies, usually in pilule form and in the 6c potency. However in emergencies and in many chronic conditions, 30c remedies should be used. Being many times more diluted, they are many times more potent.

A full range of remedies, in various potencies and also as mother tinctures, can be bought from the specialized pharmacies and manufacturers listed on p. 387–8. If you consult a homeopath, of course, he or she may dispense remedies direct.

Various other items – unmedicated pilules, phials, storage boxes, droppers, etc. – can be purchased from the Homeopathic Supply Company (see address p. 388)

In what forms are homeopathic remedies available?
Most people buy their remedies in the form of lactose (milk sugar) pilules which have been impregnated

---

BUILDING A HOME MEDICINE CHEST

Starter remedies
Aconite, Apis, Arnica, Belladonna, Cantharis, Carbo/veg., Hypericum (30c and 6c potency). Buy the 30c first.
Chamomilla, Euphrasia, Ledum, Rhus tox., Ruta (6c potency only)

Other commonly used remedies
Bryonia, Ferrum phos. (30c and 6c potency, but buy the 30c first))
Allium, Alumina, Argentum nit., Arsenicum, Calcarea, Colocynth, Gelsemium, Hamamelis, Hepar sulph., Ignatia, Ipecac., Lachesis, Lycopodium, Magnesia phos., Mercurius, Natrum mur., Nux, Phosphorus, Pulsatilla, Silicea, Sulphur, Urtica (6c potency only)

Less common but useful remedies
Glonoinum (30c potency)
Anacardium, Antimonium, Antimonium tart., Baryta carb., Calcarea phos., Causticum, Chelidonium, China, Dioscorea, Dulcamara, Graphites, Hyoscyamus, Kali carb., Natrum sulph, Opium, Phosphoric ac., Phytolacca, Sepia, Spongia, Staphisagria, Tarentula, Thuja, Veratrum (6c potency)

Mother tinctures
Calendula, Hypericum, Euphrasia (used to make up lotions for bathing, gargling, etc.)
   To make up a lotion add 10 drops of mother tincture to 0.25 litre (½ pint) boiled cooled water. If using Euphrasia to bathe eyes, add 1 teaspoon salt to solution.

Ointments
Calendula ointment (soothing ointment for sore or inflamed skin)
Hypericum and Calendula ointment (antiseptic ointment for treating grazes and wounds)
Arnica, Calendula and Urtica ointment (general purpose soothing ointment for bruises and inflammation – NOT for use on broken or cut skin)

Bach Rescue Remedy (available as a liquid or ointment, for use in emotional emergencies for effects of anguish, examinations, visits to the dentist, etc. For more information about Bach remedies, read Edward Bach's books (see bibliography p. 391.)

Tissue Salts come singly or in combinations for specific complaints. For information read Gilbert's book on Biochemic Tissue Salts (see p. 391) with a solution of the named remedy; to take the remedy one simply dissolves one or two pilules on the tongue. For babies and small children, there are also granules, which dissolve more quickly on the tongue and are less easy to spit out!

Remedies are also sold in solution form in small glass phials with screw tops. If you are allergic to lactose, one or two drops can be put directly on the tongue. The dropper should be sterilized between uses.

A few remedies are available as ointments, for topical application only, and some are available as mother tinctures, for mixing with water to make lotions for bathing, gargling, etc. Generally speaking, 10 drops of mother tincture to 0.25 litre (½ pint) of boiled cooled water are sufficient.

Can I get homeopathic remedies on the NHS?

Yes, provided they have been prescribed by a homeopath who is also a GP and working within the National Health Service, or by a homeopath working in an NHS homeopathic hospital (addresses p. 387–8).

When and how should I take homeopathic remedies?

Remedies are best taken in between meals, at least half an hour after eating, and should be dissolved or dropped on to a clean tongue. They should not be taken when your mouth tastes of toothpaste, tobacco, strongly flavoured sweets, spicy food, etc. In emergencies make sure the mouth is thoroughly rinsed before giving a remedy.

What is the correct dosage?

Frequency and duration of dosage are indicated for all the remedies mentioned in PART 4 and PART 5 of this book.

For both adults and children 'a dose' is 1 pilule or 1 drop, or just enough granules to cover the area of the small finger nail. In chronic conditions 6c is usually the most appropriate potency, but in emergencies or in acute conditions 30c may be more appropriate.

In acute conditions, doses should be taken every ½ or 1 hour to begin with, up to a maximum of 10 doses. But as soon as there is some improvement, the interval between doses should be increased to 8 or 12 hours for 2 or 3 days at most. THERE IS ABSOLUTELY NO POINT IN CONTINUING TO TAKE A REMEDY ONCE THE SYMPTOMS HAVE STARTED TO DISAPPEAR.

In chronic conditions 6c remedies are usually taken 3 times a day for up to 14 days, and 30c remedies every 12 hours for a few days. In chronic conditions the stronger the mental and emotional symptoms the higher the potency, and the stronger the physical symptoms the lower the potency.

Remember, the effectiveness of homeopathic remedies depends on matching the symptom picture to the remedy picture as precisely as you can, and then taking the smallest possible dose for the least possible time. Once the remedy has delivered its message, your Vital Force will do the rest.

Can I give homeopathic remedies to babies or very young children?

Yes, but you may find it easier to give granules rather than pilules because granules dissolve more quickly and are more difficult to spit out. If you do not have granules, you can always crush a pilule between two clean spoons.

What should I do if the symptoms get worse?

Aggravation, a temporary worsening of symptoms, is not unusual when taking homeopathic remedies. Aggravation is usually a good sign – it means that a remedy is working. If you have simply taken the wrong remedy, it will have no effect. In acute conditions, discomfort may increase for a few minutes, seldom for longer. In chronic conditions, aggravation may last longer, but very rarely for more than a day or two.

The correct thing to do in such circumstances is to stop taking the remedy and wait until your symptoms improve, as they almost certainly will. If improvement continues, there is no need to take the remedy again. If improvement stops, restart the remedy. Where improvement continues for a while, then stops, leaving you with nagging symptoms, take the remedy in a higher potency; if you are taking 6c, take up to 10 doses of 30c.

If worsening symptoms are accompanied by any of the following – a persistent temperature of 39°C [102°F] or over, spitting blood or passing blood in stools or urine, a rigid and painful abdomen, increasing breathlessness and chest pain, confusion or abnormal drowsiness – dial 999. If you have diagnosed a condition which is potentially serious, contact your GP or homeopathic physician at once.

What should I do if some symptoms improve but others don't?

If you feel better in yourself, gradually cut down the remedy dose – the physical symptoms should improve in time. If you get 'stuck', you may need another remedy, probably one that complements the previous one.

If you experience relief from physical symptoms but find that mental symptoms remain troublesome, it may mean you have suppressed symptoms, although this is quite rare with homeopathy. It is more likely that your underlying condition is changing. To be on the safe side, however, antidote whatever remedy you are taking by drinking two cups of black coffee, or by taking the specific antidote (antidotes are given under each remedy described on pp. 356*ff*).

What should I do if new symptoms appear?

First, stop the remedy. You may be proving it. The symptoms should quickly disappear. If they do not, you may have the wrong diagnosis or remedy. Recheck, and call your GP or homeopath if unsure.

What should I do if the symptoms get neither better nor worse?

Review your symptoms, being as specific as you can, and consult the General Remedy Finder (pp. 38–37) to see if you can find a more appropriate remedy.

Are there any substances I should avoid when taking homeopathic remedies?

Yes. Coffee, alcohol, tobacco, minty flavourings, highly perfumed cosmetics and toiletries, strongly smelling household cleaners, and essential oils used in aromatherapy all have the ability to antidote homeopathic remedies, and should be avoided completely in acute ailments. If you have a chronic complaint and your symptoms are steadily improving with homeopathic treatment, you could gradually reintroduce some of them, but if improvement suddenly stops they will probably be the reason why.

How should homeopathic remedies be stored?

In a cool, dry, dark place, well away from things that smell, taking care to keep the tops of phials and containers well screwed on. Stored like this, homeopathic remedies remain potent for up to 100 years. Don't transfer remedies from one container to another. And keep them out of reach of children. They aren't poisonous, however much your child may take, but a small child may experience transient diarrhoea from the lactose sugar – and your whole collection could be wiped out at one go!

Can I take homeopathic remedies as well as orthodox drugs?

Homeopathic remedies will not interfere with any drugs your GP has prescribed for you. However, many orthodox drugs – steroids, major and minor tranquilizers, oral contraceptives, sleeping pills, antihistamines – modify or completely block the effects of homeopathic remedies. If you want to come off orthodox drugs, discuss the matter with your GP first. DO NOT ON ANY ACCOUNT STOP TAKING A DRUG WITHOUT CONSULTING YOUR GP. If you have occasion to consult a homeopath, be sure to say what drugs you are taking.

How do I decide which is the right homeopathic remedy?

IN EMERGENCIES, where swift medical attention is necessary and there is no time to choose between alternative remedies, simply give the homeopathic rescue remedy which appears under the appropriate entry in PART 4: First Aid or in PART 5: Ailments and Diseases. Use the Index to find the relevant entry. If the person is in emotional shock, give 4 drops of the Bach Rescue Remedy (see p. 35) as well.

IN ACUTE CASES which are not emergencies you should have time to choose an appropriate homeopathic remedy from those listed under the relevant entry in PART 5–Ailments and Diseases and cross-check it by consulting the general Remedy Finder (pp. 38–37) but if you don't have time to draw up the kind of table shown on p. 38, don't worry. Simply choose the remedy which seems to suit the symptoms best. If the remedy does not produce some improvement you may have chosen wrong; it pays to spend 5 minutes getting it right the first time!

IN ALL OTHER CASES you should have plenty of time to track down the right remedy. This is what you do.

1 Jot down the most noticeable symptoms – these can be physical (swellings, redness, pain), mental (anxiety, irritability, grief), food-related (a dislike of milk, a craving for fatty foods) or environment-related (sensitivity to noise, symptoms which come on after getting wet) but they must be symptoms which are unusual, out-of-the-ordinary for you or for the person you want to treat.

2 Turn to the Index and see if the physical or mental symptoms have an entry in PART 5 – Ailments and Diseases. General symptoms such as COUGH, HEADACHE, FEVER, SORE THROAT, and ABDOMINAL PAIN for example appear in PART 5, with suggestions as to their possible causes. If you suspect a particular ailment or disease, refer to the Index and look up the relevant entry in PART 5.

3 Carefully read the PART 5 entry which most closely corresponds to the symptoms you have observed. It may advise you to give First Aid, dial 999, or see your GP within 2 hours, 12 hours, 24 hours, 48 hours, or as soon as convenient. If the condition is long-standing and poses no immediate or serious threat to health, it may recommend a number of homeopathic remedies for you to try at home or advise you to consult an experienced homeopath.

4 If home homeopathic treatment seems appropriate, select the remedy which most closely matches the symptoms. But if none of the remedies given seems quite right, or if you consider other symptoms to be equally or even more important than those described, consult the General Remedy Finder (pp. 38–76). Full instructions on how to use the General Remedy Finder appear on p. 38–9.

5 For further clarification, read the remedies in the 60 Remedies section (p. 356*ff*).

Note: The potencies given are only a guide. If a remedy is well indicated but you don't have the potency recommended, use whatever potency you have, obeying the given time limits or until you can obtain the indicated potency.

GENERAL REMEDY FINDER

The following pages can be used in two ways:

• to help you decide between the various homeopathic remedies recommended for the ailments and diseases in PART 5, provided you are sure of the diagnosis;

• to help you find remedies for symptoms which are at variance with normal appearance and functioning, or which reflect a low level of vitality, but which do not yet add up to any specific ailment or disease.

Symptoms are grouped under four main headings: Body, Environment, Food and Drink, and Mind and Emotions. Appropriate remedies are listed alphabetically under each symptom. Please note a remedy may appear under apparently contradictory headings.

Choosing the right remedy once you are sure of the diagnosis
Let us suppose you have a child with a sore throat and a temperature. You turn to the Index at the back of the book and look up SORE THROAT. You find it has an entry in PART 5 which tells you to contact your GP if a sore throat is accompanied by a high temperature. Your GP diagnoses TONSILLITIS, which you look up in the Childhood Ailments and Diseases section of PART 5. Seven homeopathic remedies are listed for tonsillitis in children but, on reading them through and looking in the child's throat, you cannot choose between them. This is where the General Remedy Finder becomes useful.

Carefully note down, in order of importance, any symptoms which are not part of the tonsillitis picture but which are at variance with the child's normal behaviour. You notice, for example, that he has a vacant, stupid expression on his face, which is most unusual for him. Also, despite his high temperature, he is not thirsty. Then you remember that the day before the fever came on he was playing in a very draughty corridor. When you look into his mouth, his tongue seems redder than usual. He also seems much more feverish and ill in the afternoon. These five out-of-the-ordinary symptoms – 'stupefied', 'lack of thirst', 'draughts make symptoms worse' 'tongue red all over', and 'symptoms worse in afternoon' – are all listed, with appropriate remedies, in the General Remedy Finder. You now have to see which of the tonsillitis remedies appear most frequently under those five symptoms. The easiest way to do this is to draw up a table, putting the tonsillitis remedies along the top and the five out-of-the-ordinary symptoms down the side (see below).

In this instance Belladonna emerges as clear first choice. To make doubly sure that Belladonna is the appropriate remedy, look up the general picture of Belladonna in the 60 Remedies section (pp. 356–381). If Belladonna, given in the dosage recommended under tonsillitis, fails to work, your second choice would be Apis, also given in the dosage recommended under tonsillitis.

It is best to have at least six remedies to choose from. If only one or two are recommended under the ailment or disease diagnosed, add the remedies given for the most important secondary symptom to the top line of your table, then those for the second most important, and so on, until you have at least six.

If, after having drawn up your table, no single remedy clearly emerges as more suitable than any other, see if a reading of the appropriate remedies in

Tonsillitis remedies

	Apis	Belladonna	Hepar sulph.	Mercurius	Lachesis	Phytolacca	Lycopodium
Stupefied	/	/					
Not thirsty	/						
Worse for draughts		/					
Red tongue	/	/		/			
Worse in afternoon		/					/
Total	3	4	0	1	0	0	1

the 60 Remedies section will help. If you are still stuck, consult your homeopath.

Finding an appropriate remedy for non-specific ailments
The General Remedy Finder can also be used to find remedies for general feelings of unwellness, of being out of kilter and under par, provided you can pinpoint at least six out-of-the-ordinary symptoms, six symptoms which are unusual for you or for the person you are treating. You will probably find that most of them are directly or indirectly related to an external event, either one which has just happened or one which is imminent.

Suppose, for example, you are about to sit an important exam. You are apprehensive, and also mentally exhausted because you have been studying hard. Because you have been eating badly and not getting enough exercise, you have become rather constipated and your tongue looks white and coated; you are also irritated by the slightest noise and cannot stop eating sweets. The six symptoms just mentioned – 'apprehension', 'mental exhaustion', 'hard faeces', 'tongue white and coated', 'sensitivity to noise', and 'desire for sweet foods' – all appear in the General Remedy Finder. You must decide which four or five symptoms are the most important, and their order of importance, and then draw up a table similar to the one on p. 38, putting the remedies for the most important symptom or symptoms across the top, and the other symptoms down the side. Remember, it is

important to be as specific as you can about your symptoms. The remedy that crops up most often is likely to be the one which will help you shake off the pre-exam blues. As a further check, turn to the 60 Remedies section (pp. 356–381) and see what the full picture of the remedy shows. If the cross-check is satisfactory, take the remedy in the 6c potency three times a day for up to 14 days until you detect a general upswing. Dosage should then be discontinued.

If the most important symptom only has one or two remedies, put the remedies for the second most important, and then the third most important, across the top of the table until you have at least six remedies to choose from. If the picture which emerges is inconclusive consult your homeopath.

Two things must be emphasized here. First, the General Remedy Finder is not an invitation to hypochondria, but an aid to treating imbalances before they lower vitality and resistance to the point where medically recognized ailments set in. Second, homeopathic remedies can and do relieve many vague, unspecific ailments, but their effects can be shortlived unless diet, exercise, and mental and emotional factors can be adjusted in the direction of greater vitality. Symptoms which have been present for a long time, for so long that they have become the norm rather than the exception, suggest a deep-lying imbalance. In such cases it would be better to seek constitutional treatment from an experienced homeopath than attempt to self-prescribe.

BODY

APPETITE

Appetite easily satisfied
China
Lycopodium
Platinum

Increase in appetite
Abies can.
Ammon. carb.
Argentum
Arsenicum
Calcarea
Calcarea sulph.
Cannabis ind.
China
Cina
Cinnab.
Graphites
Iodum
Lycopodium
Natrum mur.
Nux
Oleander
Petroleum
Phosphorus
Psorinum
Pulsatilla
Sabadilla
Sulphur
Veratrum

Lack of appetite
Arsenicum
Asarum
Calcarea
Chamomilla
Chelidonium
Cocculus
Cyclamen
Digitalis
Ferrum
Kali bichrom.
Lycopodium
Natrium mur.
Nux
Phosphorus
Pulsatilla
Rhus tox
Sepia
Silica
Sulphur

Lack of appetite despite hunger
Cocculus
Lachesis

Natrum mur.
Nux

Lack of appetite accompanied by thirst
Calcarea
Colchicum
Kali nit.
Phosphorus
Psorinum
Spigelia
Sulphur

Lack of appetite and lack of thirst
Argentum nit.

Ravenous appetite
Ammon. carb.
Argentum
Arsenicum
Arsenicum iod.
Calcarea
Calcarea phos.
Calcarea sulph.
Cannabis ind.
Carbon sulph.
China
Cina
Ferrum
Graphites
Iodum
Lycopodium
Natrum mur.
Nux
Oleander
Petroleum
Phosphorus
Psorinum
Pulsatilla
Sabadilla
Silicea
Sulphur
Veratrum

BODY ODOUR
   see also PERSPIRATION
Sickly
Allium
Arnica
Arsenicum
Belladonna
Bryonia
Carbo veg.
Chamomilla
Gelsemium
Hepar sulph.

Mercurius
Pulsatilla
Sulphur

Sour
Arsenicum
Bryonia
Colchicum
Hepar sulph.
Iodum
Lycopodium
Magnesia carb.
Mercurius
Nitric ac.
Psorinum
Sepia
Silicea
Sulphur
Veratrum

Sweet
Apis
Mercurius
Pulsatilla
Thuja

BREATHING
Difficult, laboured breathing
Anacardium
Antimonium
Apis
Arsenicum
Bryonia
Carbo veg.
Causticum
Chelidonium
China
Hepar sulph.
Ipecac.
Kali carb.
Lachesis
Lycopodium
Natrum sulph.
Opium
Phosphorus
Pulsatilla
Silicea
Spongia
Sulphur
Veratrum

Gasping for breath
Antimonium tart.
Apis
Colocynth

Hypericum
Ipecac.
Lycopodium
Phosphorus
Spongia

Irregular breathing
Arsenicum
Belladonna
Chamomilla
Ignatia
Nux
Opium
Pulsatilla

Rapid breathing
Aconite
Antimonium
Arsenicum
Belladonna
Bryonia
Carbo veg.
Chelidonium
Gelsemium
Ipecac.
Lycopodium
Phosphorus
Sepia
Sulphur

Sighing frequently
Bryonia
Carbo veg.
Ignatia
Ipecac.
Opium

Wheezy or asthmatic breathing
Argentum
Arsenicum
Ipecac.
Kali carb
Pulsatilla
Silicea
Spongia
Sulphur

CLOTHING
Intolerance of clothing
Argentum nit.
Calcarea
Lachesis
Lycopodium
Nux
Onosmodium
Spongia

Wanting to loosen clothing
Calcarea
Lachesis
Lycopodium
Nitric ac.
Nux

Undressing makes symptoms worse
Arsenicum
Hepar sulph.
Kali ars.
Kali carb.
Lycopodium
Magnesia phos.
Nux mosch.
Nux
Rhododendron
Rhus tox.
Sambucus
Silicea
Squilla
Zinc

COMPLEXION
Bluish
Arsenicum
Asafoetida
Baptisia
Belladonna
Bryonia
Camphor
Cannabis ind.
Carbo veg.
Conium
Cuprum
Digitalis
Hyoscyamus
Ipecac.
Lachesis
Morphine
Opium
Veratrum
Veratrum vir.

Dirty-looking
Argentum nit.
Lycopodium
Psorinum
Sulphur

Earthy
China
Ferrum
Ferrum iod.
Ferrum phos.
Graphites

Mercurius
Opium
Sepia

Pale
Anacardium
Antimonium tart.
Argentum nit.
Arsenicum
Berberis
Calcarea
Calcarea phos.
Camphora
Carbon sulph.
Carbo veg.
China
China sulph.
Cina
Clematis
Cuprum
Digitalis
Ferrum
Ferrum phos.
Graphites
Lobelia
Lycopodium
Manganum
Medorrhinum
Natrum ars.
Natrum carb.
Natrum mur.
Natrum phos.
Opium
Plumbum
Secale
Sepia
Sulphur
Tabacum
Tuberculinum
Veratrum
Zinc

Red
Aconite
Apis
Baptisia
Belladonna
Bryonia
Capsicum
Chamomilla
Chelidonium
China
Cicuta
Cina
Ferrum
Glonoinum
Hyoscyamus

Lachesis
Melilotus
Mezereum
Nux
Opium
Phosphorus
Rhus tox.
Sanguinaria
Stramonium
Veratrum vir.

Sallow
Argentum nit.
Carbo veg.
Chelidonium
Medorrhinum
Natrum mur.
Plumbum
Sulphur

Yellow
Argentum
Argentum nit.
Arsenicum
Calcarea
Calcarea phos.
Carduus
Causticum
Gelsemium
Conium
Ferrum
Ferrum iod.
Lachesis
Lycopodium
Mercurius
Natrum sulph.
Nux
Plumbum
Sepia
Sulphur

COUGHING
Coughing makes symptoms worse
Aconite
Argentum nit.
Arnica
Arsenicum
Belladonna
Bryonia
Calcarea
China
Cina
Drosera
Ipecac.
Rhus tox
Veratrum

Dry cough
Aconite
Bryonia
Spongia
Phosphorus
Nux
Sticta
Rhus tox.

Loose cough, with phlegm
Ipecac.
Hepar sulph.
Kali bichrom.

Cough dry or loose, depending on time of day
Stannum
Pulsatilla

Cough worse in evening
Belladonna

Cough worse at night
Drosera
Rhus tox.
Rumex
Spongia
Sticta

Cough worse around midnight
Arsenicum

Cough worse between 3–5 am
Kali carb.

Cough made worse by cold, dry wind
Aconite
Bryonia
Hepar sulph.
Rumex

Cough worse in cold, damp conditions
Rhus tox.

Cough made worse by change in temperature
Phosphorus

Cough made worse by draughts
Hepar sulph.

Cough worse after eating
Nux

Cough made worse by exertion
Belladonna
Ipecac.

Cough made worse by slightest movement
Bryonia

Cough made worse by laughing and talking
Stannum
Phosphorus
Rumex

Cough worse when head is down
Spongia

Cough made worse by being in warm room
Pulsatilla
Bryonia

Cough alleviated by covering head with blanket
Rumex

Cough alleviated by drinking
Causticum

Cough alleviated by eating and drinking
Spongia

Cough associated with headache
Bryonia
Belladonna
Nux

Cough causes incontinence of urine
Causticum
Pulsatilla

Cough produces stringy sputum
Kali bichrom.

Cough accompanied by thirst
Belladonna
Bryonia
Hepar sulph.
Phosphorus
Arsenicum

Cough associated with lack of thirst
Pulsatilla

Cough accompanied by vomiting
Ipecac.
Drosera

Cough associated with weak chest
Stannum
Kali carb.

DISCHARGES FROM EYES
Heavily infected
Argentum nit.
Calcarea
Hepar sulph.
Lycopodium
Mercurius
Pulsatilla

Irritating, itchy discharge
Carbon sulph.
Chamomilla
Euphrasia
Graphites
Hepar sulph.
Sulphur

Mucus or pus
Calcarea
Calcarea sulph.
Causticum
Mercurius
Pulsatilla
Tellurium

Tears
Allium
Calcarea
Belladonna
Euphrasia
Fluoric ac.
Lycopodium
Mercurius
Natrum mur.
Nitric ac.
Opium
Phosphorus
Pulsatilla
Rhus tox.
Sulphur

DISCHARGES FROM THROAT AND CHEST
(phlegm, sputum)
Clinging, difficult to cough up
Causticum
Pulsatilla
Senega

Copious
Ammonium carb.
Arsenicum

Cactus
Calcarea
Calcarea phos.
Coccus
Euphrasia
Hepar sulph.
Lycopodium
Phosphorus
Pulsatilla
Sepia
Stannum

Foul-smelling
Arsenicum
Borax
Calcarea
Guaiacum
Lycopodium
Natrum ars.
Natrum carb.
Phellandrium
Sanguinaria
Stannum

Frothy
Arsenicum

Greenish
Calcarea
Carbo veg.
Kali iod.
Lycopodium
Mercurius
Natrum sulph.
Paris
Phosphorus
Psorinum
Pulsatilla
Stannum
Sulphur

Heavily infected
Calcarea
China
Conium
Kali carb.
Lycopodium
Natrum ars.
Phosphorus
Sepia
Silicea

Rusty-looking
Bryonia
Lycopodium

Scanty
Phosphorus
Stannum

Sticky
Alumina
Argentum nit.
Coccus
Hepar sulph.
Hydrastis
Kali bichrom.
Phosphorus
Pulsatilla
Sambucus
Senega
Stannum

Stringy, ropy
Kali bichrom.

Thick
Argentum nit.
Hepar sulph.
Hydrastis
Kali bichrom.
Silicea
Tuberculinum

White, milky-looking
Lycopodium
Natrum mur.
Phosphorus
Senega
Sepia

Yellow
Calcarea
Calcarea phos.
Calcarea sulph.
Hepar sulph.
Hydrastis
Lycopodium
Phosphorus
Sepia
Silicea
Stannum
Tuberculinum

DISCHARGES FROM URETHRA
Burning, scalding
Argentum nit.
Mercurius

Greenish
Mercurius

Jelly-like
Agnus
Alum
Alumina
Benzoic ac.
Kali iod.
Natrum mur.
Petroselinum
Selenium
Sepia
Sulphur
Thuja

Discharge contains pus
Calcarea sulph.
Nitric ac.

White, milky-looking
Natrum mur.
Sepia

Yellowish
Mercurius
Natrum sulph.
Pulsatilla

DRINKING
see THIRST

EATING
Eating improves symptoms
Iodum
Natrum carb.
Phosphorus
Sepia
Spongia

Fasting makes symptoms worse
Arsenicum
Ipecac.
Ledum
Nux
Sulphur

Symptoms worse before eating
Iodum
Laurocerasus
Natrum carb.
Phosphorus

Symptoms worse after eating
Aloe
Anacardium
Arsenicum
Bryonia
Calcarea
Calcarea phos.
Causticum
Colocynth
Conium
Kali bichrom.
Kali carb.
Lachesis
Lycopodium
Natrum mur.
Nux
Phosphorus
Pulsatilla
Rumex
Sepia
Silicea
Sulphur
Zinc

Symptoms improve while eating
Anacardium
Ignatia
Lachesis
Zinc

Symptoms get worse while eating
Ammon. carb.
Carbo an.
Carbo veg.
Conium
Kali carb.
Nitric ac.
Sulphur

Eating to satiety alleviates symptoms
Arsenicum
Iodum
Phosphorus

Eating to satiety makes symptoms worse
Calcarea
Lycopodium
Pulsatilla
Sulphur

FACIAL EXPRESSION
Anxious
Aconite
Aethusa
Ailanthus

Arsenicum
Borax
Camphora
China sulph.
Lac can.
Veratrum

Confused
Aesculus
Arsenicum
Lycopodium

Distressed
Ailanthus
Arsenicum
Cactus
Croton
Iodum
Nux mosch.
Stramonium

Frightened
Aconite
Apis
Baptisia
Stramonium

Haggard
Arsenicum
Camphora
Capsicum
Carbo veg.
Kali carb.
Lachesis
Natrum mur.
Phosphorus
Silicea

Old-looking
Argentum nit.
Calcarea
Guaiacum
Natrum mur.
Opium

Sickly
Arsenicum
Arsenicum iod.
China
Lachesis
Lycopodium

Stupid, stupefied
Apis
Argentum nit.
Arnica

Arsenicum
Belladonna
Cannabis ind.
Gelsemium
Hyoscyamus
Nux mosch.
Stramonium

Sleepy
Cannabis ind.
Nux mosch.
Opium

Suffering
Arsenicum
Cactus
Kali carb.
Lyssin
Manganum
Silicea
Sulphur

FAECES
Symptoms worse before bowel movements
Kali carb.
Mercurius
Podophyllum
Rheum
Veratrum

Symptoms worse during bowel movements
China
Podophyllum
Rheum
Veratrum

Symptoms better after bowel movements
Bryonia
Natrum sulph.
Oxalic ac.
Nux

Symptoms worse after bowel movements
Causticum
China
Phosphorus
Podophyllum
Rheum
Veratrum

Frequent bowel movements
Arsenicum

Capsicum
Chamomilla
Mercurius
Mercurius corr.
Nux
Phosphorus
Podophyllum
Veratrum

Dry faeces
Bryonia
Lac deflor.
Lycopodium
Natrum mur.
Nitric ac.
Nux
Opium
Phosphorus
Silicea
Zinc

Foul-smelling faeces
Argentum nit.
Arsenicum
Asafoetida
Baptisia
Benzoic ac.
Bryonia
Carbo veg.
Carbon sulph.
Crotalus
Graphites
Kali ars.
Kali phos.
Lachesis
Mercurius corr.
Natrum sulph.
Nux mosch.
Opium
Podophyllum
Psorinum
Silicea
Squilla
Sulphur
Tuberculinum

Greenish faeces
Argentum nit.
Calcarea phos.
Chamomilla
Colocynth
Croton
Gratiola
Ipecac.
Magnesia carb.
Mercurius
Mercurius corr.

Natrum mur.
Natrum sulph.
Phosphorus
Plumbum
Podophyllum
Pulsatilla
Secale
Sulphur
Veratrum

Hard faeces
Alum
Alumina
Ammon carb.
Ammon mur.
Antimonium
Bryonia
Calcarea
Carbon sulph.
Carduus
Collinsonia
Graphites
Kali brom.
Lac deflor.
Lachesis
Lycopodium
Magnesia mur.
Mezereum
Natrum mur.
Nitric ac.
Nux
Opium
Phosphorus
Plumbum
Selenium
Sepia
Silicea
Sulphur
Veratrum
Verbascum
Zinc

Pale-coloured faeces
Arsenicum
Borax
Calcarea
Carduus
Chelidonium
China
Digitalis
Lycopodium
Mercurius
Phosphoric ac.
Sanicula
Silicea
Tabacum

Pasty-looking faeces
Bryonia
Chelidonium
Colocynth
Croton
Mercurius
Mercurius corr.
Podophyllum
Rheum
Sulphur

Faeces like sheep's droppings
Alum
Alumina
Chelidonium
Magnesia mur.
Mercurius
Natrum mur.
Nitric ac.
Opium
Plumbum
Sulphur

Faeces soft and spattery
Croton
Elaps
Gratiola
Natrum carb.
Natrum mur.
Podophyllum
Scale
Veratrum

Faeces containing undigested food
Arsenicum
Bryonia
Calcarea
China
China ars.
Ferrum
Graphites
Magnesia mur.
Phosphoric ac.
Phosphorus
Podophyllum

Watery faeces
Agaricus
Antimonium
Apis
Apocynum
Argentum nit.
Asafoetida
Benzoic ac.
Calcarea
Carbon sulph.
Chamomilla
Colchicum

Conium
Dulcamara
Iris
Kali bichrom.
Magnesia carb.
Mercurius
Natrum mur.
Natrum sulph.
Nux
Opium
Phosphorus
Picric ac.
Podophyllum
Psorinum
Pulsatilla
Secale
Sulphur
Thuja
Veratrum
Veratrum vir.

HEARING
see NOISE

LEFT SIDE/RIGHT SIDE
see also MOVEMENT AND
POSTURE p. 47/51
Symptoms worse on left side
Argentum nit.
Euphrasia
Graphites
Lachesis
Phosphorus
Sepia
Sulphur

Symptoms worse on right side
Apis
Arsenicum
Belladonna
Bryonia
Calcarea
Cantharis
Chelidonium
Colocynth
Conium
Lycopodium
Nux
Pulsatilla

MENSTRUATION
Symptoms worse before periods
Bovista
Calcarea
Calcarea phos.
Cuprum
Lachesis
Lycopodium

Natrum mur.
Pulsatilla
Sepia
Sulphur
Veratrum
Zinc

Symptoms worse after periods
Borax
Graphites
Kreosotum
Lachesis
Nux
Sepia

Symptoms worse at start of periods
Calcarea phos.
Hyoscyamus
Kali carb.

Symptoms improve during periods
Lachesis

Symptoms worse during periods
Ammon. carb.
Argentum nit.
Bovista
Carbon sulph.
Chamomilla
Graphites
Hyoscyamus
Kali carb.
Magnesia carb.
Nux
Pulsatilla
Sepia
Sulphur
Zinc

Symptoms worse at menopause
Actaea
Aloe
Argentum nit.
China
Crocus
Cocculus
Crotalus
Graphites
Ignatia
Lachesis
Lilium
Manganum
Murex
Nux mosch.
Psorinum
Pulsatilla
Sanguinaria
Sepia
Sulphur

MOUTH
Bad breath
Arnica
Arsenicum
Carbo veg.
Chamomilla
Chelidonium
Lachesis
Mercurius
Natrum mur.
Sulphur

Dry lips
Antimonium
Bryonia
Hyoscyamus
Pulsatilla
Rhus tox.
Sulphur

Pale lips
Apis
Calcarea
Ferrum phos.
Lycopodium
Opium
Pulsatilla

Red lips
Apis
Lachesis
Sulphur

Sore, cracked lips
Bryonia
Calcarea
Carbo veg.
China
Graphites
Lachesis
Natrum mur.
Sulphur

Mouth feels dry
Aconite
Arsenicum
Baryta
Belladonna
Bryonia
Chamomilla
China
Hyoscyamus
Ignatia
Lachesis
Lycopodium
Mercurius
Natrum mur.
Natrum sulph.

Nux
Phosphoric ac.
Phosphorus
Rhus tox.
Sepia
Silicea
Sulphur
Veratrum

More saliva than usual
Kali carb.
Mercurius
Natrum mur.
Nux
Veratrum

Tongue looks black
Aconite
Apis
Chamomilla

Tongue feels dry
Aconite
Apis
Arsenicum
Belladonna
Calcarea
Causticum
Chamomilla
China
Hyoscyamus
Lachesis
Mercurius
Pulsatilla
Rhus tox.
Sulphur

Tongue red all over
Apis
Arsenicum
Belladonna
Mercurius
Phosphorus
Rhus tox.

Tongue red on tip only
Arsenicum
Argentum nit.
Rhus tox.
Sulphur

Tongue red around edges
Arsenicum
Chelidonium
Mercurius
Sulphur

Tongue looks swollen
Aconite
Apis
Belladonna
Mercurius

Tongue white and coated
Antimonium
Arsenicum
Belladonna
Bryonia
Calcarea
Hyoscyamus
Mercurius
Pulsatilla
Sulphur

Tongue looks yellow
Antimonium
Chelidonium
Mercurius
Rhus tox.

Teething problems
Calcarea phos.
Chamomilla
Rheum
Silicea

MOVEMENT AND POSTURE
Moving around alleviates symptoms
Agaricus
Allium
Cedrum
Conium
Dulcamara
Iodum
Kreosotum
Lycopodium
Magnesia carb.
Magnesia mur.
Muriatic ac.
Natrum sulph.
Phosphoric ac.
Rhododendron
Rhus tox.
Ruta
Stannum

Moving around makes symptoms worse
Aconite
Actaea
Aesculus
Antimonium tart.
Apis
Apocynum

Arsenicum
Aurum
Belladonna
Benzoic ac.
Berberis
Bryonia
Cactus
Calcarea phos.
Camphora
Cantharis
Carbo veg.
Chamomilla
Chelidonium
China
Clematis
Cocculus
Digitalis
Eupatorium
Gelsemium
Glonoinum
Hydrastis
Hypericum
Iodum
Ipecac.
Iris
Kali carb.
Kalmia
Lachesis
Ledum
Magnesia phos.
Manganum
Mercurius
Mezereum
Moschus
Naja
Natrum mur.
Nux
Nux mosch.
Picric ac.
Phosphorus
Phytolacca
Plumbum
Podophyllum
Psorinum
Rheum
Salicylic ac.
Sanguinaria
Secale
Spigelia
Spongia
Stannum
Stramonium
Sulphur
Sulphuric ac.
Tabacum
Veratrum
Veratrum vir.
Zinc

Constant movement alleviates symptoms
Conium
Rhododendron
Rhus tox.
Ruta

Starting to move alleviates symptoms
Rhododendron

Starting to move makes symptoms worse
Conium
Rhododendron
Rhus tox.
Ruta

Rapid or vigorous movement alleviates symptoms
Lilium
Sepia

Rapid or vigorous movement makes symptoms worse
Ferrum
Gelsemium
Pulsatilla

Staying in same position for long periods makes symptoms worse
Thuja

Sudden movement makes symptoms worse
Ferrum

Bending backwards alleviates symptoms
Aconite
Bryonia
Calcarea
Mercurius corr.
Natrum mur.
Pulsatilla
Rhus tox.

Bending backwards makes symptoms worse
Dulcamara
Manganum

Bending forwards alleviates symptoms
Manganum

Bending forwards makes symptoms worse
Antimonium tart.
Belladonna
Spigelia

Bending double alleviates symptoms
Argentum nit.

Being carried alleviates symptoms
Antimonium tart.
Belladonna
Chamomilla
Kali carb.
Mercurius

Being carried makes symptoms worse
Arnica
Bryonia
Hepar sulph.

Changing position alleviates symptoms
Ignatia
Natrum sulph.
Phosphoric ac.
Valerian
Zinc

Changing position makes symptoms worse
Apis
Bryonia
Capsicum
Ferrum
Lycopodium
Phosphorus
Pulsatilla
Rhus tox.

Downward movement alleviates symptoms
Aesculus
Bryonia
Opium
Rhododendron
Rhus tox.
Sepia
Spongia

Downward movement makes symptoms worse
Borax
Stannum

Upward movement makes symptoms worse
Arsenicum
Bryonia
Calcarea
Spongia

Exercise makes symptoms worse
Arnica
Arsenicum

Bryonia
Cactus
Carbo veg.
Causticum
Kali bichrom.
Kali carb.
Lycopodium
Magnesia carb.
Phosphoric ac.
Sanguinaria
Veratrum

Jarring or vibration make symptoms worse
Aloe
Alumina
Arnica
Baryta
Belladonna
Berberis
Bryonia
China
Cicuta
Cina
Cocculus
Conium
Ferrum
Glonoinum
Lilium
Manganum
Natrum mur.
Nitric ac.
Sanguinaria
Phosphorus
Rhus tox.
Sepia
Silicea
Spigelia
Zinc

Kneeling makes symptoms worse
Cocculus
Magnesia carb.
Sepia

Lifting things makes symptoms worse
Ambra
Arnica
Bryonia
Calcarea
Calcarea phos.
Causticum
Cocculus
Conium
Graphites
Lycopodium
Millefolium
Natrum carb.

Phosphoric ac.
Rhus tox.
Secale
Silicea

Limbs drawn up alleviate symptoms
Calcarea
Colocynth
Hepar sulph.
Manganum
Mercurius corr.
Sepia
Sulphur

Limbs drawn up make symptoms worse
Antimonium tart.
Carbo veg.
Pulsatilla
Secale

Limbs hanging down alleviate symptoms
Conium

Limbs hanging down make symptoms worse
Calcarea
Pulsatilla
Thuja

Raising limbs alleviates symptoms
Calcarea

Raising limbs makes symptoms worse
Baryta
Conium
Phosphorus

Lying down alleviates symptoms
Antimonium
Apocynum
Arsenicum
Bryonia
Calcarea phos.
Kalmia
Manganum
Nitric ac.
Nux
Picric ac.
Plumbum
Podophyllum
Silicea
Staphisagria
Veratrum

Lying down makes symptoms worse
Antimonium tart.
Arsenicum

Belladonna
Cedrum
Chamomilla
Conium
Drosera
Ferrum
Glonoinum
Hyoscyamus
Lycopodium
Murex
Natrum sulph.
Platinum
Pulsatilla
Rhus tox.
Ruta
Sanguinaria
Stannum
Tabacum
Zinc

Lying on back alleviates symptoms
Aconite
Bryonia
Calcarea
Mercurius corr.
Natrum mur.
Pulsatilla
Rhus tox.

Lying on back makes symptoms worse
Argentum
Arsenicum
Colocynth
Dulcamara
Nux
Phosphorus
Sepia

Lying on left side alleviates symptoms
Ignatia
Muriatic ac.
Stannum

Lying on left side makes symptoms worse
Argentum nit.
Arnica
Baryta
Colchicum
Croton
Lachesis
Lilium
Naja
Natrum mur.
Phosphorus
Pulsatilla
Sulphur
Thuja

Lying on right side alleviates symptoms
Ammon carb.
Pulsatilla
Spigelia
Sulphur

Lying on right side makes symptoms worse
Benzoic ac.
Lycopodium
Mercurius
Nux
Phytolacca
Sanguinaria
Spongia

Lying on affected side alleviates symptoms
Ammon carb.
Ambra
Bryonia
Calcarea
Chamomilla
Colocynth
Pulsatilla
Sepia
Sulphur

Lying on affected side makes symptoms worse
Aconite
Antimonium tart.
Arsenicum
Baptisia
Baryta
Belladonna
Hepar sulph.
Iodum
Kali carb.
Lycopodium
Nitric ac.
Nux
Phosphoric ac.
Ruta
Silicea

Lying on unaffected side alleviates symptoms
Baptisia
Belladonna
Hepar sulph.
Iodum
Kali cab.
Nux
Ruta
Silicea

Lying on unaffected side makes symptoms worse
Ambra
Argentum
Bryonia
Chamomilla
Colocynth
Ignatia
Pulsatilla
Kali carb.
Rhus tox.
Sepia

Lying curled up alleviates symptoms
Rheum

Rising from sitting or lying position alleviates symptoms
Kali bichrom.

Rising from sitting or lying position makes symptoms worse
Antimonium
Bryonia
Digitalis
Spongia
Sulphur
Tabacum
Veratrum vir.

Getting out of bed makes symptoms worse
Bryonia
Natrum sulph.
Digitalis

Sitting up in bed alleviates symptoms
Natrum mur.

Sitting alleviates symptoms
Apis
Belladonna
Bryonia
Iodum
Nux
Staphisagria

Sitting makes symptoms worse
Agaricus
Alumina
Antimonium tart.
Ferrum
Fluoric ac.
Kali bichrom.
Murex
Natrum carb.
Phosphoric ac.
Platinum

Rhododendron
Rhus tox.

Standing alleviates symptoms
Belladonna
Cedrum

Standing makes symptoms worse
Aloe
Berberis
Cantharis
Cocculus
Conium
Fluoric ac.
Digitalis
Kreosotum
Lachesis
Phosphoric ac.
Phytolacca
Platinum
Psorinum
Rheum
Sepia
Sulphur

Stooping alleviates symptoms
Conium

Stooping makes symptoms worse
Ipecac.
Kali bichrom.
Lachesis
Millefolium
Sepia
Spigelia
Spongia
Sulphur

Stretching makes symptoms worse
Colocynth
Lycopodium

Travelling in cars, trains, etc. alleviates symptoms
Bromium
Graphites
Lycopodium
Nitric ac.

Travelling in cars, trains, etc. makes symptoms worse
Arnica
Berberis
Cocculus
Petroleum
Psorinum
Rhus tox.
Thuja
Zinc

Walking alleviates symptoms
Ambra
Arsenicum
Chamomilla
Drosera
Fluoric ac.
Murex
Natrum sulph.
Opium
Phosphoric ac.

Walking makes symptoms worse
Aconite
Aesculus
Aloe
Argentum
Baptisia
Berberis
Bryonia
Camphora
Carbolic ac.
Causticum
Conium
Hepar sulph.
Kali carb.
Ledum
Manganum
Naja
Natrum mur.
Nux
Phytolacca
Picric ac.
Podophyllum
Psorinum
Rheum
Ruta
Silicea
Spigelia
Spongia
Thuja
Veratrum vir.

MUSCLES
Tired or aching muscles
Arnica

NASAL DISCHARGE
see also DISCHARGE
FROM THROAT AND
CHEST
Bland, non-stinging
Euphrasia
Pulsatilla

Bloody
Ailanthus
Allium
Alumina
Ammonium carb.

Arsenicum
Belladonna
Calcarea sulph.
China
China ars.
Hepar sulph.
Kali iod.
Mercurius
Nitric ac.
Psorinum

Copious
Allium
Arsenicum
Kali iod.
Natrum mur.
Phosphorus

Excoriating (very irritant, causing skin to peel off)
Allium
Ammonium mur.
Arsenicum
Arsenicum iod.
Arum
Ferrum iod.
Graphites
Iodum
Kreosotum
Mercurius
Nitric ac.
Nux

Foul-smelling
Asafoetida
Aurum
Calcarea
Hepar sulph.
Kali bichrom.
Mercurius
Natrum carb.
Psorinum
Pulsatilla
Silicea
Sulphur

Greenish
Kali bichrom.
Kali iod.
Lac can.
Mercurius
Pulsatilla
Sepia

Heavily infected
Aurum
Calcarea
Calcarea sulph.

Conium
Hepar sulph.
Kali bichrom.
Kali sulph.
Lachesis
Lycopodium
Mercurius
Silicea
Tuberculinum

Thick
Arsenicum
Calcarea sulph.
Hydrastis
Kali bichrom.
Kali phos.
Lac can.
Natrum sulph.
Pulsatilla
Tuberculinum

Watery
Allium
Arsenicum
Arum
Chamomilla
Euphrasia
Graphites
Iodum
Mercurius
Natrum ars.
Nitric ac.
Nux

Yellowish
Arum
Aurum
Calcarea
Calcarea sulph.
Hepar sulph.
Hydrastis
Kali bichrom.
Kali iod.
Kali phos.
Kali sulph.
Lycopodium
Nitric ac.
Pulsatilla
Sepia
Sulphur
Tuberculinum

PAIN
Pain which comes on suddenly
Belladonna
Nitric ac.

Pain which disappears as suddenly as it comes on
Belladonna
Kali bichrom.
Nitric ac.

Pain which comes on and wears off gradually
Platinum
Stannum

Biting pain
Carbo veg.
Nux vom.
Petroselinum
Sulphur
Zinc

Boring, penetrating pain
Argentum nit.
Aurum
Belladonna
Bismuth
Pulsatilla
Spigelia

Burning pain – external
Apis
Arsenicum
Arum
Bryonia
Carbo veg.
Carbon sulph.
Causticum
Euphrasia
Iris
Mercurius
Natrum mur.
Nux
Phosphoric ac.
Phosphorus
Ratanhia
Secale
Sepia
Silicea
Stannum
Sulphur

Burning pain – internal
Aconite
Arsenicum
Arum
Belladonna
Berberis
Bryonia
Cannabis
Cantharis
Carbon sulph.

Graphites
Kali bichrom.
Mercurius
Mercurius corr.
Mezereum
Nitric ac.
Nux
Phosphorus
Prunus
Pulsatilla
Rhus tox.
Sabadilla
Sanguinaria
Secale
Sepia
Spigelia
Spongia
Sulphur
Zinc

Constricting pain – external
Platinum
Pulsatilla

Constricting pain – internal
Ambra
Ignatia
Phosphoric ac.
Platinum

Cutting pain – external
Belladonna
Calcarea
Conium
Drosera
Natrum carb.
Petroleum

Cutting pain – internal
Belladonna
Calcarea
Cantharis
Colocynth
Conium
Dioscorea
Hyoscyamus
Kali carb.
Lycopodium
Mercurius
Natrum mur.
Nux
Pulsatilla
Silicea
Sulphur
Veratrum
Zinc

Digging or gouging pain
Dulcamara
Rhododendron
Spigelia

Dragging or pulling pain
Carbo veg.
Chelidonium
Graphites
Nitric ac.
Valerian

Flitting, shifting pain
Kali bichrom.
Kali sulph.
Lac can.
Ledum
Pulsatilla

Gnawing pain
Arsenicum
Causticum
Mercurius
Silicea
Staphisagria
Sulphur

Sudden cramping pain – external
Asafoetida
Calcarea
Causticum
Menyanthes
Natrum mur
Nux
Pulsatilla
Rhus tox.
Taraxacum
Valerian

Sudden cramping pain – internal
Belladonna
China
Ignatia
Kali carb.
Nitric ac.
Pulsatilla
Silicea
Sulphur
Thuja

Numbing pain
Chamomilla
Oleander
Platinum
Sabadilla
Verbasum

Paralysing pain
Belladonna
Cina
Cocculus
Colchicum
Cyclamen
Nux
Sabina

Pinching pain
Arnica
Belladonna
Nux

Pressing, persistent pain – external
Agaricus
Apocynum
Cannabis ind.
Causticum
China sulph.
Drosera
Eupatorium
Ferrum
Kali bichrom.
Moschus
Nitric ac.
Nux
Phosphorus
Podophyllum
Pulsatilla
Rhododendron
Rhus tox.
Ruta
Sepia
Silicea
Spigelia
Stannum
Staphisagria
Sulphur

Pressing, persistent pain – internal
Argentum nit.
Arnica
Arsenicum
Asafoetida
Belladonna
Bromium
Calcarea
Cantharis
Carbo veg.
China
Cimifuga
Colocynth
Cuprum
Hamamelis
Lachesis
Lilium
Lycopodium

Menyanthes
Natrum mur.
Nux
Opium
Petroleum
Phosphorus
Pulsatilla
Ranunculus
Rhus tox.
Ruta
Sanguinaria
Secale
Senega
Sepia
Silicea
Spigelia
Spongia
Stannum
Sulphur
Valerian
Veratrum
Zinc

Heavy, pressing pain
Aconite
Belladonna
Bromium
Bryonia
Ipecac.
Lilium
Menyanthes
Nux
Pareira
Phosphorus
Ranunculus
Rhux tox.
Sepia
Sticta
Sulphur

Inward-pressing pain
Anacardium
Platinum
Stannum

Outward-pressing pain
Asafoetida
Bryonia
Cimicifuga
Pulsatilla
Sulphur
Valerian

Scraping pain
Bryonia
Drosera
Nux
Pulsatilla

Sulphur
Veratrum

Sore, bruised feeling
Argentum
Arnica
Cicuta
Cimicifuga
China
Drosera
Hamamelis
Platinum
Pyrogenium
Rhus tox.
Ruta
Silicea

Splinter-like pain
Agaricus
Argentum nit.
Hepar sulph.
Nitric ac.

Squeezing pain
Alumina
Asarum
Cocculus
Nux
Platinum
Sulphur

Stitch-like pain – external
Asafoetida
Belladonna
Bryonia
Calcarea
Carbon sulph.
Cicuta
Conium
Kali carb.
Kali sulph.
Ledum
Mercurius
Nitric ac.
Pulsatilla
Ranunculus
Rhus tox.
Spigelia
Staphisagria
Sulphur
Taraxacum
Thuja
Zinc

Stitch-like pain – internal
Asafoetida
Berberis
Borax

Bryonia
Cannabis ind.
Cantharis
Carbon sulph.
Chelidonium
China
Ignatia
Kali carb.
Kali sulph.
Lachesis
Ledum
Mercurius
Mercurius corr.
Nitric ac.
Phosphorus
Plumbum
Pulsatilla
Ranunculus
Sepia
Silicea
Spigelia
Squilla

Tearing pain – external
Aconite
Arnica
Belladonna
Berberis
Bryonia
Carbon sulph.
China
Colchicum
Hypericum
Kali carb.
Kali phos.
Kali sulph.
Ledum
Lycopodium
Natrum mur.
Natrum sulph.
Nitric ac.
Pulsatilla
Sepia
Silicea
Sulphur
Zinc

Tearing pain – internal
Belladonna
Berberis
Bryonia
Carbo veg.
Conium
Kali sulph.
Ledum
Lycopodium
Mercurius
Pulsatilla

Nux
Sepia
Silicea
Spigelia
Sulphur

Absence of pain in conditions which are usually painful
Helleborus
Opium
Stramonium

PERSPIRATION
see also BODY ODOUR
p. 40–41

Breaking into cold sweats
Ammon carb.
Antimonium tart.
Arsenicum
Camphora
Carbo veg.
China
China ars.
Cocculus
Ferrum
Hepar sulph.
Ipecac.
Lycopodium
Mercurius corr.
Secale
Sepia
Veratrum
Veratrum vir.

Breaking into hot sweats
Aconite
Chamomilla
Conium
Ignatia
Ipecac.
Nux
Opium
Psorinum
Sepia

Sweat smells offensive
Arnica
Baryta mur.
Carbo an.
Carbon sulph.
Graphites
Hepar sulph.
Lycopodium
Mercurius
Nitric ac.
Nux
Petroleum
Pulsatilla

Sepia
Silicea
Sulphur
Thuja

Profuse sweating
Antimonium tart.
Arsenicum
Belladonna
Bryonia
Calcarea
Carbo an.
Carbo veg.
Carbon sulph.
China
China ars.
China sulph.
Ferrum
Hepar sulph.
Kali ars.
Kali bichrom.
Kali carb.
Kali phos.
Lycopodium
Mercurius
Natrum mur.
Phosphoric ac.
Psorinum
Sambucus
Sepia
Silicea
Tuberculinum
Veratrum

PHLEGM
see DISCHARGES FROM THROAT AND CHEST

PULSE
Irregular pulse
Antimonium
Arsenicum
Digitalis
Lachesis
Natrum mur.
Phosphoric ac.
Secale
Stramonium
Veratrum vir.

Rapid pulse
Aconite
Apis
Arnica
Arsenicum
Arsenicum iod.
Aurum

Belladonna
Berberis
Bryonia
Collinsonia
Conium
Cuprum
Digitalis
Ferrum phos.
Gelsemium
Glonoinum
Iodum
Mercurius
Natrum mur.
Nux
Opium
Phosphoric ac.
Phosphorus
Pyrogenium
Rhus tox.
Secale
Sepia
Spigelia
Stannum
Stramonium
Sulphur
Veratrum vir.
Zinc

Slow pulse
Berberis
Cannabis ind.
Digitalis
Kalmia
Opium
Sepia
Stramonium

Strong pulse
Aconite
Antimonium tart.
Belladonna
Berberis
Bryonia
Chelidonium
Digitalis
Gelsemium
Hyoscyamus
Kali nit.
Stramonium

Weak pulse
Antimonium tart.
Arsenicum
Aurum
Berberis
Camphora
Carbo veg.
Crotalus

Gelsemium
Lachesis
Laurocerasus
Naja
Phosphoric ac.

REST
Rest alleviates symptoms
Antimonium
Arnica
Belladonna
Bryonia
Calcarea phos.
Chelidonium
China
Cicuta
Cocculus
Colocynth
Digitalis
Gelsemium
Glonoinum
Graphites
Hypericum
Ipecac.
Kalmia
Manganum
Magnesia phos.
Mercurius
Nux
Picric ac.
Plumbum
Psorinum
Sepia
Silicea
Spigelia
Sulphuric ac.
Staphisagria
Thuja

Rest makes symptoms worse
Agaricus
Allium
Anacardium
Cedrum
Conium
Drosera
Ferrum
Kali bichrom.
Kreosotum
Lilium
Lycopodium
Magnesia carb.
Muriatic ac.
Natrum carb.
Natrum sulph.
Pulsatilla
Rhododendron
Rhus tox.

Ruta
Stannum
Zinc

Being in bed alleviates symptoms
Bryonia
Cocculus
Hepar sulph.
Lachesis
Lycopodium
Nux
Psorinum
Silicea

Being in bed makes symptoms worse
Arnica
Belladonna
Chamomilla
Euphrasia
Ferrum
Hyoscyamus
Kali carb.
Magnesia carb.
Mercurius
Natrum mur.
Nux
Opium
Phytolacca
Pulsatilla
Rhus tox.
Sulphur

SEX
see also LIBIDO p. 75
Intercourse alleviates symptoms
Mercurius

Intercourse makes symptoms worse
Ambra
Agaricus
Alumina
Calcarea
Kali carb.
Kali phos.
Kreosotum
Natrum mur.
Sepia
Silicea
Staphisagria
Thuja

*Symptoms become worse during
  intercourse*
Cantharis
Graphites
Kali carb.
Selenium

*Symptoms become worse after
   ejaculation*
Kali carb.
Natrum phos.
Nux
Selenium
Sepia

SIGHT
Bright lights make symptoms worse
Belladonna
Cantharis
Stramonium

*Reading and sewing make symptoms
   worse*
Natrum mur.

Sight of blood makes symptoms worse
Nux

Sight of needles makes symptoms worse
Silicea

SKIN
Clammy skin
Arsenicum
Chamomilla
Ferrum phos.
Lycopodium
Mercurius
Phosporic ac.
Phosphorus
Veratrum

Cold skin
Arsenicum
Calcarea phos.
Ipecac.
Rhus tox.
Sepia
Sulphur
Veratrum

Cracking skin
Calcarea
Carbon sulph.
Graphites
Petroleum
Pulsatilla
Sarsaparilla
Sepia
Sulphur

Skin cracks after washing
Antimonium
Calcarea
Calcarea sulph.

Pulsatilla
Sepia
Sulphur

Skin cracks in winter
Calcarea
Calcarea sulph.
Petroleum
Psorinum
Sepia
Sulphur

Dry skin
Arsenicum
Belladonna
Bryonia
Calcarea
Chamomilla
China
Dulcamara
Kali carb.
Ledum
Lycopodium
Opium
Phosphorus
Silicea
Sulphur

Itchy skin
Agaricus
Apis
Arsenicum
Bovista
Carbo veg.
Carbon sulph.
Causticum
Chelidonium
Graphites
Lycopodium
Magnesia carb.
Mercurius
Mezereum
Natrum mur.
Psorinum
Pulsatilla
Sepia
Silicea
Spongia
Staphisagria
Sulphur
Tarentula
Urtica

Itchiness relieved by scratching
Asafoetida
Calcarea
Cyclamen
Muriatic ac.

Natrum mur.
Phosphorus

Itchiness made worse by scratching
Anacardium
Arsenicum
Capsicum
Pulsatilla
Rhus tox.

Pale skin
Belladonna
Calcarea
Ferrum phos.
Lycopodium
Pulsatilla
Sulphur
Veratrum

Red skin
Aconite
Apis
Belladonna
Graphites
Mercurius
Rhus tox.

Sensitive skin
Apis
Belladonna
China
Hepar sulph.
Lachesis
Lyssin
Mercurius
Petroleum
Phosphoric ac.
Plumbum
Silicea
Sulphur

SLEEP
Sleep alleviates symptoms
Phosphoric ac.
Phosphorus

Sleep makes symptoms worse
Lachesis
Selenium
Spongia
Stramonium
Sulphur

Symptoms worse before sleeping
Arsenicum
Bryonia
Calcarea
Carbo veg.

Mercurius
Phosphorus
Pulsatilla
Rhus tox.
Sepia
Sulphur

Symptoms get worse during sleep
Arnica
Arsenicum
Belladonna
Borax
Bryonia
Chamomilla
Hepar sulph.
Hyoscyamus
Mercurius
Opium
Pulsatilla
Silicea
Stramonium
Sulphur
Zinc

Symptoms get worse in first stages of sleep
Arsenicum
Belladonna
Bryonia
Kali carb.
Lachesis
Pulsatilla
Sepia

Symptoms worse on waking
Alumina
Ambra
Ammon. carb.
Baptisia
China
Crotalus
Iris
Kali bichrom.
Kali brom.
Lachesis
Lycopodium
Muriatic ac.
Nux
Rheum
Silicea
Spongia
Staphisagria
Stramonium
Veratrum vir.

Loss of sleep makes symptoms worse
Causticum
Cimifuga

Cocculus
Colchicum
Cuprum
Lac deflor.
Nitric ac.
Nux
Selenium
Sulphur

Overpowering desire to sleep
Nux mosch.
Opium
Pulsatilla

Sleeplessness before midnight
Ambra
Arsenicum
Calcarea
Calcarea phos.
Carbo veg.
Coffea
Conium
Kali carb.
Lycopodium
Magnesia mur.
Mercurius
Natrum ars.
Natrum carb.
Phosphorus
Picric ac.
Pulsatilla
Rhus tox.
Sepia
Silicea
Sulphur

Sleeplessness after midnight
Arsenicum
Capsicum
Coffea
Hepar sulph.
Kali ars.
Kali carb.
Nux
Phosphoric ac.
Silicea

Sleeplessness between 1 and 2 am
Kali carb.

Sleeplessness around 3 am
Magnesia carb.
Sepia
Sulphur

Sleeplessness after 4am
Sulphur

Sleeplessness due to anxiety
Arsenicum
Cocculus

Sleeplessness due to grief
Natrum mur.

Sleeplessness due to home-sickness
Capsicum

Sleepless due to joy or overexcitement
Coffea

Sleeplessness due to overwork
Nux

Sleeplessness due to racing thoughts
Arsenicum
Calcarea
Coffea
Hepar sulph.
Hyoscyamus
Nux
Pulsatilla

Inability to get back to sleep once woken
Arsenicum
Lachesis
Natrum mur.
Silicea

Talking in sleep
Arnica
Belladonna
Chamomilla
Hyoscyamus
Kali carb.
Natrum mur.
Nux
Opium
Pulsatilla
Rhus tox.

Unusual sleepiness in morning
Calcarea
Calcarea phos.
Graphites
Nux
Sepia
Sulphur

Unusual sleepiness around noon
Antimonium
Sabadilla

Unusual sleepiness in afternoon
China
Nux

Rhus tox.
Sulphur

Unusual sleepiness after meals
Agaricus
Calcarea
Nux

Unusual sleepiness after evening meal
Agaricus
Calcarea
Lycopodium
Nux

Unusual sleepiness while eating
Kali carb.

Unusual sleepiness in hot weather
Caladium
Eupatorium
Lachesis
Mezereum
Natrum mur.
Opium
Podophyllum
Robina
Sambucus

Unusual sleepiness during periods
Nux mosch.

Unusual sleepiness after mental exertion
Arsenicum

SPUTUM
see DISCHARGES FROM THROAT AND CHEST

SWELLINGS
Swelling generally
Apis
Arsenicum
Belladonna
Bryonia
Kali bichrom.
Mercurius
Nux
Pulsatilla
Rhus tox.

Swelling of affected part only
Aconite
Belladonna
Bryonia
Crotalus
Euphrasia
Gelsemium

Mercurius corr.
Pulsatilla
Rhododendron
Rhus tox.
Sepia
Silicea
Spongia
Sulphur

THIRST
Thirst makes symptoms worse
Mercurius
Natrum mur.
Opium
Phosphorus
Rhus tox.
Secale
Silicea
Stramonium
Sulphur
Tarentula
Veratrum

Lack of thirst
Antimonium
Apis
China
Colchicum
Gelsemium
Helleborus
Nux mosch.
Phosphoric ac.
Pulsatilla
Sabadilla

Wanting to drink small amounts at frequent intervals
Arsenicum
China
Helleborus
Lachesis
Lycopodium
Rhus tox.
Sulphur

Wanting to drink large amounts
Aconite
Arsenicum
Bryonia
China
Cocculus
Eupatorium
Ferrum phos.
Lac deflor.
Mercurius corr.
Natrum mur.
Stramonium
Sulphur
Veratrum

Wanting to drink large amounts at infrequent intervals
Bryonia

TONGUE
see MOUTH

TOUCH AND PRESSURE
Touching alleviates symptoms
Calcarea
Natrum mur.

Touching makes symptoms worse
Antimonium tart.
Actaea
Apis
Argentum
Argentum nit.
Arnica
Belladonna
Bryonia
Camphora
Cantharis
Capsicum
Causticum
Chamomilla
Chelidonium
China
Cicuta
Clematis
Cocculus
Coffea
Colchicum
Conium
Crotalus
Croton
Cuprum
Ferrum
Hamamelis
Hepar sulph.
Hydrastis
Hyoscyamus
Hypericum
Ignatia
Ipecac.
Kali carb.
Kreosotum
Lachesis
Lilium
Lycopodium
Manganum
Mercurius
Mezereum
Murex
Muriatic ac.
Nitric ac.
Nux
Nux mosch.

Phosphorus
Phosphoric ac.
Phytolacca
Platinum
Plumbum
Podophyllum
Psorinum
Pulsatilla
Rhododendron
Rhus tox.
Ruta
Sanguinaria
Secale
Sepia
Silicea
Spigelia
Spongia
Staphisagria
Stramonium
Sulphur
Sulphuric ac.
Terebinthus
Thuja
Urtica

Firm pressure alleviates symptoms
Ammon carb.
Bryonia
Colocynth
Ipecac.
Kali bichrom.
Kreosotum
Magnesia carb.
Magnesia phos.
Murex
Natrum carb.
Natrum mur.
Nux
Plumbum
Podophyllum
Pulsatilla
Sabina
Sepia
Stannum
Thuja

Firm pressure makes symptoms worse
Aconite
Apis
Argentum nit.
Baptisia
Belladonna
Berberis
Bromium
Calcarea phos.
Cantharis
Cicuta
Cocculus

Crotalus
Croton
Cuprum
Eupatorium
Glonoinum
Hamamelis
Hepar sulph.
Kalmia
Lachesis
Lilium
Lycopodium
Magnesia carb.
Mercurius
Mezereum
Moschus
Natrum sulph.
Silicea
Spongia
Staphisagria
Stramonium
Sulphur
Sulphuric ac.
Tabacum
Terebinthum
Zinc

Rubbing alleviates symptoms
Calcarea
Cantharis
Natrum carb.
Natrum mur.
Nux
Phosphorus
Plumbum
Podophyllum
Pulsatilla
Rhus tox.
Ruta
Tarentula
Thuja
Veratrum vir.
Zinc

Rubbing makes symptoms worse
Psorinum
Sulphuric ac.

URINE
see also DISCHARGE FROM URETHRA
Cloudy urine
Apis
Berberis
Bryonia
Cantharis
Carbon sulph.
Carbo veg.
Chamomilla

Chelidonium
Cina
China
Conium
Graphites
Mercurius
Myristica
Phosphoric ac.
Phosphorus
Sabadilla
Sepia
Sulphur

Dark urine
Aconite
Antimonium tart.
Apis
Belladonna
Benzoic ac.
Bryonia
Calcarea
Chelidonium
Colchicum
Crotalus
Equisetum
Helleborus
Lachesis
Lactic ac.
Mercurius
Mercurius corr.
Plumbum
Selenium
Sepia
Terebinthum
Veratrum

Pale, almost colourless urine
Conium
Kali nit.
Ledum
Mercurius corr.
Natrum mur.
Phosphoric ac.
Sarsaparilla

Strong- or offensive-smelling urine
Apis
Arnica
Baptisia
Benzoic ac.
Calcarea
Carbo veg.
Dulcamara
Nitric ac.
Sepia
Sulphur
Viola

Urinating very frequently
Ammonium carb.
Apis
Argentum
Argentum nit.
Baryta carb.
Calcarea
Calcarea ars.
Cantharis
Causticum
Euphrasia
Gelsemium
Graphites
Ignatia
Lachesis
Lactic ac.
Lycopodium
Mercurius
Mercurius corr.
Natrum sulph.
Nux
Phosphoric ac.
Pulsatilla
Rhus tox.
Squilla
Staphisagria
Sulphur

Feeble stream of urine
Alumina
Argentum nit.
Arnica
Clematis
Helleborus
Hepar sulph.
Mercurius
Mercurius corr.
Muriatic ac.
Opium
Sarsaparilla
Sulphur

Stream of urine slow to start
Arnica
Causticum
Lycopodium
Rhus tox.
Sepia

VAGINAL DISCHARGE
Burning, scalding
Borax
Calcarea
Calcarea sulph.
Kreosotum
Pulsatilla
Sepia
Sulphur

Creamy
Pulsatilla

Excoriating, causing skin to blister
Alumina
Borax
Carbon sulph.
Chamomilla
Ferrum
Ferrum ars.
Fluoric ac.
Graphites
Kreosotum
Lycopodium
Mercurius
Nitric ac.
Phosphorus
Pulsatilla
Sepia
Silicea

Greenish
Carbo veg.
Mercurius
Natrum mur.
Natrum sulph.
Nitric ac.
Sepia

Profuse
Calcarea
Graphites
Lycopodium
Sepia
Silicea
Stannum

Stringy or ropy
Hydrastis
Kali bichrom.
Nitric ac.
Sabina

Thick
Arsenicum
Calcarea
Hydrastis
Kali bichrom.

Transparent, like egg white
Borax
Natrum mur.
Sepia

Watery
Graphites
Nitric ac.
Pulsatilla

Unpleasant-smelling
Kali ars.
Kali phos.
Nitric ac.
Nux
Psorinum
Sepia

Yellowish
Arsenicum
Calcarea
Chamomilla
Hydrastis
Kreosotum
Sepia
Sulphur

Discharge more marked before periods
Bovista
Calcarea
Graphites
Kreosotum
Sepia

VOICE
Hoarse voice
Aconite
Allium
Argentum nit.
Arum
Belladonna
Bromium
Bryonia
Calcarea
Capsicum
Carbo veg.
Causticum
Chamomilla
Drosera
Hepar sulph.
Iodum
Kali bichrom.
Lachesis
Manganum
Mercurius
Natrum mur.
Phosphorus
Selenium
Spongia
Stannum
Stramonium

Losing voice
Alum
Antimonium
Argentum
Argentum nit.
Bromium

Carbo veg.
Causticum
Lachesis
Phosphorus
Stramonium

Nasal-sounding voice
Kali bichrom.

Weak voice
Antimonium tart.
Cantharis
Hepar sulph.
Stannum
Veratrum

Singing makes symptoms worse
Phosphorus
Spongia
Stannum

Talking makes symptoms worse
Cannabis ind.
Cocculus
Magnesia carb.
Magnesia mur.
Natrum mur.
Phosphorus
Spongia
Stannum
Silicea
Sulphur

VOMIT
Where vomiting is main symptom
Aconite
Aethusa
Antimonium
Antimonium tart.
Apis
Argentum nit.
Arsenicum
Bryonia
Cadmium
Chamomilla
China
Colchicum
Cuprum
Ferrum
Ipecac.
Iris
Kreosotum
Lobelia
Nux
Phosphorus
Plumbum

Pulsatilla
Silicea
Sulphur
Tabacum
Veratrum
Veratrum vir.

Vomiting brought on by coughing
Alumina
Antimonium tart.
Bryonia
Drosera
Hepar sulph.
Ipecac.
Kali carb.

Vomit mainly bile
Arsenicum
Bryonia
Chamomilla
Chelidonium
Eupatorium
Ipecac.
Mercurius
Mercurius corr.
Natrum sulph.
Nux
Opium
Phosphorus
Pulsatilla
Sanguinaria
Sepia
Veratrum
Colchicum

Vomit contains undigested food
Arsenicum
Bryonia
China
Eupatorium
Ferrum
Ignatia
Kreosotum
Lycopodium
Nux
Phosphorus
Pulsatilla
Sanguinaria
Veratrum

Mucus in vomit
Argentum nit.
Drosera
Kali bichrom.
Nux
Phosphorus
Pulsatilla
Veratrum

Vomit tastes sour
Calcarea
Causticum
China
Iris
Lycopodium
Magnesia carb.
Natrum phos.
Nux
Phosphorus
Psorinum
Pulsatilla
Sulphur
Sulphuric ac.
Tabacum
Veratrum

Watery vomit
Arsenicum
Bryonia
Causticum
Veratrum

WASHING, GETTING WET
   see also COLD p. 62,
   WARMTH AND HEAT
   p. 66
Symptoms alleviated by washing or
   bathing
Aurum
Fluoric ac.
Pulsatilla

Symptoms aggravated by washing or
   bathing
Aesculus
Allium
Ammon. carb.
Calcarea
Causticum
Colchicum
Dulcamara
Graphites
Mezereum
Nux
Petroleum
Phytolacca
Sepia
Silicea
Sulphur

Cold baths alleviate symptoms
Aloe
Apis
Argentum nit.
Fluoric ac.
Natrum mur.
Pulsatilla

Cold baths make symptoms worse
Antimonium
Baryta
China
Magnesia phos.
Rhus tox.

Wet applications make symptoms worse
Ammon. carb.
Antimonium
Calcarea
Chamomilla
Clematis
Rhus tox.
Sulphur

Getting wet makes symptoms worse
Calcarea
Causticum
Pulsatilla
Rhus tox.
Sepia

Wet feet make symptoms worse
Allium
Dulcamara
Pulsatilla
Rhus tox.
Sepia
Silicea

YAWNING
Yawning alleviates symptoms
Guiacum

Yawning makes symptoms worse
Cina
Ignatia
Nux

ENVIRONMENT

COLD
Cold in general makes symptoms worse
Arsenicum
Baryta
Calcarea ars.
Calcarea fluor.
Calcarea phos.
Calcarea sil.
Capsicum
Causticum
China
Dulcamara
Graphites
Hepar sulph.
Hypericum
Kali ars.

Kali carb.
Kali phos.
Lycopodium
Magnesia phos.
Moschus
Natrum ars.
Nitric ac.
Nux
Phosphorus
Psorinum
Pyrogenium
Ranunculus
Rhus tox.
Rumex
Sabadilla
Sepia
Silicea
Spigelia
Strontium

Cold air improves symptoms
Aloe
Ambra
Amyl nit.
Bryonia
Fluoric ac.
Gelsemium
Glonoinum
Iodum
Natrum sulph.
Picric ac.
Pulsatilla
Sanguinaria
Secale

Cold air makes symptoms worse
Agaricus
Allium
Arsenicum
Aurum
Badiaga
Baryta
Calcarea
Calcarea phos.
Camphora
Causticum
Cimicifuga
Cistus
Dulcamara
Helleborus
Hepar sulph.
Hypericum
Kali ars.
Kali carb.
Lycopodium
Magnesia phos.
Moschus
Nux mosch.

Nux
Psorinum
Ranunculus
Rhododendron
Rhus tox.
Rumex
Sabadilla
Sepia
Silicea
Strontium

Tendency to catch cold
Aconite
Alumina
Baryta
Bryonia
Calcarea
Chamomilla
Dulcamara
Hepar sulph.
Kali iod.
Kali carb.
Lycopodium
Mercurius
Natrum ars.
Natrum mur.
Nitric ac.
Nux
Psorinum
Rumex
Sepia
Silicea
Tuberculinum

Becoming cold improves symptoms
Iodum
Lycopodium
Pulsatilla

Becoming cold makes symptoms worse
Arsenicum
Aurum
Baryta
Hepar sulph.
Kali ars.
Kali bichrom.
Kali carb.
Lycopodium
Moschus
Nux
Phosphoric ac.
Pyrogenium
Ranunculus
Rhus tox.
Sabadilla
Sepia
Silicea
Sulphuric ac.

Symptoms come on after catching cold
Arsenicum
Baryta
Belladonna
Bryonia
Calcarea
Calcarea phos.
Chamomilla
China
Dulcamara
Hepar sulph.
Hyoscyamus
Mercurius
Nux
Phosphorus
Pulsatilla
Pyrogenium
Ranunculus
Rhus tox.
Sepia
Silicea
Sulphuric ac.

*Cold bathing and cold applications
   improve symptoms*
Aloe
Amyl nit.
Apis
Argentum nit.
Arnica
Aurum
Bryonia
Fluoric ac.
Glonoinum
Iodum
Ledum
Natrum mur.
Picric ac.
Pulsatilla
Secale

*Cold bathing and cold applications
   make symptoms worse*
Actaea
Antimonium
Antimonium tart.
Apocynum
Baryta
Belladonna
Capsicum
Causticum
Chimaphila
Kreosotum
Lachesis
Magnesia phos.
Muriatic ac.
Nitric ac.

Phosphorus
Rhus tox.
Ruta
Sepia
Spigelia

*Change from cold to warm air makes
   symptoms worse*
Bryonia
Kali sulph.
Psorinum
Sulphur
Tuberculinum

*Entering a cold place makes symptoms
   worse*
Arsenicum
Kali ars.
Ranunculus
Sepia

DRAUGHTS
Draughts make symptoms worse
Belladonna
Calcarea
Calcarea phos.
Kali carb.
Rhus tox.
Selenium
Silicea
Sulphur

Being fanned alleviates symptoms
Apis
Carbo veg.
Sulphur

HEAT AND COLD
   see also COLD and
   WARMTH AND HEAT
*Extreme heat and cold make symptoms
   worse*
Antimonium
Causticum
Fluoric ac.
Graphites
Ipecac.
Lachesis
Lycopodium
Mercurius
Natrum carb.
Natrum mur.
Nitric ac.
Phosphoric ac.
Psorinum
Sepia
Silicea
Sulphur

HUMIDITY
Damp air alleviates symptoms
Aconite
Belladonna
Bryonia
Causticum
Hepar sulph.
Ipecac.
Nitric ac.
Nux
Platinum
Spigelia
Spongia
Zinc

Damp air makes symptoms worse
Actaea
Bryonia
Dulcamara
Gelsemium
Hypericum
Sanguinaria
Thuja
Urtica

*Damp house or cellar makes symptoms
   worse*
Arsenicum
Dulcamara
Natrum sulph.
Nux mosch.
Rhus tox.
Terebinthum
Thuja
Veratrum

Dry air alleviates symptoms
Ammon. carb.
Calcarea
Dulcamara
Lycopodium
Manganum
Mercurius
Natrum sulph.
Nux mosch.
Rhododendron
Rhus tox.
Ruta

Dry air makes symptoms worse
Aconite
Belladonna
Bryonia
Causticum
Hepar sulph.
Nux

LIGHT AND DARK
see also TIME OF DAY

Light makes symptoms worse
Calcarea
Colchicum
Glonoinum
Natrum carb.

Symptoms better in dark
Calcarea
Cicuta
Hepar sulph.
Catrum carb.
Nux
Sepia

Symptoms worse in dark
Cannabis ind.
Causticum
Phosphorus
Pulsatilla
Rhus tox.
Stramonium

MOON
Full moon makes symptoms worse
Calcarea
Crocus
Graphites
Natrum carb.
Natrum mur.
Spongia
Silicea

New moon makes symptoms worse
Ammon carb.
Calcarea
Causticum
Cuprum
Crocus
Sepia
Silicea
Staphisagria

Waxing moon alleviates symptoms
Clematis

Waxing moon makes symptoms worse
Alumina
Arnica
Calcarea
China
Clematis

NOISE
Sensitivity to noise
Aconite
Asarum
Belladonna

Borax
China
Coffea
Conium
Kali carb.
Nitric ac.
Nux
Opium
Sepia
Silicea
Theridion
Zinc

Sensitivity to music
Aconite
Ambra
Chamomilla
Graphites
Kreosotum
Lycopodium
Natrum carb.
Natrum mur.
Natrum sulph.
Nux
Phosphoric ac.
Sabina
Sepia
Tarentula

Noise makes symptoms worse
Aconite
Arnica
Belladonna
Cannabis ind.
China
Cicuta
Coffea
Conium
Ipecac.
Ignatia
Kali carb.
Natrum carb.
Natrum mur.
Nux
Phosphorus
Phosphoric ac.
Picric ac.
Silicea
Spigelia
Stramonium
Zinc

OPEN AIR
Being out of doors improves symptoms
Alumina
Argentum nit.
Arsenicum
Cannabis ind.

Crocus
Kali iod.
Magnesia carb.
Magnesia mur.
Natrum sulph.
Pulsatilla
Rhus tox.
Sabadilla
Sabina

Being out of doors makes symptoms worse
China
Cocculus
Guaiacum
Hepar sulph.
Kali carb.
Mercurius
Nitric ac.
Nux
Nux mosch.
Rumex
Silicea
Sulphur

Desire to be in open air
Aurum
Aurum mur.
Calcarea iod.
Carbo veg.
Crocus
Iodum
Kali iod.
Kali sulph.
Lycopodium
Pulsatilla
Sulphur

Dislike of open air
Ammon. carb.
Baptisia
Calcarea
Calcarea phos.
Chamomilla
Cocculus
Coffea
Ignatia
Kali carb.
Natrum carb.
Nux
Petroleum
Rumex
Silicea
Sulphur

Becoming warm in open air makes symptoms worse
Bryonia
Iodum

Lycopodium
Pulsatilla

SEA
Seaside air makes symptoms worse
Arsenicum
Kali iod.
Magnesia mur.
Natrum mur.
Natrum sulph.
Sepia

Air at sea improves symptoms
Bromium
Medorrhinum
Natrum mur.

Swimming in sea makes symptoms worse
Arsenicum
Magnesia mur.
Rhus tox.
Sepia
Zinc

SEASONS
Symptoms worse in spring
Ambra
Bromium
Crotalus
Iris
Kali bichrom.
Lachesis
Lycopodium
Pulsatilla

Symptoms better in summer
Aesculus
Causticum
Silicea

Symptoms worse in summer
Antimonium
Argentum nit.
Bromium
Gelsemium
Glonoinum
Kali brom.
Lachesis
Natrum carb.
Natrum mur.
Nux
Podophyllum

Symptoms worse in autumn
Baptisia
Dulcamara
Iris

Kali bichrom.
Mercurius
Rhus tox.

Symptoms worse in winter
Aesculus
Causticum
Ipecac.
Mezereum
Nux mosch.
Rhus tox.
Silicea

TIME OF DAY
Symptoms worse during day
Sepia
Stannum
Sulphur

Symptoms worse in morning
Agaricus
Ammon. mur.
Argentum
Arsenicum iod.
Aurum
Bryonia
Calcarea
Calcarea phos.
Carbo an.
Carbo veg.
Carbon sulph
Chamomilla
Chelidonium
Cina
Crocus
Kali bichrom.
Kali nit.
Lachesis
Natrum ars.
Natrum mur.
Natrum sulph.
Nitric ac.
Nux
Onosmodium
Petroleum
Phosphoric ac.
Phosphorus
Podophyllum
Pulsatilla
Rhododendron
Rhus tox.
Rumex
Sepia
Spigelia
Squilla
Sulphur
Sulphuric ac.
Valerian

Symptoms worse just before noon
Natrum carb.
Natrum mur.
Podophyllum
Sabadilla
Sepia
Stannum
Sulphur
Sulphuric ac.

Symptoms better in late morning
Lycopodium

Symptoms worse around 10 am
Natrum mur.

Symptoms worse around 11 am
Sulphur

Symptoms worse at noon
Argentum

Symptoms worse in afternoon
Belladonna
Kali nit.
Lycopodium
Pulsatilla
Rhus tox.
Sepia
Silicea
Thuja
Zinc

Symptoms worse around 3 pm
Belladonna

Symptoms worse around 4 pm
Lycopodium

Symptoms worse between 4 and 8 pm
Lycopodium

Symptoms better in evening
Alumina
Aurum
Medorrhinum
Sepia

Symptoms worse in evening
Alumina
Ambra
Ammon. carb.
Antimonium
Antimonium tart.
Arnica
Belladonna
Bryonia
Calcarea

Capsicum
Carbo an.
Carbo veg.
Carbon sulph.
Causticum
Chamomilla
Colchicum
Cyclamen
Euphrasia
Helleborus
Hyoscyamus
Kali nit.
Lachesis
Lycopodium
Magnesia carb.
Menyanthes
Mercurius
Mezereum
Natrum phos.
Nitric ac.
Phosphoric ac.
Phosphorus
Platinum
Plumbum
Pulsatilla
Rumex
Ruta
Sepia
Silicea
Stannum
Strontium
Sulphur
Sulphuric ac.
Valerian
Zinc

Symptoms worse at twilight
Pulsatilla

Symptoms worse around 9 pm
Bryonia

Symptoms worse at night
Aconite
Argentum nit.
Arnica
Arsenicum
Arsenicum iod.
Calcarea
Calcarea iod.
Calcarea phos.
Calcarea sulph.
Carbo an.
Carbon sulph.
Chamomilla
China
Cinnabar
Coffea

Colchicum
Conium
Cyclamen
Dulcamara
Ferrum
Graphites
Hepar sulph.
Hyoscyamus
Iodum
Ipecac.
Kali ars.
Kali bichrom.
Kali carb.
Kali iod.
Lachesis
Lilium
Magnesia carb.
Magnesia mur.
Manganum
Mercurius
Nitric ac.
Phosphorus
Plumbum
Psorinum
Pulsatilla
Rhus tox.
Rumex
Sepia
Silicea
Strontium
Sulphur
Zinc

Symptoms worse before midnight
Argentum nit.
Arsenicum
Carbo veg.
Chamomilla
Coffea
Kali ars.
Ledum
Lycopodium
Phosphorus
Pulsatilla
Rumex
Sabadilla
Stannum

Symptoms better after midnight
Lycopodium

Symptoms worse after midnight
Arsenicum
Drosera
Kali carb.
Kali nit.
Natrum ars.
Nux

Phosphorus
Podophyllum
Rhus tox.
Silicea
Thuja

Symptoms worse around 1 am
Arsenicum

Symptoms worse between 2 and 4 am
Kali carb.

WARMTH AND HEAT
Warmth makes symptoms worse
Alumina
Apis
Arsenicum iod.
Glonoinum
Iodum
Kali sulph.
Lachesis
Ledum
Mercurius
Pulsatilla
Secale

Warm rooms make symptoms worse
Apis
Calcarea sulph.
Carbon sulph.
Crocus
Graphites
Iodum
Kali iod.
Kali sulph.
Lycopodium
Pulsatilla
Sabina
Secale
Senega
Sulphur

Warmth of bed improves symptoms
Arsenicum
Bryonia
Hepar sulph.
Kali carb.
Lycopodium
Nux
Nux mosch.
Rhus tox.
Silicea
Tuberculinum

Warmth of bed makes symptoms worse
Apis
Chamomilla

Drosera
Ledum
Mercurius
Opium
Pulsatilla
Sabina
Secale
Sulphur

Warm applications make symptoms worse
Apis
Iodum
Kali sulph.
Ledum
Lycopodium
Pulsatilla
Secale
Sulphur

Radiant heat improves symptoms
Arsenicum
Hepar sulph.
Ignatia
Kali carb.
Magnesia phos.
Nux
Rhododendron
Rhus tox.
Silicea

Radiant heat makes symptoms worse
Antimonium
Apis
Argentum nit.
Bryonia
Cocculus
Glonoinum
Iodum
Kali iod.
Ledum
Natrum mur.
Pulsatilla
Secale

Becoming overheated improves symptoms
Aurum
Phosphoric ac.
Sepia

Becoming overheated makes symptoms worse
Antimonium
Bromium
Bryonia
Colchicum
Graphites

Kali sulph.
Lycopodium
Pulsatilla
Thuja

Stuffy rooms make symptoms worse
Apis
Argentum nit.
Bryonia
Bromium
Lachesis
Lilium
Lycopodium
Magnesia carb.
Natrum mur.
Pulsatilla
Sepia
Sulphur

WEATHER

Changes in weather make symptoms worse
Dulcamara
Nux mosch.
Phosphorus
Psorinum
Ranunculus
Rhododendron
Rhus tox.
Silicea
Tuberculinum

Cold, dry weather makes symptoms worse
Aconite
Asarum
Causticum
Hepar sulph.
Kali carb.
Nux

Cold, wet weather makes symptoms worse
Ammon. carb.
Arsenicum
Badiaga
Calcarea
Calcarea phos.
Colchicum
Dulcamara
Medorrhinum
Natrum sulph.
Nux mosch.
Pyrogenium
Rhododendron
Rhus tox.
Silicea
Tuberculinum

Both cold and hot weather make symptoms worse
Fluoric ac.

Warm, wet weather makes symptoms worse
Carbo veg.
Gelsemium
Iodum
Kali bichrom.
Lachesis
Natrum sulph.
Silicea

Wet weather makes symptoms worse
Ammon. carb.
Arsenicum
Badiaga
Calcarea
Dulcamara
Natrum sulph.
Nux mosch.
Pulsatilla
Rhododendron
Rhus tox.

Cloudy weather makes symptoms worse
Rhus tox.

Foggy weather makes symptoms worse
Bryonia
Gelsemium
Hypericum
Manganum
Nux mosch.
Plumbum
Rhododendron
Rhus tox.
Sabina
Silicea

Snow makes symptoms worse
Calcarea
Conium
Lycopodium
Phosphorus
Phosphoric ac.
Pulsatilla
Rhus tox.
Sepia
Silicea
Sulphur

Sun makes symptoms worse
Antimonium
Glonoinum
Natrum carb.
Natrum mur.
Pulsatilla

Symptoms worse before thunderstorm
Agaricus
Calcarea
Gelsemium
Manganum
Natrum carb.
Natrum mur.
Petroleum
Phosphorus
Medorrhinum
Pulsatilla
Rhododendron
Rhus tox.
Sepia
Sulphur
Syphilinum

Symptoms worse during thunderstorm
Gelsemium
Natrum carb.
Petroleum
Phosphorus
Psorinum
Rhododendron
Silicea
Syphilinum

Wind makes symptoms worse
Chamomilla
Lycopodium
Nux
Pulsatilla
Rhododendron
Phosphorus

Cold wind makes symptoms worse
Belladonna
Hepar sulph.
Nux
Spongia

*Windy and stormy weather makes
    symptoms worse*
Aconite
Badiaga
Chamomilla
China
Hepar sulph.
Lachesis
Magnesia phos.
Muriatic ac.
Nux
Nux mosch.
Phosphorus
Psorinum
Pulsatilla
Rhododendron
Sepia

FOOD and DRINK

DRINKS
Cold drinks alleviate symptoms
Bismuth
Bryonia
Causticum
Phosphorus
Sepia

Cold drinks make symptoms worse
Cantharis
Ferrum
Rhus tox.

Warm/hot drinks alleviate symptoms
Alumina
Arsenicum
Bryonia
Carbo sulph.
Chelidonium
Graphites
Lycopodium
Manganum
Nux
Rhus tox.
Sulphur

Coffee alleviates symptoms
Chamomilla

Coffee makes symptoms worse
Cantharis
Causticum
Chamomilla
Ignatia
Nux

Tea makes symptoms worse
Aesculus
China
Ferrum
Selenium
Thuja

Vinegar improves symptoms
Asarum
Pulsatilla

Vinegar makes symptoms worse
Antimonium
Arsenicum
Belladonna
Ferrum
Natrum phos.
Sepia
Sulphur

Aversion to drinks in general
Ferrum
Hyoscyamus
Nux

Aversion to cold drinks
Caladium
China ars.
Stramonium

Aversion to warm/hot drinks
Phosphorus
Pulsatilla

Aversion to beer
Nux

Aversion to coffee
Calcarea
Nux

Aversion to water
Hyoscyamus
Lyssin
Nux
Stramonium
Staphisagria

Aversion to wine
Ignatia
Mercurius
Rhus tox.
Sabadilla
Sulphur
Zinc

Desire for cold drinks
Aconite
Arsenicum
Bryonia
China
Eupatorium
Mercurius
Mercurius corr.
Natrum sulph.
Phosphorus
Veratrum

Desire for warm/hot drinks
Arsenicum
Bryonia
Lac can.

Desire for alcohol
Arsenicum
Asarum
Capsicum
Crotalus

Lachesis
Nux
Sulphur

Desire for alcohol before periods
Selenium

Desire for beer
Aconite
Nux
Sulphur

Desire for brandy
Nux
Opium

Desire for lemonade
Nitric ac.
Sabina

Desire for vinegar
Hepar sulph.
Sepia

Desire for whisky
Lac can.
Sulphur

FOOD
Cold food makes symptoms worse
Arsenicum
Dulcamara
Lachesis
Lycopodium
Nux
Rhus tox.
Silicea

Raw food makes symptoms worse
Pulsatilla
Ruta
Veratrum

Farinaceous foods make symptoms worse
Causticum
Natrum carb.
Natrum mur.

Fatty foods make symptoms worse
Carbo veg.
Cyclamen
Ferrum
Pulsatilla
Taraxacum

Flatulent foods make symptoms worse
Bryonia
China
Lycopodium
Petroleum

Frozen food makes symptoms worse
Arsenicum
Calcarea phos.
Carbo veg.
Ipecac.
Pulsatilla

Fruit makes symptoms worse
Arsenicum
Bryonia
China
Colocynth
Natrum sulph.
Pulsatilla
Veratrum

Rich food makes symptoms worse
Bryonia
Carbo veg.
Ipecac.
Natrum sulph.
Nitric ac.
Pulsatilla
Sepia

Salty foods make symptoms worse
Alumina
Carbo veg.
Drosera
Phosphorus
Selenium

Sour foods make symptoms worse
Antimonium
Argentum nit.
Arsenicum
Belladonna
Ferrum
Natrum phos.
Sepia
Sulphur

Sweet foods make symptoms worse
Antimonium
Argentum nit.
Chamomilla
Graphites
Ignatia
Mercurius
Selenium
Sulphur

Beans, peas, and other pulses make symptoms worse
Bryonia
Calcarea
Lycopodium
Petroleum

Bread makes symptoms worse
China
Nitric ac.
Pulsatilla
Sepia

Buckwheat makes symptoms worse
Ipecac.
Pulsatilla

Butter makes symptoms worse
Carbo veg.
Pulsatilla

Cabbage makes symptoms worse
Bryonia
China
Lycopodium
Magnesia
Natrum sulph.
Petroleum
Pulsatilla

Meat which is going off makes symptoms worse
Arsenicum
Belladonna
Bryonia
Carbo veg.
Crotalus
Lachesis
Pulsatilla
Pyrogenium

Milk makes symptoms worse
Aethusa
Calcarea
Calcarea sulph.
China
Conium
Lac defl.
Magnesia mur.
Nitric ac.
Sepia
Sulphur

Onions make symptoms worse
Lycopodium
Pulsatilla

Pancakes make symptoms worse
Bryonia
Kali carb.
Pulsatilla

Pastry makes symptoms worse
Lycopodium
Phosphorus
Pulsatilla

Pork makes symptoms worse
Carbo veg.
Cyclamen
Pulsatilla
Sepia

Sauerkraut makes symptoms worse
Bryonia
China
Lycopodium
Petroleum
Phosphorus
Pulsatilla

Green vegetables make symptoms worse
Alumina
Bryonia
Helleborus
Natrum sulph.

Sight of food makes symptoms worse
Colchicum
Kali bichrom.
Lycopodium
Sulphur

Smell of food makes symptoms worse
Arsenicum
Cocculus
Colchicum
Digitalis
Ipecac.
Sepia
Thuja

Aversion to food in general
Arsenicum
China
Cocculus
Colchicum
Ferrum
Ipecac.
Lilium
Nux

Aversion to food despite being hungry
Cocculus
Natrum mur.
Nux

Aversion to warm/hot food
China
Graphites
Phosphorus
Pulsatilla

Aversion to smell of food
Arsenicum
Cocculus
Colchicum
Ipecac.
Podophyllum
Sepia

Aversion to food until tasted, then ravenous appetite
Lycopodium

Aversion to fatty and rich foods
China
Petroleum
Pulsatilla

Aversion to fish
Graphites

Aversion to fruit
Arsenicum
China
Pulsatilla

Aversion to meat
Calcarea
Calcarea sulph.
Carbon sulph.
Graphites
Muriatic ac.
Nux
Petroleum
Pulsatilla
Sepia
Sulphur
Silicea

Aversion to salty foods
Carbo veg.
Graphites
Natrum mur.
Selenium
Sepia

Aversion to sweet foods
Arsenicum
Causticum
Graphites
Mercurius
Phosphorus
Sulphur
Zinc

Aversion to beer
China
Nux

Aversion to bread
China
Natrum mur.

Aversion to butter
China
Pulsatilla

Aversion to milk
Lac defl.
Natrum carb.

Desire for cold food
Phosphorus
Pulsatilla

Desire for raw food
Sulphur

Desire for warm/hot food
Arsenicum
Chelidonium
Ferrum
Lycopodium
Phosphoric ac.
Sabadilla

Desire for fatty foods
Arsenicum
Hepar sulph.
Nitric ac.
Nux
Sulphur

Desire for fish
Natrum mur.
Phosphoric ac.

Desire for fruit
Phosphoric ac.
Veratrum

Desire for juicy things
Phosphoric ac.

Desire for salty foods
Argentum nit.
Carbo veg.
Lac can.
Natrum mur.
Phosphorus
Veratrum

Desire for spicy foods
China
Hepar sulph.
Lac can.
Nux

Phosphorus
Sanguinaria
Sulphur
Tarentula

Desire for strange foods
Bryonia
Calcarea
Calcarea phos.
Chelidonium
Cyclamen
Hepar sulph.
Mancinella

Desire for sweet foods
Argentum nit.
China
Lycopodium
Sulphur

Desire for bread and butter
Mercurius

Desire for eggs
Calcarea

Desire for herrings and other oily fish
Nitric ac.
Pulsatilla
Veratrum

Desire for ice cream
Calcarea
Opium
Phosphorus

Desire for lemons
Arsenicum
Belladonna

Desire for lime, earth, chalk, clay, etc.
Alumina
Nitric ac.
Nux

Desire for milk
Apis
Arsenicum
Aurum
Bryonia
Calcarea
Chelidonium
Lac can.
Mercurius
Natrum mur.
Nux
Phosphoric ac.
Rhus tox.
Sabadilla
Silicea

Staphisagria
Strontia

Desire for smoked meats
Calcarea phos.
Causticum
Tuberculinum

*Indistinct desires, not knowing what
    foods one wants*
Bryonia
Ignatia
Pulsatilla

TOBACCO
Aversion to tobacco
Calcarea
Ignatia
Nux

Tobacco makes symptoms worse
Arsenicum
Ignatia
Nux
Pulsatilla
Spigelia
Spongia
Staphisagria

MIND and EMOTIONS

see also BREATHING p. 40–1,
    FACIAL
    EXPRESSION p. 44–5,
    PERSPIRATION p. 54
    PULSE p. 54–5
Anger
Aconite
Arsenicum
Anacardium
Aurum
Bryonia
Chamomilla
Hepar sulph.
Ignatia
Kali carb.
Kali sulph.
Lycopodium
Natrum mur.
Nitric ac.
Nux
Petroleum
Sepia
Staphisagria
Sulphur

Anxiety
Aconite
Argentum nit.

Arsenicum
Arsenicum iod.
Aurum
Belladonna
Bismuth
Bryonia
Cactus
Calcarea
Calcarea phos.
Calcarea sulph.
Camphora
Cannabis ind.
Carbon sulph.
Carbo veg.
Causticum
China
Conium
Digitalis
Iodum
Kali carb.
Kali iod.
Kali phos.
Kali sulph.
Lycopodium
Mezereum
Natrum ars.
Natrum carb.
Nitric ac.
Phosphorus
Psorinum
Pulsatilla
Rhus tox.
Secale
Sulphur
Veratrum

Apprehension
Bryonia
Calcarea
China sulph.
Cicuta
Phosphorus

Brooding, tendency to dwell on things
Ambra
Benzoic ac.
Chamomilla
China
Cocculus
Conium
Natrum mur.
Platinum
Sepia
Sulphur

Desire for company
Argentum nit.
Arsenicum
Bismuth
Hyoscyamus

Kali carb.
Lac can.
Lycopodium
Phosphorus

Not in mood for company
Anacardium
Baryta
Carbo an.
Chamomilla
Cicuta
Gelsemium
Ignatia
Natrum mur.
Nux

Criticism makes symptoms worse
Staphisagria

*Delusions, hallucinations, overactive
    imagination*
Argentum nit.
Belladonna
Cannabis ind.
Cocculus
Hyoscyamus
Ignatia
Lachesis
Petroleum
Phosphoric ac.
Sabadilla
Stramonium
Sulphur

Depression
Aconite
Arsenicum
Arsenicum iod.
Aurum
Aurum mur.
Calcarea
Calcarea ars.
Calcarea sulph.
Carbo an.
Carbon sulph.
Causticum
Chamomilla
China
Cimicifuga
Ferrum
Ferrum iod.
Gelsemium
Graphites
Helleborus
Ignatia
Iodum
Kali brom.
Kali phos.

Lac can.
Lachesis
Lilium
Lycopodium
Mercurius
Mezereum
Murex
Natrum ars.
Natrum mur.
Natrum sulph.
Nitric ac.
Platinum
Psorinum
Pulsatilla
Rhus tox.
Sepia
Stannum
Sulphur
Thuja
Veratrum
Zinc

Despair
Arsenicum
Aurum
Calcarea
Coffea
Helleborus
Ignatia
Psorinum

Discontent, dissatisfaction
Anacardium
Calcarea phos.
Mercurius
Natrum mur.
Sulphur

*Disappointment which makes
    symptoms worse*
Ignatia

*Dullness, sluggishness, difficulty
    understanding what is going on*
Argentum nit.
Baptisia
Baryta
Baryta mur.
Belladonna
Bryonia
Calcarea
Calcarea phos.
Calcarea sulph.
Carbo veg.
Gelsemium
Graphites
Guaiacum
Helleborus

Hyoscyamus
Kali brom.
Kali carb.
Lachesis
Laurocerasus
Lycopodium
Natrum ars.
Natrum carb.
Natrum mur.
Nux mosch.
Opium
Phosphoric ac.
Phosphorus
Picric ac.
Plumbum
Pulsatilla
Senega
Silicea
Staphisagria
Sulphur
Tuberculinum
Zinc

*Embarrassment or shame makes
    symptoms worse*
Colocynth
Ignatia
Lycopodium
Natrum mur.
Palladium
Phosphoric ac.
Staphisagria

*Emotional exhaustion, apathy, and
    indifference due to grief*
Phosphoric ac.

Enthusiasm makes symptoms worse
Phosphorus

Excitement, excitability
Aconite
Argentum nit.
Aurum
Belladonna
Chamomilla
Coffea
Graphites
Hyoscyamus
Kali brom.
Kali iod.
Lac can.
Lachesis
Moschus
Natrum mur.
Nitric ac.
Nux
Opium

Phosphoric ac.
Phosphorus
Pulsatilla

*Ailments brought on by too much
    excitement or joy*
Aconite
Coffea
Opium
Pulsatilla

Fear
Aconite
Aurum
Belladonna
Borax
Calcarea
Calcarea phos.
Carbon sulph.
Cicuta
Digitalis
Graphites
Ignatia
Kali ars.
Lycopodium
Natrum carb.
Phosphorus
Platinum
Psorinum
Sepia
Stramonium

Ailments brought on by fright
Aconite
Ignatia
Lycopodium
Natrum mur.
Opium
Phosphoric ac.
Phosphorus
Silicea

Easily frightened
Arsenicum
Argentum nit.
Baryta
Borax
Graphites
Lycopodium
Natrum ars.
Natrum carb.
Sepia
Stramonium

Grief
Aurum
Causticum
Ignatia

Natrum mur.
Pulsatilla

Ailments brought on by grief
Aurum
Causticum
Cocculus
Ignatia
Lachesis
Natrum mur.
Phosphoric ac.
Staphisagria

Guilt
Alumina
Ammon carb.
Arsenicum
Aurum
Carbo veg.
Causticum
Chelidonium
Cocculus
Conium
Digitalis
Ferrum
Graphites
Hyoscyamus
Ignatia
Medorrhinum
Mercurius
Natrum mur.
Nux
Psorinum
Rhus tox.
Silicea
Sulphur
Thuja
Veratrum
Zinc

*Feeling harassed makes symptoms
    worse*
Anacardium
Cina
Colocynth
Ignatia
Ipecac.
Phosphorus
Staphisagria

Hallucinations, see *Delusions*

Haste and hurry
Lilium
Medorrhinum
Mercurius
Natrum mur.
Sulphur

Sulphuric ac.
Tarentula

Homesickness
Capsicum
Carbo an.
Ignatia
Phosphoric ac.

Impatience
Chamomilla
Ignatia
Nux
Sepia
Sulphur

*Indifference, lack of interest in people or
    things*
Apis
Carbo veg.
China
Helleborus
Lilium
Mezereum
Natrum carb.
Natrum mur.
Natrum phos.
Onosmodium
Opium
Phosphoric ac.
Phosphorus
Platinum
Pulsatilla
Sepia
Staphisagria

Indignation
Arsenicum
Calcarea phos.
Colocynth
Staphisagria

Irritability
Aconite
Alumina
Antimonium
Apis
Aurum
Belladonna
Bovista
Bryonia
Calcarea
Calcarea sulph.
Carbo veg.
Carbon sulph.
Causticum
Chamomilla
Graphites

Hepar sulph.
Kali carb.
Kali iod.
Kali sulph.
Lilium
Lycopodium
Magnesia carb.
Natrum carb.
Natrum mur.
Nitric ac.
Nux
Petroleum
Phosphoric ac.
Phosphorus
Platinum
Pulsatilla
Ranunculus
Rhus tox.
Sepia
Silicea
Staphisagria
Sulphur
Sulphuric ac.
Thuja
Veratrum vir.
Zinc

Jealousy
Apis
Calcarea sulph.
Hyoscyamus
Lachesis
Lycopodium
Medorrhinum
Pulsatilla

Can't bear to be looked at
Antimonium
Antimonium tart.
Arsenicum
Chamomilla
China
Cina
Iodum
Natrum mur.

Mental exhaustion, perhaps from
*   studying too hard*
Picric ac.

Mental exhaustion and memory
*   problems while studying for exams*
Anacardium

Can't bear to be opposed or contradicted
Aurum
Bryonia
Cocculus

Ferrum
Ignatia
Lycopodium
Nux
Sepia
Silicea

Oversensitiveness, crying when others
*   are hurt or in trouble*
Causticum
Ignatia
Natrum carb.
Natrum mur.
Nitric ac.
Nux
Phosphorus

Excessive pride
Calcarea
Lachesis
Palladium
Platinum
Silicea
Sulphur

Punishment makes symptoms worse
Argentum nit.
Capsicum
Chamomilla
China
Ignatia

Restlessness, nervousness
Aconite
Anacardium
Argentum nit.
Arsenicum
Arsenicum iod.
Baptisia
Belladonna
Calcarea
Calcarea phos.
Camphora
Cimicifuga
Colocynth
Cuprum
Ferrum
Helleborus
Hyoscyamus
Lycopodium
Mercurius
Plumbum
Pulsatilla
Rhus tox.
Sepia
Silicea
Staphisagria
Stramonium

Sulphur
Tarentula
Zinc

Rudeness
Hyoscyamus
Lac can.
Lycopodium
Nux
Stramonium
Veratrum

Rudeness makes symptoms worse
Staphisagria

Sympathy relieves symptoms
Pulsatilla

Sympathy makes symptoms worse
Ignatia
Natrum mur.
Sepia
Silicea

Can't bear being spoken to
Arsenicum
Arsenicum iod.
Carbon sulph.
Chamomilla
Gelsemium
Graphites
Hyoscyamus
Iodum
Natrum sulph.
Sulphur
Tarentula

Symptoms worse in presence of
*   strangers*
Ambra
Baryta
Bryonia
Sepia
Stramonium
Thuja

Suppressed, bottled up emotions
Aconite
Bryonia
Cuprum
Conium
Graphites
Lachesis
Natrum mur.
Opium
Secale
Sepia
Sulphur
Zinc

Tearfulness
Apis
Calcarea
Calcarea sulph.
Carbon sulph.
Causticum
Cicuta
Graphites
Ignatia
Kali brom.
Lac can.
Lycopodium
Natrum mur.
Palladium
Platinum
Pulsatilla
Rhus tox.
Sepia
Sulphur
Veratrum

Aversion to thinking
Baptisia
Carbo veg.
China
Gelsemium
Lycopodium
Phosphoric ac.
Phosphorus

Thinking about ailments tends to make them better
Camphora
Helleborus

Thinking about ailments tends to make them worse
Alumina
Baptisia
Baryta
Calcarea phos.
Causticum
Gelsemium
Helleborus
Lachesis
Medorrhinum
Nitric ac.
Nux
Oxalic ac.
Ranunculus
Sabadilla
Spongia

Timidity
Baryta
Calcarea
Calcarea sulph.
Gelsemium

Kali carb.
Lycopodium
Natrum carb.
Petroleum
Phosphorus
Plumbum
Pulsatilla
Sepia
Sulphur

Ailments brought on by unhappy love affair
Aurum
Hyoscyamus
Ignatia
Natrum mur.
Phosphoric ac.

Upset by bad news
Apis
Calcarea
Gelsemium
Ignatia
Medorrhinum
Natrum mur.
Palladium
Sulphur

LIBIDO
Diminished libido
Agnus
Baryta
Graphites
Lycopodium
Silicea
Staphisagria

Excessive libido
Phosphorus
Stramonium
Zinc

Increased libido
Baryta mur.
Calcarea
Calcarea phos.
Cannabis
Cantharis
Conium
Lycopodium
Lyssin
Nux
Picric ac.
Platinum
Pulsatilla
Silicea

Staphisagria
Tuberculinum
Zinc

Desire for sex unsatisfied
Apis
Camphora
Conium
Lyssin
Pulsatilla

TALKING
Talking very fast
Hepar sulph.
Hyoscyamus
Lachesis
Mercurius

Talking incoherently
Bryonia
Cannabis ind.
Hyoscyamus
Lachesis
Phosphorus
Rhus tox.
Stramonium

Talking obscenely
Belladonna
Hyoscyamus
Lilium
Nux
Stramonium

Extreme talkativeness
Anacardium
Bryonia
Hyoscyamus
Stramonium

Talking very slowly
Argentum nit.
Helleborus
Kali brom.
Lachesis
Opium
Phosphorus
Phosphoric ac.
Plumbum
Secale
Sepia
Thuja

Talking unintelligibly
Belladonna
Hyoscyamus
Mercurius
Phosphoric ac.

Secale
Stramonium

Straying from the point, losing the thread
Belladonna
Hyoscyamus
Lachesis

Lycopodium
Nux
Stramonium

No desire to talk
Aurum
Carbo an.
Cocculus

Glonoinum
Phosphoric ac.
Phosphorus
Platinum
Pulsatilla
Sulphur
Veratrum
Zinc

HOMEOPATHIC REMEDIES AND THEIR SOURCES

Listed below are all the remedies mentioned in this book, with their Latin and common names. The majority are derived from living organisms, sometimes from specific parts of them. Note that only very small numbers of animals and plants need to be culled to satisfy homeopathic requirements.

Abies can.   Abies canadensis   hemlock spruce, Canada pitch (fresh bark and young buds)
Abies nig.   Abies nigra   black or double spruce (gum)
Abrotanum   Artemisia abrotanum   southernwood, lad's love, old man (fresh leaves and stem)
Absinthium   Artemisia absinthium   absinth, common wormwood (fresh young leaves and flowers)
Acetic ac.   Aceticum acidum   acetic acid
Aconite   Aconitum napellus   wolfsbane, blue aconite, blue monkshood (whole plant, including root, as it comes into
   flower)
Actaea   Actaea spicata   baneberry, herb Christopher (root in autumn)
Aesculus   Aesculus hippocastanum   horse chestnut (ripe conkers)
Aethusa   Aethusa cynapium   fool's parsley (whole plant when in flower)
Agaricus   Agaricus muscarius   fly agaric (fresh fungus, or dried cap)
Agraphis   Agraphis nutans   bluebell, wild hyacinth (fresh plant and growing shoots)
Agnus   Agnus castus   chaste tree (ripe berries)
Ailanthus   Ailanthus glandulosa   Chinese sumach, tree of heaven (flowers as they begin to open)
Aletris   Aletris farinosa   stargrass, unicorn root, blazing grass, colic root (root)
Allium   Allium cepa   red onion (whole fresh plant in July/August)
Allium sat.   Allium sativa   garlic (fresh bulb)
Aloe   Aloe socotrina   common aloe (gum)
Alum   Alumen   double sulphate of aluminium and potassium
Alumina   Alumina   aluminium oxide
Ambra   Ambra grisea   ambergris, yellow-grey fatty substance from whale's intestine
Ambrosia   Ambrosia artemisiaefolia   ragweed, Roman wormwood, hogweed (fresh flower heads and young shoots)
Ammonium brom.   Ammonium bromatum   ammonium bromide
Ammonium carb.   Ammonium carbonicum   ammonium carbonate
Ammonium mur.   Ammonium muriaticum   sal ammoniac, ammonium chloride
Amyl nit.   Amyl nitrite
Anacardium   Anacardium occidentale   cashew nut (black juice between outer and inner shell of nut)
Anacardium or.   Anacardium orientale   marking nut (layer between shell and kernel)
Angustura   Angustura vera   bark of Galipea cusparia
Anthemis   Anthemis nobilis   Roman chamomile (flowers)
Anthrax   Anthracinum anthrax   poison from spleen of affected sheep
Antimonium   Antimonium crudum   black sulphide of antimony
Antimonium tart.   Antimonium tartaricum   tartar emetic, potassium antimony tartrate
Apis   Apis mellifica   honey bee (whole bee, or venom from sting)
Apocynum   Apocynum cannabinum   Indian or American hemp (whole fresh plant, including root)
Argentum   Argentum metallicum   silver
Argentum nit.   Argentum nitricum   silver nitrate
Arnica   Arnica montana   leopard's bane, Fallkraut (whole fresh plant, dried flowers or root)
Arsenicum   Arsenicum album   arsenic trioxide
Arsenicum iod.   Arsenicum iodatum   arsenic iodide
Artemisia   Artemisia vulgaris   mugwort (fresh root)
Arum   Arum triphyllum   Indian turnip (fresh tuber)
Arundo   Arundo mauritanica   an Italian grass (root sprouts)
Asafoetida   Narthex asafoetida   stinkasand (gum)

Asarum   Asarum europaeum   European snakeroot, hazelwort, wild nard (whole fresh plant, including root)
Asclepias   Asclepias cornuti or *A. syriaca*   silkweed, milkweed (root)
Astacus   Astacus fluviatilis   freshwater crayfish (whole animal)
Asterias   Asterias rubens   red starfish (whole animal)
Atropine   Atropinum   atropine, poisonous alkaloid found in deadly nightshade, see *Belladonna*
Aurum   Aurum metallicum   gold
Aurum mur.   Aurum muriaticum   gold chloride
Avena   Avena sativa   oat (fresh plant when in flower)

Bacillinum   nosode prepared from sputum of patient with tuberculosis
Badiaga   Badiaga Spongia palustris   freshwater sponge (dried sponge collected in autumn)
Baptisia   Baptisia tinctoria   wild indigo (fresh root and bark)
Baryta   Baryta carbonica   barium carbonate
Baryta mur.   Baryta muriatica   barium chloride
Belladonna   Atropa belladonna   deadly nightshade (whole fresh plant as it comes into flower)
Bellis   Bellis perennis   common daisy (whole fresh plant)
Benzoic ac.   Benzoicum acidum   benzoic acid
Berberis   Berberis vulgaris   common barberry (bark or root)
Bismuth   Bismuthum   precipitated sub-nitrate of bismuth
Blatta   Blatta orientalis   Indian cockroach (whole live insect)
Boracic ac.   Boracicum acidum   boracic acid
Borax   Borax veneta   sodium borate
Bothrops   Bothrops lanceolatus   yellow viper, fer-de-lance from Martinique (venom)
Bovista   Lycoperdon bovista   warted puffball (whole fungus)
Bromium   Bromium   bromine
Bryonia   Bryonia alba or *B. dioica*   white or common bryony (root before flowering)
Bufo   Bufo rana   common toad, Brazilian toad (venom from skin glands)

Cactus   Cactus grandiflorus   night-blooming cereus (youngest, tenderest shoots and flowers in summer)
Cadmium   Cadmium sulphuratum   cadmium sulphate
Caladium   Caladium seguinum   American arum, dumb cane (whole fresh plant)
Calcarea   Calcarea carbonica   calcium carbonate from middle layer of oyster shells
Calcarea fluor.   Calcarea fluorata   fluorspar, calcium fluoride
Calcarea hypophos.   Calcarea hypophosphorica   calcium hypophosphite
Calcarea iod.   Calcarea iodata   calcium iodide
Calcarea phos.   Calcarea phosphorica   calcium phosphate
Calcarea sil.   Calcarea silicata   calcium silicate
Calcarea sulph.   Calcarea sulphurica   gypsum, plaster of Paris, calcium sulphate
Calendula   Calendula officinalis   pot marigold (leaves and flowers)
Camphora   Laurus camphora   camphor (gum)
Cannabis ind.   Cannabis indica   Indian hemp, hashish, bhang bhanga (young leaves and twigs)
Cannabis sat.   Cannabis sativa   European or American hemp (tops of male and female flowers)
Cantharis   Cantharis Lytta vesicatoria   Spanish fly (whole live beetle)
Capsicum   Capsicum annuum   cayenne pepper (dried pods)
Carbolic ac.   Carbolicum acidum   phenol, carbolic acid
Carbo an.   Carbo animalis   animal charcoal, made from charred oxhide
Carbo veg.   Carbo vegetabilis   vegetable charcoal made from beech, birch or poplar wood
Carbon sulph.   Carbonum sulphuratum   carbon bisulphide
Carduus   Carduus mariana   St Mary's thistle, silybum (seeds)
Caulophyllum   Caulophyllum thalictroides   blue cohosh, squaw root (root)
Causticum   Causticum Hahnemanni   potassium hydrate
Ceanothus   Ceanothus americanus   New Jersey tea, red root (fresh leaves)
Chamomilla   Chamomilla vulgaris   German chamomile (whole fresh plant)
Chelidonium   Chelidonium majus   greater celandine (whole fresh plant when in flower, or root)
Chenopodium   Chenopodium anthelminticum   Jerusalem oat, wormseed (whole fresh plant, or extracted oil)
Chimaphila   Chimaphila umbellata   umbellate wintergreen, ground holly, pipsissewa, prince's pine (root and leaves, or whole fresh plant when in flower)
China   China officinalis   Peruvian bark, quinine (dried bark of *Cinchona calisaya*)

China ars.   *China arsenica*   quinine arsenate
Chininum sulph.   *Chininum sulphuricum*   quinine sulphate
Chionanthus   *Chionanthus virginica*   fringe tree (bark)
Cicuta   *Cicuta virosa*   water hemlock, cowbane (fresh root when plant is in flower)
Cimicifuga   *Cimicifuga racemosa*   black snakeroot, black cohosh (root or resinoid)
Cina   *Cina Artemisia maritima*   sea southernwood, wormseed (unopened flower heads)
Cinnabar   *Cinnabaris*   mercuric sulphide
Cistus   *Cistus canadensis*   frostweed, Canadian rock rose (whole plant)
Clematis   *Clematis erecta*   virgin's bower (leaves and stems)
Cocculus   *Cocculus indicus*   Indian cockle (seeds, which contain picrotoxine, a powerful poison)
Coccus   *Coccus cacti*   cochineal beetle (dried bodies of females)
Codeinum   prepared from codeine, an alkaloid of opium
Coffea   *Coffea cruda*   unroasted coffee (raw berries)
Colchicum   *Colchicum autumnale*   meadow saffron, autumn crocus (bulbs in spring)
Collinsonia   *Collinsonia canadensis*   stoneroot, horsebalm, richweed (fresh root)
Colocynth   *Citrullus colocynthis*   bitter apple, bitter cucumber (pulp of fruit)
Conchiolinum   mother of pearl from oyster shells
Conium   *Conium maculatum*   hemlock (fresh plant when in flower)
Convallaria   *Convallaria majalis*   lily of the valley (whole plant)
Copaiva   *Copaifera officinalis*   balsam of copaiva (seed pods)
Corallium   *Corallium rubrum*   red coral from Gorgonia nobilis (whole coral)
Crataegus   *Crataegus oxycantha*   hawthorn (ripe berries)
Crocus   *Crocus sativa*   saffron crocus (dried stigmas)
Crotalus   *Crotalus horridus*   N. American rattlesnake (venom)
Croton   *Croton tiglium*   (oil from seeds)
Cuprum   *Cuprum metallicum*   copper
Cuprum ars.   *Cuprum arsenicosum*   Scheele's green, copper arsenate
Cyclamen   *Cyclamen europaeum*   sowbread (root in spring)

Digitalis   *Digitalis purpurea*   red foxglove (second year's leaves)
Dioscorea   *Dioscorea villosa*   wild yam (fresh root or resinoid)
Drosera   *Drosera rotundifolia*   common or round-leaved sundew (active fresh plant)
Dulcamara   *Solanum dulcamara*   bittersweet, woody nightshade (fresh green stems and leaves just before plant comes into flower)

Echinacea   *Echinacea angustifolia*   purple coneflower (whole fresh plant)
Elaps   *Elaps corallinus*   Brazilian coral snake (venom)
Equisetum   *Equisetum hyemale*   scouring rush, horsetail (fresh plant, chopped and pulped)
Eupatorium   *Eupatorium perfoliatum*   boneset, thoroughwort (whole plant)
Euphorbium   *Euphorbium officinarum*   gum euphorbium (resinous juice)
Euphrasia   *Euphrasia officinalis or E. sticta*   common eyebright (whole plant)

Ferrum   *Ferrum metallicum*   iron
Ferrum ars.   *Ferrum arsenicum*   iron arsenate
Ferrum phos.   *Ferrum phosphoricum*   iron phosphate
Ferrum pic.   *Ferrum picricum*   iron picrate
Fluoric ac.   *Fluoricum acidum*   hydrofluoric acid
Fraxinus   *Fraxinus americanus*   white ash (bark)

Gelsemium   *Gelsemium sempervirens*   yellow jasmine (bark of root)
Gentiana   *Gentiana lutea*   yellow gentian (root)
Glonoinum   *Glonoinum*   trinitroglycerine
Gnaphalium   *Gnaphalium polycephalum*   sweet-scented everlasting flower (whole fresh plant)
Gratiola   *Gratiola officinalis*   hedge hyssop (fresh bulb before plant flowers)
Graphites   *Graphites*   black lead from finest English drawing pencils
Guaiacum   *Guiacum officinale*   resin from lignum vitae tree
Gunpowder   a mixture of saltpetre, sulphur, and charcoal

Hamamelis   Hamamelis virginica   common witch hazel (fresh bark of twigs and roots)
Hecla   Hecla lava   volcanic ash from Mt Hecla in Iceland
Helleborus   Helleborus niger   black hellebore, snow rose, Christmas rose (juice of fresh root)
Hepar sulph.   Hepar sulphuris calcareum   calcium sulphide
Hydrastis   Hydrastis canadensis   golden seal (fresh root)
Hyoscyamus   Hyoscyamus niger   henbane (whole fresh plant)
Hypericum   Hypericum perforatum   St John's wort (whole fresh plant)

Iberis   Iberis amara   bitter candytuft (seeds)
Ignatia   Ignatia amara or Strychnos ignatia   St Ignatius' bean (seed pods)
Iodium   Iodium   iodine
Ipecac.   Cephaelis ipecacuanha   ipecacuanha (dried root)
Iris   Iris versicolor   blue flag (fresh root in early spring or autumn)
Iris ten.   Iris tenax or I. minor   beardless iris (whole plant)

Jacaranda   Jacaranda caroba   Brazilian caroba tree (fresh flowers)
Jaborandi   Pilocarpus pinnatifolius   a S. American tree (fresh or dried leaves and stems)
Juglans   Juglans cinerea   butternut (bark or root)

Kali bichrom.   Kali bichromicum   potassium bichromate
Kali brom.   Kali bromatum   potassium bromide
Kali carb.   Kali carbonicum   potassium carbonate
Kali iod.   Kali iodatum   potassium iodide
Kali mur.   Kali muriaticum   potassium chloride
Kali nit.   Kali nitricum   potassium nitrite
Kali phos.   Kali phosphoricum   potassium phosphate
Kali sulph.   Kali sulphuricum   potassium sulphate
Kalmia   Kalmia latifolia or Ledum floribus bullatis   mountain laurel or calico bush (fresh leaves when plant is in flower)
Kreosotum   Kreosotum   creosote, oil distilled from beechwood tar

Lac can.   Lac caninum   dog's milk
Lac defl.   Lac vaccinum defloratum   skimmed cow's milk
Lachesis   Trigonocephalus lachesis   bushmaster, surucucu snake (venom)
Lacnanthes   Lacnanthes tinctoria   red root (whole plant)
Lactic ac.   Lacticum acidum   lactic acid
Lathyrus   Lathyrus sativa   chick pea (flowers or green seed pods)
Latrodectus   Latrodectus mactans   American spider (live spider)
Laurocerasus   Prunus laurocerasus   cherry laurel (young leaves)
Ledum   Ledum palustre   marsh tea, wild rosemary (leaves and small twigs dried and collected as plant comes into flower)
Lilium   Lilium tigrinum   tiger lily (fresh stalks, leaves and flower, or pollen)
Lobelia   Lobelia inflata   Indian tobacco (fresh plant when in flower, also seeds)
Lycopodium   Lycopodium clavatum   wolfsclaw club moss (spores)
Lycopus   Lycopus virginicus   bugleweed (fresh plant in flower)
Lyssin   Lyssin Hydrophobinum   saliva of dog with rabies

Magnesia carb.   Magnesia carbonica   magnesium carbonate
Magnesia mur.   Magnesia muriatica   magnesium chloride
Magnesia phos.   Magnesia phosphorica   magnesium phosphate
Magnesia sulph.   Magnesia sulphurica   magnesium sulphate
Magnetis arct.   Magnetis polus arcticus   north pole of magnet
Magnetis austr.   Magnetis polus australis   south pole of magnet
Manganum   Manganum metallicum   manganese
Melilotus   Melilotus officinalis or M. alba   sweet clover, yellow and white varieties (fresh plant when in flower)
Menyanthes   Menyanthes trifoliata   buckbean (whole plant)
Medorrhinum   Medorrhinum   urethral discharge from patient with gonorrhea
Mercurius   Mercurius solubilis Hahnemanni   mercury, quicksilver

Mercurius corr.   Mercurius corrosivus   corrosive sublimate of mercury
Mercurius cyan.   Mercurius cyanatus   mercurous cyanide
Mercurius dulc.   Mercurius dulcis   calomel, mercurous chloride
Mezereum   Daphne mezereum   spurge olive, mezereon (fresh bark before plant flowers)
Millefolium   Achillea millefolium   yarrow, milfoil (whole fresh plant)
Morbillinum   Morbillinum   nasal discharge from measles patient
Moschus   Moschus moschiferus   musk deer (musky secretion of foreskin)
Myristica   Myristica sebifera   ucuuba tree (red, acrid, poisonous gum from bark)
Murex   Murex purpurea   purple fish, a mollusc (dye)
Muriatic ac.   Muriaticum acidum   hydrochloric acid

Naja   Naja tripudians   hooded snake of Hindustan (venom)
Natrum ars.   Natrum arsenicum   sodium arsenate
Natrum carb.   Natrum carbonicum   sodium carbonate
Natrum mur.   Natrum muriaticum   salt, sodium chloride
Natrum phos.   Natrum phosphoricum   sodium phosphate
Natrum sulph.   Natrum sulphuricum   Glauber's Salts, sodium sulphate
Nitric ac.   Nitricum acidum   nitric acid
Nux   Strychnos nux vomica   poison nut tree (seeds)
Nux mosch.   Nux moschata   nutmeg, seed of *Myristica fragrans* (whole nutmeg)

Ocimum   Ocimum canum   Brazilian alfavaca (fresh leaves)
Oenanthe   Oenanthe crocata   hemlock dropwort (fresh root when plant is in flower)
Oleander   Nerium oleander   oleander, rose laurel (leaves)
Onosmodium   Onosmodium virginianum   false bromwell (whole fresh plant)
Opium   milky juice from unripe seed capsule of opium poppy *Papaver somniferum*
Oxalic ac.   Oxalicum acidum oxalic acid

Paeonia   Paeonia officinalis   paeony (fresh root in spring)
Palladium   Palladium   palladium, a rare metallic element
Pareira   Pareira brava   virgin vine (fresh root)
Paris   Paris quadrifolia   herb Paris, true love (whole plant when fruit is ripe)
Parotidinum   sputum from mumps patient
Petroleum   Petroleum Oleum petrae   rock oil, coal oil (purified oil)
Petroselinum   Petroselinum sativum   common parsley (whole fresh plant as it comes into flower)
Phellandrium   Phellandrium aquaticum   water dropwort, horsebane (fresh ripe fruit)
Phosphoric ac.   Phosphoricum acidum   phosphoric acid
Phosphorus   Phosphorus   phosphorus
Physostigma   Physostigma venenosum   Calabar bean (whole bean)
Phytolacca   Phytolacca decandra   poke root (fresh leaves or ripe berries, or root in winter)
Picric ac.   Picricum acidum   picric acid, trinitrophenol
Pilocarpin mur.   Pilocarpin muriaticum   hydrochlorate of pilocarpine (an anti-glaucoma drug)
Plantago   Plantago major   greater plantain, ribwort (root)
Platinum   Platinum metallicum   platinum
Plumbum   Plumbum metallicum   lead
Podophyllum   Podophyllum peltatum   May apple (ripe fruit, root after fruit has ripened, or whole fresh plant)
Psorinum   Psorinum   discharge from scabies blister
Pulsatilla   Pulsatilla nigricans   wind flower, pasque flower (whole fresh plant when in flower)
Pyrogenium   Pyrogenium   substance extracted from rotting meat

Quercus   Quercus robur   English oak (acorns)

Radium   Radium   radium, a radioactive metallic element
Radium brom.   Radium bromatum   radium bromide
Ranunculus   Ranunculus bulbosus   bulbous buttercup, bulbous crowfoot (whole plant)
Raphanus   Raphanus sativus   black radish (fresh roots before plant flowers in spring)
Ratanhia   Ratanhia Krameria triandra   mapato, a legume (root)
Rheum   Rheum officinale or R. palmatum   rhubarb (dried root)

Rhododendron   Rhododendron chrysanthum   Siberian rhododendron, yellow snow rose (fresh leaves)
Rhus tox.   Rhus toxicodendron   poison ivy (fresh leaves gathered at sunset just before plant comes into flower)
Rhus. ven.   Rhus venenata   poison sumach (fresh leaves and stem)
Robinia   Robinia pseudoacacia   black locust acacia, North American locust tree (beans)
Rumex   Rumex crispus   yellow or curled dock (fresh root)
Ruta   Ruta graveolens   rue (whole fresh plant)

Sabadilla   Sabadilla officinarum   seed of *Asagraea officinalis*
Sabal   Sabal serrulata   saw palmetto (juice of fresh green berries)
Sabina   Juniperus sabina   savin juniper (new leaves at tips of branches)
Salicylic ac.   Salicylicum acidum   salicylic acid, main ingredient of aspirin
Sambucus   Sambucus niger   common or black elder (fresh leaves and flowers)
Sanicula   Sanicula aqua   mineral spring water of Ottawa, Illinois, USA
Sanguinaria   Sanguinaria canadensis   bloodroot (fresh root)
Santoninum   Santoninum   santonin, substance extracted from wormseed, see *Cina*
Sarsaparilla   Sarsaparilla Smilax officinalis   wild liquorice (dried root)
Scutellaria   Scutellaria laterifolia   scullcap (whole fresh plant)
Secale   Secale cornutum   ergot, disease caused by fungus *Claviceps purpurea* (affected ears of rye before harvesting)
Selenium   selenium, a non-metallic element
Sempervivum   Sempervivum tectorium   house leek (fresh leaves)
Senega   Senega polygala   seneca, snake root (dried, powdered root)
Sepia   Sepia officinalis   cuttlefish ink
Silicea   Silicea terra   flint
Sol   lactose sugar solution exposed to concentrated sunlight
Solidago   Solidago virgaurea   common golden rod (whole fresh plant)
Spigelia   Spigelia anthelmia   pinkroot (dried plant)
Spongia   Spongia tosta   roasted common sponge
Squilla   Squilla maritima   sea onion (fresh bulb)
Stannum   Stannum metallicum   tin
Staphisagria   Delphinium staphisagria   stavesacre (seeds)
Sticta   Sticta pulmonaria or *Pulmonaria officinalis*   lungwort (whole plant)
Stramonium   Datura stramonium   thorn apple (fresh plant in flower, also seeds)
Strontium   Strontium metallicum   strontium
Sulphur   Sulphur   sublimated sulphur
Sulphur iod.   Sulphur iodatum   sulphur iodide
Sulphuric ac.   Sulphuricum acidum   sulphuric acid
Symphytum   Symphytum officinale   common comfrey, knitbone (whole fresh plant)
Syphilinum   Syphilinum   secretion from chancre of person with syphilis

Tabacum   Nicotiana tabacum   tobacco (fresh leaves before plant comes into flower)
Tamus   Tamus communis   black bryony, ladies' seal (fresh root or berries)
Taraxacum   Taraxacum officinale   dandelion (whole plant as flowers open)
Tarentula   Lycosa tarentula   Spanish spider (live spider)
Tarentula cub.   Tarentula cubensis also *Mygale cubensis*   Cuban tarantula (live spider)
Tellurium   the element tellurium
Terebinth   Terebinthinae oleum   turpentine, oleo-resin from various species of pine
Teucrium   Teucrium marum verum   cat thyme (whole fresh plant)
Theridion   Theridion curassavicum   orange spider from Curacao and W. Indies
Thlaspi   Thlaspi Capsella bursa-pastoris   shepherd's purse (fresh plant when in flower)
Thiosinaminum   alkyl sulphocarbamide, derived from mustard seed oil
Thuja   Thuja occidentalis   tree of life, arbor vitae, white cedar (fresh green twigs)
Tuberculinum   Tuberculinum of Koch   culture of tuberculosis bacilli

Uranium nit.   Uranium nitricum   uranium nitrate
Urtica   Urtica urens   small nettle (fresh plant when in flower)
Uva ursi   Arctostaphylos uva-ursi   bearberry (fresh leaves in Autumn)

Vaccinninum   smallpox vaccine
Valeriana   *Valeriana officinalis*   common valerian, all-heal (fresh root)
Variolinum   *Variolinum*   discharge from smallpox lesion
Veratrum   *Veratrum album*   white or false hellebore (roots before plant comes into flower)
Veratrum vir.   *Veratrum viride*   American white hellebore (fresh root in autumn)
Verbascum   *Verbascum thapsus*   great mullein, Aaron's rod (whole plant as it comes into flower)
Viburnum   *Viburnum opulus*   bark elder, water elder, cramp, high cranberry (fresh bark)
Viola   *Viola tricolor*   pansy, heartsease (fresh plant when in flower)
Vinca   *Vinca minor*   lesser periwinkle (whole fresh plant)
Vipera   *Vipera communis*   common viper (venom)
Viscum   *Viscum album*   mistletoe (ripe berries, bruised leaves, or whole plant)

Wyethia   *Wyethia Alarconia helenoides*   (or *Melarhiza inuloides*) poison weed (tincture of root)

Zinc   *Zincum metallicum*   zinc
Zinc sulph.   *Zincum sulphuricum*   zinc sulphate

Part 4

FIRST AID

Accidents happen. When they do, the trained first-aider can save life, limit injury, ease pain and anxiety, and summon appropriate medical help. First aid is a satisfying aspect of any therapeutic system, and every household should have at least one first-aider, trained in practice and theory.

Homeopathy has an important part to play in many accident and emergency situations, especially in the treatment of minor flesh wounds. But there is no substitute for attending a well-run first aid class and getting 'hands-on' experience. The basic information given here will help you to help others, but it is not a substitute for a practical first aid course.

Aims of first aid These are, in order of priority: to preserve life; to minimize the effects of injury; to relieve pain and distress; and to summon medical help as quickly as possible, which usually means telephoning the emergency services or taking the sufferer to hospital.

Homeopathic first aid Emergency measures following accident or injury are not intrinsically orthodox or homeopathic. They are a mixture of common sense and a modest understanding of human biology. Homeopathic remedies are only given after the threat to life has been removed. Their purpose in first aid situations is to calm the mind, relieve pain, and help the body to heal itself.

For minor injuries, choose the appropriate remedy from the alternatives given. But in a serious situation, the overriding priorities are to save life and get expert help as swiftly as possible.

Granules or drops are the easiest way of administering homeopathic remedies in emergencies: they can be put directly on the tongue and dissolve very quickly. If you only have pilules, crush one between two clean spoons and dissolve it in a teaspoon of warm water.

If the person is unconscious, pull open the lower lip and drop the remedy between lip and gum. If the person vomits immediately after you have given a remedy, repeat the dose.

Never give more than 6 doses of any emergency remedy; if the Vital Force is able to respond, it will rapidly do so. Dose frequency depends on the severity of the situation. If the dose frequency recommended does not seem to be stabilizing the situation, shorten the time between doses. In most cases, 30c remedies are more appropriate than 6c.

If the person concerned is very emotionally upset, worried, or panicking, give 4 drops of the Bach Rescue Remedy (see p. 35) as well.

For more information about homeopathic remedies and how to use them, turn to p. 77*ff.*

For cleaning wounds use Hypericum and Calendula Solution (5 drops of mother tincture of each in 0.25 litre [½ pint] of boiled cooled water). Arnica ointment is useful for bruises.

The basics of a first aid kit are:

sterile gauze
crepe roller bandages
butterfly sutures
sling or triangular bandage
roll of sticking plaster
scissors
safety pins

If these are not to hand, you will have to improvise. Shirts, sheets, tights, belts, tissues, etc. all have their uses in emergencies.

(For details of a special homeopathic first aid kit, contact the British Homeopathic Association – *see under* 'Useful Addresses', p. 385.)

Priorities in an Emergency

1 Don't become a casualty yourself. This may sound facetious, but you cannot help anyone if you yourself are *hors de combat*. Don't jump into the water to save someone if you cannot swim. Think twice about dragging someone clear of a burning car – the petrol tank may be about to explode. Cool logic is often forgotten in emergencies.

2 Remove the casualty and yourself from immediate danger. If there is no danger, do not move the casualty – you may cause further injury. The condition which is most life-threatening is the condition which should be dealt with first.

3 Make sure that the person is breathing and that the heart is beating. If not, give artificial respiration and/or cardiac resuscitation (see BREATHING below and CIRCULATION p. 88).

4 Check for and stop severe BLEEDING.

5 If the person is unconscious or shows signs of failing consciousness, put him or her in the recovery position and check the pulse at regular intervals (see UNCONSCIOUSNESS p. 90). Never leave an unconscious person alone unless this is unavoidable.

6 Treat any serious WOUNDS or BURNS and immobilize any FRACTURES or DISLOCATIONS.

7 When the casualty's condition is stable, take steps to prevent SHOCK and place in the recovery position (see UNCONSCIOUSNESS p. 90). Keep the person warm but not too hot. Do not give anything to eat or drink, except in specific situations such as BURNS, HEATSTROKE or HYPOTHERMIA, There may be internal injury, or the person may need a general anaesthetic in hospital later.

Getting medical help Away from home, dial 999. Otherwise try and get hold of your GP; if he is not immediately available, dial 999. Only if you are in an isolated situation, and there is likely to be considerable delay before help can get to you, should you consider taking the casualty to hospital yourself.

If possible, get someone else to phone the emergency services, otherwise dial 999 at the first opportunity. Usually the person who answers the telephone will ask a series of questions designed to extract the most vital information first. Respond calmly, answer clearly, and be prepared to give details of how many casualties are involved, the types of injuries, the kind of help needed, the exact location, and your phone number.

If the emergency services are not required, arrange for transport to the nearest Accident and Emergency (formerly 'Casualty') department, or ring your local GP.

Examining the casualty Check immediately for breathing and pulse (see BREATHING p. 86), and continue to check and record the pulse every 5 minutes. Try to find out from the casualty, or from a witness, exactly what happened. If the injured person is conscious, ask if there is pain and where, and examine the body very gently but firmly for bleeding, bruising, or limb deformities, comparing both sides of the body.

Note the colour of the person's skin. Pallor may indicate SHOCK. Feel the forehead with the palm of your hand. If it feels very hot, the casualty may have a fever; if it feels cold, he or she may be going into shock. Examine the pupils of the eyes. Are they very large or unequal in size? Smell the breath for alcohol. Look for any 'Medic-alert' cards, bracelets, or neck chains which warn of a medical condition such as EPILEPSY, DIABETES, or HAEMOPHILIA; these usually indicate the kind of help that is required.

Record the results of your examination if you can, and pass them on to the medical helpers when they arrive.

BREATHING

If the airway to the lungs (mouth, throat, or windpipe) is obstructed, the person will not be able to breathe (see ASPHYXIA p. 90). Breathing can also cease because the lungs are damaged or full of fluid, or contain gases other than air. Or there may be a brain or heart malfunction. If breathing stops, the brain becomes starved of oxygen and irreversible damage may occur.

Hold your ear close to the casualty's nose and mouth. If he or she is breathing you should hear or feel the movement of air. While you are doing this, look at the chest wall to see if it is rising and falling. If the skin looks very pale, or bluish, especially around the lips, this is more evidence that breathing has stopped or that circulation is impaired.

Artificial respiration If breathing has stopped, place the casualty on his or her back on a firm surface. Tilt the head backwards and bring the lower jaw upwards and forwards to open the throat and keep the tongue from blocking the airway. Clear out any material from the mouth and throat.

Pinch the casualty's nose. Take a deep breath, seal your mouth around the casualty's mouth and blow strongly into the lungs. Watch the chest rising as you blow in, then take your mouth away and watch the chest fall. If the heart is beating, the casualty should regain a healthy colour after the first few inflations. Give the first 6–12 breaths quickly, then slow down to a rate which is enough to keep the casualty's colour normal-looking – about the same as your own breathing rate.

Once the casualty is breathing strongly and unaided, place him or her in the recovery position (see UNCONSCIOUSNESS p. 90 and monitor breathing until medical help arrives. If breathing falters or does not continue unaided, carry on giving artificial respiration until medical help arrives.

If, after 6 breaths of artificial respiration, the casualty does not respond, give cardiac resuscitation (see CIRCULATION p. 88).

Homeopathic remedies If you are on your own, do not give any remedies until the casualty is breathing regularly and unaided. However, if there is someone else present who can carry on with the resuscitation, select a remedy from the list below.

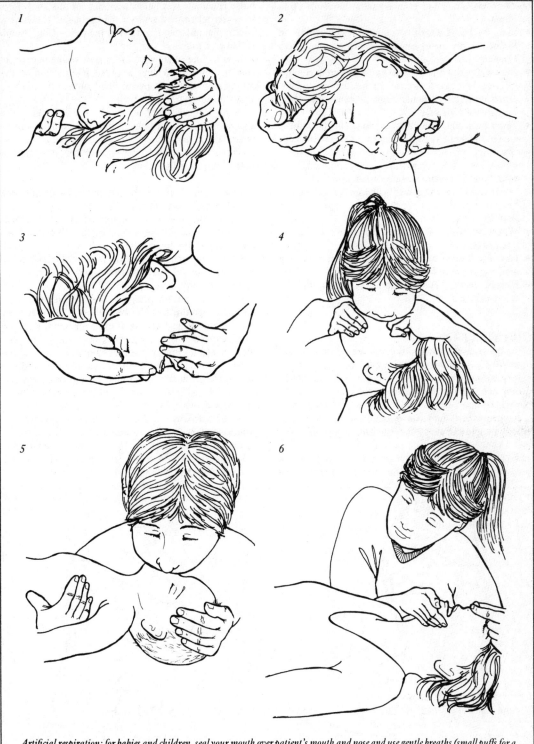

Artificial respiration: for babies and children, seal your mouth over patient's mouth and nose and use gentle breaths (small puffs for a baby)

Specific remedies to be given every 60 seconds for up to 10 doses

- Skin cold and marbled-looking, cold sweat on forehead, face pale, casualty retches on recovery *Veratrum 30c*
- Face puffy and bluish, cold sweating, great hunger for air (yawning), desire to be fanned with cold air, especially after carbon-monoxide poisoning from car exhaust *Carbo veg. 30c*
- Person unconscious, noisy or irregular breathing, face hot and puffy, pupils very small *Opium 30c*
- Breathing difficulties due to bubbling oral or nasal secretions, rattly breathing, frothy phlegm, face cold, blue, and clammy *Antimonium tart. 30c*
- Obstructed breathing due to severe reaction to a bee sting or insect bite, throat or tongue swollen *Apis 30c*
- Where breathing difficulties come on after injury *Arnica 30c*
- Casualty panicky and afraid once normal breathing is re-established *Aconite 30c*
- If none of the remedies above seem appropriate *Carbo veg. 30c*

CIRCULATION

If the heart stops beating, blood flow to the brain and other vital organs ceases. With each heartbeat blood surges through the arteries, giving a pulse or throb, which can be felt at various points on the body. Normal pulse rate is 60–80 beats per minute in adults; in infants and young children it is faster, in elderly people and very fit people somewhat slower.

Taking the pulse You can hear a person's heart by pressing your ear to his or her chest. The strongest pulse is usually just below the angle of the jaw, where the external carotid artery runs up beside the larynx. The radial pulse in the wrist at the base of the thumb is also easy to feel.

Feel for the pulse with the tips of your fingers (not your thumb, as it has a pulse itself). Count the number of beats per minute and note if it is fast or slow, full or weak.

If the heart is not beating, there will be no pulse and no detectable breathing, and the casualty will be unconscious, and either pale or blue, especially round the lips. As soon as you are sure the heart is not beating, give cardiac resuscitation.

Cardiac resuscitation Put the patient on his or her back and give a sharp thump to the chest, about half way down the breastbone and slightly to the left (this is where the heart lies, protected by the rib cage). This often starts the heart again. Follow up with 6–12 breaths of artificial respiration (see BREATHING p. 86 and you should see the person's colour return to normal.

If this does not happen, press the heel of your hand on the lower third of the breastbone, and place the heel of your other hand on your lower hand. Keeping your arms straight, rock backwards and forwards three times, springing the breastbone down by about 5 cm (2 in) each time. Do three pushdowns and five breaths of artificial respiration, three pushdowns and five breaths, and so on, until you can detect the pulse or hear the heart.

If the casualty is a child, use less pressure or you may cause internal injury. Continue artificial respiration until the casualty is breathing again unaided, then put him or her in the recovery position (see UNCONSCIOUSNESS p. 90).

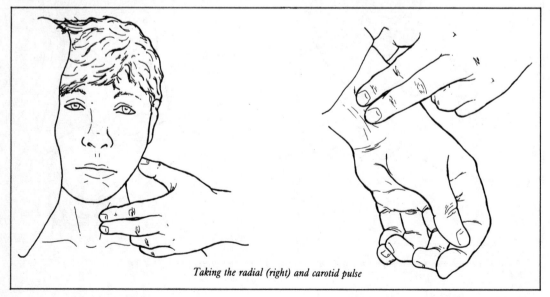

Taking the radial (right) and carotid pulse

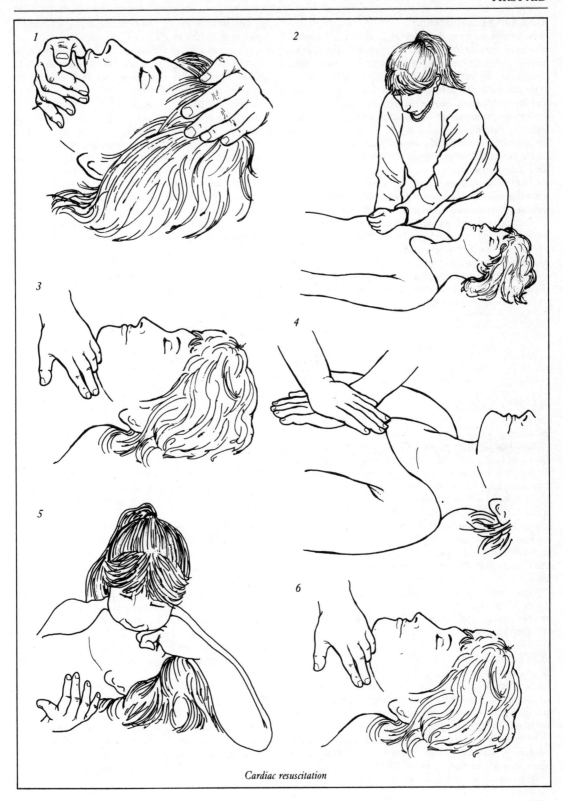

Cardiac resuscitation

UNCONSCIOUSNESS

Any departure from full alertness after an accident is cause for worry. An injured person who seems dazed and confused can be regarded as not fully conscious. In reality, there are different levels of consciousness from fully alert, through drowsiness (where the casualty can be roused) and stupor (where he or she responds only to pain) to coma (where the casualty cannot be roused at all). Unconsciousness may be the result of brain damage, loss of blood, lack of oxygen to the brain, chemical changes in the blood, or a drug overdose.

The main danger in an unconscious person is choking, so the first aider's immediate task is to relieve or prevent any obstruction to breathing.

Clear the mouth of debris. If the casualty is not breathing, start artificial respiration (see BREATHING above). When breathing and pulse are stable, put the casualty into the recovery position. Loosen tight clothing at the neck and waist, and check the pulse at 5-minute intervals. Do not leave the person alone.

Recovery position In this position, the airway cannot be obstructed by the tongue or by vomit. The aim is to get the person lying almost on his or her front, with the face turned to one side, the jaw pointing upwards and outwards, with one knee and one elbow half propping up the weight of the body.

If you suspect a SPINAL INJURY, do not place the person in the recovery position unless there is vomiting, and even then, try to move the person without bending, twisting, or jolting the spine. In such cases, choking and being unable breathe are the immediate threats to life, not the spinal injury.

If you suspect broken bones (see FRACTURES), put the person in the nearest approximation to the recovery position, but avoid putting any weight on the broken part. Use rolled-up blankets or coats to support the person in the recovery position if necessary.

Anyone who becomes unconscious for more than a few seconds, even though apparently recovered, should be seen by a doctor.

FIRST AID A-Z

AMPUTATION

Accidents in which limbs are completely severed are mercifully rare.

Get the casualty to lie down, raise the affected limb, and tie a bandage tightly around and over the stump. If the wound continues to bleed, add another bandage, applying as much pressure as you can. Put the severed limb in a clean container or plastic bag, and if possible pack the container in ice. Watch carefully for symptoms of SHOCK.

Take the casualty and the amputated limb to the nearest hospital as quickly as possible. Make sure the staff know that the severed part has come with the casualty.

Specific remedy to be given every minute for up to 6 doses

● To relieve pain after a limb has been severed *Hypericum 6c*

ASPHYXIA

Starved of oxygen, tissues rapidly die. Oxygen may be prevented from diffusing into the lungs because of CHOKING, DROWNING, suffocation, strangulation, paralysis, or injury to the lungs or chest. Lack of oxygen in the air also causes asphyxia.

Symptoms include an increased rate and depth of breathing, noisy breathing, frothing at the mouth, blue lips, unconsciousness, and cessation of breathing.

Remove whatever is causing the asphyxia, or move the casualty into the fresh air. Begin artificial respiration (see BREATHING p. 86) if necessary, place in the recovery position (see UNCONSCIOUSNESS p. 90), and dial 999.

BITES AND STINGS

For bites which cause deep puncture WOUNDS, severe BLEEDING, or AMPUTATION, turn to the relevant entry in this section.

The bites of animals carry two main dangers: TETANUS and RABIES. In the UK at the moment we are lucky not to have rabies, but it is present in many other countries. Orthodox immunization against rabies may be advisable if you make frequent trips abroad or your job involves animals. While visiting countries where rabies is endemic, take *Hydrophobinum 30c* daily for 7 days, followed by *Belladonna 6c* twice daily for 6 months. Any bite that punctures the skin should be checked by a doctor. Human bites carry even greater danger of infection than animal bites.

Tetanus, or lockjaw, is a potentially fatal infection which can enter the body through any dirty wound. Orthodox immunization has to be repeated every 5 years. If you have not received a booster injection in the last 5 years, take *Hypericum 6c* three times daily for 3 weeks as a preventive.

Bathe any wounds with Hypericum and Calendula solution.

RECOVERY POSITION

1

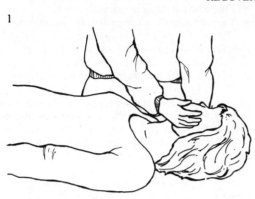

Kneel by the casualty's side, turn head towards you and tilt it back, keeping jaw forward

2

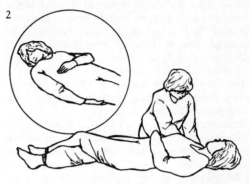

Place the arm nearer you by casualty's side; place casualty's hand under buttock, palm upwards if possible. Bring other forearm over the front of chest. Hold far leg by knee or ankle and bring it towards you over near leg

3

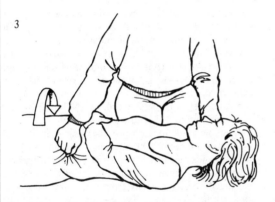

Support casualty's head with one hand; with the other, grasp casualty by clothing at farther hip and pull quickly towards you. Support casualty against your knees

4

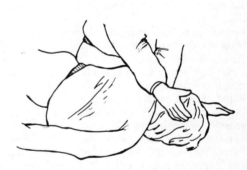

Move head to ensure airway is open. Bend casualty's arm to support upper body

5

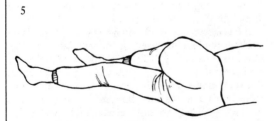

Bend casualty's uppermost leg at the knee, bringing thigh well forward to support lower body

6

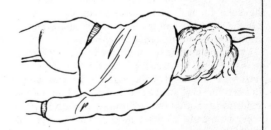

Carefully pull other arm from under casualty, working from shoulder down. Leave it lying parallel to the body to prevent casualty rolling on to the back

Poisonous bites and stings In Britain there is only one poisonous snake, the adder, not counting escaped pets or zoo animals. But abroad, especially in hot countries, scorpions and venomous snakes and spiders are common. As a repellant to such animals, apply Pyrethrum solution (10 drops of mother tincture in 0.25 litre (½ pt) boiled cooled water) to vulnerable parts of the body.

The symptoms of poisoning are blurred vision and nausea, difficult breathing, increased salivation and sweating, and sometimes SHOCK.

Reassure the casualty and keep him or her still. Apply an ice pack to the site of the bite. If the person loses consciousness or stops breathing, place in the recovery position or give artificial respiration or cardiac resuscitation (see UNCONSCIOUSNESS p. 90 and BREATHING p. 86). Dial 999 or take the person to hospital yourself. Try to describe the animal which bit the person, or if you can, capture it in a safe container and retain to show medical attendant.

Specific remedies to be given every 5 minutes for up to 10 doses
- Where there is swelling, bruising and pain *Arnica 30c*
- Person faints, has difficulty breathing, becomes hypersensitive to draughts and cold air *Moschus 6c*
- Purple discoloration around bite, with seepage of dark blood, person feels worse after sleep (this last symptom is typical of a tarantula bite) *Lachesis 6c*
- Rapid onset of swelling and subcutaneous bleeding, skin around bite discoloured, casualty very sensitive to jarring *Crotalus 6c*
- Vomiting, feeble pulse, slow, shallow breathing, torpor, band-around-the-head feeling, face dusky and congested-looking, with pale nose and mouth, abnormally acute sense of smell *Carbolic ac. 6c*
- Violent pains, skin around bite erupts in rash or streaks, person feels cold and numb, tremor in hands and feet *Oxalic ac. 6c*
- If person has been stung by a jellyfish *Apis 30c*

Wasp and bee stings should be removed with tweezers as quickly as possible. Do not suck out the poison. If the sting is inside the mouth or throat, rinse the mouth with iced water to discourage swelling, and get the person to hospital as quickly as possible.

Undiluted mother tinctures can be dabbed directly on insect bites. Pyrethrum mother tincture is good for most bites and stings. Otherwise use Ledum mother tincture for bee stings, Arnica or Ledum mother tinctures for hornet or wasp stings, and a mixture of Hypericum and Calendula mother tinctures for gnat bites.

Specific remedies to be given every 15 minutes for up to 6 doses
- Weakness and collapse *Carbolic ac. 6c*
- Rapid swelling *Apis 30c*
- Redness and burning *Cantharis 30c*
- Blueness and burning *Tarentula cub. 6c*
- Shooting pains in affected limb *Hypericum 30c*

Anaphylactic shock is a rare and very severe reaction to being bitten or stung. See SHOCK p. 103 and POISONING p. 102 for symptoms and treatment.

Poisonous plants If skin has been in contact with plants such as poison ivy, bathe the area with milk and give *Anacardium 6c* every 15 minutes until inflammation abates. In severe cases give 1 gm of Vitamin C hourly.

BLEEDING

Occurs when blood vessels are damaged. External bleeding often looks more dramatic than INTERNAL BLEEDING, but the latter can be more serious.

In a minor graze or bruise only the smallest blood vessels, the capillaries, are broken; blood seeps slowly into the surrounding tissues but soon clots, resealing the capillaries and stopping further leakage. If a vein is broken, dark red blood flows steadily from the wound; if the vein is large, blood loss must be stopped as it will not seal itself. If an artery is broken, bright red blood spurts from the wound in time with the pulse; arterial blood is under pressure because it is being pumped directly from the heart; loss of blood from an artery must be stopped, or it will quickly lead to excessive blood loss and SHOCK.

Bleeding often looks more alarming than it is. A very small amount of blood goes a long way. Most adults can lose up to 1 litre (2 pints) of blood without danger to life. However, this amount can easily be lost into the tissues, especially from a fracture of a large bone, so the blood loss that one can see is not always the true picture.

Treatment of bleeding Only treat bleeding if you have established that the injured person has a pulse and is breathing.

Check for, and remove, any foreign bodies in the wound, and apply pressure directly over the site of bleeding using the thumb or squeezing the edges of the wound together. Cover with a clean dressing, and secure firmly with bandages.

If bleeding from a limb will not stop, apply pressure to either the brachial artery or the femoral artery (see illustration opposite). N.B. This procedure drastically cuts blood flow to distal tissues and can damage them if it is continued for more than 15 minutes at a time. Rest the patient and keep him or her still – this aids the body's natural clotting mechanism. Raise the legs to maintain blood flow to the heart and brain if you estimate that more than 1 litre (2 pints) of blood has been lost.

Emergency bandages can be made from sheets, towels, pillowcases, scarves, cotton clothes, clean

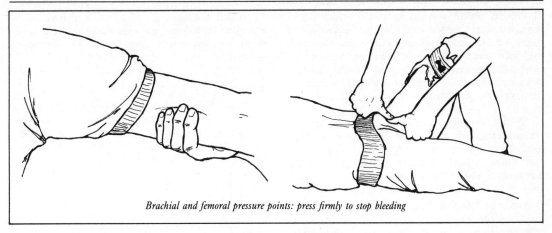

Brachial and femoral pressure points: press firmly to stop bleeding

blankets, paper hankies, and many other items. If blood seeps through them, do not take them off; keep adding more layers. Check the person's pulse every 5 minutes and jot it down. If the pulse rate is increasing, check for other sites of external bleeding. If external bleeding has been controlled, increased pulse indicates internal bleeding.

Specific remedies to be given every 10–15 minutes for up to 10 doses once bleeding has been brought under control

- Bleeding follows injury, with extensive or serious bruising *Arnica 30c*
- Person restless, anxious, chilly, and exhausted *Arsenicum 6c*
- Bright red blood, pulse full and laboured, face red and hot *Belladonna 30c*
- Person collapsed, hungry for air (yawning), wanting cool air to be fanned across the face *Carbo veg. 30c*
- Bright red blood, person nauseous, cold and sweaty, gasping for air *Ipecac. 6c*
- Casualty can't stand warmth or tight clothing around neck or waist *Lachesis 6c*
- Bleeding difficult to stop, blood bright red and flows in fits and starts, casualty thirsty for ice-cold drinks *Phosphorus 6c*

BLISTERS
Blisters are bubbles of fluid (blood serum) which form under the skin due to friction or BURNS AND SCALDS.

Do not burst blisters – they may get infected. Put a plaster over them if necessary. Bathe burst blisters with Hypericum and Calendula solution, and expose them to the fresh air.

Specific remedy to be given every 4 hours until pain wears off

- Itchy, burning blisters, relieved by cold applications *Cantharis 30c*
- Red, swollen, intensely itchy blisters *Rhus tox 6c*

BRUISING
see BLEEDING, INTERNAL BLEEDING

BURNS AND SCALDS
Burns are caused by heat, friction, or chemicals (see CHEMICAL BURNS); scalds are caused by hot liquids. If severe, either may affect the whole body, not just the burnt or scalded part. The main dangers from large burns are fluid loss leading to SHOCK, and infection. Deep burns are less painful than superficial ones; this is because in deep burns the nerves have been destroyed. Any burn bigger than the palm of the hand needs urgent medical attention.

Fire This is what you should do to help someone who has been burned in a fire.

1 Prevent further damage by removing the cause of the burn, or pulling the casualty clear of the fire, taking great care not to get burned yourself. If someone is on fire, push him or her to the ground and smother the flames with a rug, heavy coat, curtains, or any heavy fabric that happens to be nearby, but take great care not to burn your hands in the process. Dial 999 at the first opportunity.

2 Having removed the casualty from danger, immerse any burnt areas, provided the skin is not broken, in cold water for at least 10 minutes, or until the pain dies down. Hypericum and Calendula mother tinctures added to the water (20 drops of each per litre [2 pints] of water) enhance its pain-relieving effect. Cooling also reduces the severity of the burn, and in the case of chemical burns washes off the chemical and dilutes any that is left. Remove rings, bracelets, and any other jewellery from burnt areas – they will be difficult to remove once the skin swells. If there is burnt clothing sticking to the skin, leave it; immerse skin and clothing in cold water.

3 Prevent infection. Apply non-fluffy, clean dressings. Do not use cotton wool, lint, or adhesive tape. If there is burnt clothing sticking to the skin, leave it – it will have been sterilized by the heat; put the dressing over it. If the area of burnt skin is extensive, cover it with lots of small dressings; this makes them easier to remove in hospital later.

4 Do not burst blisters or apply any lotions, greases, or antiseptics. Be careful not to breathe or cough over the burnt area and do not touch it. You should not handle a burn victim more than is absolutely necessary. Do not attempt to remove any dressings.

5 Minimise fluid loss. If the casualty is conscious, give frequent sips of water, especially if he or she is vomiting. Keep this up until you get to hospital. Fluid loss into the tissues may cause a person suffering from severe burns to go into SHOCK; be alert for this.

Specific remedies to be given every 15 minutes as soon as burn or scald has been cooled and emergency help has been summoned
- *Arnica 30c* (3 doses only) followed by *Cantharis 30c* (up to 6 doses)
- If the burn continues to sting *Urtica 6c* (up to 6 doses)

Specific remedies to be given every 4 hours for up to 10 doses
- Where burns are second degree burns, looking like ulcers *Kali bichrom. 6c*
- If burns become infected *Hepar sulph. 6c* and clean with Hypericum and Calendula solution

Recovery from burns can be helped by taking 1 gm of Vitamin C every hour. If burn scars remain painful, take *Causticum 6c* four times a day for up to 7 days.

Sunburn and superficial burns can be soothed by applying Aloe vera gel or Urtica urens ointment. Excessive blistering due to sunburn may need medical attention. *Sol 30c* can be taken every 4 hours as a preventative, especially in people sensitive to sunlight. Also 4-hourly for sunburn, for up to 10 doses.

CARBON MONOXIDE POISONING see POISONING, CHEMICALS (INHALED)

CHEMICAL BURNS

Caustic or corrosive chemicals can badly damage the skin, especially the eyes. Industrial chemicals are not the only culprits; many potentially dangerous chemicals are used in the home.

Be sure not to contaminate yourself when dealing with chemical burns. Damaged skin will be red, stinging, and may erupt in blisters. A damaged eye will be painful, red, swollen, and watering. Wash away the chemical by holding the affected part or eye under gently running water. Then treat as for BURNS AND SCALDS.

CHEMICALS, INHALED

If there are poisonous substances in the air, these will be breathed in. Thick smoke causes the muscles lining the airways to go into spasm; the victim begins to choke and suffocate. Carbon monoxide (from vehicle exhausts) replaces oxygen in the blood, causing oxygen deficiency in the tissues. Other gases, such as those given off by burning foam rubber and other plastics, are toxic and can cause paralysis of the muscles involved in breathing.

Someone who has inhaled a poisonous chemical fights for air, goes cherry-pink in the face, becomes confused, complains of a headache, and may eventually become paralysed and unconscious.

The first thing to do is to remove the person from the chemical fumes or contaminated area without exposing yourself to danger. Give artificial respiration and cardiac resuscitation if necessary (see BREATHING p. 86 and CIRCULATION p. 88), and place in the recovery position (see UNCONSCIOUSNESS p. 90) so that the airway is open. Then dial 999.

CHEST INJURIES

Chest injuries usually fall into one of three categories: penetrating wounds, blast injuries, and broken bones.

Penetrating wounds allow air from the outside to enter the lungs directly. This causes breathing difficulties similar to those of ASPHYXIA; blood may be coughed up; the wound itself may make sucking noises.

The first thing to do is cover the hole in the chest to prevent the air from getting in; polythene and adhesive tape make an effective seal, and will make breathing easier. Then sit the casualty upright, leaning his or her body to one side so that the undamaged lung is uppermost. Dial 999.

Blast injuries are caused when the chest is compressed by a sudden increase in air pressure due to an explosion. Again, there may be signs of ASPHYXIA; there may be other internal injuries, and the person may also be in a state of panic, which further interferes with breathing.

Do not move the casualty unless it is absolutely necessary, to avoid further danger, for example. Examine him or her and treat the most serious condition first. Then dial 999.

Specific remedy to be given every 15 minutes for up to 10 doses
- *Aconite 30c*, followed by *Arnica 6c* four times a day for up to 7 days

Fractures of the ribs or breastbone, usually due to falls, blows, or crushing injuries, cause intense pain at the slightest movement. A stove-in chest, in which several ribs may have been broken, causes 'paradoxical' breathing – the ribs are sucked in on inhalation and out on exhalation, the opposite of what normally happens. Breathing will be difficult; there may also be INTERNAL BLEEDING.

Fold the arm across the chest on the injured side and bandage it in place. Position the casualty in a half-sitting position with the uninjured side uppermost. Dial 999.

Specific remedies
- *Bryonia 30c* every ¼ hour until pain begins to wear off, followed by *Symphytum 6c* twice daily for up to 3 weeks to speed healing

CHOKING

Food, vomit, and the tongue itself can obstruct the airway to the lungs and cause choking. The signs of choking are difficulty breathing and speaking, and sometimes coughing. If the obstruction cannot be removed, the person will turn blue and clutch at the throat; after a minute or so, he or she will become unconscious. Choking while remaining conscious is a frightening experience, but usually the obstruction clears itself before serious harm is done.

The logical first step is to try to clear the mouth and throat of blood, vomit, foreign bodies such as dentures, and so on. If this does not work, or if the choking person stops coughing and begins to turn blue, bend the body over slightly (or get the person to lie on his or her side) and sharply thump the back between the shoulder blades three or four times, using the heel of your hand. If the casualty is a child, hold him or her upside down or face-down over your knee and strike with less force. If the obstruction is not dislodged, repeat after a few seconds. This 'shock treatment' usually works even when obstruction is caused by spasm of the muscles lining the windpipe.

If the obstruction remains, try once again to remove it with fingers or tweezers. If this fails, carry out the Heimlich or 'abdominal thrust' manoeuvre.

Abdominal thrust Grasp the casualty from behind, tucking one of your fists underneath the breastbone and grasping it with your other hand. Pull sharply inwards, thrusting in and up beneath the breast bone. This produces a sudden increase of pressure in the chest cavity, which should expel the obstruction. Repeat up to three times if necessary. If the obstruction persists, or if the person becomes unconscious, commence artificial respiration, or put the person in the recovery position (see BREATHING p. 86 and UNCONSCIOUSNESS p. 90), and dial 999.

With a child, use just two fingers under the breastbone rather than your whole fist, and pull upwards and inwards more gently.

The Heimlich manoeuvre is not without risk itself. After using it, the casualty should be examined in hospital to make sure no internal damage has been done.

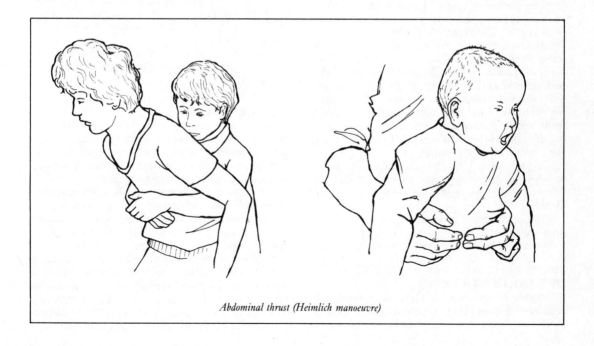

Abdominal thrust (Heimlich manoeuvre)

COMA
see UNCONSCIOUSNESS, DIABETIC
COMA

CRUSH INJURIES

Severe crush injuries cause extensive damage to skin, muscle, nerves, and bone. There may be internal and external bleeding, or blood supply to a limb may be cut off for some time. Large quantities of plasma may leak from the blood vessels into the damaged tissues, causing swelling and SHOCK. When the crushed part is released, toxic chemicals produced by damaged muscles get into general circulation, leading to kidney failure in severe cases.

If the crushed part has been trapped for more than 30 minutes, do not attempt to release the casualty before medical help arrives. If release is immediate, raise the affected limb, but keep the victim still. Try to prevent bleeding (see BLEEDING p. 92), dial 999, and give as much comfort and reassurance as you can.

Minor crush injuries, such as slamming a finger in a car door or dropping a hammer on a toe, hurt because of the high concentration of nerve fibres in the extremities.

Specific remedy to be given every 15 minutes to begin with, then three or four times daily until recovery is well established
- *Hypericum 30c*

CYANOCRYLATE GLUES

These are fast-setting, 'superglue' adhesives that bond anything, including human skin, in seconds. In rare cases a large drop will cause a burn (see BURNS AND SCALDS p. 93), since cyanocrylates heat up as they set.

Immerse the bonded sections of skin in warm soapy water. Peel or roll the surfaces apart with the aid of a teaspoon handle, then remove the glue from the skin with soapy water. Don't try to pull the surfaces apart.

If an eye or eyelid is involved, wash it thoroughly with warm water and apply a gauze patch. The eye will open, without further action on your part, in a day or two. Do not try to force the eye open. In doubtful cases, see a doctor as soon as possible.

If the lips are accidentally stuck together, apply lots of water and encourage salivation inside the mouth. Peel or roll the lips apart – do not pull them apart directly.

It is almost impossible to swallow 'superglue' but if a drop does enter the mouth, position the casualty so that it does not cause choking when it detaches.

DENTAL OPERATIONS

If a tooth socket starts to bleed after extraction, encourage the person to spit the blood out rather than swallow it. Place a clean pad of gauze over the socket and ask the person to bite on it for 15–20 minutes. Once the bleeding has stopped, rinse the mouth with Hypericum and Calendula solution; this can be repeated every 30 minutes. If severe bleeding persists, go back to the dentist.

Specific remedies to be taken every 5 minutes for up to 10 doses after dental treatment
- Where there is a lot of pain *Hypericum 30c*
- Where there is a lot of bleeding *Phosphorus 6c*
- Where hypericum fails *Staphysagria 6c*

Specific remedies to be taken hourly for up to 6 doses before going to the dentist
- Fear and panic *Aconite 6c*
- Great apprehension, knees feel weak and wobbly *Gelsemium 6c*

DIABETIC COMA

Both diabetes insipidus and diabetes mellitus can, if incorrectly managed, lead to unconsciousness and even death. For more information, see DIABETES p. 257–8.

The symptoms of hyperglycaemia (too much blood sugar) come on gradually, while those of hypoglycaemia (too little blood sugar) can be sudden and dramatic. Diabetics usually carry a card or bracelet warning of their condition, and giving instructions about what to do in emergencies.

If the concentration of sugar in the blood drops suddenly, the diabetic becomes faint and appears to be drunk; there is sweating, shallow rapid breathing, and a rapid pulse. Give sugar in any form, unless the person is already unconscious, in which case place him or her in the recovery position (see UNCONSCIOUSNESS p. 90) and dial 999.

NB Patients on the new generation of Human Insulins may not show the classic early symptoms of hypoglycaemia.

DISLOCATIONS

Dislocation occurs when the bones at a joint are forcibly knocked or twisted apart; this causes severe pain, sometimes nausea, inability to move the joint, swelling, bruising, and obvious deformity. For more information, see DISLOCATIONS p. 204.

For the first aider, dislocations are often difficult to distinguish from a FRACTURE, so should be treated as such. Do not attempt to straighten or realign the joint; simply support the affected joint as comfortably as possible with cushions or coats, and dial 999.

If the jaw or shoulder is dislocated, and dislocation has occurred before (jaws and shoulders have a tendency to keep dislocating), take the person to the nearest Accident and Emergency department; bandage the jaw, or apply a sling (see p. 105) to the arm to minimize jolting and jarring during the journey.

DROWNING

Do not attempt to drain fluid from the lungs of someone who has nearly drowned. Start artificial respiration (see BREATHING p. 86) as soon as possible – at the water's edge or in the boat – and dial 999. Continue artificial respiration for up to 1 hour if necessary.

On recovery, the victim should be seen by a doctor because of the danger of respiratory infection.

EAR INJURIES

Ears are very delicate, and only the gentlest measures should be taken to dislodge foreign bodies from the outer ear canal.

Foreign body in the ear If a small bead or insect gets into the ear, wash out the ear with tepid Hypericum and Calendula solution. Tilt the person's head so that the affected ear is uppermost, gently pull back the ear lobe to straighten the ear canal, and pour the solution into the ear. With luck, the object will float out. If not, see a doctor as soon as possible.

Specific remedies
- Continuing pain after removal of foreign body *Hypericum 30c* potency every 30 minutes, for up to 10 doses
- After an operation to remove a foreign body from the ear *Arnica 30c* every 4 hours for up to 6 doses

Bleeding from the ear This may be due to laceration of the external part of the ear or the ear canal, perforation of the eardrum due to a sudden increase in pressure (caused by diving or a nearby explosion), or a fracture of the skull (see HEAD INJURIES), in which case there may be leakage of a clear fluid instead of blood. Bleeding may also be accompanied by earache, headache, deafness, and loss of consciousness.

Place the casualty in a half-sitting position, with the head tilted towards the side that is bleeding. This allows blood, etc. to drain out of the ear. Cover the ear with a sterile dressing, but do not restrict the drainage of fluids. Check breathing, pulse, and state of alertness, and dial 999.

Specific remedy to be taken every 15 minutes for up to 10 doses
- Where bleeding is caused by a blow to the ear, person panicky *Aconite 30c*

ELECTROCUTION AND ELECTRICAL INJURIES

Electrical shocks can stop a person's breathing or heart, and also cause burns (see SHOCK p. 103, BURNS AND SCALDS p. 93).

If the victim is still in contact with the electricity source, be extremely careful that you don't become the next casualty. Switch off the current if you can. If this is not possible, push the casualty away from the electricity source using some form of insulated or non-conducting lever (a wooden chair, a broom handle). Remember that water is an extremely good conductor, so beware of wet hands, wet floors, and anything damp.

High-voltage electricity – the kind carried by power lines or railway cables – is usually instantaneously fatal. Never go near such a casualty; high voltage electricity can 'arc' several metres through the air.

As soon as you have switched off the electricity or separated the victim from the faulty appliance, check for breathing and pulse, and give artificial respiration (see BREATHING p. 86) or cardiac resuscitation (see CIRCULATION p. 88) as necessary, place in the recovery position (see UNCONSCIOUSNESS p. 90), and dial 999.

Specific remedy to be given every 30 minutes for up to 6 doses after an electric shock
- *Phosphorus 6c*

EPILEPSY

Major epileptic fits come on suddenly, although sometimes there may be warning symptoms (see EPILEPSY p. 127). Epileptics usually carry a card or bracelet warning of their condition. In *grand mal* epilepsy the person loses consciousness and may fall to the ground; then the body stiffens and starts to jerk; bladder and bowel control may be lost; breathing may become noisy or stop altogether, resulting in blue lips and congestion of the face. The seizure may last for several minutes.

The most important thing is to prevent injury, and remove the person from danger. Do not try to restrain the person while convulsions continue, and do not put anything in the mouth. A bitten tongue (which heals quite quickly) is preferable to choking on objects placed in the mouth. Once the convulsions subside and the body loses its rigidity, place the person in the recovery position (see UNCONSCIOUSNESS p. 90). He or she should regain consciousness in a few minutes, but may be dazed and confused. Stay with the person until he or she is fully recovered. Advise the person to see a doctor if it is a first attack.

Specific remedy to be given every 10 minutes for up to 10 doses after seizure has worn off
- *Hyoscyamus 6c*

EYE INJURIES

Generally speaking, first aid for all eye injuries (other than the removal of small foreign bodies) should be followed up by expert examination of the eyes. The surface of the eye is very delicate, easily damaged.

Foreign body in the eye Small items such as dust and grit can be washed from the eye with gently running water. The eye should then be bathed with Hypericum and Calendula solution. Larger objects can be dabbed off the eyeball with a clean handkerchief dipped in the same solution; you may have to lift the upper lid to encourage the natural tear fluid to wash the object to the front of the eyeball.

If pain persists after removal of a foreign body, bathe the eye with Euphrasia solution (10 drops of mother tincture to 0.25 litre [½ pint] of warm water) every 4 hours, and give Euphrasia 6c every 2 hours for up to 3 doses.

If pain persists for more than 12 hours after removal of a foreign body, see a doctor as soon as possible.

If the eye is penetrated by glass or splinters, do not try to remove them. Dial 999, and put a pad of gauze over both eyes to discourage eye movements (if the uninjured eye moves, the injured eye moves with it).

Bruising around the eye A single black eye is usually the result of a hard knock on the nose. If the skin around both eyes is bruised and blackened, the person may have sustained a fracture of the skull (see HEAD INJURIES p. 102).

Specific remedies to be given every 15 minutes (or less often as pain diminishes) for up to 10 doses
- Immediately after injury *Arnica 6c*
- Immediately after injury caused by a blunt object *Symphytum 6c*

Specific remedy to be given every 2 hours for up to 10 doses
- If pain persists after Arnica but is eased by cold applications *Ledum 6c*

Cuts near the eye If the cut is small, bring the edges together and apply butterfly sutures. If the cut is large, soak a pad of gauze in Hypericum and Calendula solution, wring it out, bandage it tightly over the cut, and take the person to the nearest Accident and Emergency department to have it stitched.

Specific remedies
- For minor cuts *Calendula 6c* every 8 hours for up to 3 days
- For deeper cuts caused by sharp objects *Aconite 30c* every 5 minutes (or less often as pain eases) for up to 10 doses

Chemicals in the eye Chemical accidents involving the eyes call for very swift action indeed. As well as causing excruciating pain, they can lead to permanent blindness.

Turn the head so that the affected eye is lower than the other – this prevents the offending chemical from trickling into the uninjured eye. Hold the person's face and eye under a gently running tap for 10–15 minutes, separating the eyelids with your fingers. Then cover the eye with sterile gauze and a bandage. Take the person to the nearest Accident and Emergency department to have the eye checked.

Specific remedy to be given every 5 minutes until pain begins to ease
- *Aconite 30c*

Snow blindness This is the result of over-long exposure to snow glare without the benefit of sunglasses or ski goggles. The eyes become puffy, painful, and water profusely.

Bathe the eyes frequently with Euphrasia solution (10 drops of mother tincture to 0.25 litre [½ pint] boiled cold water), cover the eyes with sterile pads, and seek expert medical help.

FAINTING
Temporary loss of consciousness caused by disruption of blood flow to the brain, brought on by emotional upset, pain, or hunger. Some people are particularly prone to fainting, but usually recover rapidly and completely. However, if a faint lasts for longer than a few minutes, internal or external BLEEDING should be suspected; this in turn may lead to SHOCK.

If the person has fainted but is breathing normally, put him or her in the recovery position (see UNCONSCIOUSNESS p. 90). When he or she comes round, give reassurance, and a few sips of cold water. If internal bleeding is suspected, call 999, check the pulse at 5-minute intervals, and be prepared to give artificial respiration (see BREATHING p. 86) or cardiac resuscitation (see CIRCULATION p. 88) if necessary.

If the person is feeling faint – the signs are nausea, unsteadiness, pallor, and a slow or weak pulse – sit him or her down, encourage a few deep breaths, and gently push the head towards the knees. Alternatively, get the person to lie down in the recovery position (see UNCONSCIOUSNESS p. 90). Loosen any tight clothing and allow plenty of fresh air. Lift up to increase blood flow to brain.

Specific remedies to be given every 5 minutes for up to 10 doses
- Fainting due to intense emotion *Ignatia 6c*
- Fainting due to over-excitement *Coffea 6c*
- Fainting due to over-exertion *Nux mosch. 6c*
- Fainting due to fright *Aconite 30c*
- Fainting caused by loss of blood *China 6c*
- Fainting caused by severe pain *Chamomilla 6c*
- Fainting caused by minor pain *Hepar sulph. 6c*
- Fainting in hot, stuffy surroundings *Pulsatilla 6c*
- Fainting at sight of blood *Nux 6c*
- Fainting at sight of needles *Silicea 6c*
- Fainting brought on by strong perfumes or odours *Nux 6c*

FISH HOOKS
Do not attempt to remove a fish hook unless it is impossible to get medical aid within an hour or two.

However, if help is far away, remember it is easier to *push* the point of the hook through and out of the skin by the shortest possible route than attempt to *pull* it out and rip the skin with the barb, unless you know how to do it using a piece of string and downward pressure. Remove the line from the hook first. Alternatively, if wire cutters are available, cut off the exposed barb and pull the hook back through the skin. Wash the area thoroughly (bathe with Hypericum and Calendula solution if possible). To prevent tetanus and other infections, get medical attention as soon as possible.

FITS AND CONVULSIONS

The symptoms of a fit, convulsion, or seizure include any or all of the following: jerky, uncontrolled movements; rigid limbs; foaming at the mouth; loss of bladder or bowel control; coughing and choking; and, in rare cases, cessation of breathing and unconsciousness. Fits can be caused by EPILEPSY (see p. 127), high fever, brain tumours, and other disorders which upset the electrical functioning of the brain.

If someone is having a fit, make sure that he or she does not suffer injury. Gently lead the person out of any possible danger, and clear the area of objects that may cause harm if the person falls or collapses. When the rigid phase has passed, place the person in the recovery position (see UNCONSCIOUSNESS p. 90). Give reassurance and advise a visit to a doctor, especially if there is no history of fits.

Febrile convulsions (see FEBRILE CONVULSIONS p. 320) These are most common in children, and are brought on by a high temperature during fevers and infections. First aid consists of bringing temperature down by undressing the child and sponging the body with tepid water, or wrapping the child in a wet sheet. Usually the situation is not as serious as it seems, but if convulsions continue for more than a few minutes, dial 999.

Specific remedies to be given every 5 minutes for up to 10 doses once the jerky phase is over
- Fit brought on by fright *Aconite 30c*
- Fit brought on by heat or a hot bath, casualty emits a high-pitched cry and bends head back *Apis 30c*
- Fit comes on suddenly, skin hot and dry, pupils fixed and staring, extreme sensivity to cold, light, jolting, and jarring once fit is over *Belladonna 30c*
- Fit brought on by anger or teething, one cheek red, the other pale *Chamomilla 6c*
- Fit brought on by too much sun *Glonoinum 30c*
- Where fit has a hysterical or emotional component *Ignatia 6c*
- Face dark red and mottled, pupils very small, violent muscle spasm, head bent back *Opium 6c*
- Face bluish, cold sweat on forehead, body icy cold *Veratrum 6c*

FRACTURES

A broken bone may be just cracked or broken right through (see FRACTURES p. 205). In an open fracture, the skin is broken and infection can enter the wound; in a closed fracture, the skin is unbroken. In either case, matters may be complicated by internal bleeding, or injury to nerves and internal organs. Open fractures can lead to heavy blood loss.

Some fractures can only be confirmed by X-ray. But if someone has sustained a fall or an impact injury of some kind, says that he or she felt or heard something snap or give way, and is obviously in great pain and unable to move the affected part of the body, a fracture is almost certain. Sometimes, though not always, there is a visible deformity if you compare both sides of the body. There may also be swelling, bruising, or blood loss.

Do not move the casualty any more than is absolutely necessary. Severe bleeding (see BLEEDING p. 92), difficulty breathing (see BREATHING p. 86), and loss of consciousness (see UNCONSCIOUSNESS p. 88) should be dealt with *before* the suspected fracture.

Bleeding can be controlled by applying pressure to the sides of the fractured bone. Cover the broken skin or protruding ends of bone with sterile gauze. Place a ring dressing over the site to prevent it being knocked or touched, and secure it with a bandage. Dial 999.

In isolated situations where the journey to hospital may take some time, immobilize the affected part as best you can to prevent further damage and bleeding. For example, bandage the arm against the chest, the jaw to the head, one leg to the other. Pad the bandaging above and below the fracture so that clothes and blankets cannot touch it.

Do not move the casualty any more than is absolutely necessary to stop bleeding and cover the wound. Check the extremities of the injured limb for circulation, colour, and feeling, and loosen bandages if necessary. Watch for signs of SHOCK.

Specific remedies
- *Arnica 30c* every 10 minutes until shock of wound passes off, then every 8 hours for up to 4 days
- After Arnica, and to promote healing *Symphytum 6c* every 8 hours for up to 3 weeks

FROSTBITE

Caused by freezing conditions which cut off circulation, usually in extremities (hands, feet, ears, nose), which may be permanently affected. Frostbitten areas are cold, pale or marbled-looking, solid to the touch, and painless (until circulation is restored). Most at risk are people who already have circulation problems and people taking beta-blockers to lower blood pressure. If deep tissues are damaged, gangrene may set in.

First aid consists of moving the casualty to shelter, giving warm drinks, and covering with blankets. Warm the injured part with body heat only – put a hand under an armpit, for example. Do not rub the skin or apply direct heat to the injured area. There will be redness and considerable pain as the affected part thaws. Keep the casualty warm, and get him or her to hospital.

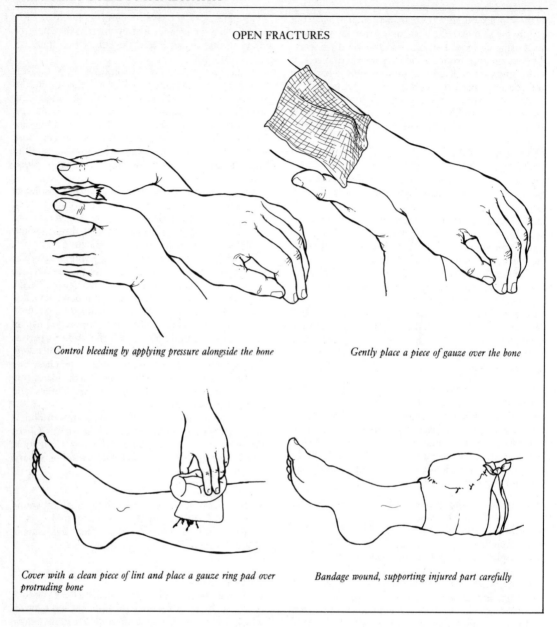

OPEN FRACTURES

Control bleeding by applying pressure alongside the bone

Gently place a piece of gauze over the bone

Cover with a clean piece of lint and place a gauze ring pad over protruding bone

Bandage wound, supporting injured part carefully

Specific remedies to be given every 15 minutes for up to 6 doses
- Frostbitten skin which looks like chilblains *Agaricus 6c*
- Severe burning pain *Apis 30c*
- Purple discoloration of skin *Lachesis 6c*

Frostbite can be prevented by wearing waterproof garments with several layers of dry clothing underneath, and making sure the hands, feet, ears, and nose are well protected.

HEAD INJURIES

After an accident, any departure from full awareness, even for a few minutes, suggests that the brain has been damaged, if only temporarily. Anyone who passes out or feels dazed or confused after a blow to the head should see a doctor.

Concussion is usually the result of a blow to the head. Symptoms include shallow breathing, cold, clammy, pale skin, nausea, temporary loss of consciousness (a few seconds), and sometimes temporary loss of memory.

Compression is a serious condition in which internal bleeding or a cranial fracture causes increased pressure inside the skull, and therefore pressure on the brain. Compression sometimes follows concussion, but symptoms may not appear for up to 24 hours. Breathing becomes noisy, temperature rises but the person does not sweat, the pulse is full but slow, the pupils of the eyes dilate to different degrees, and one side of the body may become paralysed; eventually the person lapses into unconsciousness.

The first thing to do is check the person's breathing and pulse (see BREATHING p. 86, CIRCULATION p. 88) and if necessary put the person in the recovery position (see UNCONSCIOUSNESS p. 90) and treat for SHOCK (see p. 103). Then dial 999. Check the pulse every 5 minutes while waiting for help, and give a full account of your observations when help arrives.

Specific remedy to be given every 15 minutes for up to 10 doses once casualty regains consciousness
- Arnica 30c

Other remedies
- Rigid back and general muscle spasm, dilated pupils, mental confusion *Cicuta 30c* every 6 hours until person recovers
- Where the person claims he or she has never fully recovered from a head injury *Natrum sulph. 30c* every 8–12 hours for up to 10 doses

HEART ATTACK
The symptoms of a heart attack can be dramatic: severe constricting or bursting pain in the chest, sometimes spreading to the arms, neck, and back; faintness and shortness of breath; irregular pulse; blue lips; collapse and unconsciousness. Breathing and heartbeat may stop. For more information, see HEART ATTACK p. 192.

If the victim remains conscious, prop him or her up in a half-sitting position with knees bent. Dial 999. Calm and reassure the person as much as you can, keep him or her warm and comfortable, loosen any tight clothing, and keep a careful watch on breathing and pulse.

If the casualty is unconscious, check breathing and pulse, and if necessary give artificial respiration and cardiac resuscitation (see BREATHING p. 86, CIRCULATION p. 88). As soon as you judge breathing and heartbeat to be regular, put the person in the recovery position (see UNCONSCIOUSNESS p. 90). Then dial 999.

Specific remedies to be given every 2–5 minutes (depending on severity of attack) for up to 6 doses
- Fear of dying, restlessness, numbness *Aconite 30c*
- Chest feels as if there is an iron band around it, pain in left arm, feeling of weight on chest makes breathing difficult *Cactus 6c*

- Violent chest pain which extends into fingers, gasping for breath, numbness, pulse rapid and feeble *Latrodectus 6c*
- Heart throbs and surges as if about to burst through chest wall, faintness, anxiety, sweating *Spongia 6c*

HEATSTROKE AND HEAT EXHAUSTION
Heatstroke is caused by excessive fluid and salt loss in hot or humid conditions; this leads to general dehydration and exhaustion. Predisposing factors include general fatigue or ill health, too much alcohol, and wearing too many clothes. As heatstroke develops, the person complains of feeling hot, headachy, dizzy, and nauseous, and begins to breathe fast and noisily; the skin remains dry, although the face may be flushed; there may be cramps or muscle twitches. If temperature is allowed to rise above 40°C (104°F), the person eventually collapses and becomes unconscious.

First aid priorites are to bring the person's temperature down and prevent further dehydration. Undress the person, wrap him or her in a wet sheet, and create a draught by fanning or switching on an electric fan; as the water in the sheet evaporates, it will cool the skin beneath. Keep the sheet well wetted. Sponge the face. Give only water to drink, with a little salt dissolved in it (½ teaspoon of salt to 0.5 litre [1 pint] water – these quantities are important as too much salt will cause vomiting and further dehydration). Once the person has cooled down, cover them with a dry sheet. If temperature starts to climb again, dial 999.

Specific remedies to be given every 5 minutes for up to 10 doses
- Muscle cramps *Cuprum 6c*
- Skin flushed, hot, and dry, pulse strong and rapid, pupils fixed and dilated *Belladonna 30c*
- Throbbing, bursting headache, hot face, sweaty skin *Glonoinum 30c*
- Severe headache made worse by slightest movement, nausea *Bryonia 30c*

HYPOTHERMIA
Sets in when core body temperature falls below 35°C (95°F); if cooling continues to 25°C (77°F) or below, recovery is unlikely. As temperature dips, the person becomes dreamy, unresponsive, and reluctant to move; hands, feet, and abdomen feel cold to the touch; there may also be cramp, numbness, or paralysis, causing falls and accidents if the person tries to move.

First, check breathing and pulse, and if necessary give artificial respiration and cardiac resuscitation (see BREATHING p. 86, CIRCULATION p. 88). Do not give cardiac resuscitation unless you are absolutely sure there is no heartbeat.

Bring the person into the warm, and give sips of hot, sweet drinks, but *no alcohol*. Warm the person up gently, to avoid overstraining the heart. Place warm, not boiling, hot water bottles, well wrapped up, against the person's body if you like, but not against the extremities. Do not rub or massage the limbs or encourage the person to do warm-up exercises. DO NOT PUT THEM IN THE BATH.

Babies and old people are most vulnerable to hypothermia. A hypothermic baby will be unusually limp and drowsy, and refuse feeds, although face, hands, and feet may appear normal. The most effective way of rewarming a baby is to hold him or her against your skin in a warm bed or bath, or put to the breast if nursing. In the elderly, it is sometimes difficult to distinguish hypothermia from a STROKE or HEART ATTACK. Call your GP within 2 hours.

Specific remedy to be given every 10 minutes for up to 10 doses
- If hypothermia is accompanied by cramp *Cuprum 6c*

INTERNAL BLEEDING
Internal bleeding, often more serious than external bleeding, is usually the result of CRUSH INJURIES, FRACTURES, or a burst peptic ulcer. Blood lost internally can pool in connected tissues and cause a build-up of pressure on vital organs; a haemorrhage inside the skull, for example, can lead to compression of the brain (see HEAD INJURIES). Both internal and external bleeding can reduce blood pressure and cause SHOCK.

Internal bleeding should be suspected if the person has pale, clammy skin, and a rapid, feeble pulse. (Note that the pulse may be slow if bleeding inside the skull has occurred.) Breathing may become shallow, with air hunger (yawning), restlessness, and thirst. Coughing or vomiting blood is another sign. There may also be pain and swelling at the site of bleeding, or bruising under the skin.

First, encourage the person to rest quietly with legs raised, unless of course there is a chest injury, in which case he or she should sit propped up. Dial 999 and keep the person warm until help arrives. There is nothing else you can do, unless you have special training.

Specific remedy to be taken every 2–5 minutes for up to 10 doses
- Internal bleeding, collapse, air hunger (yawning), forehead cold *Veratrum 6c*

NOSEBLEEDS
Lean the casualty over a basin, pinch the lower part of the nose for 10 minutes, then release slowly. If blood starts to flow again, pinch the nose for another 5 minutes. If bleeding persists, take the person to a doctor. Do not allow the person to lie down. The nose should not be forcibly blown for 2–3 days after a nosebleed. If the remedies below produce no improvement, try one of the remedies listed under BLEEDING p. 92.

Specific remedies to be taken every 2 minutes for up to 10 doses
- Nosebleed follows injury *Arnica 6c*
- Where blood is bright red *Ipecac 6c*
- Bleeding brought on by violent nose-blowing *Phosphorus 6c*
- Nosebleed accompanied by a headache which gets worse if head is bent forwards *Hamamelis 6c*
- Bright red blood, person feels faint, especially if he or she usually looks rather pale *Ferrum phos. 6c*
- In all other cases *Vipera 6c*

PANIC
Panic makes pain and fear worse, and hinders first aid. Give as much reassurance to the casualty as you can.

Specific remedies to be given every few minutes for up to 10 doses
- Remedy of first resort *Arnica 30c*
- Paralysing fear *Opium 6c*
- If person still feels weak and shaky after panic has subsided *Gelsemium 6c*

POISONING
Poisoning involving household chemicals is one of the most preventable of emergencies. Poisons can enter the body through the mouth or skin, or they may be inhaled (see CHEMICALS, INHALED p. 94). They can do temporary or permanent damage, and may be fatal. Corrosive poisons cause burns; neurotoxins damage the nervous system; other poisons prevent blood carrying oxygen to the tissues; others damage the digestive system. Symptoms vary enormously, from nausea and vomiting to dizziness, paralysis, numbness, convulsions, and collapse. If possible, take some evidence of the cause of poisoning – pill box, medicine bottle, fluid container, sample of vomit – to the hospital with the casualty.

Poisons absorbed through the skin, for example pesticides and insecticides, can cause convulsions (see FITS AND CONVULSIONS p. 99). Wash the chemical from the skin with large amounts of water, and make sure the contaminated water drains away safely. Do not contaminate yourself. Dial 999.

Poisons taken by mouth include proprietary and prescription drugs and medicines, household and garden chemicals, food contaminated with dangerous bacteria, and poisonous plants, especially fungi and berries. Symptoms include convulsions, retching or vomiting, abdominal pain, and unconsciousness. In the case of household and garden chemicals, there may be burns around the mouth; with food poisoning, symptoms come on 2–6 hours after eating contaminated food, and usually include diarrhoea; with drug abuse, there may be injection marks and swollen veins on the inside of the forearm.

Try to find out what has caused the poisoning. If the casualty is unconscious, check breathing and pulse, give artificial respiration and cardiac rescuscitation if necessary (see BREATHING p. 86, CIRCULATION p. 88), and then place in the recovery position (see UNCONSCIOUSNESS p. 90). Dial 999.

Do not try to induce vomiting or 'neutralize' the poison with anything by mouth, unless the lips and mouth are burned, in which case give sips of water or milk. Poisoning with Paracetamol (e.g. Calpol, Panadol) can cause liver damage. If in doubt, see your GP within 2 hours.

SHOCK

Sets in when blood flow through vital organs becomes inadequate due to loss of body fluids (see BLEEDING, INTERNAL BLEEDING, FRACTURES, BURNS and SCALDS), a HEART ATTACK, or a sudden drop in blood pressure in response to an allergen or infection (anaphylactic shock). Symptoms include pallor, cold clammy skin, anxiety, nausea, thirst, and faintness. Breathing becomes rapid and shallow, and the pulse 'thready' (weak and fast). In some people insect BITES AND STINGS cause a shock reaction, accompanied by swelling of the throat and difficult breathing.

When a person is in shock, every second counts. Dial 999 immediately.

Check breathing and pulse and quickly assess any injuries to see if there is preventable blood loss. If possible, lie the casualty on his or her back and raise the legs slightly (unless injury prevents this) to improve blood flow to the heart, lungs, and brain. Keep the head tilted to one side, with the chin up, to keep the airway open.

If the person becomes unconscious or vomits, put him or her into the recovery position (see UNCONSCIOUSNESS p. 90) and, if possible, raise the feet. Loosen any tight clothing and cover with a blanket or coat. Do not move the person; do not give anything to drink; and do not apply direct heat.

Specific remedies to be given every 60 seconds for up to 10 doses
- Person extremely fearful and restless *Aconite 30c*
- Person yawning and hungry for air, face bluish and puffy, collapse *Carbo veg. 30c*
- Skin cold and mottled, forehead cold and sweaty *Veratrum 6c*
- Shock brought on by injury *Arnica 30c*

SLIPPED DISC

Occurs when an intervertebral disc impinges on a ligament or narrows the space through which a nerve leaves and enters the spine; overuse or degenerative change precedes most disc problems, the awkward bend or twist being the final straw. In most cases, symptoms are sudden, severe pain, usually in middle or lower back, and inability to straighten up or bend the neck forwards; there may be severe pain down one or both legs. Sometimes, however, symptoms onset gradually. For more information, see PROLAPSED DISC p. 210.

Let the person lie down in whatever position feels most comfortable; lying on the side, with the knees tucked up and a cushion between them, is sometimes more comfortable than lying flat on the back with the knees flexed. See your doctor within 12 hours. Rest is usually the best medicine; the back should not be manipulated until pain has abated.

Specific remedy to be given ½ hourly for up to 10 doses, then every 4 hours for up to 5 days
- *Arnica 30c*

SNAKEBITE
see BITES AND STINGS

SPINAL INJURY

Since the spinal cord consists of nerves which carry messages from the brain to the body and vice versa, injury at any point in its course through the canal formed by the vertebrae is potentially serious. Fracture or dislocation of the vertebrae can cause loss of movement and sensitivity in those parts of the body below the point of injury. Damage may be caused directly, by a blow to the spine, or indirectly, by landing heavily on the feet or buttocks. Whiplash injury to the neck (when the neck is flung violently backwards or forwards) is common in car accidents and falls from motorbikes. For more information, see SPINAL CORD INJURY p. 134.

The casualty may complain of severe pain in the back or of feeling 'cut in half'. There may be loss of feeling and control in the limbs supplied by the nerves below the level of the injury. With lower back injuries, bladder or bowel control may be lost.

In such cases, the aim of first aid is to prevent further injury. Inability to move fingers or toes is an indication that the spine may be injured. Do not move the person unless he or she is in immediate, serious danger. Prevent movement by placing rolled blankets alongside the head and trunk; cover with coats or blankets and give comfort and reassurance. Dial 999.

Specific remedies
- *Arnica 30c* every 5 minutes for up to 10 doses, followed by *Hypericum 30c* every 4 hours for up to 3 days

SPLINTERS

The main danger from splinters of wood or metal is tetanus.

If the splinter is protruding from the skin, remove it

carefully with tweezers. If it is just underneath the skin, heat a needle tip (this sterilizes it), let it cool, then gently slit the skin over the end of the splinter until you can get hold of it with tweezers. If the splinter is deeply embedded, bathe with Hypericum and Calendula solution, and seek medical help.

Specific remedy to be given 4 times daily for up to 2 weeks
- *Silicea 6c*

SPRAINS AND STRAINS

Sprains – technically the overstretching or tearing of ligaments which bind joints together – can be mild or severe, and sometimes difficult to distinguish from FRACTURES and DISLOCATIONS. A strain is something similar in a muscle; a few or many muscle fibres may be torn. The symptoms are similar – swelling, stiffness, and pain when the joint or muscle is used. If questioning of the casualty leads you to suspect a fracture, treat the injury as such.

Otherwise, support the injured part in the most comfortable position. Reduce swelling by applying a cold compress – soak the compress in Arnica solution made by mixing 10 drops of mother tincture with 0.25 litre (½ pint) cold water. Light bandaging will also help to reduce swelling. Remove the shoe if the ankle is sprained (ankle sprains are caused by 'going over' on the outside of the ankle), but bandage the joint firmly to give support. Take the person to hospital if pain and swelling do not subside within 24 hours.

Specific remedy to be given every ½ hour for up to 10 doses
- *Arnica 30c*

After Arnica, the following may be given 4 times daily until pain and stiffness wear off
- Where tendons, ligaments, or periosteum (tissue covering bone) are involved *Ruta 6c*
- Muscles torn, joint swollen, hot, and painful, pain intensifies when person starts to move but wears off

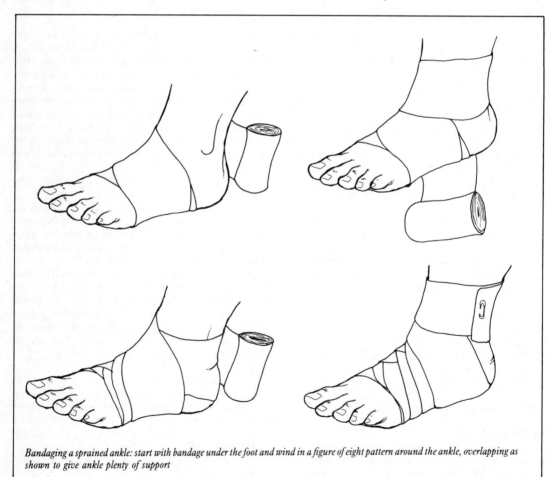

Bandaging a sprained ankle: start with bandage under the foot and wind in a figure of eight pattern around the ankle, overlapping as shown to give ankle plenty of support

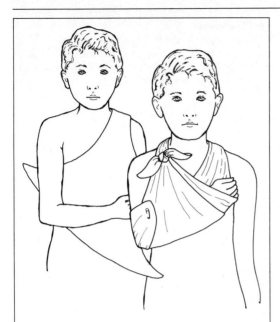

Making a sling: use a triangular bandage, passing longest edge over uninjured shoulder and under injured arm, tying at injured shoulder. Raise injured arm, and pin for support

with continued movement *Rhus tox. 6c*
- Joint very swollen, slightest movement causes pain *Bryonia 6c*
- Joint swollen, cold, and numb, but cold applications have a beneficial effect *Ledum 6c*

STROKE
Strokes occur when part of the brain's blood supply is cut off. This can be caused by a local haemorrhage or a blood clot in one of the arteries supplying the brain. For more information, see STROKES p. 135.

Stroke symptoms include inability to speak, severe headache, confusion, and a pounding pulse. There may be weakness and numbness on one side of the body and unequal dilation of the pupils. In a major stroke, the casualty quickly becomes unconscious.

Check breathing and heartbeat and if necessary give artificial respiration (see BREATHING p. 86) and cardiac resuscitation (see CIRCULATION p. 88). If the person is unconscious, place him or her in the recovery position (see UNCONSCIOUSNESS p. 90). If the person remains conscious, prop him or her up in a half-sitting position and give as much comfort and reassurance as you can. Dial 999.

Specific remedies to be given every 5–10 minutes for up to 10 doses
- Person very fearful *Aconite 30c*
- Person has collapsed, face dark and flushed, loud 'snoring' breathing, cheeks puff out as person exhales *Opium 6c*

Once the person's condition is stable, give *Arnica 6c* every 4 hours for up to 3 days.

SURGICAL OPERATIONS
Homeopathic remedies have their uses before and after surgical operations, especially when admission to hospital is unexpected and traumatic. After surgery, wounds can be kept clean by bathing with Hypericum and Calendula solution.

Specific remedies to be given ½ hourly for up to 10 doses
- Person panicking, in great fear of surgery *Aconite 30c*
- Person very apprehensive, weak, and trembling *Gelsemium 6c*
- To relieve vomiting after anaesthetic *Phosphorus 6c*
- To relieve pain and prevent infection after surgery *Arnica 30c*
- After Arnica. *Staphysagria 6c*

WOUNDS
A wound is any break in the skin which allows blood to escape and infection to enter; surrounding or underlying tissues may be bruised or torn as well.

The aim of first aid is to stop bleeding and prevent infection. Avoid touching wounds as much as possible. If it is necessary to clean a wound, wipe it with a sterile pad soaked in Hypericum and Calendula solution, always wiping outwards from the wound, never towards it. All kinds of wounds, from minor grazes to gaping cuts, can be cleaned with Hypericum and Calendula solution.

Minor wounds should then be covered with a sterile dressing, and the dressing left undisturbed for 2–3 days. Sizeable cuts and gashes will need stitching, so take the person to hospital. If the casualty has not had a tetanus injection in the last 5 years, make sure he or she is given one. This is particularly important if the wound involves old machinery or garden implements, or has dirt in it.

Specific remedies to be given every 30 minutes for up to 6 doses
- If wound is deep and requires stitching *Arnica 30c*
- If wound is very painful *Staphisagria 6c*, followed by *Calendula 6c* every 6 hours for up to 3 days

Specific remedies to be given every 2 hours for up to 6 doses, then 3 times daily for up to 3 days
- Moderate or severe bruising *Arnica 30c*
- If wound feels numb and cold but is better for cold applications *Ledum 6c*
- Shooting nerve pains after stitching *Hypericum 30c*

Puncture wounds, from rusty nails, or animal bites, become infected quite easily as there is little bleeding to remove foreign bodies and bacteria. Check for tetanus immunity. There may also be damage to underlying blood vessels, tissues, or organs. Wash with Hypericum and Calendula solution immediately, and see a doctor if the wound becomes more painful within the next 24 hours. Pus oozing from the wound, or red streaking of the skin around it, is a sure sign of trapped infection.

Specific remedies
- *Hepar sulph. 6c* every 2 hours for up to 6 doses, followed by *Ledum 6c* every 8 hours for up to 3 days
- If wound gives nervy, shooting pain *Hypericum 30c* every 8 hours for up to 3 days

Part 5

AILMENTS AND DISEASES

How to use this section

Ailments and diseases are divided into sections referring to parts of the body, systems or 'special problems' (e.g. 'Skin, Nails and Hair', 'Mind and Emotions' or 'Special Problems in Infancy'). Within each section ailments are listed alphabetically. Cross-references in SMALL CAPITALS should be looked up in the index: page numbers are only given when the same ailment occurs twice (e.g. bronchitis appears in 'Ailments and Diseases in Childhood' and the reader is referred to 'BRONCHITIS page 178' in 'Lungs and Respiration').

The most likely causes of an ailment or symptoms are underlined.

If specific remedies but not specific symptoms are given, try the remedies in the order listed: the one given first is most likely to be effective.

In cases of sudden or acute illness, prompt action may be necessary. The symbols used in the text are:

- (999) Emergency – call GP, but if not immediately available, dial 999 and ask for ambulance
- (2) Consult your doctor if there is no improvement in 2 hours
- [12] Consult your doctor if there is no improvement in 12 hours
- [24] Consult your doctor if there is no improvement in 24 hours
- [48] Consult your doctor if there is no improvement in 48 hours

MIND AND EMOTIONS

AS you read through the ailments described in the following pages, remember that 'depression', 'anxiety' and 'grief', and the symptoms which constitute them, are only labels of convenience. Psychology and psychiatry have divided and sub-divided human behaviour into hundreds of categories, and gained valuable knowledge by doing so. Homeopathy makes use of such labels because they are common currency, but never loses sight of the whole individual behind the label.

Very few diseases are wholly psychological or wholly physical. 'Mind' and 'body' affect one another interminably. The dichotomy is convenient, even useful in some circumstances, but it is false – who can say where the one begins and the other ends? Homeopathy treats only one entity, the Vital Force, the engine which drives every aspect of individual behaviour, and as clues to the state of that force, thoughts and feelings are just as important as lumps and bumps.

It is impossible to draw a line between balance and imbalance on the mental and emotional level. Mental health is a relative thing, depending entirely on what is acceptable or tolerable to the individual and to the community he or she lives in. If you find your thoughts and emotions uncomfortable, or are worried by certain aspects of your behaviour, that in itself is a recognition of imbalance; if your family, or society at large, finds your behaviour outrageous or damaging you may be labelled as mentally ill whether you agree with the label or not.

If you recognize in yourself, or in members of your family, tendencies which are life-denying – unsociability, apathy, insecurity – go and see a homeopathic physician. The earlier such tendencies are treated constitutionally the better; untreated they may deepen or interfere permanently with your enjoyment of life. The remedies given during constitutional treatment will act on your Vital Force, giving you more energy and more confidence to sort out your problems. You may, in addition, be advised to make changes in diet, exercise, and lifestyle.

More than anything else, try to be kind to yourself and accept the way you are. Try to accept that there is a place inside you which has remained unchanged since babyhood. It is innocent, it trusts, it knows no fear, and needs only love. If that sounds saccharine and woolly-minded, perhaps you are not allowing yourself to get in touch with those feelings. At a very early age we learn that love is not always returned. Indeed it often has to be earned. This hurts, and so we close up and pretend that we do not want to love or be loved. In later life these dammed-up feelings prevent us opening up to other people, and lead to fear, anxiety, insecurity, loneliness, and depression.

Whenever you feel tempted to close down, shut off, hide away, give up . . . try to open up. *There are always alternatives*. A lot of problems are the result of getting it into our heads that there is no alternative, no escape, and we are left feeling helpless and hopeless. This has a profoundly weakening effect on the whole mind-body continuum. Try to give priority to your creative, life-seeking instincts; try to focus on other people's problems for a change. If you are unable to sit down and clear your mind and experience the contentment of just being alive, then you should consider learning some form of relaxation or meditation (see PART 2) which will give you that experience.

Although most mental and emotional problems are rooted in upbringing and childhood experiences, illness and various stressful life events also take their toll. Depression is quite common after viral illnesses such as influenza, glandular fever, shingles, and hepatitis. Bereavement, redundancy, family pressures, and pressures at work also place a severe strain on a person's ability to adapt.

Orthodox treatment of emotional and mental problems consists of drugs, often combined with some form of psychotherapy. If you wish to switch to constitutional homeopathic treatment, consult your GP first.

Severe mental problems requiring psychiatric treatment in hospital are rare, but if you find yourself in this situation and wish to have homeopathic treatment – homeopathically-trained psychiatrists being very few and far between – ask your psychiatrist if he or she would have any objections to your taking homeopathic remedies or extra vitamins; these will not interfere with any drugs you are taking. When you are discharged, your psychiatrist may rarely agree to tail off your drugs so that you can switch fully to constitutional homeopathic treatment.

Addiction see also DRUG ADDICTION, ALCOHOLISM

An inability to do without something on the physical or psychological level, to the point where craving for it begins to destroy or dominate family, social, or working life.

We begin wanting things as soon as we are born – food, warmth, love – and we want them instantly. As children we exist in a broil of anticipation, of the next birthday, of the next trip to the seaside. As adults our needs are more varied and complex, but the world no longer revolves around us as it did when we were children; unsatisfied, those needs make us vulnerable to palliatives such as alcohol, drugs, tobacco, and so on. Not everyone succumbs, not because they are models of morality, or will-power, or emotional stability, or cushioned by circumstances, but because their brain chemistry is not affected by them in a sufficiently rewarding way.

The brain is receptive to pain-relieving and pleasure-giving substances because it manufactures similar substances itself; if the manufacture of these substances, collectively known as endorphins, is low, for congenital reasons or because their production has been depressed or disordered by drug-taking, the conditions exist in which drugs and other addictive substances will be gratifying. Unfortunately, the highs produced by most substances of abuse are shortlived, quickly followed by lows. The higher the highs, the lower the lows. The only cure for a low is another high . . . and so the destructive spiral of addiction sets in. So-called addictions to television, sweets, coffee, and so on are not in the same league as dependence on drugs or alcohol, but like life-threatening addictions they are often substitutes for needs which are not being met.

Patterns of addiction, and attitudes towards it, are changing. In the last 25 years, for example, the proportion of female to male alcoholics has increased from 1 in 8 to 2 in 5. The prevailing view today is that dependence on alcohol or drugs is a disease, precipitated by social and emotional factors certainly, but due primarily to constitutional factors.

The first step towards fighting addiction is to recognize that you are becoming addicted. Since addicts in bud have a great capacity for denying the truth, the first alarm bells are usually sounded by friends, relatives, or colleagues at work.

There is no definite point at which a casual drug user becomes an intensive user or a heavy social drinker becomes an alcoholic, so it is no use saying to yourself: 'I'll stop when such and such happens'. When it becomes difficult to do without, physically or psychologically, you are already becoming dependent; the substance is controlling you, not you it. The only way to prevent dependence increasing, as it almost certainly will, is to stop now, with the help of family, friends, and support organizations.

Agoraphobia see also PHOBIA

Extreme ANXIETY attached to being in public or crowded places. By avoiding such places anxiety is reduced to a tolerable level, but the anxiety is also reinforced. Since panic feelings can be made worse by HYPERVENTILATION or HYPOGLYCAEMIA, simply treating these may help to keep phobia under control. If not, behaviour therapy may be effective.

Specific remedies to be given 4 times daily for up to 7 days, or ½ hourly for up to 10 doses if phobia is acute and disabling

- Person terrified of dying or collapsing if he or she goes into a shop, gets onto a bus, etc. *Aconite 6c*
- Fear brought on by an accident *Arnica 6c*
- Person chilly, exhausted, restless *Arsenicum 6c*
- In an emergency, where no other remedy seems to be indicated *Sulphur 6c*

Alcoholism see also ADDICTION

The modern concept of alcoholism is that it is a disease which is curable. Individual tolerance to alcohol varies widely, even among alcoholics, but tolerance increases as drinking gets heavier. Patterns of drinking also vary; some alcoholics drink constantly, others have binges lasting for several days and then don't touch a drink for a week.

In the early stages, it may be difficult to tell whether someone is an alcoholic. There is no convenient borderline between 'social drinking' and alcoholism. Social drinkers, even heavy social drinkers, may be correct in assuming that they drink simply to be sociable; they may *not* be constitutionally predisposed to addiction. But alcohol is no respecter of motives. It is a powerful poison, affecting every cell in the body, especially those in the liver, heart, and brain, and it produces increasing tolerance. It also causes nutritional deficiencies because it disrupts appetite and destroys nutrients in the gut. It can also cause foetal abnormalities. If a person is drinking more than 20 (for women) or 30 (for men) units of alcohol per week (1 unit is equivalent to ½ pint of beer, or 1 glass of wine, or 1 measure of spirits), the chances are that he or she has a drink problem.

Among the signs of growing dependence are a tendency to start drinking earlier and earlier in the day, and not just in public but also secretly; increasing irritability and aggression, blurred recall of events in the immediate past, even blackouts, unreliability, and a general drop in performance at all levels. At this stage the person usually denies that he or she has a problem.

The later signs of dependence are more difficult to deny. At the psychological level there may be DEPRESSION, PARANOIA, marked difficulties with memory and concentration, and at the physical level a husky voice, flushed, red face with prominent veins, bruises and contusions from falls, trembling hands, chronic stomach ache due to GASTRIC EROSION AND GASTRITIS, and CIRRHOSIS OF THE LIVER. If the craving for alcohol is not satisfied, withdrawal symptoms set in (see DELIRIUM TREMENS for description and treatment).

Various studies of twins have shown that heredity plays a more powerful part in alcoholism than environment. Most at risk are people who have a parent, or parents, with a drink problem. However, a diet poor in certain vitamins and minerals, or a tendency to HYPOGLYCAEMIA, also poses a risk, and recently it has been suggested that excess lead in the diet or environment may be a predisposing factor. Alcoholism is most common among people aged 35–50, but is not unknown among adolescents. The extent of the problem is not precisely known, since far more people are affected than are diagnosed or treated, but estimates range from 1 to 4 per cent of the population.

Alcoholism requires professional medical help. It is possible to wean a person off alcohol in the short term by using vitamins, tranquilizers, various forms of aversion therapy, counselling, and so on, but that is only the first step. As most ex-alcoholics will confirm, the hard work starts when a person leaves the hospital or clinic after detoxification, and realizes that he or she must never touch alcohol again. The right amount of alcohol for an ex-alcoholic is no alcohol. This is where Alcoholics Anonymous provides invaluable support.

Homeopathy does not offer treatment for alcoholism as such, although in emergencies various homeopathic remedies can be used to relieve the symptoms of withdrawal. However, it does offer constitutional treatment to boost general health, vitality, and self-confidence once the habit has been broken. The author unhesitatingly recommends such treatment as part of staying alcohol-free.

That said, homeopathy can offer a number of remedies for the effects of occasional over-indulgence in alcohol.

Specific remedies to be taken ½-hourly, or more frequently if necessary, for up to 12 doses
- Hangover in morning, especially after drinking spirits, person 'burning the candle at both ends' *Nux 6c*
- Stomach pain after heavy drinking *Capsicum 6c*
- Social bingeing, person talks too much and hates tight clothing *Lachesis 6c*
- Person more depressed and irritable than usual, near end of tether *Avena 6c*
- Person apprehensive, trembling, lethargic, sensitive to noise *Zinc 6c*
- Solitary drinking, abnormal flatulence, nervous exhaustion *Sulphur 6c*
- Nausea and vomiting after drinking beer, tendency to profuse, stringy catarrh *Kali bichrom. 6c*

Self-help The role of Alcoholics Anonymous (address p. 384) has already been referred to; meetings take place most nights of the week in most towns of any size, and anyone who thinks he or she has a drink problem can attend. There is a sister organization, Al-Anon Family Groups UK & Eire (address p. 384), which offers support and counselling to the families and friends of alcoholics.

After stopping drinking it is important to eat a healthy, varied diet and to make up deficiencies of Vitamins A, B, C, D, K, folic acid, bioflavinoids, iron, manganese, potassium, and cysteine (an amino acid found in dairy products, whole grains, nuts and seeds). A high-dose multivitamin and mineral supplement would be the most convenient way of doing this in the first month after stopping drinking. Regular intake of all the nutrients mentioned above is advised even for moderate social drinkers. Evening primrose oil would also be beneficial.

Amnesia see MEMORY LOSS

Anger

An emotional and physiological response to events which are seen as psychologically or physically threatening. Pulse rate and skin conductivity increase, the stomach feels tight or fluttery, and various muscle groups tense up. Bottled up anger lies at the root of much DEPRESSION, especially if self-esteem is shaky and many situations are seen as threatening.

Specific remedies to be taken ½-hourly for up to 10 doses
- Person extremely critical of everyone and everything, very impatient and irritable, always ready to flare up, may have been overworking or overindulging in food and alcohol *Nux 6c*
- Sudden violent outbursts of anger which stem from feelings of insecurity and apprehension *Lycopodium 6c*
- An angry, bad-tempered child who pulls away from touching and hugging, constantly demands things but throws them aside as soon as they are given *Cina 6c*
- An irritable child who insists on being carried around and starts screaming the moment he or she is put down, especially during teething if one cheek is red and the other pale *Chamomilla 6c*
- Anger brings on spasms of stomach pain *Colocynth 6c*
- Anger brings on a high fever, or anger triggered off by a bad fright *Aconite 30c*
- Anger brings on hysterical symptoms (such as vomiting, blacking out, temporary loss of memory, sight, speech or hearing, paralysis) *Ignatia 6c*

Self-help Vitamin B complex, Vitamin C, bioflavinoids, calcium and magnesium all help to soothe jangled nerves. Exercise, relaxation, and meditation can also help to dissolve the physical tensions which accompany anger. If anger is rooted in fragile self-esteem and INSECURITY, assertiveness training may be useful.

Anniversary reaction see also DEATH, GRIEF
Very few people who have lost a loved one are immune from painful thoughts when the anniversary of their loss comes round. Over the years the reaction tends to fade, but it can give rise to chronic or recurrent DEPRESSION.

Specific remedies to be taken 4 times daily for up to 14 days, or every hour for up to 10 doses if feelings are particularly painful

- Great sadness, person emotionally self-contained, refuses sympathy *Natrum mur. 6c*
- Hysterical laughter or weeping *Ignatia 6c*
- Fear of dying, sudden feelings of panic *Aconite 30c*
- Person angry, irritable, overcritical *Nux 6c*

Anorexia see also BULIMIA
Not usually diagnosed until at least 10 per cent of body weight has been lost due to persistent fasting or food abuse. It is important to seek help early, since disorder becomes less easy to reverse the more weight is lost. Incidence among girls is about 20 times higher than among boys.

Some experts distinguish between *primary anorexia*, which occurs in adolescence and seems to be brought on by a crisis reaction to the sexual and emotional changes which adolescence involves, and *secondary anorexia*, which occurs later and is more likely to be due to a weight PHOBIA, social inadequacy, DEPRESSION, or general inability to cope. Other experts distinguish between anorexia and BULIMIA (bingeing and starving), or regard bulimia as a variant of anorexia, or look on both as part of a whole spectrum of 'eating disorders'. Significantly, most anorexics are girls or young women, more vulnerable than other members of society to messages which tell them that to be loved and accepted they have to be perfect.

Anorexia begins as normal dieting, which then becomes obsessive and compulsive. The less you eat, the less you want to eat; the more weight you lose, the more terrified you are of putting on weight. Anorexics go to extraordinary lengths to avoid eating, making all sorts of excuses for not appearing at meals, eating alone so that they can throw food away, and so on. When they can no longer deny themselves food, they may binge, and then attempt to undo the imagined consequences by self-induced vomiting and taking laxatives.

The resulting symptoms are those of severe malnutrition and DEHYDRATION. As body fat is lost, hormone balance is disrupted and periods cease (see amenorrhea – MENSTRUAL PROBLEMS); then the protein in muscles is broken down to provide energy; complications include swelling and occasionally rupture of the stomach, lung damage from inhaling vomit, over-alkalinization of the blood, low levels of chlorine and potassium in the blood, tooth decay and tooth loss, swelling of the parotid glands, and inflammation and rupture of the oesophagus. Appearance becomes sallow and skeletal, and behaviour apathetic, depressed, and even suicidal.

Severe anorexia requires expert medical attention, usually in hospital. Eating is voluntary, except as a last resort. Psychotherapy appropriate to the underlying causes is also given.

If you have a tendency to diet strictly and often, when family and friends see no need for you to do so, or a tendency to binge and starve rather than eat regular meals, constitutional treatment from an experienced homeopath would be a wise precaution.

Self-help Zinc is recommended.

Anxiety

Both an emotional and a physiological state, in which subjective feelings are apprehension and worry, and physical symptoms are increased pulse rate, clammy skin, and disturbed sleep and appetite. In some people physical symptoms can be severe enough to mimic a HEART ATTACK. Take no chances; if someone is breathless, sweating, complains of pains in the chest, or looks as if they are about to collapse, give First Aid as if for a heart attack (see p. 102).

In most people anxiety prompts some kind of action to counter a perceived threat. In this sense anxiety is helpful, of survival value. But if anxiety becomes a permanent state because almost everything is perceived as a threat, DEPRESSION and other psychosomatic illnesses can set in. A PHOBIA is an acute, disabling anxiety state attached to a certain object, animal, or situation. COMPULSIONS and OBSESSIONS are attempts to defuse anxiety. Anxiety can also be a symptom of HYPOGLYCAEMIA, withdrawal from drugs (see DRUG ADDICTION), or, if accompanied by WEIGHT LOSS and bulging eyes, of thyrotoxicosis (see THYROID PROBLEMS). HYPERVENTILATION and FOOD ALLERGY also raise anxiety levels. It is often a way of dealing with hidden DEPRESSION.

Conventional medicine offers drugs (benzodiazepines and other minor tranquillizers, beta blockers in certain circumstances) and psychotherapy. Homeopathic medicine offers constitutional treatment where anxiety is chronic, but also a number of emergency remedies.

Specific remedies to be taken every 2 hours for up to 10 doses if anxiety is acute or if constitutional treatment is awaited
- Anxiety about a new situation, or any situation that involves performing in front of an audience, especially if person craves sweets and feels worse in hot, stuffy rooms *Lycopodium 6c*
- Feeling restless, insecure, chilly, tired, and fending off anxiety by being meticulously tidy *Arsenicum 6c*
- Feeling as nervous as a racehorse, extremely sensitive to the thoughts and feelings of others, grateful for reassurance, twice as nervy during thunderstorms *Phosphorus 6c*
- Person fears for his or her sanity, forgets things, easily becomes overweight, feels the cold *Calcarea 6c*
- Person apt to dwell on morbid topics, hates fuss or sympathy *Natrum mur. 6c*
- Anxiety follows loss of a loved one or break-up of a love affair *Ignatia 6c*
- Nervous system revving out of control due to overwork, person finds it difficult to let go and relax, even in bed *Tarentula 6c*

Self-help Vitamin B complex, Vitamin C, calcium, and magnesium are recommended.

If anxiety is caused by specific situations, try to avoid them, at least for a while. Avoid tea and coffee. Relaxation and meditation (see PART 2) can also help.

Bereavement see DEATH AND DYING, GRIEF, ANNIVERSARY REACTION

Bulimia see also ANOREXIA p. 110

Compulsive eating of huge quantities of food, usually of the sweet kind, followed by guilt, self-induced vomiting and/or abuse of laxatives, and a period of normal eating or total abstinence from food. Gorging (bulimia comes from two Greek words, *bous* meaning 'ox' and *limos* meaning 'hunger') is sometimes a feature of ANOREXIA, but many bulimics are not anorexic in appearance, nor are most of them in their teens or still living under their parents' roofs, and so the true extent of the condition is not known.

For bulimics themselves, the problem is more psychological than medical; they know that bingeing is a form of consolation – perhaps for loneliness or lack of affection – but they also know that it is a form of self-punishment, like the vomiting and laxatives afterwards. If the root of the problem is DEPRESSION, INSECURITY, or a general feeling of inadequacy, psychotherapy or constitutional homeopathic treatment is recommended. Some bulimics find that vigorous exercise helps them keep their appetite under control. If no emotional cause can be established, the possibility of a food ALLERGY or nutritional deficiency should be investigated.

Specific remedies to be taken every 12 hours for up to 1 week when the urge to binge is very strong
- Person lacks emotional outlets, dislikes sympathy, puts on weight on buttocks and thighs, has a thin neck *Natrum mur. 30c*
- Person overweight, always feeling chilly, apprehensive and timid, craves eggs *Calcarea 30c*
- Person has anaemic pallor but flushes easily, oversensitive, physically weak *Ferrum 30c*
- Person timid and weeps easily, feels uncomfortable in stuffy surroundings *Pulsatilla 30c*

Claustrophobia see also PHOBIA

Acute ANXIETY about being in enclosed spaces with no means of escape, typically experienced as a feeling of suffocation. HYPERVENTILATION or HYPOGLYCAEMIA can make the experience worse, so treatment of these may reduce anxiety to an acceptable level. If not, behaviour therapy may be effective.

Specific remedies to be taken 3 times daily for up to 14 days, or ½-hourly for up to 10 doses in emergencies
- Person afraid that tall buildings will fall in on him or her, fear intense enough to cause diarrhoea *Argentum nit. 6c*

For explanation of other symbols, see page 107

- Person feels worse in hot, stuffy rooms, and weeps easily *Pulsatilla 6c*
- In an emergency, when no other remedy seems appropriate *Sulphur 6c*

Compulsions see OBSESSIONS AND COMPULSIONS

Confusion

Partial loss of contact with reality, not knowing what time of day it is, what is going on, or where you are. If a first occurrence, and not obviously related to any known physical problem, 24.

In elderly people, confusion may be a symptom of SENILE DEMENTIA, HYPOMANIA or of physical problems such as HYPOGLYCAEMIA (if no food has been eaten for some time), HYPOTHERMIA (if home is inadequately heated and person's stomach feels very cold – see First Aid p. 100), coughing, or INCONTINENCE of urine may mean there is an underlying chest or urinary infection which requires treatment.. It can be dangerous to leave a confused person, especially an elderly person, living alone; forgetting to turn off gas and electrical appliances, for example, can be disastrous. Medical supervision is essential in such cases.

If confusion comes on after a head injury, the cause may be a subdural haemorrhage (see BRAIN HAEMORRHAGE); if it is associated with weakness and DIZZINESS, NUMBNESS or tingling, blurred vision or difficulty speaking, the cause may be a STROKE or transient ischaemic attack (TIA). If brain haemorrhage, stroke, or TIA is suspected, ②.

Confusion can also accompany FEVER, and in some cases may be due to lead poisoning or drug side effects, or abuse of drugs e.g. solvents.

In both conventional and homeopathic medicine confusion is treated, in the first instance, by treating discernable physical causes. Thereafter conventional medicine offers drugs and homeopathy offers constitutional treatment.

Specific remedy
- Person confused, hasty, in a hurry in the mornings, calmer and more lucid as day goes on, constipated *Alumina 6c*, 4 times daily for up to 14 days

Self-help Supplements of potassium and Vitamin B_3 may be beneficial. Also check for lead in food and environment.

Death and dying see also GRIEF, ANNIVERSARY REACTION

The clinical signs of death are the cessation of breathing and heartbeat, and dilation and fixing of the pupils; the skin becomes pale, and the body starts to cool. If a person is on a life support system, he or she cannot be considered dead until brain death has been established; this is done by a series of tests which have to be carried out by at least two doctors. Only then may the life support system be switched off.

What we know of the subjective experience of death

we know from people who have been very near death. Most people who have had near-death experiences describe a sense of timelessness, an awareness of their own death, a strong sense of having reached reality. One of the 116 critically ill patients described in Dr Michael Sabom's study *Recollections of Death* said: 'That was the most beautiful instant in the whole world, when I came out of that body.' He remembered the experience as an absence of physical pain, a feeling of tranquillity, even of delight. If such reports are true, then the moment of death must often be more distressing for friends, relatives, and carers than for the dying person. Yet something of the quality of the moment of death seems to transmit itself to certain people; far from feeling a sense of desolation, they feel uplifted, at peace, affected by a powerful sense of awe.

The realization that death is inevitable comes to most of us around the age of nine; before the age of three we have no concept of death at all. Fear of dying is probably the most primitive and potent of all human fears. Some people come to terms with it through religion, spiritual experience, or a near-death experience. Others block off the fear, hoping that death, when it comes, will be quick and painless; when the inevitable happens, they may refuse to believe it, or go into shock, or into a state of panic, which can be very unpleasant and difficult to deal with. Most of us occasionally allow our fear to seep through to consciousness, particularly as we get older, but only partly cope with it, and get depressed and anxious.

As a general rule, it is important for people to know that they are dying, so that they have time to sort out their emotions, their spiritual understanding, and their worldly affairs. It is important that relatives and friends know too; they also need time to adjust.

For three people out of four, dying is a process rather than an event, a process that takes weeks or months. If someone asks you if he or she is dying, answer truthfully, if you know, but never force the knowledge onto someone who does not wish to know. 'How long have I got?' is a more difficult question, since it can only be answered with approximations such as days, weeks, or months. Most people who are dying are, at some level, aware of the fact even though they may deny it; denial is an attempt to hang on to independence and dignity.

Care of the dying Home care may be feasible if the carer has the support of GP, nurses, relatives, and friends, but it is important that he or she has time off to sleep and relax. The first duty of anyone caring for a dying person is to alleviate physical pain and discomfort but not, if it can be helped, at the cost of affecting the dying person's awareness. So whether homeopathic remedies or orthodox drugs are used, small doses at frequent intervals may be better than large doses at long intervals. Your GP will be able to advise on this.

In the terminal stages of dying, restlessness and

noisy breathing are quite common. This is because secretions in the lungs are no longer being coughed up. At this time emotional comfort may be even more important than physical comfort; holding a person's hand communicates sympathy and reassurance in a way which drugs and remedies cannot.

If home care is out of the question, or no longer practical, admission to a hospice may be possible; hospices specialize in care of the dying and allow people to die with more dignity than can be catered for in a busy hospital ward.

Homeopathic treatment of the dying requires considerable skill. If at all possible, consult an experienced homeopath. However, the two remedies below may be helpful.

Specific remedies to be given as often as symptoms recur or worsen
- Person very afraid of dying, very restless, thirsty for sips of water, wants to sit up *Arsenicum 30c*
- Lungs very congested, person literally drowning in own phlegm *Antimonium tart. 30c*

Legalities of death A Death Certificate must be issued. This is the duty of the dead person's GP, unless death occurs in unusual circumstances or the GP has not seen the person for some time, in which case a Coroner's Report is required. When issuing the Death Certificate, the GP will explain what you should do next. Contact an undertaker to arrange the funeral, and get in touch with the dead person's solicitor.

Bereavement It is important to have an outlet for GRIEF. True mourning cannot begin until we realize that a loved one is really and truly dead. One of the functions of a burial or cremation ceremony is to bring that realization home to us. It also allows us to express grief. If weeks or months pass and your feelings of loss are still bottled up inside you, a memorial service, or just a visit to the grave or crematorium, may help you to get in touch with emotions you have suppressed. See GRIEF for homeopathic remedies.

Specific remedy
- Where death has been particularly violent or terrible, and relatives or witnesses go into a state of shock *Aconite 30c* to be taken every 5 or 10 minutes until shock wears off

Delirium see also DELIRIUM TREMENS
Extreme confusion, in which person is completely out of touch with reality, disoriented, excited, incoherent, unaware of surroundings or of other people, and possibly having HALLUCINATIONS. Can be brought on by FEVER or withdrawal from drugs or alchohol (see ALCOHOLISM, DRUG ADDICTION); delirium brought on by withdrawal from alcohol is known as DELIRIUM TREMENS. The wisest course, regardless of the cause, is ②, then select a from the list below.

Specific remedies to be given every 15 minutes for up to 10 doses while waiting for help
- Fever, face flushed and hot, eyes wide and staring *Belladonna 30c*
- Person very restless, terrified of being left alone, whole body icy cold *Arsenicum 6c*
- Delirium comes on suddenly, person obsessed with death and dying *Aconite 30c*
- Delirium accompanied by foolish laughter and obscene talk or gestures *Hyoscyamus 6c*
- Great muttering and writhing, tendency to be violent *Stramonium 6c*
- Delirium in someone who has heart disease *Lachesis 6c*
- Delirium in someone who has lung disease *Bryonia 6c*
- Delirium in someone who has diabetes *Opium 6c*

Delirium tremens see also ALCOHOLISM
The result of ADDICTION to alcohol or barbiturates. When physical craving is not satisfied, withdrawal symptoms set in; these include muscular tremors and twitching, INSOMNIA, PALPITATIONS, and HALLUCINATIONS. Condition requires professional medical treatment, so ②. Person will probably be admitted to hospital, sedated, and given injections of Vitamin B.

Specific remedies to be given every 15 minutes until help arrives
- Flushed face, staring eyes *Belladonna 30c*
- Hallucinations about insects *Stramonium 6c*
- A lot of muttering and obscene talk *Hyoscyamus 6c*
- Person excessively restless and agitated *Arsenicum 6c*

Delusions see PARANOIA, SCHIZOPHRENIA

Depression see also POSTNATAL DEPRESSION, MANIC DEPRESSION
A small word that describes a huge range of negative thoughts and feelings from sadness to utter hopelessness, and an equally broad spectrum of physical symptoms. If the cause is a specific external event, such as bereavement, depression is usually temporary; it has a natural timespan, and after a while life regains its interest and colour. Depression can also follow childbirth (see POSTNATAL DEPRESSION). It can also occur after GLANDULAR FEVER and other viral infections (see POST-VIRAL SYNDROME), or be brought on by changes in body chemistry produced by ADDICTION to drugs or alcohol. Occasionally it is a symptom of developing SCHIZOPHRENIA. But far more often it is the mind which manufactures causes for depression, in the form of rather fixed, life-denying attitudes and beliefs which lead to fear, ANGER, guilt, frustration, a sense of persecution, loneliness, hopelessness. . . These then affect the body, which in turn affects the mind, and so the vicious circle is established. One person in twenty-five feels depressed enough to seek professional help at some point in his or her life, and on average twice as

many women seek help as men. Depression is not something to be ashamed of; it is a recognized illness.

Depression is diagnosed when a person has been feeling down for a significant length of time, for months rather than weeks, and when some of the following symptoms are also present: a significant increase or decrease in appetite or weight, excessive sleep or an inability to sleep, a marked slowing down of movement and thinking, a marked lack of energy, inability to concentrate or make decisions, general loss of interest in activities once considered enjoyable, recurrent thoughts of DEATH or SUICIDE. If several of these symptoms are present, don't delay in seeking professional help. Severe or prolonged depression yields more surely to professional help than to self-help or help from friends or relatives; the sufferer (and to some extent those around him or her) is too locked inside the depression to be objective about it.

It is not true that people who talk of suicide do not attempt suicide; they can and do. If you feel that life is no longer worth living, and start thinking about suicide and the methods you are going to use, call the Samaritans or your doctor immediately. You need help, fast.

The symptoms described above are one aspect of a form of depression called MANIC DEPRESSION, in which mood alternates between depression and mania. In manic phases the person is reckless and impulsive, highly energetic, even euphoric.

If your GP diagnoses mild depression, he or she will probably prescribe antidepressants or refer you to to a psychotherapist. Antidepressants do not cure depression; they merely relieve distressing symptoms until the underlying causes resolve themselves. If depression is severe you will be referred to a psychiatrist; again the options are antidepressants and psycho-therapy, and in extreme cases ECT (electroconvulsive therapy) which requires a stay in hospital, and perhaps occupational therapy to re-establish a normal pattern of life. You should think long and hard before agreeing to ECT as it can impair long-term memory and its effects may not be permanent. Where there is a marked chemical component to depression a change in diet may be recommended (excess Vitamin D, zinc, copper, and lead are known to contribute to depression).

Both chronic and acute depression will respond to constitutional treatment from an experienced homeo-path, but if you, or a friend or a relative, feel suicidal, call the Samaritans or your doctor immediately.

Specific remedies to be taken 3 times daily for up to 14 days during episodes of mild or moderate depression or while waiting for constitutional treatment
- Person restless, chilly, exhausted, obsessively neat and tidy *Arsenicum 6c*
- Feeling chilly, suffering from wind, on edge, over-sensitive to noise, light and other stimuli, racing thoughts get in the way of sleep, vivid dreams leave

you exhausted on waking *China 6c*
- Lack of energy and stamina after viral illness such as flu or glandular fever *Cadmium phos. 6c*
- Feeling totally worthless, suicidal, disgusted with oneself and *Aurum 6c* (if suicidal, also phone the Samaritans or your doctor).
- Depression follows deep grief or heartbreak after a love affair *Ignatia 6c*
- Bottling up emotions, rejecting sympathy because it embarrasses you and makes you want to break down and cry, wanting to hide away *Natrum mur. 6c*
- Bursting into tears at the slightest provocation, wanting a lot of reassurance and attention *Pulsatilla 6c*
- Extremely irritable, finding fault with everyone around you *Nux 6c*
- Feeling irritable, tearful, chilly, very turned off even by the idea of sex *Sepia 6c*

Self-help Mild depression can often be relieved by making minor changes in lifestyle. If you feel under too much pressure, give up one or two activities that are not essential. If you feel isolated or out of touch, try to get out more or take up a new interest so that you meet other people. If you have children, organize a baby sitter so that you can have at least one night a week to yourself. Make sure your diet does not include excessive amounts of Vitamin D, zinc, copper, or lead, and avoid tea and coffee. In some women, oral contraceptives seem to contribute to depression; the obvious course is to discuss alternatives with your GP. Increase your intake of Vitamins B_1, B_2, B_3, B_5, B_6, and C, folate, biotin, bioflavinoids, calcium, potassium, and magnesium.

Drug addiction see also ADDICTION

Addictive drugs may be legal and prescribed by a doctor, or illegal and 'recreational'. The longer a drug is taken for, the more the body adapts to it; when the drug is stopped, the adaptive mechanisms continue to operate, unopposed by the drug, usually producing unpleasant rebound effects such as restless-ness, trembling, nervousness, and ANXIETY.

Among the prescription drugs the benzodiazepines or Valium-type tranquilizers (especially Lorazepam or Ativan) are the most addictive and the most commonly prescribed; they should not be taken for longer than 2–3 weeks; if taken continuously for 3 months or more, the person taking them is likely to have become addicted to them. The main effect of benzodiazepine drugs is ABNORMAL SLEEPINESS OR DROWSINESS. If you suspect an overdose, but the person is still conscious, give First Aid (see Poisoning p. 102) and take him or her to your local casualty department; if unconscious, (999) put him or her in the recovery position (see First Aid p. 90–91) and take any tablets, powders, or drug-taking equipment along to the hospital for identification.

Illegal drugs include marijuana, LSD, cocaine, opiates such as heroin, and various solvents taken by sniffing. As with alcohol, there is no easy demarcation line between social use and addiction, or casual use and intensive use. Unfortunately in a book of this scope it is not possible to describe each drug and the kind of addiction it causes. But if you are a parent and are worried about your child taking drugs, write to the DHSS Leaflet Unit (address p. 385) and ask for the leaflet 'Drugs: what you can do as a parent'; it describes the effects of all the commonest substances of abuse, what the symptoms of addiction are, and how to get help.

If you yourself have a problem, seek expert help, initially through your GP or homeopath.

There are many reasons why people turn to drugs, why they 'escape into failure' – they may be insecure and unhappy, bored, fed up with establishment values, or simply copying their peers and unable to resist the urge to experiment.

Whether a drug is regarded as 'soft' or 'hard', 'recreational' or 'social', or taken casually or intensively, it is *illegal*. Some of the consequences of taking drugs – the hassle, the fines, the imprisonment, the social stigma – may well endorse the user's low opinion of society, but it is the user, and his or her family and friends, who will be damaged, not society. Also, drugs popularly seen as harmless may be more damaging than was once thought; recent reports suggest that frequent marijuana abuse causes irreversible brain damage.

Coming off prescription drugs If you feel you are becoming addicted to a drug, go and see your doctor and explain your feelings. If he or she advises you not to come off it, ask why (the effects of coming off some prescription drugs, Ativan for example, can be very unpleasant). If you are not satisfied with the explanation, you are entitled to seek a second opinion, but make sure the person you seek it from is medically qualified. There may be a tranquilizer addicts' support group in your area (Citizens' Advice Bureau will give you the address) through which you can find sympathetic help, or perhaps assurance that the symptoms you are experiencing are nothing to worry about. A medically qualified homeopath may or may not recommend constitutional treatment, but will almost certainly prescribe vitamins and mineral supplements (especially Vitamins B and C, and calcium and magnesium) to aid recovery from the drug.

To put your system in a fit state to do without the drug, reduce your consumption of tea, coffee, cigarettes, and alcohol before you start to come off; come off the drug gradually rather than suddenly, unless you are on a very small dose; and take more exercise – it will increase the general efficiency of your metabolism.

Coming off illegal drugs Living without drugs, once the habit has developed, takes a lot of courage, discipline,

and perseverance, and the chances of coming off and staying off are better with professional help than without it. This is especially true of opiate drugs such as heroin. However, there is great controversy as to whether the short-term 'cold turkey' (detoxification) approach or the long-term 'maintenance' approach is more effective/ethical/socially responsible. Maintenance, on synthetic opiates such as methadone, may cut down burglary and theft as a means of financing drug-taking, but it does not 'cure' addiction; in fact many addicts find methadone harder to kick than heroin. Detoxification treatment is given on an in-patient basis, maintenance by a GP or a local drug clinic. Most large towns have a branch of Narcotics Anonymous, which offers support and counselling to anyone who has a drug problem; Families Anonymous is a sister organization which offers support to the relatives and friends of addicts.

Addiction cannot be treated homeopathically, but constitutional treatment can prevent drug-taking progressing beyond the experimental stage. There are also a number of specific remedies which antidote the effects of first time use. However, if a person becomes violent, suicidal, or appears to be losing consciousness, ⑨⑨⑨; if possible, gently restrain the person, but without putting yourself in danger, or, if appropriate, put him or her in the recovery position (see First Aid p. 90–91).

Specific remedies to be taken every 15 minutes for up to 10 doses or until the effects of first time use wear off
- Great anxiety, restlessness, fear of being alone *Arsenicum 6c*
- Person depressed or very talkative, feeling persecuted *Lachesis 6c*
- Sudden panic, fear of dying, feeling chilly *Aconite 30c*
- Person depressed, dizzy, disorientated, having hallucinations *Absinthium 6c*
- Marked paranoia (person feels persecuted or controlled by external forces), muttering, obscene talk and behaviour *Hyoscyamus 6c*

Self-help A course of multivitamins and minerals is recommended.

Drug withdrawal see ADDICTION

Fears see PHOBIAS, AGORAPHOBIA, CLAUSTROPHOBIA, INSECURITY

Fright see also SHOCK
An extreme reaction to a threatening event. Breathing rate speeds up, sometimes leading to HYPERVENTILATION; adrenaline pours into the bloodstream, speeding up heartbeat, felt in extreme cases as PALPITATIONS; digestion slows down, causing a churning sensation in the stomach; blood vessels in the skin constrict, causing the skin to turn pale.

If any of the above symptoms follows injury, or is

accompanied by NAUSEA AND VOMITING, severe pain, FAINTING, or clouding of consciousness, the person may be in shock, in which case ⑨⑨⑨ and give First Aid (see p. 103).

Specific remedies to be given 4 times daily for up to 14 days, or ½-hourly for up to 10 doses in extreme cases
- Marked palpitations, fear of dying *Aconite 30c*
- Person scared stiff, numb and dozy with fright *Opium 6c*
- Person hysterical, weeping one minute and laughing the next *Ignatia 6c*
- Inability to get to sleep because mind is racing *Coffea 6c*

Grief see also DEATH AND DYING

A natural reaction to the loss of a person, animal, or object in whom or in which one has invested much love and affection; not a reaction to be underestimated or bottled up. Grieving is a process which has several fairly distinct stages. First, there may be a sense of unreality, numbness, a refusal to believe that the loved one is dead; then there may be a mixture of complex emotions such as guilt (at not having been close enough to the person or done enough for them, for example) and ANGER (that the hospital or doctor did not do enough, that the person had no right to die, etc.). Then DEPRESSION may set in. Finally, life becomes bearable again, even enjoyable. The whole process may take from one to two years, and even then there may be a painful ANNIVERSARY REACTION when the anniversary of the person's death comes round.

How well we cope with grief depends partly on our relationship with the dead person; if there were elements in the relationship that gave rise to strong feelings of guilt or anger, grief may be blocked. A lonely, isolated person may also find grief difficult to cope with; he or she has no one to express grief to. There is also a theory that in grieving we relive the experience of being separated from the nipple; if our infantile reaction was rage and desolation, our adult reaction to the loss of love may be the same, making it very difficult to progress through the various stages of grief to full recovery. If grief lasts for longer than about 18 months, professional help may be necessary to prevent depression becoming chronic.

Most people receive a lot of attention and kindness in the weeks immediately after bereavement, but it is often four or five months later that they need most support; that is often the worst time, when they finally accept that the person is dead. Give as much practical help as you can, and allow the person to talk about his or her loss even if it is painful; if he or she so much as hints at SUICIDE, seek professional help. And continue your support for as long as you can.

Orthodox treatment of grief is based on anti-depressants and psychotherapy, or both. Homeopathy offers specific remedies during the various stages of grief, and also constitutional help if there is a failure to progress from one stage to the next.

Early stages *Specific remedies* to be taken 4 times daily for up to 14 days, or every hour for up to 10 doses if feelings of grief are overpowering
- Person wants to be left alone, insists that he or she feels all right, doesn't want to be touched, reactions are those of someone in shock *Arnica 30c*
- Person fearful, on verge of collapse *Aconite 30c*
- Person very frightened by death of loved one, numb with grief *Opium 6c*

Later stages *Specific remedies* to be taken 3 times daily for up to 14 days, or every 2 hours for up to 10 doses if feelings are disrupting normal life
- Person extremely angry and critical of others *Nux 6c*
- Person very depressed and apathetic *Phosphoric ac. 6c*
- Sleeplessness, helpless weeping, catarrh *Pulsatilla 6c*
- Person rejects consolation and sympathy because it makes him or her cry, prefers to hide feelings *Natrum mur. 6c*
- Person finds emotions difficult to control, and laughs, sighs, or cries at inappropriate moments *Ignatia 6c*

Final stages See remedies listed under DEPRESSION.

Self-help Talk, say how you feel, ask for help. A stiff upper lip may look dignified, but the cost may be chronic depression and lowered resistance to illness. Organizations such as Cruse (address p. 387) offer counselling and support to the bereaved. Your homeopath or GP may be able to recommend a psychotherapist who can help you to get over the worst. Some people seek comfort in spiritualism, but it takes an experienced spiritualist, and one who has some knowledge of basic psychotherapy, to assist a person through the mourning process; satisfying a desire to communicate with the dead may prolong grief rather than assuage it and make it difficult to move on. Above all, be patient with yourself.

Hallucinations

In the normal waking state our perceptions are real in the sense that they are caused by external stimuli, but if we are under hypnosis, or suffering from lack of food or sleep, or deprived of normal stimuli, or experiencing great emotional stress, or taking hallucinogenic drugs, or drinking large quantities of alcohol ... the mind begins to manufacture its own stimuli, as it does in dreams, and we hallucinate. It is not unusual for someone who has just been bereaved, for example, to see or hear the person who has died. Hallucinations can also accompany DELIRIUM brought on by FEVER, ALCOHOLISM, or DRUG ADDICTION; hallucinogenics

---

⑨⑨⑨ Emergency – call GP (or dial 999) immediately. ② Consult your doctor if no improvement within 2 hours

like LSD tend to cause visual rather than auditory sensations. Accusing, persecuting voices may be a sign of DEPRESSION or PARANOIA. Physical sensations such as animals wriggling about in the stomach, or complaints that food has been poisoned, may be early signs of SCHIZOPHRENIA.

Orthodox treatment is by drugs in the first instance, followed by treatment of the underlying cause. Homeopathy offers constitutional treatment, and also the emergency remedies listed below.

If hallucinations are accompanied by CONFUSION, extreme agitation, or physical symptoms, ②.

Specific remedies to be given every 10–15 minutes for up to 10 doses in acute situations or while waiting for help
- Terrifying visions, loss of memory, giddiness and a tendency to fall backwards, particularly if person has taken LSD or other hallucinogenic drugs *Absinthium 6c*
- Hallucinations which transform even a spoonful of water into a huge lake, or a small crack into a gaping chasm, person shaking and trembling *Agaricus 6c*
- Hallucinations mainly visual, usually of monsters with hideous mouths and eyes, person has hot, red face and staring eyes *Belladonna 30c*
- Slowed sense of time in which seconds seem like hours, uncontrollable laughter *Cannabis ind. 6c*
- Hallucinations accompanied by great suspiciousness, quarrelsomeness, and obscene behaviour *Hyoscyamus 6c*
- Person drowsy, lapses into heavy sleep *Opium 6c*
- Person very talkative, says prayers, hears voices, sees ghosts and spirits *Stramonium 6c*

Hypochondria

Obsessive ANXIETY about the workings of one's own body; buying lots of medicines and consulting one doctor after another are attempts to keep the anxiety at bay. Constitutional treatment from an experienced homeopath may help. The structure of the homeopathic consultation is likely to encourage the person to think of himself or herself as a harmonious entity rather than as a collection of parts to be tinkered with.

Specific remedies to be taken 4 times daily for up to 14 days while waiting for constitutional treatment
- Person obsessed with heart disease, skin dry and scaly *Kali ars. 6c*
- Person complains of burning pains, feels anxious, restless, and chilly, thirsty for small sips of water *Arsenicum 6c*
- Person constipated, depressed, has a muddy complexion *Natrum mur. 6c*
- Where main symptom is disordered digestion, person also irritable, angry, and behaving violently *Nux 6c*
- Person fears for his or her sanity *Calcarea 6c*
- Where cause is enforced abstinence from sex *Conium 6c*

Self-help Exercise, relaxation, meditation, in fact any activity which encourages body and mind to work in harmony, is almost sure to be beneficial. Vitamin C is also recommended.

Hysteria

Symptoms brought on by severe STRESS, ranging from inability to control emotions normally to partial PARALYSIS or loss of various sensory functions. Even a very stable person can become hysterical under extreme stress. If you are prone to stress and find your emotions difficult to control, constitutional homeopathic treatment could help.

Extreme hysterical reactions, such as AMNESIA, paralysis, or loss of speech, hearing, or sight require professional treatment, so 12 . In the meantime, one or other of the remedies listed below may be helpful.

Specific remedies to be given once every 15 minutes or once every 2 hours for up to 10 doses depending on severity of symptoms
- Symptoms brought on by grief or break up of a love affair, sudden changes of mood, person complains of lump in throat and other inappropriate symptoms (such as a sore throat made better by swallowing) *Ignatia 6c*
- Symptoms accompanied by sensations of floating, levitating, or losing identity, sleeplessness *Valeriana 6c*
- Person haughty and contemptuous, feels numb and cold *Platinum 6c*
- Person becomes manipulative and over-dramatic, has palpitations, complains of difficult breathing and tightness in chest, even asthma *Moschus 6c*
- Person becomes asthmatic, develops hysterical cough, feels as if body is about to explode, gullet and stomach tend to work in reverse, rejecting food and causing retching *Asafoetida 6c*

Self-help Vitamin C is often helpful.

Insecurity see also ANXIETY

Now and then almost everyone feels insecure, often with good reason; insecurity often prompts us to put our affairs in order and make contingency plans. Chronic insecurity, which can manifest itself as DEPRESSION, SHYNESS, LACK OF CONFIDENCE, or inability to form stable relationships, has less to do with external events than with unrealistic expectations and a rather gloomy view of self. Homeopathy regards such tendencies as symptoms of constitutional imbalance; treatment is therefore long-term and constitutional. In acute circumstances, one of the remedies below should be tried.

Specific remedies to be given 4 times daily for up to 14 days
- Insecurity brought on by a traumatic or near-death experience *Aconite 30c*

- Insecurity after bereavement or break-up of love affair *Ignatia 6c*
- Person nervous and highly strung, comforted by sympathy and reassurance *Phosphorus 6c*
- Person shy, tearful, feels worse in hot, stuffy rooms *Pulsatilla 6c*

Insomnia see SLEEP PROBLEMS

Irritability *see ANGER*

Manic depression (bipolar depression) see also DEPRESSION

Inexplicable and extreme mood swings, from joy and elation to gloom and apathy, interspersed with periods of normal functioning. Changes of mood are part of normal human functioning, but they last only a short while and have fairly obvious causes. For someone who is a manic-depressive, the highs are very high and the lows are very low, and can last for weeks, and neither seem to be linked with obvious external causes. This has prompted some psychiatrists to suggest that an imbalance in body chemistry is the cause: according to one theory, over-sensitivity to light may disrupt production of hormones by the pineal gland. Studies of the Amish community in the United States suggest that manic depression runs in families. Whatever the cause, the condition affects three times as many women as men, often after childbirth or during the MENOPAUSE.

In deep depression SUICIDE is unlikely, but the risk of suicide increases as mood begins to swing up again. In the manic phase the person is frenetically active, full of plans and projects, few of which get accomplished; behaviour may also be reckless or socially unacceptable. Some psychiatrists distinguish between full blown *mania*, in which behaviour is outrageous and often violent, and *hypomania*, in which behaviour is less extreme. In between alternating episodes of depression and mania there may be very long periods, sometimes years, of normal functioning.

Manic depression is conventionally treated by a combination of drugs, especially lithium and psychotherapy, and in extreme cases may require admission to hospital. Homeopathy offers constitutional treatment, and also a number of remedies for use during manic episodes (for remedies during depressive bouts, see DEPRESSION). If person is suicidal, (999); if hallucinating or uncontrollably violent during manic episodes, (2).

Specific remedies to be given every 4 hours for up to 10 doses, or ½-hourly for up to 6 doses if mania is extreme
- Person convinced he or she is going to die, not thirsty, very jealous *Apis 30c*
- Person hallucinating, quarrelsome, making obscene remarks, afraid of being poisoned (2) and *Hyoscyamus 6c*

- Person looks as if he or she has high fever, face red, eyes wild and staring *Belladonna 30c*
- Sense of time awry, everything very slowed down, uncontrollable laughter, exalted ideas *Cannabis ind. 6c*
- Flashes of temper, mood goes up and down like a yoyo, reassurance has calming effect *Phosphorus 6c*

Self-help Take extra Vitamin C but avoid dairy products, grains, refined carbohydrates, tea, coffee, and food additives.

Memory loss

Brief loss of memory is not uncommon after drinking alcohol, or after a high FEVER, an operation, an epileptic fit (see EPILEPSY), or a diabetic coma (see DIABETES). DEPRESSION and ANXIETY can also cause temporary memory loss. In these circumstances, inability to remember is not something to worry about; nor is everyday forgetfulness, which tends to increase as we get older; most of us cope by using mnemonic aids such as lists and diaries. We also tend to forget unpleasant things, a mechanism which psychoanalysts call repression; hysterical amnesia is partial or total repression of memories that are too threatening to live with. Memory loss can also follow an accident or injury, temporarily wiping out the events which led up to it. BRAIN INJURY, especially after a blow to the head or a STROKE, can cause irreversible memory loss, affecting intelligence, personality, speech, and movement. PRE-SENILE and SENILE DEMENTIA involve progressive loss of short-term memory until, eventually, the person is quite unable to remember what he or she did or said or heard or saw a moment before; the first signs may be a decline in personal appearance and cleanliness, or difficulty following conversations or instructions. Memory difficulties can also be a side effect of some prescription drugs.

If memory loss occurs after a head injury, (2); if after taking a new drug, 48.

Memory difficulties are often associated with symptoms which benefit from constitutional homeopathic treatment, and are therefore best treated constitutionally.

Specific remedies to be given 4 times daily for up to 14 days
- Person elderly, behaviour childish, attention wandering, finds words most difficult to remember *Calcarea 6c*
- Words cause most difficulty, person anaemic, colicky, or suffering from a nervous complaint *Plumbum 6c*
- Person absent-minded because of inner conflict between two seemingly different personalities, memory for names most affected *Anacardium 6c*
- Difficulty remembering words and names *Sulphur 6c*

---

(999) Emergency – call GP (or dial 999) immediately. (2) Consult your doctor if no improvement within 2 hours

Specific remedies after head injury
- Person forgets what he or she had just heard, read, or said, or is about to say, also slow in answering questions *Arnica 30c* every 2 hours for up to 10 doses
- If memory difficulties persist after taking Arnica *Helleborus 6c* every 8 hours for up to 14 days

Self-help Take extra Vitamin B_3, B_6 and B_{12}.

Mental exhaustion see also STRESS

Also referred to as nervous exhaustion or nervous breakdown, a catch-all term not used by psychiatrists but meaningful to the ordinary person, signifying a sudden inability to cope, usually due to overwork or other forms of pressure. Just as ligaments and tendons can be stretched beyond their elastic limit, so can emotional and mental resources. Some people have more resilience and stamina, more ability to absorb STRESS for longer periods, than others. If it takes very little to topple you into ANXIETY or DEPRESSION, constitutional homeopathic treatment could help.

Specific remedies to be taken every 2 hours for up to 10 doses
- Feeling emotionally drained by grief, very apathetic, physically exhausted *Phosphoric ac. 6c*
- Lack of will-power or determination *Picric ac. 6c*
- Feeling mentally exhausted after working hard for exams *Anacardium 6c*
- Headache and exhaustion from overwork *Silicea 6c*
- Great sensitivity to noise, forgetfulness, a tendency to repeat everything *Zinc 6c*

Mourning see GRIEF

Nervous breakdown see MENTAL EXHAUSTION

Nightmares see SLEEP PROBLEMS

Obsessions and compulsions

An obsession is a thought or idea that seizes the mind and won't let go; a compulsion is an irresistible urge to act out a thought or idea, however absurd. HYPOCHONDRIA, for example, is an obsession with health which is translated into buying cupboardfuls of medicines; ANOREXIA is an obsession with physical appearance which translates itself into self-starvation. Most people develop relatively harmless obsessions and compulsions at some time or other, commonly to do with diet, health, hygiene, and personal safety. But if certain thoughts or actions begin to dominate behaviour and disrupt work, family, and social life, treatment should be sought, initially through your GP. A combination of psychotherapy and drugs is the conventional solution, although in extreme cases surgery may be used to cut certain nerve pathways in the brain. Homeopathic treatment is constitutional and long-term, and compatible with psychotherapy but not always with psychoactive drugs.

Specific remedies to be taken every 2 hours for up to 10 doses only if an obsession or compulsion becomes overwhelming.
- Thoughts of death and dying, feeling utterly worthless (999), then *Aurum 30c*
- Person feels as if body and mind are separate, or that his or her mind is being controlled by some superhuman agency *Anacardium or. 30c*
- Unshakeable feelings of inadequacy, overwhelming urge to sit on floor and count small objects *Silicea 30c*
- Person convinced there are live animals wriggling round in stomach, or that limbs are made of glass and so brittle they will break, especially if he or she has warts *Thuja 30c*

Organic psychosis see PSYCHOTIC ILLNESS

Panic see PANIC p. 102; also FRIGHT, PHOBIA, ANXIETY

Paralysed wakefulness see SLEEP PROBLEMS

Paranoia see also SCHIZOPHRENIA, PSYCHOTIC ILLNESS

Persistent delusions about being persecuted, occasionally accompanied by HALLUCINATIONS. The behaviour of the person concerned is usually completely consistent with his or her delusions of being followed, spied on, picked upon, singled out for destruction. Full-blown paranoia is classed as a psychotic illness, as are SCHIZOPHRENIA and MANIC DEPRESSION, and is conventionally treated by drugs. If person attempts to harm himself or herself, or others, in an effort to evade persecution, or begins to hallucinate, (2).

Constitutional homeopathic treatment is only appropriate in less severe cases.

Specific remedies to be given every 12 hours for up to 10 doses while professional treatment is being sought
- Symptoms fairly mild *Lachesis 30c*
- Symptoms acute and severe *Hyoscyamus 30c*

Self-help Vitamin B_3 may be beneficial.

Phobia see also AGORAPHOBIA, CLAUSTROPHOBIA, ANXIETY

A phobia is a more or less disabling fear attached to a specific object or situation which is, on the face of it, not at all threatening. A fear of snakes is reasonable in the middle of Africa, less so in Britain, but when a picture or even a shape suggestive of a snake causes intense physical loathing, the fear is irrational, phobic. Most of us have a phobic reaction to something, but in the normal course of events either manage to avoid it or to keep our fear in check.

A phobia may be the result of an unpleasant personal experience, but it can also be a fear copied from parents, a fear transferred from quite another object or set of circumstances, or a fear dredged up from the deepest levels of consciousness where Jung imagined the collective memory of the human species to exist. More prosaically, though rarely, phobias can be due to organic disease, to EPILEPSY, BRAIN TUMOURS, or BRAIN INJURY. Acute panic states can also be brought on by HYPOGLYCAEMIA (low blood sugar levels) or HYPER-VENTILATION (fast, shallow breathing which starves the brain of oxygen).

Where no organic cause can be found, conventional treatment is by drugs (to control the anxiety), and various forms of behaviour therapy, notably desensitiz-ation (step by step exposure to the feared object or situation, coupled with relaxation techniques) and flooding (very unpleasant, full-scale exposure to it). Homeopathy offers constitutional treatment, and a number of remedies for specific situations. See also remedies listed under FRIGHT.

Fear of heights   Specific remedies to be taken 4 times daily for up to 14 days, or ½-hourly for up to 10 doses if fear is intense
- Fear associated with impulse to jump *Argentum nit. 6c*
- Fear associated with sensation of falling *Borax 6c*
- Fear associated with extreme giddiness *Sulphur 6c*

Fear of the dark   Specific remedies to be taken 4 times daily for up to 14 days, or ½-hourly for up to 10 doses if fear is acute
- Person talks and prays continuously *Stramonium 6c*
- Person nervous and highly strung, responds immedi-ately to affection and reassurance *Phosphorus 6c*

Stage fright, fear of performing in public   Specific remedies to be taken 4 times daily for up to 14 days, or ½-hourly for up to 10 doses if fear is acute
- Great apprehension, although person performs well once he or she has started, or person who, when eating in company, feels full after a small amount of food and socially inadequate *Lycopodium 6c*
- Person feels weak at the knees *Gelsemium 6c*
- Where person is a musician and prone to stomach upsets *Anacardium 6c*
- Fear acute enough to cause flatulence and diarr-hoea *Argentum nit. 6c*

Self-help With certain phobias, if motivation is strong enough, it is possible to desensitize yourself to some extent; this is true of some animal phobias, and of CLAUSTROPHOBIA and AGORAPHOBIA. Take things very slowly, exposing yourself to the thing you fear step by step; learn a few simple breathing and relaxation techniques (see PART 2) so that you can defuse anxiety each time it threatens to get the better of you.

Psychopathic behaviour see also HYPERACTIVITY

Usually starts at a young age, with the person concerned failing to learn the social and moral lessons which stop most of us from giving way to our more violent and destructive impulses; he or she is emotion-ally unstable, irresponsible, perhaps violent, un-touched by the hurt and harm caused to others, and often unable to form steady relationships or hold down a job for very long. Most psychopaths eventually fall foul of the law, often with repeated convictions for assault or vandalism. Somewhere in the immediate family background of most such offenders is mental instability, ALCOHOLISM, and criminality, providing support for both genetic and environmental theorists, but there may be other causes. It has now been shown, for example, that some forms of violent behaviour are caused by food ALLERGY. If a youngster suddenly becomes very restless and destructive, but otherwise seems to understand and abide by basic social rules, it would be sensible to consult a nutritionally trained physician. Drugs and alcohol, HYPOGLYCAEMIA and some forms of BRAIN DAMAGE, can also remove inhibitions and lead to antisocial behaviour.

Psychopathy is treated, in the context of a high security psychiatric hospital if the person is extremely violent, by the use of tranquillizers, although the nutritional approach is slowly gaining ground, parti-cularly in the United States, thanks to the work of Alexander Schauss.

Extreme anti-social behaviour is not treatable homeopathically, but a tendency towards emotional instability can be treated constitutionally.

Psychotic illness see also MANIC DEPRESSION, SCHIZOPHRENIA, PARANOIA

Severe disturbance of thoughts and emotions in which person is completely out of touch with reality as other people perceive it. Symptoms include complete social withdrawal, profound apathy, delusions, HALLUCIN-ATIONS and other sensory distortions, and wildly inappropriate speech, behaviour, thoughts, and feel-ings. MANIC DEPRESSION, SCHIZOPHRENIA, and PARA-NOIA are classed, by the psychiatric profession, as psychoses or psychotic illnesses. There is much debate about causes, ranging from the genetic and biochemi-cal to the environmental and frankly existential. Some psychotic states, however, can be fairly clearly related to damage or injury to the brain. These are known as *organic psychoses*, to distinguish them from other forms of psychosis which appear to have no physical cause. Psychotic behaviour can be triggered off, for example, by an impact injury to the brain, by a BRAIN TUMOUR, by toxic metals (lead, mercury, copper), by certain prescrip-tion drugs, or by lung infections such as PNEUMONIA. In such cases, treatment or removal of the apparent cause may relieve psychotic symptoms. Conventional treatment of non-organic psychoses is by antipsychotic drugs, with or without admission to hospital.

Once the cause has been found and treated, or once orthodox drugs have stabilized behaviour, constitutional homeopathic treatment and nutritional manipulation are recommended.

Psychosomatic illness
As Hahnemann pointed out, there is no such a thing as a one-sided ailment, an ailment purely of the body (*soma* in Greek) or purely of the minde (*psyche*). Even something as obviously physical as an accident may have an emotional cause, such as worry or inattention. Psychosomatic ailments are physical conditions which seem to be caused, or maintained, or significantly aggravated by emotional factors; into this category come HIGH BLOOD PRESSURE, HEART ATTACK, ASTHMA, ECZEMA, PSORIASIS, ALLERGY, MIGRAINE, PEPTIC ULCERS, and OBESITY. The homeopathic approach is constitutional, aimed at treating mind and body as a whole.

Schizophrenia
A severe and disturbing illness in which normal patterns of thought and feeling appear to break down. Symptoms are highly variable, and a number of different forms of schizophrenia are recognized. Some sufferers experience thought blocking as well as great pressure of thought; at one moment they feel utterly overwhelmed and bombarded by thoughts and images and sensations, and the next blank out completely. For others the main features are gradual social withdrawal, and a slowing up and general disorganisation of thinking. Another form of schizophrenia is characterized by stupor and immobility, with the emotions becoming dull and flat, or at times wildly inappropriate. In some cases PARANOIA – delusions of grandeur, of persecution, of being controlled from another planet, of having thoughts stolen and thought by others – takes the leading role. HALLUCINATIONS, more often auditory than visual, are quite common.

The causes of schizophrenia are not known, although most psychiatrists believe that the answer lies somewhere in the chemistry of the brain. Many social workers and psychologists, however, point to problems in the family as the cause or trigger. Nutritionists point to food ALLERGY as a possible cause. Recently, some researchers claim to have identified a substance in the urine of schizophrenics which can be made to disappear by giving large doses of vitamins and minerals, with some remission of symptoms, but not all schizophrenics respond to such treatment or even agree to it. Drugs, especially the phenothiazaines, still constitute the main form of treatment.

Schizophrenia is relatively rare, and those most at risk, whether for genetic or environmental reasons, are likely to have a mother or father who is schizophrenic. Schizoid tendencies, however, are more common; 1 person in a 100 has a tendency towards shyness and withdrawal, INSECURITY, or PARANOIA.

Because of its complex and disturbing nature, diagnosed schizophrenia should be treated by a psychiatrically trained homeopath.

Specific remedies to be given every hour for up to 10 doses in acute situations while waiting for professional help, but if person concerned becomes violent or threatens to commit suicide, (999).
- Main feature is paranoia (person acutely suspicious and mistrustful), worst after sleep and first thing in morning, also depression, constricted feeling in throat, desire not to wear clothes *Lachesis 6c*
- Person red in face, eyes wild and staring, delirious *Belladonna 30c*
- Person violent, talkative, overactive, swearing or praying, hearing voices and talking to them, loathes the dark *Stramonium 6c*
- Paranoia and suspicion, inappropriate laughter, tendency to obscene talk and behaviour *Hyoscyamus 6c*
- Person very agitated, always bustling and busy, very affected by music *Tarentula 6c*
- Strange sensations (such as bones being made of glass or animals writhing in stomach) accompanied by depression and anxiety *Thuja 6c*
- Person feels as if two selves are battling for control *Anacardium 6c*

Self-help The nutritional approach – extra Vitamin B_1, B_2, B_3, B_5, B_6, B_{12}, C, folate, E, zinc, and manganese, and evening primrose oil – might be of benefit, so ask your GP or homeopath for referral to an 'orthomolecular' or nutritionally trained psychiatrist. Also check for excessive amounts of copper in diet or environment. Family therapy can be especially valuable if schizophrenia is diagnosed in the early stages.

Sexual problems see pp. 264–270

Sleep problems see also SLEEP PROBLEMS
p. 308–9, ABNORMAL SLEEPINESS OR DROWSINESS
The purpose of sleep is not fully understood; certainly lack of sleep, especially of dreaming sleep, leads to lapses in concentration, irritability, irrationality, HALLUCINATIONS, and even death. Though sleep seems to be essential to the brain, it seems less so to the body. What sends us to sleep is also a puzzle; it could be a decrease in oxygen supply to the brain, a decrease in sensory input to the brain, fluctuation of certain chemicals in the brain, or simply a conditioned response. Most adults need 7 or 8 hours' sleep, even as they get older.

There are between 10 and 12 million poor sleepers in the United Kingdom alone, with women outnumbering men by 8 to 1 in the over-40 age group; only 22 per cent of people aged between 60 and 80 say they get a good night's sleep. Being highly strung or having a poor self-image seems to be quite a common denominator among poor sleepers.

For explanation of other symbols, see page 107

Insomnia is not a single night or even several nights of disturbed sleep, but a persistent pattern of short-sleeping which leaves the sufferer feeling unrested, worn out, and ragged round the edges. Most people who complain of insomnia do in fact get some sleep, but clearly not enough. Insomnia can be due to physical problems such as BREATHLESSNESS brought on by heart or lung disease, PROSTATE PROBLEMS, discomfort during pregnancy, or having to get up during the night to pass urine; or the cause may be too many late meals, too much caffeine, a food ALLERGY, overindulgence in alcohol or drugs, or something as simple as an airless or overheated bedroom. More often the causes are emotional – ANXIETY caused by pressure of work or financial problems, DEPRESSSION, GRIEF, too much excitement. Coming off sleeping pills or tranquillizers can also cause insomnia. In fact one of the commonest causes of insomnia is fear of not being able to sleep. The drugs most commonly used to treat insomnia today are the benzodiazepines, which have a sedative, anti-anxiety, muscle relaxing action; they also have side-effects.

Other sleep disorders include nightmares, night terrors, sleepwalking, sleep-talking, rocking, head banging, GRINDING TEETH, paralysed wakefulness, RESTLESS LEGS (a creeping sensation under the skin of the legs, or twitching of the leg muscles, which disturbs sleep but does not necessarily cause the person to wake), and disturbed breathing (breathing may cease for anything from 10 seconds to 3 minutes, occurring perhaps hundreds of times a night, followed by snorts or gasps for breath, during which the person partially wakes).

Nightmares and night terrors are more common in children than adults, possibly because adults have developed other mechanisms for coping with anxiety, than insomnia; during a nightmare heart rate climbs from about 64 beats per minute to 80, or during a night terror to 150, often causing the person to wake up; as well as being manifestations of anxiety, bad dreams can be a symptom of MENTAL EXHAUSTION, FEVER, over-indulgence in food or alcohol, withdrawal from sleeping tablets, or a side effect of certain prescription drugs.

Sleepwalking, sleep-talking, and making repetitive movements during sleep are also less common in adults than children. The muscles and senses concerned are, as it were, on automatic pilot, the person's conscious mind not being involved; he or she has no memory of the night's activities. Psychologists believe that dissociation of behaviour from consciousness is an attempt to resolve conflict. Interestingly, this kind of behaviour does not occur during dreaming, when all muscle movements, except those around the eyes, are inhibited. The important thing is to prevent the person concerned from coming to harm.

Paralysed wakefulness is an unpleasant state in which the person is awake but cannot move; it most often occurs, very briefly, on waking, but is not a cause for worry.

Chronic sleep problems require constitutional treatment, but in the short-term the remedies below may help. If no improvement is discernable within 3 weeks, consult your GP or homeopath.

Specific remedies to be taken 1 hour before going to bed for 10 nights running; repeat dose if woken by a nightmare or if you wake and cannot get to sleep again

- Mind overactive as the result of good or bad news, inability to switch off *Coffea 30c*
- Sleeplessness due to great mental strain, over-indulgence in food or alcohol, or withdrawal from alcohol or sleeping tablets, person wakes around 3 or 4 am then falls asleep just as it is time to get up, has nightmares, is irritable during day *Nux 30c*
- Person restless in first sleep, feels too hot and throws covers off, then feels too cold and lies with arms above head, not thirsty, insomnia worse after rich food *Pulsatilla 30c*
- Sleep problems worse after shock or panic, restlessness, nightmares, fear of dying *Aconite 30c*
- Feeling wide awake and irritable during first part of night, especially if person is a child and wants to be carried around *Chamomilla 30c*
- Mind very active at bedtime, going over and over work done during day, person aware of dreaming a lot, talks and laughs in sleep, wakes around 4 am *Lycopodium 30c*
- Person used to being up at night, perhaps looking after an invalid, feels too tired to sleep, giddy, irritable *Cocculus 30c*
- Person yawns a lot but cannot sleep, dreads not being able to sleep, especially after emotional upset; when sleep comes nightmares come too *Ignatia 30c*
- Bed feels too hard, person overtired, fidgety, dreams of being chased by animals *Arnica 30c*
- Feeling sleepy but unable to get to sleep, senses feel so sharp a fly can be heard walking on the wall, bed too hot, or else sleep comes but is so heavy that the person snores and cannot be roused *Opium 30c*
- Waking between midnight and 2 am, restless, worried, apprehensive, foreboding dreams of fire or danger *Arsenicum 30c*
- Person cannot sleep, is irritable, restless and walks about, especially if there is pain or discomfort *Rhus tox. 30c*
- Dreams about dying, hunger, or problems at work, descent into profound depression *Aurum 30c*

Self-help Insomnia is one ailment that can be very successfully tackled by self-help methods. Try whichever of the following measures seem most appropriate.

1 Stop working an hour before bedtime and read something light.
2 Take more exercise, preferably earlier in the day.
3 Avoid meals late at night and eat at the same times each day to establish body rhythms.

4 As a bedtime drink, try a herbal infusion (chamomile, valerian, passionflower, skullcap) or a hot milky drink which contains tryptophan (thought to help sleep); but avoid cocoa, tea, and coffee, and over-the-counter sleep remedies.

5 Take a warm bath.

6 Sexual release has a tension-reducing effect.

7 Learn some form of relaxation or meditation (see PART 2).

8 Don't lie tossing and turning if you cannot get to sleep; switch the light on and read, or do the ironing, then go back to sleep; resist tea, coffee, and other stimulants.

9 If you are overtired when you go to bed, take an afternoon nap (no longer than 15 minutes) to try and break the cycle.

10 Get your partner to give you a massage.

11 Wake up at the same time each day.

12 Remove the clock from your bedroom.

13 Make sure the room is not too hot or too cold (15-19°C [60-65°F] is about right) and minimize noise and light.

14 Increase your intake of Vitamin C, B_1, biotin, folate, and zinc, and if you are taking supplements of Vitamin A reduce your intake. Also check for excess lead and copper in your diet or environment.

Stress

Notoriously difficult to define since similar events affect people differently; one person's 'enjoyable challenge' may be another's 'last straw'. Psychologist Hans Seyle has theorized that we all make some attempt to improve performance under pressure, but that at some point we all begin to suffer from overload; if the pressure continues, we lose our resilience, tire, and fall into ill health.

In homeopathic medicine, ailments such as as food ALLERGY, ASTHMA, HYPOGLYCAEMIA, digestive disorders, HIGH BLOOD PRESSURE, etc., are looked on as manifestations of stress. Accordingly, treatment is long-term and constitutional. However, in acute circumstances, one of the remedies below may be appropriate.

Specific remedies to be given every 4 hours for up to 10 days

• Stress due to grief or bad news *Phosphoric ac. 30c*

• Stress due to overwork *Picric ac. 30c*

• Stress following emotional upset, a broken love affair, etc. *Ignatia 30c*

• Stress brought on by 'burning candle at both ends',

especially by smoking, eating, or drinking too much, person irritable *Nux 30c*

Self-help Learn some form of relaxation or meditation (see PART 2), even if it is only 10 minutes a day. Shed one or two burdens/obligations and don't take on any new ones until you feel better – learn how to say no. Eat at regular times, and get a proper night's rest. Take Vitamin B complex. Take more exercise, but don't exercise to the point of tiredness. If you need emotional support, try counselling; the counsellor's job is to work *with* you, pinpointing areas of stress and helping you deal with them.

Suicidal tendencies see also DEPRESSION, MANIC DEPRESSION, SCHIZOPHRENIA

Thoughts of suicide, and talk of suicide, are danger signals which should never be ignored. If someone is feeling suicidal, give *Aurum 6c* once every 5 minutes for up to 10 doses. Phone Samaritans or your doctor immediately.

Suicide is less frequent among married people than among single, widowed or divorced people, which clearly suggests that the factors leading to it – DEPRESSION, ANXIETY, INSECURITY, GRIEF – are aggravated by loneliness, or at least by the lack of close, continuing relationships.

Tension see ANGER

Unusual behaviour

Changes in behaviour can be symptomatic of CONFUSION (not knowing what time or day it is or where you are), ADDICTION to drugs or alcohol (short spells of very odd behaviour), DEPRESSION (withdrawal, apathy, disturbed appetite or sleep), OBSESSIONS AND COMPULSIONS (a single idea or activity becomes all important), ANXIETY (inability to concentrate, disturbed sleep), and MANIC DEPRESSION (marked mood swings). See relevant entry for homeopathic treatment.

Unusual thoughts or feelings

These too may be medically significant, perhaps symptoms of underlying conditions such as DEPRESSION (feeling worthless, that life is futile) and ANXIETY (feeling tense, aggressive, on edge), or of more serious illnesses such as SCHIZOPHRENIA (delusions, hallucinations, jumbled thoughts and feelings). Sexual fantasies are part of normal sexual functioning; treatment is not appropriate unless they become obsessive or threaten to damage a valued relationship (see Sexual Problems pp. 264–270).

BRAIN AND NERVOUS SYSTEM

THE human brain contains between 10 and 14 thousand million neurons or nerve cells, far more it seems than any of us ever use, and weighs about 1.5 kg (3 lb 5 oz). It generates consciousness and all mental and physical behaviour; rather like a central executive committee, it evaluates stimuli from inside and outside the body and issues orders to the body to adapt in ways which are likely to ensure survival.

The brain, together with its spinal extension, the spinal cord, is known as the central nervous system, as distinct from the peripheral nervous system, which consists of the 31 pairs of nerves which branch off from the spine. Those which leave the spine in the neck region go to the head and arms, those in the thoracic region go to the rib cage and abdomen, those in the lumbar region to the legs, and the lowest of all to the bowels and bladder. The peripheral nerves contain nerve fibres (very elongated nerve cells) which are either sensory or motor in function; if you trap your finger in a door, a sensory nerve fibre shoots a pain signal up to the brain, and the brain sends back the message 'Remove finger from door' via a motor nerve fibre.

Unlike most other cells in the body, nerve cells have only a very limited capacity for self-repair. They are so specialized and have such delicate junctions with other nerve cells that, once damaged, they lose their ability to transmit nerve impulses, or minute voltage electrical signals, and they can be quite easily damaged, by compression, injury, surgery, viral or bacterial infections, or oxygen starvation. The brain is plentifully supplied with arteries – about one eighth of the oxygenated blood leaving the lungs goes to the brain – but if any area of it is deprived of blood for more than a few minutes it ceases to function, and the result is a stroke.

Fortunately, every nerve cell in the brain has so many connections that the effects of damage to a small area may be insignificant or not noticed at all; connected areas may take over the function of the damaged area. Obviously the smaller the area devoted to a particular function, the more severe the effects of damage. Injury to the spinal cord may be much more disabling, because sensation and movement in every part of the body supplied by nerves entering and leaving the spine below the point of injury may be lost or severely impaired. However, both the brain and the spinal cord are well protected, the brain by the skull and the spinal cord by the vertebrae; both are also enclosed in three delicate membranes, the meninges, and bathed in shock-absorbing fluid. The nerves themselves are protected and insulated by a fatty substance called myelin; the biggest nerve fibres have the thickest insulation and conduct nerve impulses at

about 500 km (300 miles) per hour; the smallest fibres have no myelin covering, and so conduct impulses much more slowly.

In evolutionary terms the cerebellum and brain stem are more primitive than the much folded rind, or cortex, of the brain. The cortex is concerned with higher mental functions such as memory and learning, planning, intellectual effort, and integrating activities with movement, speech, sight, and hearing. Beneath the cortex lies the sub-cortex, containing structures concerned with more fundamental aspects of behaviour. The thalamus, for example, relays sensory information to appropriate areas of the cortex and also enables us to concentrate on one thing at a time; the hypothalamus regulates hunger, thirst, sleep, body temperature, and basic emotions such as fear and anger, as well as controlling the secretions of the pituitary gland beneath it, which in turn controls growth and stimulates other glands in the body to produce hormones.

The cerebellum or hind-brain acts as a non-stop monitor of all movements commanded by the motor area of the cortex, ensuring precision, smoothness, coordination and balance; nerve impulses from the semicircular canals in the inner ear go to the cerebellum for interpretation.

The brain stem is the most primitive part of the brain; from being little more than a terminus for all the ascending and descending nerve tracts in the spinal cord, it has evolved into a very complex relay station, with connections to all parts of the cortex; it controls automatic functions such as heartbeat and breathing, and also consciousness as we know it; without a particular clump of neurons at its core, we would be in a state of perpetual somnolence.

Rather like a walnut, the brain has two obvious halves – these intercommunicate very extensively through a stout bridge of nerve fibres called the corpus callosum – with the right half controlling the left side of the body and vice versa. Much has been made of the division of higher mental labour between the two halves of the brain. In most people the left hemisphere specializes in logical, analytical, and verbal activity, which is why so many people write with their right hand, while the right hemisphere is predominantly 'artistic', better at associative, intuitive, imaginative thought, more concerned with processing spatial information.

Between them the two halves daily impose order and meaning on an avalanche of information coming from specialized nerve endings all over the body – these detect heat, cold, pain, pressure, even texture – and of course from the eyes, ears, nose, and tongue. However, the processing power required to make visual information meaningful is greater than that required to interpret all other forms of sensory information put together; next in terms of sensory importance, but a long way behind the eyes, come the hands and feet, lips and tongue, ears and genitals. When it comes to moving different parts of the body, the hands, feet, mouth, and tongue – all capable of very precise movements – account for the largest areas in the motor cortex.

Abnormal sleepiness or drowsiness

When not due to tiredness or lack of sleep, sluggish drowsy, drugged behaviour may be a sign of BRAIN INJURY, POISONING (drugs, alcohol, poisonous plants or berries, garden or household chemicals), MENINGITIS (if accompanied by fever, vomiting, headache, aversion to light, a stiff neck), dehydration due to DIARRHOEA or VOMITING, DIABETES (if person is thirsty and passing large quantities of urine, with or without recent weight loss), or DRUG ADDICTION (prescription or recreational drugs). Occasionally, abnormal drowsiness may be due to an excess of Vitamin D or lithium. Narcolepsy, which causes sudden lapses into sleep for no apparent reason, is an extremely rare and not fully understood disorder, usually treated by stimulant drugs, but it may respond to diet and constitutional treatment.

If drowsiness follows a head injury or suspected POISONING, ⑨⑨⑨, and see First Aid p. 102 for treatment of poisoning. If meningitis, diabetes, or dehydration are suspected, ②.

Specific remedy to be given every 10 minutes for up to 10 doses while waiting for medical help
• If drowsiness follows recent head injury *Arnica 30c*

Bell's palsy

Temporary PARALYSIS of the muscles on one side of the face due to swelling of the facial nerve as it exits from the skull. Sometimes accompanied by ear pain on the affected side. If the eye cannot be closed, a patch should be worn. Condition usually clears up of its own accord within 2 weeks. Conventional treatment is by steroids. Homeopathy offers two home remedies, but if symptoms persist see your homeopath.

Specific remedies
• If onset follows exposure to cold, dry winds *Aconite 30c* to be taken hourly for up to 6 doses
• If condition persists despite Aconite *Causticum 6c* to be taken 4 times daily for up to 5 days.

Brain damage

Can occur at all stages of life and for a variety of reasons, causing various degrees of intellectual or physical impairment. Faulty development of the brain may be preordained if, before conception, the sperm or ova of the parents have been damaged by toxic metals or grossly inadequate nutrition (see Preconceptual Care p. 23).

In the womb, damage may be caused by infection, poor nutrition, or conditions such as ANTE-PARTUM HAEMORRHAGE and PLACENTA PRAEVIA which impair the placenta's ability to provide the foetus with oxygen and nutrients. At birth, a baby's brain can be damaged by a difficult or too hasty delivery (see EMERGENCY CHILDBIRTH p. 295). At birth also some degree of HYDROCEPHALUS (a larger than normal skull due to faulty drainage of cerebrospinal fluid from the brain) may be apparent, signifying some degree of under-development.

In children and adults brain damage can be caused by head injuries, infections such as ENCEPHALITIS, a STROKE (which disrupts oxygen supply to the brain), EPILEPSY, BRAIN TUMOURS, MULTIPLE SCLEROSIS, and surgery to the brain. Drugs and heavy metals (aluminium, lead, mercury) can also cause damage. Symptoms include CONFUSION, MEMORY LOSS, SPEECH DIFFICULTIES, PARALYSIS, and poor coordination, depending on site of damage.

For description and treatment, see entries for each of the conditions mentioned above.

Brain haemorrhage see also STROKE

Caused by blood leaking out of blood vessels in the brain itself or out of blood vessels in the various layers of tissue between the brain and the skull; the result is a slow or sudden pooling of blood in a confined space and pressure on the sensitive tissues of the brain.

There are four main types of haemorrhage: *cerebral vascular haemorrhage*, a kind of STROKE, which occurs inside the brain, causing sudden loss of speech, NUMBNESS or loss of movement down one side of the body, CONFUSION, and sometimes unconsciousness; *subdural haemorrhage*, relatively rare and usually caused by an injury to the head, in which there is a slow seepage of blood from the vessels between the dura and arachnoid membranes, and a slow onset of ABNORMAL SLEEPINESS OR DROWSINESS, CONFUSION, blurring of vision, weakness or NUMBNESS on one side of the body, and a persistent or recurrent HEADACHE, symptoms which are very difficult to distinguish from SENILE DEMENTIA; *subarachnoid haemorrhage*, usually caused by a blood vessel bursting and flooding the space between the pia and arachnoid membranes, causing a sudden HEADACHE, a very stiff and painful neck, intolerance of light, FAINTING, DIZZINESS, CONFUSION, ABNORMAL SLEEPINESS OR DROWSINESS, VOMITING, and loss of consciousness; and *extradural haemorrhage*, usually the result of a head injury, in which the larger vessels between the meninges and the skull are ruptured, causing a sudden and severe HEADACHE, NAUSEA, ABNORMAL SLEEPINESS OR DROWSINESS, and loss of consciousness.

If a subarachnoid or extradural haemorrhage is suspected, ⑨⑨⑨, put person in recovery position (see First Aid p. 90–91) if necessary, and if possible give *Arnica 30c* every 5 minutes for up to 10 doses or until help arrives; once in hospital, an operation may be necessary to seal off haemorrhaging blood vessels. If a cerebral vascular or subdural haemorrhage is suspected, ②, and select a remedy from those listed under STROKE.

Brain injury

A blow to one side of the skull can cause the brain to hit the other side of the skull inside, whether or not the skull is fractured at the point of impact, resulting in two areas of injury, primary and secondary. A severe impact can cause concussion (loss of consciousness for a few seconds) or coma (days or weeks of unconsciousness), or rupture blood vessels and cause BRAIN HAEMORRHAGE or MENINGITIS. Permanent effects from coma and concussion are rare, but brain haemorrhage or meningitis can cause residual physical or mental damage.

If someone has received a severe blow to the head, ⑨⑨⑨ and give First Aid (see HEAD INJURIES p. 99); if person is unconscious put him or her in recovery position. If possible, give *Arnica 30c* every 5 minutes.

The remedies listed below are for the after effects of head injury; if they do not seem to help, see your homeopath.

Specific remedies to be taken every 4 hours for up to 6 doses once person is out of danger but suffering from after-effects
- Persistent headache, reactions slow and stupid, person picks at his or her clothes *Helleborus 6c*
- Head feels very sensitive, tingling and drowsiness *Hypericum 30c*
- Person seems depressed, indifferent to what is going on, gets upset when sympathy is offered *Natrum sulph. 6c*

Brain tumour see also CANCER

Abnormal growth of tissue in the brain; may be benign (non-cancerous) or malignant (cancerous). As tumour grows, the adjacent tissues of the brain become dangerously compressed, resulting in such symptoms as HEADACHE (made worse by lying down), NAUSEA AND VOMITING (or more often vomiting without the nausea), blurred or double vision, weakness down one side of the body, unsteadiness, loss of sense of smell, MEMORY LOSS, personality changes, and FITS. If several of these symptoms are present, ⟨24⟩ your GP will refer you to a neurologist for tests. Benign tumours can sometimes be completely removed by surgery; cancerous tumours are very often secondary, arising from a tumour somewhere else in the body, and require drugs and radiotherapy as well as surgery.

The homeopathic remedies listed below are recommended while tests are being carried out or where surgery is not appropriate.

Specific remedies to be taken 4 times daily for up to 2 weeks
- Symptoms made worse by exertion, or by cold or damp, person apprehensive, confused and frightened *Calcarea 6c*
- Swollen glands (lymph nodes) throughout body, facial neuralgia *Kali iod. 6c*
- Symptoms onset after injury to head *Hypericum 30c*
- Painful, persistent headaches, alleviated by warmth and pressure *Magnesia phos. 6c*

Carpal tunnel syndrome

Loss of sensation in the palm, thumb, and first two fingers of the hand, and pains which shoot up the arm from the wrist; caused by pinching of the median nerve as it passes through the carpal tunnel, a tunnel of tissue beneath the bones of the wrist. Symptoms worse at night, often relieved by hanging arm over side of bed. Cause may be hormonal. Conventionally treated by diuretics and steroids, or by surgery if condition is severe.

Specific remedies to be taken 4 times daily for up to 2 weeks
- Person has a great craving for salt *Natrum mur. 6c*
- Pain relieved by warmth and rubbing *Magnesia phos. 6c*
- Pain severe enough to wake person up at night *Aconite 30c*

Self-help Vitamins B_2 and B_6 may give some relief.

Cerebral vascular accidents see STROKE, BRAIN HAEMORRHAGE

Convulsions see FITS, EPILEPSY

Dizziness see also DIZZINESS p. 339

A sensation of being unbalanced and spinning, often associated with a STROKE (if there is also weakness, numbness or tingling in arms and legs, blurred vision, difficulty speaking), MENIERE'S DISEASE (loss of hearing, noises in the ear), LABYRINTHITIS (especially after a cold or 'flu) and other ear problems, HYPOGLYCAEMIA (sweating, unsteadiness, headache, hunger, tingling in lips or hands), CERVICAL SPONDYLOSIS (stiff, painful neck, dizziness worse when head is turned slowly), a subdural BRAIN HAEMORRHAGE or BRAIN TUMOUR (recurrent headaches, especially in the morning, nausea or vomiting), travel sickness (see p. 219), or CLAUSTROPHOBIA (worse in hot, crowded rooms or confined spaces). May also be a side effect of drugs

---

⑨⑨⑨ Emergency – call GP (or dial 999) immediately. ② Consult your doctor if no improvement within 2 hours

such as quinine, salicylates (including aspirin), non-steroidal anti-inflammatory drugs, and some anti-biotics, diuretics, and hypertensives.

Specific remedies to be taken as often as necessary for up to 10 doses when attack comes on

- Symptoms made worse by loud noise (airports, factories, discos) *Theridion 6c*
- Symptoms made worse by downward motion *Borax 6c*
- Symptoms made worse by looking up *Calcarea 6c*
- Symptoms made worse by lying down *Conium 6c*
- Person feels trembly as well as dizzy *Gelsemium 6c*
- Person feels better in open air, but worse if he or she tries to walk, turn, or read *Kali carb. 6c*
- Symptoms made worse by flickering lights (television, strobe lighting) *Nux 6c*

Self-help Take Vitamins B$_2$ and B$_3$, and extra salt if working in hot climates and sweating profusely, and check for a possible excess of lead, mercury, bismuth, or iron in diet or environment.

Drowsiness see ABNORMAL SLEEPINESS AND DROWSINESS

Encephalitis

Inflammation of the brain, usually caused by a viral infection, sometimes by the viruses responsible for MUMPS, MEASLES, or GLANDULAR FEVER, which of course affect other parts of the body in preference to the brain, but more often by viruses which affect only the brain. In the latter event, symptoms are FEVER, HEADACHE, loss of energy, loss of appetite (see APPETITE CHANGES), irritability, restlessness, ABNORMAL SLEEPINESS OR DROWSINESS, intolerance to light and, in severe cases, muscular weakness, DOUBLE VISION, loss of speech and hearing, and finally coma and death. A very dangerous condition in babies and the elderly. Appropriate action is ②.

Specific remedies to be taken every 15 minutes for up to 10 doses while waiting for help

- Flushed face, staring eyes, person delirious *Belladonna 30c*
- Marked drowsiness, especially in an infant *Nux mosch. 6c*
- Person feels dizzy, complains of tight band around forehead, wants nothing to drink, feels weak and trembly *Gelsemium 6c*

Self-help Take extra Vitamin C.

Epilepsy see also FITS

Recurrent excessive electrical discharge from groups of nerve cells in the brain, overwhelming normal functioning in neighbouring cells. Epilepsy affects 1 person in every 200, and appears to run in families, but in two cases out of three no obvious physical cause (i.e. brain damage due to injury or infection) can be found. However, there is a slight danger that repeated fits may cause BRAIN DAMAGE. Diagnosed epileptics must report their condition when applying for a driving licence – the consequences, to themselves and to others, of an attack occurring at the wheel are too unpleasant to need spelling out.

There are four main types of epilepsy: petit mal and grand mal epilepsy; and focal epilepsy and temporal lobe epilepsy, which are less common. *Petit mal epilepsy* mostly occurs in children and usually disappears in adolescence. There is no loss of consciousness or falling to the ground; the child just stares blankly for a few seconds, perhaps makes swallowing movements or jerks his or her head or arms, and then comes back to normal, often without realising what has happened. In *grand mal epilepsy* the person loses consciousness and falls to the ground, and the body stiffens and starts jerking; this generally lasts for a few minutes, after which the person either regains consciousness and is very confused or falls into a deep sleep. Many sufferers experience strange sensations affecting smell, sight, or hearing just before a fit comes on; these are known as an 'aura'. In *focal epilepsy* just one part of the body starts to twitch and jerk, but there is no loss of consciousness. In *temporal lobe epilepsy*, so called because the lobes of the brain just behind the temples are the site of abnormal electrical activity, there is a brief aura followed by behaviour which is bizarre or totally out of character.

The first thing to do when someone has a fit is to remove dangerous objects and make sure the person is not in danger (in the middle of the road, for example). A baby having a fit should be wrapped in a sheet or blanket to prevent injury. If the person passes out, put him or her in the recovery position (see First Aid p. 90–91). If the fit continues for more than 3 minutes, or stops and then starts again, ⑨⑨⑨. Once the fit is over, allow the person to sleep. Most authorities now advise against putting objects in the mouth to prevent the tongue being bitten as this can cause broken teeth; a bitten tongue heals very quickly.

Orthodox management of diagnosed epilepsy is by anti-convulsant drugs, some of which have unpleasant side effects; only in rare cases can the condition be cured. Depending on the nature of the attacks and the potential hazards, constitutional treatment from an experienced homeopath might also be appropriate, although certain prescription drugs are known to antidote homeopathic remedies. For specific remedies, see FITS; these should be given immediately after an epileptic fit wears off.

Self-help If taking a prescription drug, make sure you follow your GP's instructions exactly. Carry a tag or card telling people what to do if you have a fit – some people have the information engraved on a bracelet or pendant. Tell friends and work colleagues that you have epilepsy, so that they are not frightened and know what to do when you have a fit. Vitamin B$_6$, magnesium, calcium, and zinc prove beneficial in some cases. Evening primrose oil is *not* suitable for self-treatment; it has been known to aggravate rather than alleviate the condition. Lastly, join the British Epileptic Association (address p. 383); they will keep you up to date on research and treatment.

Extradural haemorrhage see BRAIN HAEMORRHAGE

Fainting

Suddenly feeling weak and unsteady, and momentarily passing out; caused by a momentary shortfall in oxygen supply to brain. In fact, fainting is the body's way of getting you to lie down so that blood, and the oxygen it carries, can reach the brain more easily.

Fainting can be a symptom of LOW BLOOD PRESSURE (if it happens after a few days in bed, or as you stand up from a stooping or sitting position), HYPOGLYCAEMIA (if you are diabetic or have not eaten for some time), HYPERVENTILATION (after fasting or prolonged shallow breathing), CERVICAL SPONDYLOSIS (if person is over 50 and has only to turn head slowly to feel faint), ANAEMIA (increasing shortness of breath and tiredness), or HEAT EXHAUSTION (after several hours in sun or in hot, stuffy surroundings); can also be a side effect of drugs given for high blood pressure; coughing, stretching, breath-holding, and unusually strenuous exercise can also cause fainting, as can CONSTIPATION, menstruation, and pregnancy. If person is unconscious, put in recovery position (see First Aid pp. 90–91); if person feels faint, get him or her to lie down with legs raised or sit with head between knees (see First Aid p. 98); if heat exhaustion is suspected, see First Aid p. 101.

If faints last for more than a minute or two, or occur quite frequently, see your GP.

There are also a number of acute conditions which cause fainting or faintness, together with other symptoms; these require urgent action. If person suddenly feels faint and weak, looks very pale, and gasps for air, there may be internal bleeding; appropriate action is ⑨⑨⑨, with doses of *Arnica 30c* every 2 minutes until help arrives. If there is NUMBNESS and tingling, blurred vision, CONFUSION, difficulty speaking, or loss of sensation in limbs, person may be having a STROKE;

appropriate course is ②, and *Arnica 30c* every 15 minutes until help arrives. If person has a history of heart disease, loss of consciousness may be a STOKES ADAMS ATTACK; again, ② is the appropriate action, with *Aconite 30c* every 15 minutes until help arrives.

Constitutional homeopathic treatment may be appropriate if fainting is recurrent and related to emotional stress.

Specific remedies to be given every 5 minutes for up to 7 doses when faintness comes on or immediately after fainting
- Faintness associated with shortness of breath and unaccustomed exercise *Nux mosch. 6c*
- Brought on by fright, person pale, tense, scared of dying *Aconite 30c*
- Brought on by fright, person feels weak and shaky *Gelsemium 6c*
- Brought on by fright, person numb with shock *Opium 6c*
- Brought on by emotional shock *Ignatia 6c*
- Brought on by anger *Veratrum 6c*
- Brought on by excitement *Coffea 6c*
- Faintness associated with racing thoughts, person very thirsty for ice-cold water *Phosphorus 6c*
- Faintness caused by loss of blood *China 6c*
- Faintness caused by lack of sleep *Cocculus 6c*
- Person faints at sight of blood *Nux 6c*

Self-help Get the person to sit down and gently push their head down towards their knees, or better still get the person to lie down, then put a cushion or two under their ankles; both measures encourage blood to flow towards the head. Loosen clothing around the neck, give the person as much fresh air as possible, and stop people crowding round.

Fits see also FITS pp. 321–22

Can take different forms depending on the part of the brain affected; for reasons which are not clear, the electrical signals sent out by nerve cells in the affected part of the brain suddenly become very strong, disrupting the function of surrounding cells and causing uncontrollable jerking and twitching of various parts of the body. In two-thirds of cases, no physiological cause can be found; in other cases, the cause may be BRAIN DAMAGE, either sustained at birth or the result of a head injury, brain infections such as ENCEPHALITIS, or a BRAIN TUMOUR. One fit does not constitute EPILEPSY, which is a recurrent condition; in children, fits may be due to breath-holding, infantile spasm (see FITS pp. 321–22), or FEBRILE CONVULSIONS.

However, if you or a member of your family have had a fit, for whatever presumed reason, you should consult your GP; after a first occurrence, medication may or may not be recommended, depending on the nature of the fit and the circumstances in which it occurred. If

---

⑨⑨⑨ Emergency – call GP (or dial 999) immediately. ② Consult your doctor if no improvement within 2 hours

more fits occur, you will be referred to a neurologist and probably put on anti-convulsants.

Specific remedies to be taken every 60 seconds for up to 10 doses immediately after person stops twitching and jerking
- Fit brought on by fright or fever *Aconite 30c*
- Fit follows an attack of gastroenteritis, particularly in infants allergic to cow's milk, with drowsy spells after vomiting or passing stool, pupils dilated, teeth clenched, thumbs clenched inside fists *Aethusa 6c*
- Person red-faced, feverish, eyes wide and staring, symptoms made worse by jolting or jarring *Belladonna 30c*
- Brought on by teething or after outburst of anger, especially if one cheek is red and the other white, greenish watery stools, thumbs clenched inside palms *Chamomilla 6c*
- Fit very violent, face and lips turn blue, thumbs clenched inside fists *Cuprum 6c*
- Fit brought on by exposure to sun or intense heat, head hot and congested, fingers and toes spread wide *Glonoinum 30c*
- Fit brought on by emotional upset, face pale, twitching starts in face *Ignatia 6c*
- Person, especially a child, in pre-rash stage of an infectious illness, head rolling from side to side, fidgety movements of feet and legs, very bad-tempered before attack comes on *Zinc 6c*

Friederich's ataxia
An extremely rare inherited disease in which certain groups of nerve fibres slowly degenerate, causing loss of coordination of movement and balance; walking is affected first, then there may be difficulty with arm movements, speaking, or just standing still; typically, the intention to move a limb is accompanied by a tremor. Age of onset is between 5 and 15. Anyone who has the disease and who wants children should seek genetic counselling.

The cause of the condition is not known, and doctors generally consider that very little can be done. However, the traditional homeopathic view is that the condition is due to inherent weakness in the nervous system, aggravated by wrong diet, injury, or acute infectious diseases such as SCARLET FEVER, WHOOPING COUGH, TYPHOID, and DIPHTHERIA. Fortunately the condition is so rare that the author has had no personal experience of treating it; however the homeopathic literature suggests that expert constitutional treatment, at as early an age as possible where a child is known to be at risk, might help to postpone or minimize disability. Foods high in calcium and iron are also recommended.

Guillain Barre Syndrome
Sudden inflammation of the peripheral nerves of the body (those outside the brain and spinal cord), thought to be an allergic reaction to a viral illness or to vaccination. In the United States in 1976, for example, there were hundreds of adverse reactions to 'swine' 'flu vaccine. Symptoms onset rapidly a few days after infection or vaccination, beginning as tingling, NUMBNESS, weakness or PARALYSIS in the hands and feet, then spreading to the rest of the body; if paralysis begins to affect breathing, ⑨⑨⑨ as intensive care in hospital will be necessary.

Specific remedies
- If symptoms onset after vaccination and person has no difficulty breathing *Thuja 30c* every 12 hours for up to 6 doses
- If symptoms onset after viral infection and person has no difficulty breathing *Aconite 30c* ½-hourly for up to 10 doses

Hangovers see HEADACHE

Headache see also MIGRAINE
Most headaches are due to strain on the muscles in the neck or head, or congestion of the blood vessels which supply them; the brain itself cannot feel pain because it contains no pain receptors.

Headaches can be a symptom of ANXIETY, STRESS, physical tension (especially in the back and shoulders), lack of sleep, over-consumption of caffeine in tea or coffee or suddenly cutting down caffeine intake, food ALLERGY, EYESTRAIN, FEVER, HYPOGLYCAEMIA (low blood sugar, especially if you have not eaten for some time), MIGRAINE (recurrent one-sided headaches, with nausea, vomiting, and bivisual disturbances), drug side effects (especially if you have started a new drug), SINUSITIS (especially after a cold, if there is dull pain or tenderness in the cheeks or around the eyes which gets worse when you bend forwards), CERVICAL SPONDYOSIS (stiff neck, an ache which extends from spine to top of head, headache made worse by lifting, driving, or turning head slowly) and other spinal problems, PREMENSTRUAL TENSION (headache comes on before a period), post-herpetic NEURALGIA following SHINGLES, malocclusion or sepsis after dental treatment (see your dentist), and HIGH BLOOD PRESSURE. That very common form of headache, the hangover, is mainly caused by DEHYDRATION (alcohol is a powerful diuretic). TEMPORAL ARTERITIS (dull, throbbing headache behind one or both temples) is caused by inflammation of the arteries which supply the scalp.

Headaches can also be a symptom of damage to the blood vessels in and around the brain itself, or of infection to the tissues surrounding the brain and spinal cord. In such cases prompt action and close observation are required.

If a headache follows a head injury, and the person is drowsy, nauseous, and vomiting, the cause may be an extradural BRAIN HAEMORRHAGE; if there has been no injury, but symptoms are headache, nausea, vomiting, drowsiness, and intolerance of light, cause may be a subarachnoid BRAIN HAEMORRHAGE; in either case ⑨⑨⑨ and give *Arnica 30c* every 15 minutes until help arrives.

A bad headache, with a temperature of more than 100°F or 38°C and intolerance of light, may be MENINGITIS; pain behind one eye, with blurred vision, may be ACUTE GLAUCOMA or IRITIS; if any of these conditions is suspected, ②.

Where a headache has lasted for several days, seems worse in the mornings, and is accompanied by nausea or vomiting, |12|; high blood pressure, stress, or a BRAIN TUMOUR may be the cause.

Constitutional treatment is recommended for recurrent headaches caused by stress, anxiety, or tension. However, if you know or suspect that a headache is a symptom of another condition, one which does not require prompt medical attention, look up the remedies for that condition, then compare the symptoms listed with those given against the remedies below. If you still draw a blank, refer to the General Remedy Finder (pp. 38–76). Remedies for severe, one-sided, sick headaches are given under MIGRAINE.

Specific remedies to be taken every 10–15 minutes for up to 10 doses
- Headache comes on suddenly, feels worse in cold or draughty surroundings, person apprehensive, headache feels like a tight band around head or as if brains are being forced out of head *Aconite 30c*
- Head feels bruised and aching, pain occasionally sharp, made worse by stooping *Arnica 30c*
- Stinging, stabbing or burning headache, rest of body feels bruised and tender, symptoms worse in hot, stuffy surroundings *Apis 30c*
- Throbbing, drumming headache, flushed face, dilated pupils, distinctly worse in hot sun *Belladonna 30c*
- Head feels bruised, sharp, stabbing pain made worse by slightest eye movement *Bryonia 30c*
- Head feels full and swollen, face purple and congested-looking, expression dull and heavy, dilated pupils, limbs weak and shaky *Gelsemium 6c*
- Violent headache in which every heartbeat sets up an answering thump and throb in the head, made worse by stooping or shaking head *Glonoinum 30c*
- Bursting, aching headache, hypersensitive scalp, worse in damp, foggy weather *Hypericum 30c*
- Headache described as tight band across forehead or as nail being driven out through side of head *Ignatia 6c*
- Person often irritable, prone to dull, dizzy, bruising headaches which are rather like being beaten around the head, worse first thing in morning but better when person gets up *Nux 6c*
- Pressing, bruising headache associated with fatigue, made worse by reading, alleviated by rest *Ruta 6c*

Specific remedies for hangovers, to be taken hourly for up to 6 doses, with copious glasses of water between doses (where headache is main feature, see also ALCOHOLISM).
- For the proverbial 'bear with a sore head' who wants to be left alone *Chamomilla 6c*
- Head feels super-sensitive, mind in overdrive, tea and coffee make things worse *Coffea 6c*
- Head aches as if it has been beaten, feeling dull, dizzy, and irritable *Nux 6c*
- Feeling weepy and miserable, hangover due to rich food as well as alcohol *Pulsatilla 6c*

Self-help If taking supplements of Vitamin A, stop them for a while and see if the headaches stop – overdosing with Vitamin A does occasionally cause headaches. Take extra Vitamin B$_3$ and potassium for a while. Osteopathy, in particular cranial manipulation, would be well worth trying.

Huntington's chorea
A rare inherited degenerative disease which does not declare itself until middle age. Symptoms are swift, jerky movements which become increasingly uncontrollable, and mental deterioration, including MEMORY LOSS; the whole personality of the sufferer also changes. Remedies given for MULTIPLE SCLEROSIS may also be beneficial. If there is a history of the condition in your family and you want to have children, ask your GP about genetic counselling; this will help you to evaluate the risks.

Self-help The best course is to get as much sleep as possible and not to overtax the nervous system. Supplements of choline may be helpful, but these should only be given under medical supervision as very high doses are required.

Migraine
Occasional severe headaches, usually confined to one side of head, associated with NAUSEA AND VOMITING, blurred vision, and other visual disturbances, intolerance to light, and occasionally NUMBNESS and tingling in the arms. In a severe attack, the only thing to do is lie down in a darkened room until the symptoms wear off. Attacks are often heralded by abnormal tiredness, nausea, or flashing, shimmering or distortion of objects towards edge of visual field; once the headache comes on, these symptoms tend to disappear.

The immediate cause of migraine headaches is constriction, then swelling of the arteries which supply the brain, but why the arteries suddenly behave in this way is not known. STRESS, HYPOGLYCAEMIA, and certain foods are the most frequently cited 'trigger factors' of this miserable complaint, which affects 1 person in 10, and three times as many women as men, and are often worse round period time. Incidence and frequency of attacks tend to tail off in middle age, though they may worsen during the menopause in women.

Taken early enough, vasoconstrictors, antihistamines, and anti-emetics can minimize the symptoms of an attack; alternatively, combinations of antihypertensives, tranquilizers and anti-depressants can be taken on a permanent basis to prevent attacks. A few hospitals offer biofeedback treatment, in which sufferers are trained to control their blood pressure and body temperature by relaxation. Osteopathy, in particular cranial manipulation, may also offer relief.

Homeopathic treatment of migraine is constitutional; however, the remedies listed below are recommended for use in emergencies.

Specific remedies to be taken ¼-hourly for up to 10 doses, if possible at the first signs of an attack
- Blurring of vision before headache comes on, tight feeling in scalp, headache right-sided but less insistent if person moves around, vomit mostly bile *Iris 6c*
- Headache worse on right side, feels as if temples are being screwed into each other, trying to concentrate makes pain worse, dizziness *Lycopodium 6c*
- Throbbing, blinding headache, warmth and moving around make headache worse, head feels overstuffed and congested, attack preceded by numbness and tingling in lips, nose, and tongue *Natrum mur. 6c*
- Headache worse in evening or during a period, aggravated by rich, fatty food, head feels as if it is about to burst, person easily bursts into tears *Pulsatilla 6c*
- Headache worse in morning, bursting pain which is right- sided and seems to start at back of head, with pain extending into right shoulder, some improvement later in day *Sanguinaria 6c*
- Pain starts at back of head, then shifts and settles above one eye, aggravated by cold, alleviated by wrapping head up warmly and tightly, person prone to head sweats *Silicea 6c*
- Sharp, darting, severe pain over left eye, pain seems to pulse with every heartbeat, stooping or moving suddenly makes pain worse *Spigelia 6c*
- Left-sided headache, as if head is being pierced by a nail *Thuja 6c*

Self-help In addition to avoiding stress, tension, and tiredness, and learning some form of relaxation or meditation (see PART 2), try eliminating certain foods from your diet and then reintroducing them, to see what effect they have. Foods known to trigger off migraines are, in order of their attack-producing potential: chocolate (and other forms of concentrated sugar), cheese and dairy products, citrus fruit, alcohol (especially red wine), greasy fried foods, some vegetables (especially onions, broad beans, and Sauerkraut), tea, coffee, cocoa, and cola (all of which contain caffeine), wheat and yeast extracts, meat (especially pork, liver, sausages, and cured meats such as bacon and salami), and shellfish. Stay off these, one at a time, for about 4 weeks, then reintroduce them. Alternatively, consult a dietary therapist; he or she may be able to help you pinpoint the offending food more quickly.

Food additives – notably E101, 210-219, 321, and 621–can also act as migraine triggers, as can smoking, perfumes, and some oral contraceptives. Excessive TV watching is not a good idea either.

Positive measures include taking extra Vitamin B_6, C, and E, and also evening primrose oil, and also adding fresh root ginger to cooking.

Some sufferers swear by the herb feverfew, but in the opinion of the author it should only be taken on a 5 days out of 7 basis, and then only if constitutional treatment is not working; feverfew can cause griping abdominal pain, heavier than normal periods, mouth ulcers, and swelling of the tongue if taken too enthusiastically.

If you sense an attack coming on, splash your face with cold water for a few minutes, then lie down somewhere quiet for an hour or so; for some sufferers this has the effect of fending off an attack altogether. For more information about research and treatment write to the Migraine Trust (address p. 383).

Meningitis see also MENINGITIS p. 326

Viral or bacterial infection of the delicate membranes, the meninges, surrounding the brain; the disease organisms responsible spread to the brain via the blood from sinus, ear, and lung infections, or can be introduced directly as the result of head injury. Symptoms are FEVER, NAUSEA AND VOMITING, a stiff neck, a severe HEADACHE made worse by bending forwards, intolerance of light, possibly CONFUSION and DELIRIUM, then ABNORMAL SLEEPINESS OR DROWSINESS and perhaps coma; in babies, symptoms may be different (see p. 307). Recovery from viral meningitis takes 2–3 weeks, and is usually complete, but the consequences of the bacterial form (same bacilli which cause TUBERCULOSIS, for example, also cause meningitis) can be more serious – loss of hearing, BRAIN ABSCESS, BRAIN DAMAGE, and even death.

If meningitis is suspected ②, and choose one of the emergency remedies from the list below. Diagnosis will be confirmed by lumber puncture (taking a sample of fluid from the spine); antibiotics are given if infection is bacterial, with bed rest and drugs to ease fever and pain.

Specific remedies to be taken every 10 minutes for up to 10 doses while waiting for help
- Symptoms onset after head injury *Arnica 30c*
- Symptoms accompanied by restlessness, fear, dry skin, great thirst *Aconite 30c*
- Person very hot, delirious, with staring eyes *Belladonna 30c*
- Severe headache made worse by slightest eye movement, person becoming steadily more depressed and comatose *Bryonia 30c*

Motor neurone disease

Progressive degeneration of the nerves which deliver movement messages to the muscles of the body, causing wasting, weakness, and difficulty swallowing, walking, breathing, etc. Usually fatal within 5–10 years, but rare under age of 50. Unfortunately the condition is not really understood, and there is no cure. The aim of treatment, homeopathic as well as conventional, is to maintain mobility and independence for as long as possible. Homeopathy can help with some of the symptoms, but the person concerned should be under the care of an experienced homeopath. High dose specific amino acids are currently under trial to try and slow down the progression of the disease.

Multiple sclerosis (MS)

Damage to nerve fibres in the central nervous system caused by inflammation of the fatty tissue (myelin) which sheathes and insulates them. Symptoms vary depending on the site of the damage. The first signs, often noticed after a hot bath or exercise, may be tingling, NUMBNESS, or weakness affecting a hand, foot, or one side of the body, DOUBLE VISION, or things suddenly looking misty or blurred; after a day or two these symptoms disappear, and for some people they never return. For others, however, attacks are repeated and lead to some measure of disability, depending on severity and frequency; in only a minority of cases is MS crippling.

The cause of MS is not known; one line of research points to a virus, another to congenital defects in the myelin coating of nerves. In older homeopathic textbooks MS is attributed to inherent weakness of the nervous system aggravated by trauma, shock, infection, or toxic metals. There also appears to be a link with solar radiation.

Conventional treatment is to give ACTH (adreno-corticotrophic hormone) to encourage the adrenal glands to produce more steroids to combat inflammation, and also physiotherapy. The homeopathic approach is constitutional.

Specific remedies to be given 4 times daily for up to 2 weeks while waiting for constitutional treatment
- Exaggerated reflexes, episode linked to some kind of emotional upset, person tends to faint easily *Phosphorus 6c*
- Very jerky movements of hands, feet, and tongue *Tarentula 6c*
- Sharp, shooting pains, movements very weak and shaky *Agaricus 6c*
- Weakness in back and limbs, made worse by exercise, leaving person very fatigued and in pain; perhaps complete paralysis of affected limb *Kali phos. 6c*
- Painful spasms of twitching and jerking, soothed by warmth, pressure, and friction *Magnesia phos. 6c*

Self-help A diet low in animal fats and high in gamma linoleic acid (a fatty acid found in sunflower seeds and safflower oil) is recommended; a gluten-free diet can also be beneficial. Make sure your body knows what rest and exercise feel like; take three 10–20 minute rest periods every day, spaced out through the day, and do some form of fairly vigorous exercise every day – walking, press-ups, lifting weights (lie on your back, and lift a 3 kg [7 lb] weight up and down above your chest or to and from your hips and shoulders). As with all forms of exercise, start slowly and build up gradually. As far as vitamins and minerals are concerned, make sure you get plenty of Vitamin B_6, B_3, B_{12}, folate, C, and E, and also zinc and magnesium; evening primrose oil is also recommended. Check the possibility of excess mercury in your diet or environment.

Neuralgia and neuritis

Pain or tingling from damaged or inflamed peripheral nerves (nerves not in the brain or spinal cord); some forms are mild or temporary, others recurrent or severe, such as SCIATICA (affecting the sciatic nerve in leg) and TRIGEMINAL NEURALGIA (shooting pains in the main facial nerve). Nerves can be damaged by alcohol, drugs, too much glucose in the blood (as in one form of DIABETES), too much Vitamin B_6, arsenic, mercury, lead, and organo-phosphate residues (from weed-killers); they can also be damaged by vitamin deficiencies, especially of the B vitamins; or damage may be a consequence of infections such as SHINGLES, DIPTHERIA, POLIO, TETANUS, or leprosy, or vaccines, as in GUILLAIN BARRE SYNDROME. Some form of neuropathy affects 1 person in 400; symptoms vary from mild tingling to agonising or shooting pains, and from pins and needles to complete NUMBNESS and wasting of unused muscles. Weakness and loss of sensation can easily result in injury.

Neuralgia and neuritis should be treated by an experienced homeopath. Your GP may recommend analgesics or painkillers if the pain is severe, and perhaps physiotherapy.

Specific remedies to be given 4 times daily for up to 2 weeks while constitutional help is being sought
- Nerves flare up after exposure to cold, affected part of body feels congested as well as numb *Aconite 30c*
- Attack brought on by dry cold, person feels chilly, exhausted, restless, burning or searing pains *Arsenicum 6c*
- Attack brought on by cold or damp, pain violent and lacerating, and better for application of heat, especially if person is suffering from facial neuralgia *Colocynth 6c*
- Pain worse after sleep *Lachesis 6c*
- Pain alleviated by heat and pressure *Magnesia phos. 6c*
- Neuralgia affecting rib cage or located above right eye *Ranunculus 6c*
- Pain above left eye, made worse by movement *Spigelia 6c*

---

⑨⑨⑨ Emergency – call GP (or dial 999) immediately. ② Consult your doctor if no improvement within 2 hours

Self-help Vitamins B_1, B_2, and biotin are good for nerves generally; for neuralgia after shingles, take extra Vitamin E as well; for diabetic neuritis, take extra B_{12} and chromium in addition to the general nerve vitamins mentioned above.

Numbness

Under this general description come tingling and pins and needles as well as complete loss of sensation. Usually caused by <u>pressure on a nerve</u> or poor blood supply to a nerve. Not uncommon after sleeping or <u>sitting in an awkward position</u>, but may also be a symptom of <u>CERVICAL SPONDYLOSIS</u> (pressure on nerves in neck, causing numbness in hands, stiff neck, headaches), <u>CARPAL TUNNEL SYNDROME</u> (numbness in thumb side of hand, sharp pain at night), or <u>RAYNAUD'S SYNDROME</u> (fingers and toes go blue in cold weather, then become red and painful as sensation returns).

Numbness associated with blurred vision, difficulty speaking, CONFUSION, DIZZINESS, or weakness in the arms and legs could be a STROKE; appropriate action is ②.

See NEURALGIA AND NEURITIS for specific homeopathic remedies.

Paralysis

Individual muscles or groups of muscles capable of little or no movement are said to be paralysed; in *flaccid paralysis* the nerves fail to stimulate contraction of the muscles, and in *spastic paralysis* they fail to stimulate relaxation. Paralysis may be temporary or permanent, depending on the nature of the damage to the nerves; prolonged disuse causes muscles to waste.

Nerves supplying muscles can be damaged by impact injuries (especially those involving the brain or spinal cord), by infections (POLIO and TETANUS, for example), by oxygen starvation (as in a STROKE), by pressure or compression (caused by a tumour or a PROLAPSED DISC, for example), or simply by the process of ageing. Nerve damage may also be congenital, as in SPINA BIFIDA or CEREBRAL PALSY.

Conventional treatment is to encourage the person to be as mobile as possible; support measures include physiotherapy and other manipulative therapies (chiropractic, osteopathy), and various mobility aids. Homeopathy can offer constitutional treatment and also remedies for use in acute cases.

Specific remedies to be given every hour for up to 8 doses
- Movement difficulty after an accident *Arnica 30c*
- If Arnica produces no improvement *Hypericum 30c*
- Loss of movement in a hand or foot (provided not due to lead poisoning) *Plumbum 6c*
- Paralysis of eye muscles *Conium 6c*
- Writer's cramp *Gelsemium 6c* or *Cuprum 6c*

Self-help Extra vitamin B_1 may be beneficial. Check possibility of excess mercury, lead or iron in diet or environment.

Parkinson's disease (Parkinsonism) see also
TREMBLING AND TWITCHING
Gradual deterioration of nerve centres in brain responsible for controlling movement; as degeneration proceeds, the delicate balance between two chemicals (neurotransmitters) which ensure transmission of nerve impulses is also upset. In most cases no obvious cause can be found, but in a few the culprit has been found to be carbon-monoxide poisoning, poisoning by heavy metals such as mercury or manganese (see pp. 30–31, 348, 349), a rare form of ENCEPHALITIS, or drugs, particularly the phenothiazines used in the treatment of SCHIZOPHRENIA; if drug-related, the condition usually disappears when the drug is stopped.

Early symptoms of Parkinson's disease are an involuntary tremor of the hands or head which more or less stops when the person consciously decides to move them. Gradually, movements which are only just under voluntary control – keeping one's balance or swinging one's arms when walking, writing legibly, talking clearly – are affected; then voluntary movements are affected, becoming slow and difficult to initiate; gait becomes shuffling, and the person tends to fall easily; other problems are excessive salivation (see SALIVATION DISORDERS), abdominal cramp, MEMORY LOSS, and patchy concentration. The condition is not fatal in itself, nor is it painful; it affects 1 person in 1000 and slightly more men than women, seldom starts before the age of 50, and may have a minor hereditary component.

In orthodox medicine Parkinsonism is usually controlled by anticholinergic drugs (drugs which counteract the dominance of one of the neurotransmitter chemicals referred to earlier), but these can have unpleasant side effects. Although homeopathy can offer a number of specific remedies for occasional use, the condition really requires the ongoing care of an experienced homeopath. A 'designer' recreational drug, MTPP, is known to produce Parkinsonian symptoms; prepared in a homeopathic potency, it could be used to treat people genuinely afflicted with the condition.

Specific remedies to be given 4 times daily for up to 2 weeks when symptoms are particularly bad, or while waiting to see a homeopath
- Over-production of saliva, sweet/metallic taste in mouth, trembling hands, tremor accompanied by perspiration and made worse by it, equal sensitivity to heat and cold, patchy memory and concentration, loss of will-power *Mercurius 6c*
- Person restless, twitching in every muscle, very suspicious and jealous, inclined to behave obscenely *Hyoscyamus 6c*

For explanation of other symbols, see page 107

- Limbs tremble, twitch, and jerk, person complains of stiffness and itchiness in affected limbs, spine feels extremely sensitive *Agaricus 6c*
- Where main complaint is stiffness or cramp, made worse by damp or immobility but alleviated by moving, tremor not very marked *Rhus tox. 6c*
- Excessive trembling and weakness affecting mainly tongue, eyes, and attempts to swallow, staggering gait *Gelsemium 6c*
- Where none of the above remedies is effective *Manganum 6c*

Self-help Extra Vitamin B$_6$ and C may be beneficial, but if person is on orthodox drugs, consult GP first, as dosage may need to be changed.

Peripheral neuropathy see NEURALGIA AND NEURITIS

Pins and needles see NUMBNESS

Polio (poliomyelitis)
A virus disease which attacks motor nerves, causing wasting and PARALYSIS; now rare in the West thanks partly to polio oral vaccine, but still endemic in some tropical countries. Virus is spread by personal contact or through faecal-oral route. First symptoms are those of acute INFLUENZA, accompanied by HEADACHE and FEVER. If suspected, 12

Specific remedies to be taken every 30 minutes for up to 10 doses
- Early stages of polio, person restless, scared, and very thirsty, skin dry, early signs of meningitis, including neck rigidity *Aconite 30c*
- Early stages of polio, high fever and delirium, staring eyes, stiff neck *Belladonna 30c*
- Early stages of polio, severe headache made worse by slightest eye movement, person becoming more and more depressed and lapsing into coma *Bryonia 30c*

Specific remedy to be taken 4 times daily for up to 2 weeks after initial attack
- Spastic paralysis with rigid legs, numbness in fingers, inability to place heels on ground because of tension in calves *Lathyrus 6c*

Post-herpetic neuralgia see SHINGLES

Presenile dementia see also SENILE DEMENTIA
Comparatively swift deterioration of mental and physical powers at a relatively young age or before the age of 60, causing death within about 5 years. Unlike dementia in the elderly, presenile dementia progresses fairly quickly and sometimes has a removable cause – a BRAIN TUMOUR, HYPOTHYROIDISM, or aluminium poisoning, for example. In some cases deterioration may be genetic or due to a slow virus infection. If no obvious cause can be established, constitutional care from an experienced homeopath is recommended. In addition to the specific remedy given below, the remedies listed under SENILE DEMENTIA would be appropriate.

Specific remedy to be given every 12 hours for up to 2 weeks
- When confusion gets suddenly worse *Alumina 30c*

Self-help Encourage person to use his or her senses – especially taste, smell, and touch – to the full. Pets and music also have a positive effect on mood and help to keep blood pressure down. Avoid cooking in aluminium utensils or using aluminium foil, and remove as many other sources of aluminium from the environment as possible (see p. 349 for list); it might also be worth having aluminium levels assessed by hair analysis. Extra Vitamin C and Vitamin B complex, calcium, magnesium, and zinc are recommended, as is evening primrose oil.

Spinal cord injury
Usually caused by falls or traffic accidents, especially by whiplash injuries in which the head is suddenly thrown backwards or forwards. Immediate symptoms depend on which part of the spine is injured; neck injuries can be fatal if the nerves that control breathing are damaged; injuries further down the spine can cause loss of sensation in or control over limbs, inability to control bladder and bowel movements, severe pain, or the sensation of being 'cut in half'.

If the spinal cord is merely bruised, recovery can be complete. If there is more serious damage, surgery may be necessary to maintain stability of the spine, followed by physiotherapy and occupational therapy, and it may take 3–4 months to assess whether disability will be lasting or not. Some of the secondary effects of spinal injury may be urinary infections if the bladder is paralysed, inability to achieve an erection, and pressure sores if immobility is prolonged.

If you are confronted with someone who has been in an accident, and he or she is conscious but cannot feel or move arms or legs, or complains of numbness, (999), but do not move them; ambulances have special equipment for lifting spine-injured casualties. If, however, the person starts to vomit, put him or her in the recovery position (see First Aid pp. 90–91); in such circumstances the risk of further damage to the spinal cord is less than the risk of dying from inhaled vomit. For further First Aid measures see p. 103.

Specific remedies
- Person suffering from spinal shock (after a fall, or after jumping and landing badly) *Arnica 30c* every 15 minutes for up to 10 doses, followed by *Hypericum 6c*, 4 times daily for up to 3 weeks

Spinal cord tumour see also CANCER

Similar to a BRAIN TUMOUR, but much rarer; as tumour begins to press on spinal nerves, there may be persistent BACK PAIN, NUMBNESS, coldness or weakness in one or more limbs, or difficulty urinating or defaecating. Investigation is by myelography (X-raying spinal cord after injection of special fluid into spine), CAT scan (computerised axial tomography, in which hundreds of X-ray pictures of tiny slices of the spine are taken by a revolving camera) or NMR (nuclear magnetic resonance, in which the tumour is imaged by a highly sophisticated form of magnetic current). Where the tumour is benign, surgery may be successful; if malignant, chemotherapy and radiotherapy may also be necessary. For homeopathic treatment, see CANCER p. 273.

Stroke

Occurs because blood supply to the brain is disturbed or insufficient; depending on the part of the brain affected, there may be sudden loss of speech or movement, sudden heaviness in the limbs, NUMBNESS, blurred vision, CONFUSION, DIZZINESS, or loss of consciousness. If symptoms last for 24 hours or longer, a full stroke has occurred; if they last for a few hours only, then a *transient ischaemic attack* or TIA has occurred. Appropriate action, in either case, is ②; if the person loses consciousness, put him or her in the recovery position (see First Aid pp. 90–91). In fact any of the above symptoms should reported to a GP; they can be early warnings of a stroke or TIA.

The particular event which starves the brain of vital oxygen (ischaemia literally means 'keeping back blood') may be a THROMBOSIS, an EMBOLISM, or a haemorrhage. Cerebral thrombosis usually occurs because the arteries which supply the brain have become narrowed or damaged by ATHEROSCLEROSIS or hardened by ARTERIOSCLEROSIS; blood flow becomes so sluggish that a clot forms, creating a partial or total blockage. A cerebral embolism is caused by a blood clot which breaks away from an artery wall somewhere else in the body and lodges in an artery supplying the brain. A cerebral haemorrhage occurs when blood leaks or bursts out of a weak-walled artery in the brain; pressure of blood in a confined space eventually slows down the bleeding and a clot is formed. In each case, the result is the same: some part of the brain has its blood and oxygen supply cut off. Once damaged, brain cells do not regenerate, although their function may be taken over by uninjured cells.

More people die of CORONARY ARTERY DISEASE every year than die of strokes, but hardened, furred up arteries are the immediate cause of both. Factors which contribute to artery disease are HIGH BLOOD PRESSURE, SMOKING, and raised cholesterol levels; the latter are, in turn, the result of eating too much animal fat, not taking enough exercise, and STRESS.

One in three first strokes is fatal; for those who survive, full recovery is as likely as some degree of impairment, though much depends on the severity of the stroke and the kind of care and rehabilitation given afterwards. Speech therapy and physiotherapy can improve talking and walking; anticoagulants such as aspirin can prevent further blood clots, but should not be prescribed to anyone who has a history of stomach ulcers (see PEPTIC ULCER), or who develops sensitivity to aspirin (see TINNITUS); surgery can also remove obstructions from arteries.

Constitutional treatment from an experienced homeopath can aid recovery after a stroke; changes in diet, exercise, and lifestyle will almost certainly be recommended too. In addition there are specific remedies which can be given during and immediately after a stroke, and during recovery.

Specific remedies to be given every 15 minutes for up to 10 doses during a stroke while medical help is being sought
- Face hot and flushed, headache, eyes wide and staring *Belladonna 30c*
- At first signs of attack, especially if brought on by heavy meal or alcohol *Nux 6c*
- Person panicky and afraid of dying once he or she realises what is happening *Aconite 30c*
- In later stages, person lapsing into unconsciousness, face bluish and congested, breathing heavy and laboured *Opium 6c*

Specific remedy to be taken 4 times daily for up to 2 weeks immediately after a stroke
- *Arnica 6c*

Specific remedies to be taken 4 times daily for up to 3 weeks during recovery
- Person elderly, physically and mentally weak *Baryta 6c*
- Where main after effects are numbness and trembling, inability to speak, pain at back of head *Gelsemium 6c*
- Speech very slow *Lachesis 6c*
- Speech unintelligible, tendency to clutch private parts *Hyoscyamus 6c*
- Person clearly depressed *Aurum 6c*

Self-help To prevent a stroke in the first place or to prevent recurrence, cut down on animal fats (including dairy products) and protein, increase fibre intake, eat fresh fruit and vegetables every day, try to lose some weight, or at least take more exercise, STOP SMOKING, and learn to relax or meditate if you suffer from stress or high blood pressure (preventive lifestyles are discussed in PART 2). Extra vitamin C can do no harm, but Vitamins E and B_6 should only be taken under medical supervision.

Subarachnoid haemorrhage see BRAIN HAEMORRHAGE

Transient ischaemic attach (TIA) see STROKE

Trembling and twitching
In the absence of other symptoms, involuntary trembling and twitching may be due to drug side effects (especially if you have just been put on a new drug), withdrawal from alcohol (see DELIRIUM TREMENS), or caffeine poisoning (after drinking too much tea or coffee), or a symptom of PARKINSON'S DISEASE (tremor worse when resting), THYROTOXICOSIS (excessive sweating or fatigue, bulging eyes, weight loss), or RHEUMATIC FEVER (involuntary jerking of hands, arms and face, joints painful and swollen).

If shakiness is part of a general picture of nervousness and tension, constitutional treatment could be helpful.

Specific remedies to be taken 3 times daily for up to 2 weeks
- Person jerks during first sleep, has frightening anxiety dreams *Belladonna 30c*
- Violent jerking or great restlessness during sleep *Sulphur 6c*
- Marked twitching, rhythmic spasms *Agaricus 6c*
- Involuntary writhing movements, person wakes up in a fright, especially after receiving a terrible shock *Stramonium 6c*
- Person weak and shaky as if with flu *Gelsemium 6c*
- Trembling gets worse with strong emotion *Ignatia 6c*
- Excessive saliva, stammering, trembling of tongue and fingers *Mercurius 6c*

Self-help Vitamins B_2 and B_6, and choline are recommended, as are zinc, magnesium, and lecithin. Reduce intake of caffeine (in tea, coffee, cocoa, and cola), and check diet and environment for excess mercury and bismuth. If taking lithium as an antidepressant, ask your GP if you could reduce the dosage.

Vertigo see DIZZINESS

SKIN, NAILS AND HAIR

The skin accounts for 16 per cent of total body weight and is therefore the largest organ in the body. Stretched out, it would cover 2.0-2.6 m^2 (15–20 ft^2). Skin is lost and renewed at the rate of 30 g (1 oz) a month, which adds up to about 18 kg (40 lb) in an average lifetime. The outer layer, the epidermis, is effectively lifeless; it consists of flattish cells which are dying or already dead. These cells waterproof the skin and protect it from infection, and are continuously manufactured in the underlying layer of skin, the dermis. In this deeper, living layer lie blood vessels, lymph vessels, nerve endings sensitive to heat, cold, pain, and pressure, glands which manufacture sebum to keep the skin supple and waterproof, follicles which manufacture hair and nails, glands which eliminate toxins and wastes as perspiration, cells which synthesise vitamin D if the skin is exposed to sunlight, and cells which contain the dark pigment melanin which protects the skin from harmful wavelengths in sunlight. Binding them all together, and giving the skin its softness and resilience, are two more kinds of tissues, fatty (adipose) tissue and elastic connective tissue. Wrinkles represent a loss of fat and elasticity. Beneath the dermis and attached to it by flexible fibres lie muscles, tendons, ligaments, and bones.

In homeopathic medicine skin conditions, which include conditions affecting hair and nails, are viewed as manifestations of general imbalance, of poor metabolic function. Rather than treating the obvious and visible symptoms – itchiness, blisters, scaliness, etc. – the whole constitution is treated. Suppressing symptoms at skin level may cause the underlying imbalance to express itself in an internal, and often more important, organ. Skin tone and colour tells a trained homeopath a great deal about a person.

In general, skin problems are not helped by sugar, refined carbohydrates, chocolate, tea, coffee, alcohol, spices, or perfumed cosmetics, or by constipation and lack of exercise, both of which slow down the elimination of toxins.

To moisturize dry skin, use pure olive oil or Calendula cream; if using these on the face, apply them very sparingly. Excessive washing tends to dry the skin, but skin brushing – with a dry loofah or soft bristle brush – is very beneficial; it removes dead cells from the epidermis and because it gently massages the blood and lymph vessels in the dermis it speeds up the elimination of toxins. Always brush towards the heart, with a brisk, flicking motion. Avoid brushing the face. Facial gymnastics – systematically exercising the main muscle groups in the face – also help to keep the skin youthful and supple.

Abscess
Often the result of a puncture wound (unsterilized needles, animal bites, etc.). Effectively sealed inside the skin, bacteria multiply, producing toxins which cause heat, swelling, and pain; to prevent toxins entering the bloodstream, surrounding tissues wall off the infected area, which becomes filled with pus (a mixture of defending white blood cells, dead bacteria, and blood serum). Eventually abscess bursts, and pus drains out, or surrounding tissues gradually digest and dispose of abscess contents; occasionally, however, an

abscess becomes chronic – infection continues to smoulder because the body is unable to deal with it.

Given early enough, homeopathic remedies or antibiotics can prevent abscess formation; later, surgical incision may be necessary to drain pus.

Specific remedies to be given every hour for up to 10 doses
- A slow-forming abscess located fairly deep, with swelling of surrounding lymph glands, or a chronic abscess which neither goes away nor comes to a head, or to aid healing after abscess has been incised and cleaned *Silicea 6c*
- A suppurating abscess which is tender to the slightest touch and causes sharp, stabbing pain, chilliness, irritability *Hepar sulph. 6c*
- Abscess in early stage, especially if perspiration is smelly and person cannot tolerate heat or cold *Mercurius 6c*
- Abscess in early stage, angry red, throbbing, tender, and very sensitive to cold air *Belladonna 30c*

Self-help Hot compresses may help to bring abscess to a head and then encourage discharge of pus. Once abscess is open, bathe with Hypericum and Calendula solution (5 drops of each in 0.25 litre ([½] pint boiled cooled water).

Acne see also ACNE ROSACEAE
Mainly an affliction of adolescence, but can persist into middle age. In adults, condition requires constitutional homeopathic treatment, a careful watch on diet, perhaps with extra vitamins and minerals, and changes in hygiene routines and lifestyle. For full description and treatment see ACNE p. 336.

Acne Rosaceae
Produces ACNE-like symptoms, but occurs in middle age; cheeks and nose flush easily, becoming permanently red, with small pus-filled spots; usually aggravated by hot spicy foods, tea, coffee, and alcohol (see also ALCOHOLISM), and by STRESS, but causes are thought to be oral contraceptives, steroid ointments, and possibly a deficiency of Vitamin B_2 (riboflavin). Antibiotics are usually prescribed.

If stress is the major factor, homeopathic treatment is constitutional. However, the remedies listed below may be beneficial.

Specific remedies to be taken 3 times daily for up to 3 weeks
- Face dry and burning, cold applications only make things worse, skin flakes and scales, restlessness, chilliness *Arsenicum 6c*
- In early stages, face red, dry, and burning hot *Belladonna 6c*
- Face always red and dry, with pimples and pus-filled spots *Sulphur iod. 6c*
- Burning and itching aggravated by heat, especially in women with scanty periods *Sanguinaria 6c*

- Condition made worse by alcohol, tea, and coffee, person constipated, irritable, and chilly *Nux 6c*
- Red, painful, or itchy spots, face puffy and swollen, cold or wet weather makes condition worse *Rhus tox. 6c*
- Condition markedly worse in morning and aggravated by alcohol, face reddish-purple and mottled *Lachesis 6c*

Self-help Take extra Vitamin B_2 and try the Liver Diet (pp. 352–3) for 1 month. If you are on steroids, stop taking them if possible. Discuss with your GP.

Alopecia see HAIR LOSS

Athlete's foot
Fungal infection in which skin round toes becomes red and itchy, then white and soggy, and flakes or peels off; in severe cases toenails become yellow and distorted. *Jock itch* (similar symptoms around groin) and RING-WORM (red, itchy rash on scalp) are caused by the same fungus, which likes warmth and moisture found in swimming pools and changing rooms. Most GPs prescribe anti-fungal ointments, powders, or tablets. As with many skin conditions, homeopathic approach is to boost immune system generally, so treatment is constitutional.

Self-help Wash feet regularly and dry them thoroughly (a hair dryer is good for drying between toes). Let as much air get to your feet as possible; if you must wear socks, wear cotton rather than nylon, and if you must wear shoes, wear sandals. Over-the-counter anti-fungal powder should only be used if condition is very persistent.

Baldness see HAIR LOSS

Birthmarks see BIRTHMARKS p. 300

Blushing see BLUSHING p. 337

Boils and carbuncles
Infections of the hair follicles, usually the work of *Staphylococcus* bacteria, also responsible for FOOD POISONING; a carbuncle is a particularly large boil or a close-knit group of boils sited somewhat deeper in the dermis than the average boil. As white cells attack bacteria, thick white or yellow pus accumulates, causing pain and swelling, and boil develops a head; after a day or two boil either bursts or slowly reduces and heals. Recurrent boils can be a symptom of DIABETES. Orthodox treatment is antibiotics and, if necessary, lancing. Homeopathic treatment is constitutional, but the remedies below can be used to relieve pain and swelling.

Specific remedies to be given every hour for up to 10 doses

- Boil in early stage, skin very red and tender *Belladonna 30c*
- If boil weeps easily and is sensitive to the slightest touch, or to bring boil to a head *Hepar sulph. 6c*
- To cleanse a boil which has burst, or to help heal a boil which has been slow to develop and slow to disperse *Silicea 6c*
- Skin over boil bluish, blistered, and very angry-looking, with a black centre *Anthracinum 6c*
- Skin over boil burning hot, aggravated by application of heat *Arsenicum 6c*
- Boil weeps but causes little pain *Gunpowder 6c*

Self-help At first sign of inflammation, bathe affected area with Hypericum and Calendula solution (5 drops of mother tincture of each to 0.25 litre [½ pint] boiled cooled water). A pad of cotton wool soaked in hot salt water (1 teaspoon to 0.25 litre [½ pint]) and applied to the boil every few hours reduces pain. Never squeeze a boil. If it bursts, let it drain by itself. If possible, avoid handling food.

Bruising see BRUISING p. 189

Burning feet
Continuous burning and smarting of the feet, possibly due to vitamin deficiency, but in most cases no cause can be found.

Specific remedies to be taken 3 times daily for up to 3 weeks; if no improvement within 1 month, see your homeopath
- Feet burn and sting, and look puffy *Apis 6c*
- Burning worse at night, person puts feet out of bed to cool them, tendency to feel hot most of time *Sulphur 6c*
- Feet hot and sweaty, anger seems to make things worse *Chamomilla 6c*
- Burning sensation made worse by walking *Graphites 6c*
- Burning sensation made worse by heat and by letting legs hang down, relieved by lying down *Pulsatilla 6c*
- Burning sensation worse at night, though feet are cold and clammy, feet sweat and smell unpleasant during day *Silicea 6c*

Self-help Take Vitamin B complex. Soak feet in cold water occasionally, and go barefoot or wear sandals whenever possible.

Burns see First Aid pp. 93–4

Cancer of the skin see also CANCER
Skin cancer can take the form of a rodent ulcer, a squamous cell carcinoma, or a malignant melanoma. Of these, rodent ulcers are the most common, and malignant melanomas potentially the most serious.

Most at risk are people over 50, people with fair skins, and people who have had long exposure to strong sunlight. Any lump or 'bite' which does not heal within a week or two, or any change in a mole or wart, should be investigated by your GP.

Malignant melanomas are usually confined to the legs although they can also occur on soles of feet; unfortunately, chances of this form of cancer spreading to other parts of the body are high, unless it is caught in very early stages. Judging by doubling of number of deaths from this form of cancer since 1950, short intense exposure to strong sun, the kind of exposure many people get on holidays abroad, may be a significant factor. Malignant melanomas develop from pigment cells, usually from pre-existing moles – see MOLES for danger signs. If you notice changes in a mole, or a new mole or new patch of pigment, [48]. If mole is malignant, immediate surgery and perhaps radiotherapy will be necessary. If cancer has already spread, alternative therapies, especially Gerson therapy, may be more beneficial than chemotherapy – see CANCER for details.

Rodent ulcers almost always appear on the face, especially on the nose or around the eyes; they grow very slowly, and seldom if ever spread to other parts of the body, although they can be locally invasive and destroy an eye or ear, or erode a major artery, if not treated early. Some rodent ulcers are merely raised lumps with a scabby crust, others are like bright pink warts with a fissured centre, and others look like small fleshy cushions; they may bleed from time to time, but they never heal. Routine treatment is to freeze ulcer and remove it, or destroy it by radiation. A rodent ulcer is not a sign that cancer is likely to develop elsewhere.

Squamous cell carcinomas most commonly appear on the lips, near the ears, or on the hands, and may take the form of enlarging open sores or wart-like lumps; sunlight, tars, and in some cases SOLAR KERATOSES are thought to be triggers. This form of cancer can metastasize, so early treatment is essential; options, depending on size and site of carcinoma, are freezing, radiotherapy, or surgical removal.

For all three forms of skin cancer constitutional homeopathic treatment is recommended in addition to orthodox treatment.

Carbuncles see BOILS AND CARBUNCLES

Cellulite
Unsightly 'orange peel' skin and dimpling, especially on thighs and upper arms; due to fluid retention and hard accretions of fat cells; culprits are insufficient exercise, poor elimination of fluids and wastes through lymphatic vessels, being overweight, and not eating enough raw vegetables and fruit. Persistent, unsightly fat is often a depot for toxins, either environmental or dietary. Exercise, skin brushing, massage, and eating as many organic and as few processed foods as possible can help a lot.

Cellulitis see ERYSIPELAS

Chilblains see CHILBLAINS p. 189

Chloasma

Patches of darker skin on face, especially on cheeks, which appear during pregnancy or while on the pill; once hormones settle down after childbirth or discontinuation of the pill, patches usually fade. If the remedy below produces no improvement within 1 month, consult your homeopath.

Specific remedies to be taken every 12 hours
● *Sepia 6c*

Self-help Take extra Vitamin C and E.

Cold sores see COLD SORES p. 171

Corns and calluses

Under constant or repeated pressure, skin thickens and hardens; calluses are patches of hard skin on hands or feet, and are quite common with BUNIONS; corns occur on the toes and are small areas of hard skin which have been pressed inwards. When pressed, both corns and calluses feel tender; ULCERS can develop beneath calluses in DIABETES. Culprits are ill-fitting shoes and high heels, or heavy manual work. If corns are very painful, your GP will refer you to a chiropodist.

Specific remedy to be taken 4 times daily for up to 2 weeks
● *Antimonium 6c*

Self-help Corns and calluses will not go away if you continue to wear the shoes which caused them. Wear flat, comfortable shoes – sandals would be better – and as a temporary measure place felt or rubber rings over the corns to relieve pressure. Regularly soften hard skin with Calendula ointment or cut it away with a corn file. To strengthen your arches and prevent your untramelled feet from splaying, try picking up rubber squash balls with your toes!

Cracks and fissures

For reasons which are not fully understood but which are generally labelled 'constitutional', some people are prone to cracked lips, finger tips, etc. If the remedies below do not improve matters, constitutional homeopathic treatment should be sought.

Specific remedies to be taken 3 times daily for up to 2 weeks
● Cracks at corner of mouth, skin rough and red *Petroleum 6c*
● Cracking in folds of skin, especially if complicated by fungal infection in areas which are kept warm and moist, skin dirty-looking and very itchy, symptoms aggravated by washing *Sulphur 6c*
● Cracking in nostrils, on lips, behind ears, on nipples, or on fingertips *Graphites 6c*
● Cracking worse in winter, person overweight, chilly and sweaty *Calcarea 6c*
● Cracks on finger tips become deeper in cold weather and are slow to heal, sweaty hands and feet *Silicea 6c*

Self-help Apply Calendula ointment. Vitamin B complex, Vitamins A and C, zinc, and essential fatty acids should be beneficial.

Cysts see SEBACEOUS CYSTS

Dandruff

Excessive amounts of flaking skin on scalp, sometimes with itchiness and redness; may be a symptom of SEBORRHOEIC ECZEMA, a mild form of eczema which can also affect face and chest; more rarely, condition is a feature of PSORIASIS, involving knees and elbows as well, or a sign of a fungal infection. Hair growth is not usually affected. If possible, try the homeopathic remedies and self-help measures given below before resorting to scalp preparations containing steroids. If appropriate, use remedies given for SEBORRHOEIC ECZEMA and PSORIASIS

Specific remedies to be taken 3 times daily for up to 2 weeks
● Scalp dry, sensitive, and very hot, unbearably itchy at night, round bare patches of scalp show through hair *Arsenicum 6c*
● Scalp moist, greasy, and sensitive around hair roots *Sepia 6c*
● Dandruff thick, a lot of scratching at night, which causes skin to burn, scalp made even drier by washing hair *Sulphur 6c*
● Intense itching, thick leathery crusts with pus underneath and white scabs on top *Mezereum 6c*
● Flaky scalp, hair loss *Fluoric ac. 6c*
● Scalp moist, encrusted, and smelly, crusting worse behind ears *Graphites 6c*
● Itching like insect bites all around hairline of forehead, moist, smelly spots behind ears, itchiness made worse by heat *Oleander 6c*
● White crusting around hairline, hair lank and greasy *Natrum mur. 6c*

Self-help In addition to the remedies above, take Kali Sulph (see Tissue Salts p. 388) 3 times daily for up to 1 month, then 3 times daily for only 5 days out of 7 until scalp improves. Reduce intake of refined carbohydrates and animal fats, and take extra Vitamins B,C, and E, and zinc.
   Dandruff which sticks to the hair and scalp can be loosened by rinsing scalp with sour milk or a mild solution of lemon juice (2 tablespoons lemon juice to 0.5 litre [1 pint] boiled cooled water). As for shampoo, use pure soap. Apply Calendula ointment to itchy areas

around hairline. If whole scalp itches, apply cold-pressed linseed oil overnight (sleep on an old towel) and wash it off with pure soap shampoo in the morning. If all else fails, wash hair in shampoo which contains selenium, but follow the instructions carefully.

Darkening of the skin

When not due to SUNBURN, may be a symptom of CHLOASMA (if you are pregnant or on the pill) or ADDISON'S DISEASE (a permanent tanned look), WEIGHT LOSS, loss of appetite (see APPETITE CHANGES), tiredness, ANAEMIA, bouts of CONSTIPATION and DIARRHOEA, NAUSEA AND VOMITING). A greyish tinge to the skin is sometimes a sign of excess iron.

Dermatitis see ECZEMA

Eczema (dermatitis) see also ECZEMA IN CHILDREN p. 320, SKIN PROBLEMS pp. 341–2

Local inflammation of the skin, accompanied by ITCHING, redness, weeping, blistering, and bleeding if scratched.

Contact eczema is caused by allergies to plants, fabrics, and metals (poison ivy, tomato or primula leaves, chrysanthemums, wool, nickel, for example), and is often associated with ASTHMA, HAY FEVER or ALLERGIC RHINITIS. *Seborrhoeic eczema* seems to be inherited, not linked to any allergy; it causes flakiness and itching in smile lines between nose and mouth, in beard area, around hairline, on scalp (see DANDRUFF), on chest, and also in the groin or armpits, or between or under the breasts. *Detergent eczema* is an occupational hazard of housewives, catering workers, hairdressers, nurses, mechanics . . . anyone in fact who comes into daily contact with household cleaners, washing-up liquid, shampoos, grease removers, all of which contain detergents; hands become rough, red, scurfy, sore, and itchy, especially on knuckles. *Pompholyx eczema* causes itchy, weeping blisters on palms of hands and soles of feet, and is thought to be due to STRESS or poor diet; it is uncommon, and usually clears up of its own accord after 2 or 3 weeks. *Discoid eczema* appears on arms or legs as itchy, round, red patches which proceed to flake, blister, weep, and form crusts; condition may last for several months, but it is rare and its cause is not known.

The orthodox approach to eczema is to prescribe steroid ointments to relieve inflammation, and if necessary antihistamines and antibiotics to control itching and infection; to discover the allergen(s) involved in contact eczema, a patch test may be necessary. However, steroid preparations should be avoided unless eczema is so bad that it is causing miserable, sleepless nights, which in turn are causing stress and aggravating the eczema.

Homeopathic treatment for eczema is constitu-tional, but the following remedies may be used while help is being sought or when itching is very bad.

Specific remedies to be taken 4 times daily for up to 2 weeks
- Eczema mainly affects palms and area behind ears, honey-like discharge from skin *Graphites 6c*
- Skin red, dry, rough, and itchy, aggravated by heat and washing, especially if person has diarrhoea which gets worse early in morning *Sulphur 6c*
- Affected skin cracks easily *Petroleum 6c*
- Blisters itch more at night or in damp weather, but improve with warmth *Rhus tox. 6c*
- Skin dry and itchy, person constipated *Alumina 6c*
- Skin very sensitive and easily infected, feeling generally chilly and worse in cold *Hepar sulph. 6c*
- Skin dry and burning, but aggravated by cold applications *Arsenicum 6c*
- Skin irritated, dirty-looking, and prone to infection, general chilliness *Psorinum 6c*

Self-help Obviously, known irritants should be avoided. Wear rubber gloves for gardening, housework, washing-up, etc. If rubber gloves are the culprits, wear cotton gloves inside them. Always dry hands thoroughly after washing, and use Calendula cream as a moisturizer. If culprit is stress, exercise, relaxation, or a simple form of meditation (see PART 2) may help.

You could also try rubbing evening primrose oil on to unaffected areas of skin. Take extra Vitamins B and C, and also zinc. Add safflower oil capsules to diet. Going on the Liver Diet (pp. 352–3) for 1 month would do no harm either.

Erysipelas (cellulitis)

Streptococcus infection of broken skin, usually on face or lower leg, causing mild FEVER, redness, tenderness, and swelling, sometimes with red lines (inflamed lymph vessels) radiating from site of infection towards nearest lymph gland (see LYMPHANGITIS). Untreated, bacteria may enter general circulation and cause SEPTICAEMIA. Orthodox treatment is antibiotics.

Specific remedies to be taken every hour for up to 10 doses; if fever and swelling do not abate within 24 hours, see your GP
- Skin burning hot, watery swelling under skin *Apis 30c*
- Bluish-purple tinge to skin around infected area, perspiring more than usual *Lachesis 6c*
- Infected area blistered and intensely itchy, general restlessness *Rhus tox. 6c*
- Lesions bright red, throbbing and tender, cold air intensifies discomfort *Belladonna 30c*
- Nearby glands swollen, sweat smells unpleasant, heat and cold equally uncomfortable *Mercurius 6c*

Self-help If a limb is affected, keep it raised as much as possible.

Excessive perspiration see PERSPIRATION
PROBLEMS

Facial hair problems

In men, facial hair is a secondary sex characteristic
marking the transition from juvenile to adult; in
women, facial hair commonly increases after the
menopause or it may run in the family. Excessive
hairiness generally may be a sign of HYPOPITUITARISM,
which is usually accompanied, in women, by WEIGHT
GAIN, deepening of the voice, and cessation of periods.
Certain drugs can also cause facial and body hair to
increase; if this is the case, see your GP.

If facial hair causes embarrassment, plucking,
waxing, shaving, or special depilatories will temporarily
remove it; electrolysis may or may not remove hair
permanently, and needs to be done by an expert.
Constitutional homeopathic treatment may help, but
there are no specific remedies apart from the one given
below.

Specific remedy to be given every 12 hours for 3 doses
and observe for 1 month
- Hair confined to upper lip, especially if growth
  increases after vaccination against smallpox or after
  a bad reaction to some other vaccine *Thuja 30c*

Flushing see also BLUSHING p. 337

Flushing of the face, typically of the nose and cheeks,
can be brought on by STRESS, hormone changes during
MENOPAUSE, alcohol, or spicy food; in middle age it
may be a prelude to ACNE ROSACEAE; it can also be a
drug side effect, or a symptom of thyrotoxicosis (see
THYROID PROBLEMS), food ALLERGY, or excessive
consumption of Vitamin B$_3$. It is quite natural for the
face and sometimes the thighs to turn bright red during
strenuous exercise.

Self-help If flushing come on during menopause, take
Vitamin E, but check with your doctor first if you have
high blood pressure or are taking anticoagulants.

Greasy hair

Caused by overactivity of the sebaceous glands, which
produce a waxy substance called sebum to keep hair
supple and waterproof; often associated with other skin
problems, and in youngsters either with ACNE or the
general hormonal upheaval of adolescence. Can be
aggravated by over-frequent washing with strong
shampoos which destroy acid balance of scalp.
Constitutional treatment is recommended if the
specific remedies and self-help measures below do not
improve matters.

Specific remedies to be given every 12 hours for up to
1 month
- As first resort *Bryonia 6c*

- Greasiness associated with tight sensation in scalp,
  which feels sweaty, over-production of saliva,
  intolerance of heat and cold *Mercurius 6c*
- Greasiness associated with thinning hair, especially
  after prolonged emotional stress or grief *Phosphoric
  ac. 6c*

Self-help Cutting down on refined carbohydrates
(sweets, chocolates, soft drinks) often helps, and so
does frequent washing with mild or very dilute
shampoo (try a herbal shampoo such as seaweed or
rosemary).

Greasy or oily skin

Greasy skin, caused by overactive sebaceous glands,
tends to run in families, but is usually worst during
adolescence when it conspires with rapid production
and shedding of epidermal cells to produce ACNE –
blackheads, whiteheads, and infected pimples. Similar
problems occur with greasy skin alone. Hormone
imbalances, oral contraceptives, and steroids increase
sebum secretion. Constitutional treatment is recommended, but the remedies below should be tried first.

Specific remedies to be given every 12 hours for up to
1 month
- Face oily and shiny, oiliness worse on hairy parts,
  person constipated *Natrum mur. 6c*
- Oil on face smells unpleasant, oiliness worse in cold
  and hot weather, trembling, increase in saliva
  production, sticky perspiration *Mercurius 6c*

Self-help Greasy skin should not be cleansed more
frequently than night and morning; use Hamamelis
solution (10 drops of mother tincture fo 0.25 litre [½
pint] boiled cooled water) as a cleanser. Sun also helps
to clear up a greasy skin, provided complexion is dark
or sallow, and tans rather than burns. Avoid taking
steroids and oral contraceptives. Try the Liver Diet
(p. 352–3) for 1 month, and take Vitamin B complex.

Greying hair

Essentially, we all go grey when our genes say so, when
they turn off the pigment-producing cells in our hair
follicles. However, premature greying may be due to a
lack of Vitamin B$_5$ or PABA (para-aminobenzoic acid),
or to severe STRESS; it can also be an indicator of
increased risk of AUTOIMMUNE DISEASE. If associated
with ECZEMA or HAIR LOSS, constitutional treatment
would be appropriate, but the remedies given below
should be tried first.

Specific remedies to be given every 12 hours for up to
1 month
- Greying associated with hair loss, especially after
  grief or prolonged mental stress *Phosphoric ac. 6c*
- Greying associated with baldness and eczema
  behind ears *Lycopodium 6c*

- Greying associated with hot flushes and painful scalp *Sulphuric ac. 6c*

Self-help Vitamin B$_{12}$ and B complex and also zinc are recommended.

Hair loss

A natural process, since hair is continuously growing, but if hair growth temporarily slows down, as is quite common <u>after childbirth or after a feverish illness,</u> hair is lost faster than it is replaced. <u>Slight thinning is also common in men and women as they get older.</u> Baldness is predominantly a male phenomenon, tending to run in families; in men a receding hairline generally meets a thinning crown, producing a tonsure effect; in women only the crown thins. In babies, rubbing can cause hair loss, but the hair regrows.

Rarely hair loss is caused by deficiency ailments such as hypothyroidism (see THYROID PROBLEMS) or iron-deficient ANAEMIA, by a lack of zinc or B vitamins, especially biotin, and inositol, or by cytotoxic drugs used to treat CANCER; too much Vitamin A or selenium, and also oral contraceptives and anticoagulant drugs, can have the same effect. Generally speaking, once the cause is removed, hair starts growing again. Conditions which destroy hair follicles, however, such as RINGWORM and LICHEN PLANUS, cause permanent patches of baldness. In *alopecia areata* patches of baldness appear quite suddenly, with all but a few hair follicles becoming inactive; the cause is not known.

The pharmaceutical industry has recently come up with a new drug which stimulates hair growth, but it has to be taken on a permanent basis and may have long-term side effects.

Constitutional treatment can be helpful for thinning hair, giving a boost to the metabolism generally, but the remedies below should also be tried.

Specific remedies to be taken every 12 hours for up 1 month
- Hair loss after childbirth, or premature baldness and greying *Lycopodium 6c*
- Hair loss associated with boils on scalp and headaches which become more insistent at night, person very depressed *Aurum 6c*
- Hair is brittle and falls out in little tufts *Fluoric ac. 6c*
- Scalp feels painful when touched, loss of body hair as well *Selenium 6c*
- Hair loss related to hormone changes after childbirth or at menopause, indifference towards loved ones *Sepia 6c*
- Hair loss after grief or extreme emotion, predominant feelings are indifference and exhaustion *Phosphoric ac. 6c*
- Hair loss follows severe injury *Arnica 6c*
- Hair loss associated with dryness of hair and scalp *Kali carb. 6c*

- Hair loss in an elderly person who has poor circulation and is mentally slow *Baryta carb. 6c*
- Hair loss associated with dandruff and white crusts on scalp, especially around hairline *Natrum mur. 6c*
- Hair falls out in handfuls *Phosphorus 6c*

Self-help Hair which is regularly bleached, dyed, permed, or straightened is more fragile than untreated hair. Over-frequent washing and conditioning encourage dryness and make the hair look greasy quickly. One application of shampoo is quite enough to remove dirt and grime; if possible let hair dry naturally. Scalp massage may be beneficial in some cases since it encourages circulation. Vitamin B complex, Vitamin C, zinc, and iron are recommended. Also, make sure diet contains sufficient protein (from vegetable as well as animal sources).

Head lice see HEAD LICE p. 323, PUBIC LICE

Herpes see COLD SORES

Hives see URTICARIA

Icthyosis

A rare inherited condition in which skin is very dry and flakes off in diamond-shaped scales rather like those of a fish, especially in winter; condition begins in early childhood but usually gets better during teens. If the remedies given below produce no improvement within 1 month, see your homeopath.

Specific remedies to be given every 12 hours for up to 1 month
- Extensive scaling, leaving skin beneath raw and weepy *Arsenicum iod. 6c*
- Skin burning, itchy, dry, rough, and scaly, and markedly worse in cold weather *Arsenicum 6c*
- Skin rough, with a grey, bluish, or yellow tinge and dark brown patches *Plumbum 6c*
- Scaling skin made worse by touching, warts, brittle and deformed nails *Thuja 6c*

Impetigo

Contagious bacterial infection of the skin, more common in children than adults, but not serious except in newborn babies; in a baby, bacteria may spread to kidneys and cause GOMERULONEPHRITIS. Symptoms are small patches of tiny blisters which then burst and form a crust like brown sugar; these can occur anywhere on body, but most commonly affect area round nose and mouth. Bacteria are spread by touching blisters, then touching another part of body, or by using towels or flannels used by an infected person. If remedies below do not clear up infection, see your GP; he or she will prescribe antibiotic tablets or ointment, after which general immunity should be boosted by constitutional homeopathic treatment, especially if contact with infected individuals is still likely.

Specific remedies to be given every hour for up to 10 doses
- Blisters round nostrils and mouth, especially in children *Antimonium 6c*
- Scalp most affected, blisters thickly encrusted and oozing pus which irritates surrounding skin *Mezereum 6c*
- Scrotum most affected, blisters inflamed and oozing pus *Croton 6c*
- Blisters accompanied by physical exhaustion, chilliness, and mental restlessness *Arsenicum 6c*

Self-help Bathe affected areas with Hypericum and Calendula solution (5 drops of mother tincture of each to ½ pint boiled cooled water) or dilute TCP (follow instructions on bottle) several times a day, and keep towels and flannels away from other members of the household. Always wash hands thoroughly before preparing food. A child with impetigo should be kept away from school until blisters heal.

Itching
If accompanied by a *rash*, may be due to ECZEMA (extensive patches of red, sore skin), URTICARIA (light red, raised weals), scratching (raised red weals following line of scratch), PSORIASIS (red patches covered in silvery scales), RINGWORM (red, ring-shaped patches fading in centre), SCABIES (red rash on trunk, also on hands and wrists, or genitals, with scabies mite burrows visible under magnifying glass), OR LICHEN PLANUS (small, shiny, violet spots).

Among the conditions which cause itching, but no obvious rash, are THREADWORMS, PRURITIS ANI, ANAL FISSURE, PILES, and sometimes DIARRHOEA (itching confined to anal area), JAUNDICE (general itchiness, eye whites yellowish), ICTHYOSIS (skin dry and scaly, especially in cold weather), HEAD LICE, and DANDRUFF.

If itchiness is accompanied by fever, with or without a rash, see FEVER pp. 305–6 for possible causes. Otherwise see conditions mentioned above for suitable homeopathic remedies.

Keloid see also SCARRING
Excessive and sometimes unsightly growth of scar tissue after an injury, burn, vaccination, or operation, or after ear-piercing, most common in dark-skinned people; wound appears to heal normally at first, then scar begins to grow; occasionally, keloids develop from old scar tissue or from unscarred skin. Orthodox treatment is by steroid injections, freezing, radiotherapy, or cosmetic surgery. If specific remedies given below do not halt or reduce growth within a month or so, see your homeopath.

Specific remedies to be taken 3 times daily for up to 3 weeks

- Keloid in early stages *Graphites 6c*
- Long-standing keloid *Silicea 6c* followed by *Fluoric ac. 6c*

Lichen planus
An itchy outbreak of small, shiny, purplish-red lumps, often on arms and legs, but occasionally on scalp, causing HAIR LOSS; can also lead to nail deformities (see NAIL PROBLEMS), or cause white lacy pattern inside mouth. Cause is not known, but majority of people affected are over 50; condition is harmless, if annoying, and onsets suddenly, with spots fading to brown before disappearing. Conventionally treated with steroid tablets or ointment. Constitutional homeopathic treatment is recommended if condition recurs, as it sometimes does once steroid treatment stops; however, the remedies below should be tried first.

Specific remedies to be given 4 times daily for up to 3 weeks
- Remedy of first resort, whether condition is acute or chronic *Sulphur iod. 6c*
- Rash burns and itches *Arsenicum 6c*
- Outbreak worse on face and neck, spots feel prickly and itchy *Juglans 6c*
- Undressing makes itching worse *Rumex 6c*

Lumps or swellings
Innocuous bumps on hands or feets may be WARTS, CORNS OR CALLUSES, OR GANGLIA; painful swelling may be an ABSCESS or the after-effect of a vaccine; BOILS AND CARBUNCLES and BITES AND STINGS (see First Aid p. 90–92) also cause painful swellings; potentially more serious are lumps in the lymph glands of the armpit, breast, or groin, suggesting the possibility of infection or irritation from anti-perspirants CANCER OF THE BREAST, HODGKIN'S DISEASE, OR LYMPHOMA, and moles or warts which suddenly enlarge or become more prominent, suggesting some form of CANCER OF THE SKIN; swelling of the lymph glands at the back of the skull may be a symptom of GERMAN MEASLES (with a pink rash and fever); if lymph glands in the neck are swollen, PHARYNGITIS, TONSILLITIS, OR GLANDULAR FEVER (with sore throat) may be the cause; swelling between ear and jaw on one side of face may be MUMPS (sometimes glands under jaw swollen too, pain on swallowing, fever), a TOOTH ABSCESS (jaw aches or throbs), or a salivary duct tumour; an unfamiliar small bulge on the abdomen or groin may be a HERNIA; swellings around joints, accompanied by stiffness, pain, and tenderness, may be BURSITIS, RHEUMATOID ARTHRITIS, OR OSTEOARTHRITIS; fluid retention or OEDEMA may be due to kidney problems such as GLOMERULONEPHRITIS OR KIDNEY FAILURE (swollen ankles, passage of small amounts of urine, nausea and vomiting, drowsiness).

If you suspect a lump or swelling may be malignant, 48; if either of the kidney problems mentioned above is suspected, 12. Otherwise see entries above for homeopathic remedies.

Malignant melanoma see CANCER OF THE SKIN

Moles

Dense collections of cells containing the skin pigment melanin – the rest of the pigment cells are evenly distributed and are only stimulated to produce melanin when the skin is exposed to the sun's ultraviolet rays. Moles can be flat, raised, or hairy, and usually develop in childhood; moles which develop later should be regarded with suspicion as they may be an early sign of malignant melanoma (see CANCER OF THE SKIN), a form of cancer which develops in pigment cells. Other danger signs in moles are, a diameter of more than 1 cm, an increase in size, an irregular notched outline, inflammation in or around a mole, an irregular dark area within a mole, crusting or oozing, bleeding, or itching, or other change in sensation. Occasionally a seborrhoeic wart (see WARTS) may be mistaken for a mole.

Nail problems

Disorders specifically affecting the nails are few; more often, discolouration or deformity is the result of injury, or of nutritional, respiratory, or heart disorders.

Deformed nails have a variety of causes, including iron deficiency (nails become spoon-shaped), respiratory or heart problems (nails become clubbed, growing round swollen ends of fingers and sometimes toes), PSORIASIS (nails become pitted), injury and infection (nails develop horizontal ridges), or simply old age (nails develop vertical ridges, possibly due to malabsorption of Vitamins A, B complex, and C, calcium, magnesium, zinc, and essential fatty acids).

Self-help Preventive measures include keeping nails short, wearing gloves for gardening and rubber gloves if hands are repeatedly immersed in water, trimming toenails straight across to prevent them ingrowing (see below), and wearing shoes which do not press on toenails.

Discoloured nails can be telltales of a variety of conditions, including ANAEMIA (nails very pale), liver problems (nails whitish) BACTERIAL ENDOCARDITIS (nails have dark flecks in them which look like splinters), and fungal infections (nails turn whitish and soft or crumbly); nails also turn purplish or black when hit (see sub-ungual haematoma below) or put under gentle but constant pressure for any length of time. White spots on nails are often a sign of zinc or Vitamin A deficiency.

Fungal infections turn the nails white and crumbly, causing ridging and thickening afterwards. Orthodox medicine prescibes antifungal drugs or ointments. However, the homeopathic remedies below should be tried first.

Specific remedies to be taken 4 times daily for up to 3 weeks

- Nails brittle, with horny thickening *Antimonium 6c*
- Nails deformed, with white spotting *Silicea 6c*
- Nails thickened, deformed, brittle or crumbly, inflamed and painful, with blackening *Graphites 6c*
- Nails brittle, with skin at base red and swollen *Thuja 6c*

Self-help Soak nails twice a day in Calendula solution (10 drops mother tincture fo 0.25 litre [½ pint] boiled cooled water) or apply Calendula ointment.

Ingrowing toenails are usually caused by ill-fitting shoes or by tapering nails at sides instead of cutting them straight across; occasionally they can be due to problems in the nailbed. As the sides of the nail curve under, surrounding skin becomes inflamed and tender. Orthodox treatment is minor surgery. In early stages, process can be arrested by working a small piece of lint between side of nail and skin over top of nail and nailbed underneath) after thoroughly bathing toe with Hypericum and Calendula solution (5 drops of mother tincture of each in 0.25 litre [½ pint] boiled cooled water). If nail becomes infected, use remedies given for paronychia (see below).

Specific remedies to be given every 12 hours for up to 1 month, then see your GP if no improvement
- To strengthen nails which repeatedly ingrow *Magnetis austr. 6c*
- If nails are very brittle *Thuja 6c*

Paronychia is an acute bacterial or yeast infection which attacks growing tissue at base of nails, causing red, swollen cuticles, and sometimes blisters of pus (whitlows) alongside nails; can result in deformed or discoloured nails.

Specific remedies to be given hourly for up to 10 doses
- Early stage, skin at base of nails hot, red, tender, and throbbing *Belladonna 30c*
- Base of nails yield pus when pressed, skin around nails very tender *Hepar sulph. 6c*
- Infection slow to heal *Silicea 6c*

Self-help See fungal infections (above). Also, take zinc, Vitamin C, and Vitamin B complex.

Sub-ungual haematoma is a very painful condition caused by crushing or trapping injuries; nail rapidly blackens as blood accumulates beneath it; only way to relieve pain is to relieve pressure of blood under nail. Your GP will do this by lancing the nail, but if medical help is not available, you can lance the nail yourself by heating a straightened paper clip with a match or lighter and plunging it through the nail in the centre of the blackened area until blood appears. Also, immediately after the injury, take *Arnica 30c* every hour for up to 10 doses.

Whitlows see Paronychia

Nettle rash see URTICARIA

Oedema see also PULMONARY OEDEMA

Abnormal accumulation of fluids in body tissues, showing as puffiness under the skin, especially around ankles; occurs in heart, liver, and kidney disease, and in protein malnutrition; many women, especially before periods (see PREMENSTRUAL SYNDROME), in hot weather, and as result of prolonged standing, develop a minor form of oedema. Exact cause of condition is not known; probably a combination of factors – hormonal, metabolic, nervous – is responsible, and in some cases ALLERGY may play a role. *Angioneurotic oedema* is a complication of URTICARIA, an allergic reaction to nettles and other plants, and is thought to be caused by STRESS; swelling rapidly affects eyes and lips, and may extend to throat, obstructing breathing; appropriate action is ⑨⑨⑨ and *Apis 30c* every 5 minutes for up to 10 doses. PULMONARY OEDEMA (breathlessness and coughing, with blood-flecked sputum, dramatically worsening in space of a few hours) is also life-threatening; again, appropriate action is ⑨⑨⑨.

Severe chronic oedema causes swelling of ankles, legs, abdomen, face, and hands; weight fluctuations during course of day; intense thirst and frequent urge to urinate, especially when lying down; bowel and bladder upsets; HEADACHE, visual disturbances, FAINTING; mental function may also be impaired. Orthodox treatment is restriction of carbohydrates, especially refined carbohydrates; diuretics are also used, but can cause dependency and further fluid retention. Homeopathic treatment is constitutional; in meantime, choose a remedy from the list below.

Specific remedies to be taken 3 times daily for up to 2 weeks
- Swelling of feet and ankles, chilliness, restlessness, thirst for hot beverages taken in small quantities at frequent intervals *Arsenicum 6c*
- Swelling accompanied by inflammation and stinging pains, discomfort made worse by heat and even light pressure *Apis 6c*
- Mild swelling in hot weather or hot rooms *Natrum mur. 6c*

Self-help Cut down on salt and try to lose weight. Take extra Vitamin B_6 and B complex, and magnesium. If swelling occurs mainly in hot weather, take **Natrum Mur.** tissue salt (see p. 35) 3 times a day while weather remains hot.

Perspiration problems

Sweat glands (eccrine glands) are most plentiful on forehead and scalp, palms of hands, soles of feet, in groin and armpits, and around nipples; sweating reduces body heat and gets rid of various wastes. Naturopathically speaking, it is not healthy to suppress perspiration with anti-perspirants.

Excessive perspiration (hyperhidrosis), if not obviously due to hot surroundings or exertion, may be a sign of FEVER, OBESITY, thyrotoxicosis (loss of weight despite increased appetite, bulging eyes, trembling – see THYROID PROBLEMS), HODGKIN'S DISEASE (swollen glands, especially in neck, itchy skin), or TUBERCULOSIS (night sweats despite few bedclothes, weight loss, coughing); tuberculosis and Hodgkin's disease require prompt medical attention.

Body temperature, and therefore sweating, can also be increased by alcohol or withdrawal from alcohol (see ALCOHOLISM), aspirin, Vitamin B_1 deficiency, or wearing man-made fibres; ANXIETY produces sweating on forehead, upper lip, soles, and palms; hot flushes – suddenly feeling very hot and sweaty – are a common symptom of the MENOPAUSE; cold sweats can be a symptom of HYPOGLYCAEMIA. Adolescent concerns about increased sweating and BODY ODOUR are related to the fact that sweat glands under arms and in groin do not become active until adolescence. Appreciable amounts of sodium and zinc are lost in perspiration.

If excessive sweating is causing embarrassment, and does not seems to have any clear cause, constitutional homeopathic treatment may help. In the meantime, the remedies below should be tried; they should produce some improvement within about 2 weeks.

Specific remedies to be taken 4 times daily for up to 2 weeks
- Person overweight, cold and clammy, sweat smells sour, head sweats worse at night *Calcarea 6c*
- Person thin, chilly, prone to sweaty feet which smell unpleasant *Silicea 6c*
- Hot sweating on head, with diarrhoea first thing in morning *Sulphur 6c*
- Sweating worse on head, sweat profuse and sour-smelling, cold weather and walking reduce sweating *Fluoric ac. 6c*
- Perspiration very pungent and sticky, made worse by heat or cold *Mercurius 6c*
- Perspiration smells unpleasant and is worst on feet and under arms, right foot may be hot and left foot cold *Lycopodium 6c*

Lack of perspiration (anhidrosis) is probably due to some fault in the autonomic nervous system (part of nervous system which is not under voluntary control); overheating and possibly HEAT STROKE are risks in hot weather. Constitutional treatment is recommended, but one or both remedies below should be tried first.

Specific remedy to be taken 3 times daily for up to 3 weeks
- *Aethusa 6c* or, if no improvement, *Alumina 6c*

Self-help If you suffer from excessive perspiration, shower night and morning to remove stale sweat (body odour is mostly caused by bacteria, which thrive on sweat), and wear cotton underwear and shirts, and change them daily. The answer to smelly feet is to wash and dry them thoroughly at least once a day, avoid nylon socks and tights, and wear sandals rather than shoes. If you must use a deodorant/anti-perspirant, use one which does not contain aluminium (look in your local healthfood shop).

Pityriasis rosea
A skin rash, probably caused by a virus, which mainly affects children and young adults, especially in spring and autumn; often starts as single ring-shaped, reddish brown, scaly patch – a 'herald' patch – on trunk, then in space of 7–10 days smaller patches appear on trunk, neck, upper arms, and thighs; usually clears up of own accord within 2–3 months; may cause minor ITCHING and a mild SORE THROAT. Conventional treatment, if rash is bad, is steroid cream and antihistamine. If the remedies given below are not effective within a week or two, see your homeopath or GP.

Specific remedies to be given 4 times daily for up to 3 weeks
- Anxiety, restlessness, wanting sips of water all the time *Arsenicum 6c*
- Spots fiery red, burning, and painful *Radium brom. 6c*
- Spots show red under thin white scales, warmth or exercise makes itchiness worse *Natrum mur. 6c*

Self-help Apply Urtica ointment to affected areas.

Prickly heat
Acute itchiness most common among fair-skinned people in tropical or sub-tropical climates (dark-skinned people are not affected); due to a combination of damp heat, wearing clothes, being overweight, using soap too often, and a tendency to produce too much sebum (see GREASY OR OILY SKIN). Itchy, prickling sensation is due to inflammation caused by bursting of sweat gland ducts blocked by sebum; if many sweat gland ducts are blocked, result may be HEAT STROKE. If condition is particularly troublesome, constitutional treatment would be appropriate.

Specific remedy to be taken every 2 hours for up to 10 doses as soon as prickling sensation starts, but not more frequently; if necessary, repeat dose daily.
- *Apis 30c*
- As preventative, take *Sol 30c* 3 times daily during exposure for up to 3 weeks in every 4

Self-help Avoid hot baths and showers, use soap once a day only, and try to acquire a protective tan (see SUNBURN). Avoid hot drinks, spicy foods, and meat extract. Increase Vitamin C intake.

Psoriasis
An inherited skin condition in which the epidermis produces new cells too fast for keratin formation to take place – keratin is a fibrous protein that forms a tough, protective covering over skin, nails, and hair. As a result, unsightly patches of flaking skin develop, on knees, elbows, sacrum, or scalp behind ears; patches are well-defined, slightly raised, deep pink beneath their silvery scaling, and not necessarily sore or itchy. Nails may also be affected, becoming thick, rough, or pitted, or separating completely from the nailbed (see NAIL PROBLEMS). In a few sufferers, joints of hands, fingers, knees, and ankles may become inflamed and swollen. Condition is chronic, flaring up at intervals; it is rare before age of 5, and most common between age of 15 and 30; can be precipitated by infections (especially those caused by *Streptococcus* bacteria), by drugs such as chloroquine (used in treatment of rheumatism and malaria), and also by STRESS or injury.

Orthodox treatments include steroid and coal tar ointments, cytotoxic drugs which slow down cell division, Vitamin A and D derivatives (which can be highly toxic), and special ultraviolet therapy. Condition can be managed each time it recurs, but not cured. Constitutional homeopathic treatment, and the self-help measures below, usually prove beneficial. If the remedies given below do not produce some improvement within 2 weeks, see your homeopath.

Specific remedies to be taken 4 times daily for up to 2 weeks
- Affected areas of skin burning hot, mentally restless but physically exhausted, feeling chilly *Arsenicum 6c*
- Dry, red, scaly, itchy patches worse after baths, especially if person often feels too hot *Sulphur 30c*
- Skin behind ears affected, exuding honey-coloured pus *Graphites 6c*
- Affected areas extremely scaly, aggravated by warmth *Kali ars. 6c*
- Condition aggravated by cold and worse in winter *Petroleum 6c*

Self-help Provided you do not have a sensitive skin, careful sunbathing (6 sessions starting at 10 minutes and increasing to 60 minutes) or several 10-minute sessions under an ultraviolet lamp may help to clear up an outbreak. To reduce stress, learn to relax or meditate (see PART 2). Try the Liver Diet (pp. 352–53) for 1 month, and take extra zinc.

Puffiness and swelling of the skin see OEDEMA

Rodent ulcers see CANCER OF THE SKIN

Scarring see also KELOID
Once blood clotting has effectively sealed a wound, and special white blood cells have disposed of bacteria and other wound debris, cells called fibroblasts start to repair the wound internally, producing scar tissue; this consists of very strong but relatively inelastic fibres of

protein which tend to shrink with age. Uncontrolled production of scar tissue leads to a KELOID.

Homeopathic treatment can help scars to fade, or prevent them thickening; if the remedies below produce no improvement within a month or so, see your homeopath.

Specific remedies to be given every 12 hours for up to 1 month
- To minimize scarring or remove superficial scars *Thiosinaminum 6c*
- Old scars which suddenly become itchy, painful, or inflamed *Silicea 6c*
- Scar beginning to thicken or with a tendency to weep *Graphites 6c*

Self-help Some people report that external application of Vitamin E during healing makes scars less visible.

Sebaceous cysts (wens)
Smooth, yellowish lumps under the skin, especially on the scalp, with small sacs of whitish fluid inside; painless and harmless unless infected by bacteria, in which case they may burst, releasing pus; if infection recurs, as it tends to, surgical removal may be recommended, otherwise conventional treatment is antibiotics. If remedies below do not clear up infection within 5 days, see your homeopath.

Specific remedies to be given every 8 hours for up to 5 days
- Cyst on scalp which is sensitive and flaking *Baryta 30c*
- Cyst producing pus *Hepar sulph. 30c*

Solar keratoses
Rough red patches on skin which develop as result of prolonged exposure to strong sunlight; most common in people with fair or sensitive skin, and sometimes a precursor of squamous cell carcinoma (see CANCER OF SKIN).

If the homeopathic remedies given below do not reduce redness and roughness within 1 month, see your GP.

Specific remedies to be taken every 12 hours for up to 1 month
- A general tendency to feel hot, fair skin which burns easily in sun, a tendency to bleed easily *Phosphorus 6c*
- Red patches which are dry, flaky, and burning hot, but rest of body feels cold *Arsenicum 6c*

If you are fair-skinned and about to take a holiday in the sun, take *Sol 30c* as a preventive; correct dosage is three times daily for 3 weeks out of 4 while exposed to the sun.

Self-help The only sensible precaution, if you have a fair or sensitive skin, is to stay out of the sun or use high factor sun creams.

Squamous cell carcinoma see CANCER OF THE SKIN

Sunburn
The sun's ultraviolet rays can cause a lot of damage to skin. Even dark skins wrinkle badly after prolonged exposure to the sun (ultraviolet light actually breaks down the elastic tissues). In skins unused to the sun, reckless exposure produces heat and redness – the boiled lobster look – and even blistering. Gradual exposure, however, encourages the skin to step up melanin production, giving natural protection against sunburn. In fair skins which have little melanin-producing capacity, exposure can produce SOLAR KERATOSES and malignant changes (CANCER OF THE SKIN).

Sensible sunbathing means exposing yourself to the sun gradually so that your skin has time to produce more melanin; sunbathe for 15 minutes on the first day, then increase sun time by 15 minutes each day. Suntan lotions without a screening factor – the factor which minimizes burning – are useless; buy one with a screening factor that suits your skin type.

For treatment of sunburn, see FIRST AID pp. 93–94.

Swellings see LUMPS AND SWELLINGS

Ulcers see VARICOSE ULCERS, CANCER OF THE SKIN

Urticaria (nettle rash, hives)
Raised red patches or weals, sometimes with paler areas in centre, which cause intense itching; can be caused by food ALLERGY (to shellfish, strawberries, nuts, etc.), food additives, certain drugs (notably aspirin), scratching, insect bites, and extreme STRESS (grief at the death of a loved one, for example); in people with sensitive skin, heat, cold, or sunlight may raise weals. Regardless of the cause, stress and tension usually make condition worse. Conventional treatment is by antihistamines. In a few cases, eyes, lips, and throat may swell dramatically (see angioneurotic OEDEMA), leading to suffocation; this is an emergency situation, so ⑨⑨⑨ and give *Apis 30c* every minute until help arrives.

If, after avoiding known causes, condition recurs, constitutional homeopathic treatment would be worthwhile.

Specific remedies to be taken every hour for up to 10 doses during attack or while constitutional help is being sought
- Burning and swelling of lips and eyelids, made worse by warmth *Apis 30c*
- Rash caused by stinging nettles or some other plant, made worse by touching, scratching, or bathing with water *Urtica 6c*

- Chronic urticaria, made worse by exercise and stress *Natrum mur. 6c*
- Rash appears after becoming overheated in damp weather *Dulcamara 6c*
- Rash burns and itches, blisters develop, person very restless *Rhus tox. 6c*
- Skin red, itchy, and puffy, made worse by heat and bathing with water *Sulphur 6c*
- Rash made worse by fatty foods or stuffy rooms, person rather weepy *Pulsatilla 6c*
- Weals accompanied by stomach upset and white-coated tongue *Antimonium 6c*
- With restlessness and anxiety *Arsenicum 6c.*

Self-help Apply ice pack to affected area, or take a cold shower. Urtica ointment also relieves itchiness.

Varicose ulcers (venous ulcers)
In older people with POOR CIRCULATION or VARICOSE VEINS, even a tiny crack or injury to the skin can be slow to heal; without a good supply of fresh blood to bring in infection-fighting white blood cells or take away toxins, the injury site may become ulcerated and take months to heal; a typical varicose ulcer has a pale, weeping centre, a red, itchy surround, and brown mottling around that; commonest site is on legs, just above ankles. Routinely treated by applying antiseptic dressings to prevent infection, and support bandaging to speed up blood flow; in severe cases, GP may recommend hospitalization, and vein surgery or a skin graft may be necessary.

The remedies given below promote healing, but if there is no improvement within 14 days, see your homeopath.

Specific remedies to be taken 4 times daily for up to 14 days
- General remedy for varicose ulcers *Hamamelis 6c*
- Ulcers bleed easily and cause splinter-like pains *Nitric ac. 6c*
- Ulcers burn, especially between midnight and 2 am, but are less painful when heat is applied *Arsenicum 6c*
- Skin around ulcers bluish-purple *Lachesis 6c*
- Ulcers which are slow to form and equally slow to heal, with chronic mild infection *Silicea 6c*
- Early stages, before ulcer forms, when skin is hot, red, and throbbing *Belladonna 30c*
- Edges of ulcers clear-cut, as if made with a hole punch, white discharge *Kali bichrom. 6c*
- Ulcers oozing unpleasant-smelling pus and serum *Mercurius 6c*
- Ulcers form reddish scabs with pus beneath *Mezereum 6c*
- Ulcers bleed easily *Phosphorus 6c*
- Varicose ulcers in an elderly person *Carbo veg. 6c*
- Ulcers at site of injury *Arnica 6c*

Self-help If ulcers are due to varicose veins, raise legs above hip level when resting, avoid standing for any length of time, and go for a daily walk. Take extra Vitamin C and zinc. Apply Hypericum and Calendula ointment to dressings, and change them daily.

Verrucas see WARTS

Vitiligo
A rare condition in which white patches appear on skin due to a shutting down of pigment (melanin) production; since it occurs frequently in conjunction with pernicious anaemia (see ANAEMIA) and hypothyroidism (see THYROID PROBLEMS), it may be a disorder of the autoimmune system (see AUTOIMMUNE DISEASE), but nutritional deficiencies or tropical fungal disease may also be responsible.

There are no specific homeopathic remedies for vitiligo, but constitutional treatment may help. If pigment loss is extensive and embarrassing, your GP may refer you to a dermatologist.

Warts
Caused by viruses which invade the skin and cause the cells to multiply rapidly, forming raised lumps; unable to kill the viruses, the body walls them off. In susceptible individuals, warts are contagious: touching warts can quite easily transfer viruses to new sites, and new warts develop (see vulval and penile warts – VAGINAL AND VULVAL PROBLEMS, PENIS PROBLEMS).

Common warts are small, horny, and flesh-coloured or whitish, and most commonly occur on hands; on soles of feet, where they are called *verrucas*, constant pressure causes them to harden and burrow inwards, making walking quite painful. Two other types of wart, most common in children, are *plane warts* (which usually occur in groups, and look like tiny, brownish, fleshy blisters) and *molluscum contagiosum* (small, pearl-like warts with depressed centres, which seldom occur singly). Persistent warts are conventionally treated with wart paint, or they can be burnt or frozen off, or dug out. Warts which form after the age of 45, particularly *seborrhoeic warts*, which look like large, rough-surfaced moles, should be shown to your GP as soon as possible; they may be completely innocuous, or they may be malignant (see CANCER OF THE SKIN).

Homeopathic medicine offers a number of specific remedies for warts, but if home treatment does not produce improvement within a month or so, consult your homeopath. Long-term constitutional treatment may be necessary to tackle the underlying problem.

Specific remedies to be given every 12 hours for up to 3 weeks
- Soft, fleshy, cauliflower-like warts – chiefly on back of head – which ooze and bleed easily *Thuja 6c*
- Many warts, chiefly on face, eyelids, and fingertips, also painful verrucas *Causticum 6c*
- Cauliflower-like warts which itch and sting, and sometimes ooze and bleed, or become large and jagged-edged, upper lip most affected *Nitric ac. 6c*

- Many small, horny warts which itch, sting, weep, and bleed *Calcarea 6c*
- Horny warts associated with a callus *Antimonium 6c*
- Hard, smooth, fleshy warts, chiefly on back of hands *Dulcamara 6c*
- Warts on hands *Kali mur. 6c*
- Weeping, ulcerated warts on tips of toes *Natrum carb. 6c*

- Warts on palms of hands, tendency to sweaty palms *Natrum mur. 6c*
- Large black warts with hairs in them *Sepia 6c*
- Hard warts which burn and throb *Sulphur 6c*

Self-help Apply *Thuja* mother tincture twice daily and cover with a plaster. Over-the-counter wart preparations can also be used, but never on facial warts; apply them to the wart only, not to the surrounding skin, and be careful not to get them in your eyes.

EYES

THE eye is designed to bend (refract) light rays and bring them to a focus on the retina. When we want to focus on near objects, tiny circular muscles around the lens contract, making the lens fatter; when we focus on distant objects, another set of muscles, radial muscles, contracts and pulls the lens flatter. All the transparent elements of the eye – the conjunctiva, the cornea, the fluid-filled chamber in front of the lens and the gel-filled chamber behind it – contribute something to refraction but only the lens is capable of 'accommodation', changing its focusing power.

In a person who is short-sighted images of distant objects are brought to a focus just in front of the retina. This happens if the eyeball is too long from back to front, or if the ligaments which attach the radial muscles to the lens become slack. In a long-sighted person, the opposite occurs; near objects are focused just behind the retina, either because the eyeball is too short from back to front or because the radial muscles become lazy. In either case, the result is a fuzzy image. These and other refractive errors are relatively easy to correct.

The eyeball consists of three distinct layers of tissue: a tough, opaque outer layer called the sclera, in which the cornea is a transparent window; the choroid layer, liberally supplied with tiny blood vessels and heavily pigmented to stop light escaping through the back of the eye or setting up reflections within the eyeball; and the light-sensitive retina, literally a carpet of nerve fibres with specialized endings. Pigments in these nerve endings (photoreceptors) change their chemical composition in response to various wavelengths and intensities of light, and as these changes take place electrical impulses are generated and transmitted to the optic nerve and then to that part of the brain which makes sense of visual stimuli. Objects are upside down when projected on to the retina, but 'seen' the right way up because certain fibres in the optic nerve cross over before they reach the brain. The retina is easily damaged – by leaking blood vessels in the choroid, for example, or by a build-up of pressure within the eye.

In dim light, which stimulates the 125 million or so rod receptors around the edge of the retina, we see things in monochrome, in shades of black, white, and grey. In bright light, which stimulates the 7 million or so cone receptors packed in the central area of the retina, we see things in colour and with great sharpness. There are three kinds of cones, sensitive to the red, blue, and green wavebands of the visible spectrum; the marvellous variety of colours we see are the result of differential stimulation of these three kinds of receptors. The light sensitive pigment inside them, called rhodopsin, is replaced during sleep, a process which requires Vitamin A. Whereas rod receptors, which contain a different pigment, wear out every 2 weeks or so, cones remain functional for 9–12 months. At the end of their useful life, rods and cones are replaced, but after the age of 40 cone replacement becomes less efficient, leading in severe cases to macular degeneration.

The pigmented, muscular iris controls the amount of light reaching the retina. In dim light the iris aperture, the pupil, is large; in bright light it shrinks to pinhead size. Iridologists diagnose many different ailments from the state of the iris. Eye movement is controlled by three pairs of muscles originating from the bony orbit of the eye and attached to the sclera. Under normal circumstances both eyes swivel in unison, receiving two almost identical pictures of the world which we 'see' as one.

The conjunctiva, a continuation of the epidermis, is continuously cleansed and lubricated by salty, bactericidal fluid produced in the tear glands just above the eye. If dust, bacteria, and irritants are not constantly removed, the conjunctiva becomes scratched and sore, and sometimes infected. The duct which drains away this cleansing fluid opens into the back of the nose. Small wonder that our noses run when we start slicing onions! The fluid in the front chamber of the eye nourishes both lens and cornea; it too is constantly replenished. Blockage of the duct through which it drains can lead to glaucoma, a rise in pressure inside the eyeball.

For explanation of other symbols, see page 107

Astigmatism

Uneven curvature of the lens causing distorted vision; either vertical or horizontal lines are out of focus, depending on which rays of light are abnormally bent. Usually present from birth and accompanied by some degree of SHORT SIGHT or LONG SIGHT. Correctable by a cylindrical lens shaped to compensate for the un-evenness of the natural lens. Constitutional homeopathic treatment is also recommended; eye exercises can also be helpful.

Black eye

Rupture of small blood vessels around eye causing blood to leak into surrounding tissues, rapidly showing as red, purple, then nearly black bruising. After HEAD INJURY, may be due to bleeding from a fracture at base of skull; if a skull fracture is suspected, or both eyes turn black, (999). More frequently, black eyes are caused by hitting or punching. Where fracture or haemorrhage is suspected, give *Arnica 30c* immediately and then every 15 minutes until help arrives.

Specific remedies to be taken every 4 hours for up to 10 doses
- If black eye follows blow to head or eyes *Arnica 30c*
- If pain is relieved by applying cold compress *Ledum 6c*

Self-help An ice pack (a packet of frozen peas will do!) applied to the eye will help to constrict local blood vessels and staunch bleeding.

Blepharitis see EYELID PROBLEMS

Blurred vision see LOSS OF SIGHT AND BLURRED VISION

Cataract

Gradual clouding of the lens due to changes in its protein make-up; result is misty or distorted vision, usually affecting both eyes but one more than the other; most common in old age but occasionally seen in newborn babies; may also be a consequence of IRITIS, DIABETES, EYE INJURY, steroids (taken orally or applied as eye drops), or faulty microwave ovens. If cataract is bad enough to prevent normal functioning, surgical removal of the affected lens may be necessary; this makes the eye long-sighted, but this can be corrected by placing a plastic lens in the eye or wearing spectacles or contact lenses.

Specific remedies to be taken 3 times daily for up to 7 days, then twice a day for up to 1 month if you notice an improvement; if vision continues to improve, have a 2-day break, then take the remedy twice a day for another month
- Sensation of mist or veil before the eyes, or of something being pulled tightly over the eyes *Phosphorus 6c*
- In early stages, with circular lines visible in lens *Calcarea 6c*
- In later stages, with cataract beginning to interfere severely with sight *Silicea 6c* If no improvement within 2 months, consult your homeopath.

Self-help Take Vitamin E, bioflavinoids, potassium, and selenium.

Choroiditis

Inflammation of choroid layer (layer of blood vessels) directly behind retina; can lead to scarring of both choroid and retina, permanently impairing vision, especially if central area of retina is affected. Condition is painless, but should be suspected if there is blurred vision in centre of visual field and person has been exposed to *Toxocara* infection from close handling of dogs and cats and contact with their faeces (see TOXOCARIASIS). Choroiditis is also seen in babies whose mothers are infected with syphilis (see SEXUALLY TRANSMITTED DISEASES), though very rarely. Your GP will arrange for blood tests and X-rays, then prescribe steroids or, in severe cases, immuno-suppressive drugs to prevent further damage to choroid and retina. If you are unable to take these drugs, or if condition recurs after stopping them, consult your homeopath.

Specific remedies to be taken every ½ hour for up to 10 doses when disturbance to vision is most acute, or while waiting to consult a homeopath
- Congestive headache with flashing lights *Belladonna 30c*
- When everything seems green *Arsenicum 6c*
- Symptoms improve by wearing sunglasses or shading eyes *Phosphorus 6c*

Conjunctivitis

Inflammation of the conjunctiva, the transparent covering of the eye, due to infection or ALLERGY; uncomfortable but not serious except in newborn babies. Gummy, yellow discharge on waking in the morning is usually a sign of infection. When caused by HAY FEVER AND ALLERGIC RHINITIS, or by a food allergy, the whites of the eyes become red and gritty (the 'ground glass in the eyes' feeling) but there is no discharge. Occasionally condition is caused by cleaning solution used with soft contact lenses (see CONTACT LENS PROBLEMS).

Specific remedies to be taken every hour for up to 10 doses; if condition does not improve within 24 hours, see your homeopath or GP
- Symptoms come on after injury or exposure to cold *Aconite 30c*
- Copious discharge *Argentum nit. 6c*
- Little or no discharge *Euphrasia 6c*

Self-help Bathing the eyes with *Euphrasia* (10 drops of *Euphrasia* mother tincture and 1 level teaspoon salt to 0.25 litre [½ pint] warm water) is very soothing, whether condition is caused by infection, allergy, or lens cleaner; bathe them every 4 hours, but not more than 4 times a day, and use a disposable eye bath. Never use anyone else's face cloth or towel on your face, and be scrupulous about washing your hands before and after touching your eyes.

Contact lens problems
Contact lenses do not suit all eyes; if you suffer from HAY FEVER or bouts of CONJUNCTIVITIS, for example, spectacles may be more suitable. Many people find soft contact lenses more comfortable than hard ones; they can be left in for several days at a time or alternated with spectacles, but they usually need replacing within a couple of years. The softest kind can be worn continuously for days or weeks. Hard lenses are less comfortable and take some getting used to, but they are cheaper and last for 6 to 8 years; they also tend to give better vision, are prescribed for a wider range of sight problems, and are easier to keep sterile.

One you have become used to wearing contact lenses, the main problems are irritation and infection. Foreign particles trapped between the lens and the conjunctiva can cause irritation; so can hot, dry, or smoky atmospheres. Infection of the conjunctiva is usually caused by poor hygiene or by wearing lenses for too long. Always wash your hands before putting lenses in or taking them out, and always follow your optician's instructions about cleaning and soaking your lenses. A few people, especially if they have some form of ALLERGY already, become allergic to contact lenses or to soft lens cleaning solutions, in particular those containing the preservative Thiomersal; in such cases, alternative cleaning methods are available.

See CONJUNCTIVITIS for specific remedies and self-help measures.

Corneal ulcer
A sore on the cornea, the tough, transparent covering of the eye between the conjunctiva and the lens; usually the result of a scratch or foreign body in the eye, and subsequent infection, but occasionally a direct infection. *Herpes simplex*, the virus which causes COLD SORES, causes *dendritic ulcers* on the cornea, so called because they have a branching pattern. Symptoms are pain and watering of the eye, with the white of the eye becoming pink or red. Prompt treatment is required, so

24; antibiotic or antiviral drops or ointments will probably be prescribed.

Specific remedies to be taken every hour for up to 10 doses in addition to medication prescribed by GP
- As a first resort *Hepar sulph. 6c*
- If cornea damaged by being too near heat or flames, burning discharge from eyes *Mercurius 6c*
- Thick green or yellow discharge from eye, no burning sensation *Pulsatilla 6c*
- If above remedies do not work, and if ulceration is severe, light hurts eye, discharge is yellow, and lids are inflamed and stuck together *Rhus tox. 6c*
- Extreme intolerance to light, eye watering profusely, neck glands swollen *Conium 6c*
- Nausea when looking at moving objects *Ipecac. 6c*
- Eye sensitive to slightest touch *Hepar sulph. 6c*

Detached retina
The retina can detach itself from the underlying choroid layer for a variety of reasons: most common cause is perforation of the retina due to injury; retina may also be stretched too tight if eyeball is too long from back to front, as in SHORT SIGHT, or if lens has been removed because of a CATARACT; detachment can also occur if the vitreous fluid in the inner chamber of the eye shrinks away from the retina and tears it. Once detachment starts, vitreous fluid quickly seeps between the retina and choroid, lifting more and more of the retina away from the choroid. Symptoms are flashes of light, and black, floating, cobweb-like shapes, followed by a loss of peripheral vision in the affected eye, as if a curtain were being drawn; if left untreated, central vision will also be impaired. By the time symptoms appear, the retina has already detached, so ②; surgery under anaesthesia may be necessary. There is a small risk of recurrence after surgery, but a greater risk that the other eye will be affected, so have both eyes checked regularly. Constitutional treatment can help to prevent recurrence.

Specific remedies to be taken every 15 minutes for up to 10 doses while waiting for specialist help
- Early symptoms (as fluid seeps between retina and choroid) *Apis 30c*
- If Apis does not stabilize eye within 2 hours *Gelsemium 6c*
- If there is a history of injury to the eye *Arnica 30c*

If detachment has occurred before, *Aurum mur. 30c* taken every 12 hours for up to 10 doses may exert a protective effect.

Self-help Zinc and Vitamin A may be beneficial.

Diabetic retinopathy
Vascular damage to the retina associated with DIABETES, especially in diabetics who do not control

---

blood glucose levels properly; leakage of blood from the retinal blood vessels can cause scarring of the retina or clouding of the vitreous humour, or new blood vessels, also liable to leak, can form on the surface of the retina; result is a reduction in sharpness of vision or permanent loss of vision. All diabetics should have their eyes checked regularly. Condition requires prompt treatment, so 24. Formation of new, leaky blood vessels can be prevented by laser surgery, and by proper control of blood glucose levels. Homeopathic approach is to give constitutional treatment for diabetes.

Specific remedies to be taken every 2 hours for up to 6 doses
- As soon as floaters are seen *Arnica 30c*
- If Arnica does not stabilize condition within 12 hours *Conium 6c*

To help prevent further leakage of blood vessels in retina, once condition is stable, take *Lachesis 6c* every 4 hours for up to 6 doses.

Self-help Sensible measures include increasing intake of Vitamins C, E, and B$_6$, bioflavinoids, selenium, and zinc. Evening primrose oil is also beneficial.

Double vision
Seeing two images rather than one is sometimes a feature of EXOPHTHALMOS; an adult who develops a SQUINT also sees double. In exophthalmos the external muscles of the eyes are affected, preventing eyes from swivelling in unison; a squint in an adult is usually a complication of DIABETES or HIGH BLOOD PRESSURE, ailments which affect the eye muscles, or the nerves controlling them, and impair coordination. The brain, instead of receiving two very similar pictures, receives two very different ones; unable to integrate them, it 'sees' both. Excessive alcohol and some drugs can also cause double vision. Also BRAIN INJURY may cause double vision after severe blow to head. 999 and give *Arnica 30c* every 15 minutes. See also MULTIPLE SCLEROSIS and drooping eyelids under EYELID PROBLEMS.

Drooping eyelids see EYELID PROBLEMS

Dry eye
Lack of lubrication from the tear glands above the eyes, causing eyes to feel gritty and the whites to turn red; mainly affects women, usually in middle age; sometimes linked to RHEUMATOID ARTHRITIS or to an ALLERGY (especially to gluten, house dust, and pets), but can also be a drug side effect. Your GP will prescribe artificial tear drops. Hot rooms filled with cigarette smoke should be avoided.

Self-help Euphrasia eye baths (see CONJUNCTIVITIS) can relieve soreness temporarily, but extra Vitamin C,

B$_2$, B$_6$, and A, and evening primrose oil, may have longer-lasting effects.

Ectropion see EYELID PROBLEMS

Entropion see EYELID PROBLEMS

Exophthalmos
Bulging of the eyeballs due to abnormal swelling of soft tissues which line eye sockets; often a complication of overactivity of the thyroid gland (see THYROID PROBLEMS), but also a symptom of ORBITAL CELLULITIS (severe pain, eye filmed over with pus), or a TUMOUR OF THE EYE. Eyes tend to feel dry and gritty, lids may be unable to close, and vision may be blurred or double; corneas may also become infected (see CORNEAL ULCER). If condition persists despite treatment of underlying problem, steroids or surgery may be necessary to relieve pressure on eyeball. Homeopathic treatment is constitutional.

Eyelid problems see also LUMP ON EYELID, STYE
Blepharitis Crusting and redness around the edge of the eyelids, often associated with DANDRUFF. Untreated, flakes of skin may enter the eye and cause CONJUNCTIVITIS, or the eyelashes may fall out. Like dandruff, condition is deep-rooted and best treated constitutionally. Orthodox treatment is by antibiotic or steroid ointments which suppress rather than cure the condition.

Specific remedies to be taken every 4 hours for up to 2 weeks
- Eyelids red and gummy *Hepar sulph. 6c*
- Eyelids red and swollen, gummy in morning *Graphites 6c*
- Where itchiness is main complaint *Calcarea 6c*
- Lids sore and burning, with tiny ulcers, made worse by bathing eyes in water *Sulphur 6c*

Self-help Last thing at night, bathe eyelids with saline solution (1 teaspoon salt to a glass of warm water) and lightly apply *Calendula* ointment. Reduce intake of animal fats, and take 1 tablespoon cold-pressed linseed oil daily. Vitamins B and C, and zinc may also be beneficial.

Drooping eyelids (ptosis) Caused by damage to the lid muscle or to the nerve controlling it; damage may be a consequence of injury, MYASTHAENIA GRAVIS, DIABETES, or an ANEURYSM within the skull, or simply the result of ageing. Can block vision, and is often accompanied by DOUBLE VISION; sometimes correctable by surgery. Constitutional homeopathic treatment should certainly be tried.

Specific remedy to be taken every 12 hours for up to 10 doses while constitutional treatment is being sought
- *Gelsemium 30c*

Ectropion A turning outwards of the lower lid as the lid muscles become lax, exposing the lower part of the eyeball and preventing tears from draining into tear duct; tears run down cheek instead, lower lids become dry and sore, and lower part of conjunctiva thickens, pushing lid further away from eyeball; usually a complaint of old age. Untreated, a CORNEAL ULCER may form; in severe cases, minor surgery may be necessary.

Specific remedy to be taken 4 times daily for up to 2 weeks
• *Borax 6c*

Self-help Bathe eye with *Euphrasia* solution (see CONJUNCTIVITIS).

Entropion A turning inwards of the lower lid due to contraction of the muscles around the lid margin, causing CONJUNCTIVITIS or a CORNEAL ULCER as inturned lashes irritate and scratch the eyeball; condition mainly affects old people, and can be caused, and made worse, by screwing up and rubbing eyes. Can be corrected by minor surgery.

Specific remedy to be taken every 4 hours for up to 2 weeks
• *Borax 6c*

Self-help Bathe eyes with *Euphrasia* solution (see CONJUNCTIVITIS).

Eyestrain

If you are aware of tightness around the eyes, or if you habitually screw up your eyes or have difficulty focusing on distant objects after focusing on near ones for any length of time, or vice versa, have your eyes tested by a qualified optician. If you wear spectacles or contact lenses, your eyesight should be tested once a year.

Specific remedies to be taken 4 times daily for up to 7 days
• Ciliary muscles tired from looking into distance for a long time *Arnica 6c*
• Eyes ache when you look up, down, or sideways *Natrum mur. 6c*
• Eyes burn and feel strained after close work or reading *Ruta 6c*
• Tired eyes associated with great nervousness and apprehension, or with sexual overindulgence *Phosphorus 6c*

Floaters

Small objects which seem to drift across field of vision when eyes or head are turned; in the elderly, cause may be degeneration of vitreous humour inside the eyeball; other causes may be DETACHED RETINA or bleeding into the eye. In naturopathy, if the above causes have been ruled out, floaters are taken to be a symptom of a sluggish liver and a build up of toxins in the body. If condition worsens, or if vision starts to blur, ②.

Specific remedies to be taken 3 times daily for up to 7 days
• If symptoms come on after an accident *Arnica 6c*

• Where specialist has diagnosed bleeding from back of eye *Hamamelis 6c*
• Floaters associated with misty vision *Phosphorus 6c*

Self-help If the above remedies do not help, and if retinal detachment has been ruled out, follow the Liver Diet (pp. 352–3) for 1 month.

Glaucoma

Build-up of fluid in front chamber of eye (space between cornea and lens) due to sudden or gradual blockage of the channel or tissues through which fluid normally drains; pressure in the eyeball increases, causing collapse of tiny blood vessels at back of eye where nerve fibres from the retina enter the optic nerve; starved of nourishment, these fibres die, causing loss of vision.

Blockage of the channel between the iris and the cornea is known as *angle closure glaucoma*; this occurs mainly in elderly people who are long-sighted, onsets fairly suddenly, and usually affects only one eye at a time. First symptoms, lasting an hour or two at most, may be blurred vision or haloes round lights, especially in evenings when iris opens wide to let in as much light as possible; the eye may also be red and painful. At this stage, no permanent damage has been done. But if symptoms persist and worsen, pressure can irreversibly damage nerve fibres at back of eye; cornea becomes cloudy and grey-green as fluid is forced into it, pressure in the eyeball is felt as pressure in the head, causing vomiting, exhaustion, and intolerance of light, and the eyeball itself feels very hard and tender. One person in 20 over the age of 65 suffers from this acute form of glaucoma, which should be treated as early as possible. If you have any of the symptoms above, ②. Conventional treatment is to reduce pressure in the eye by drops or dehydrating agents, then to snip away a small piece of the iris beneath the upper eyelid (an iridectomy) to re-establish a drainage channel.

Specific remedy to be taken every 15 minutes for up to 10 doses when symptoms start
• Blurred vision, pain in one eye, made worse by bright light *Belladonna 30c*

In *open angle glaucoma*, which usually affects both eyes equally, the network of tissue in the drainage angle between the iris and cornea becomes blocked; over a period of years field of vision imperceptibly narrows to straight ahead only, then even this is lost. Open angle glaucoma tends to run in families, so if you have a parent or grandparent who is affected, have your own eyes checked every year. Conventionally, pressure within eyeball is kept at a non-dangerous level by use of eye drops. However, if sight is not yet at risk, a combination of constitutional homeopathic treatment and a cleansing diet such as the Liver Diet on pages 352–3 may be helpful; if, on checking with an eye

For explanation of other symbols, see page 107

specialist these measures seem to be controlling the condition, drops may not be necessary.

Hypermetropia see LONG SIGHT

Injury to eye see also BLACK EYE

Most eye injuries are caused by foreign bodies becoming lodged in the eye, or by blows to the eye or nose. If the eye has been cut or perforated, or if you suspect fragments of metal, grit, or glass may be embedded in it, (999) give First Aid (see page 98), and tell the person not to move his or her good eye, as the injured eye will inevitably move with it. Very prompt First Aid is necessary if corrosive chemicals enter the eyes. If, after a blow to the eye, the person cannot see properly or complains of pain, (2) and give one of the rescue remedies listed below.

Specific remedies to be taken every 5–10 minutes for up to 10 doses in emergency
- *Arnica 30c*
- Injury caused by a blunt object, pain felt deep in eyeball *Symphytum 6c*
- If pain persists after treatment from GP *Hypericum 30c*
- If Hypericum does not ease pain *Aconite 30c*

Iritis

Inflammation of the iris of one or both eyes; if acute, may give rise to GLAUCOMA, either because white cells produced in response to inflammation build up and block channel which drains fluid from front chamber of eye, or because iris sticks to front of lens, which also prevents drainage of fluid; if long-standing, may give rise to CATARACT. Condition mainly affects young adults, but is not at all common; occasionally it is a complication of RHEUMATOID ARTHRITIS, ANKYLOSING SPONDYLITIS, SARCOIDOSIS, or even syphilis (see SEXUALLY TRANSMITTED DISEASES), but more often it has no obvious cause. Symptoms are redness and discomfort, slight blurring of vision, and sometimes a HEADACHE. If symptoms include headache and pain in affected eye, (2). Because of the risk of glaucoma, an eye specialist should be seen as soon as possible; steroid drops may be necessary to reduce inflammation and prevent iris sticking to lens, but they do not get to the root of the problem. Iritis tends to be a recurrent, constitutional problem, so constitutional treatment from an expert homeopath should be sought.

Specific remedies to be taken ½-hourly for up to 10 doses in acute attack
- At first signs of inflammation *Aconite 30c*
- If back of iris threatens to stick to lens *Mercurius corr. 6c*
- If inflammation occurs after an eye operation *Rhus. tox. 6c*

Self-help If iritis is associated with autoimmune disease (rheumatoid arthritis, for example), changing to a more alkaline diet (see p. 350) may prevent recurrence.

Long sight (hypermetropia)

Difficulty bringing both near and distant objects into focus either because eyeball is too short from front to back or because lens and cornea do not bend light sufficiently; in either case, rays of light from near and distant objects converge not on the retina but some way behind it, producing a blurred image. Condition tends to run in families, and is usually diagnosed in childhood when child starts to read and complains of EYESTRAIN or eye ache. Long sight can also develop from middle age onwards as lens loses its elasticity (see PRESBYOPIA). Convex spectacles or contact lenses solve the immediate problem, but do not prevent the ciliary muscles getting weaker; this is where constitutional homeopathic treatment or eye exercises can help.

Specific remedies to be given 4 times daily for up to 2 weeks while waiting for constitutional treatment
- Eyes sore, smarting and aching after reading or doing close work for only an hour or two *Ruta 6c*
- If above remedy is not effective *Jaborandi 6c*

Loss of sight and blurred vision

Sudden loss of sight in one or both eyes, or in part of the visual field, is almost always caused by a sudden decrease in blood flow to the retina or choroid layer, or to the part of the brain which interprets visual information; the specific event causing loss of sight may be RETINAL ARTERY OCCLUSION or a transient ischaemic attack (see STROKE) or RETINAL VEIN OCCLUSION causing blurring over a period of hours. Slow deterioration of sight may be due to a CATARACT on the cornea, MACULAR DEGENERATION, DIABETIC RETINOPATHY, chronic GLAUCOMA, or age-related refraction problems such as PRESBYOPIA. Sudden blurring of vision after a head injury may be the result of a subdural BRAIN HAEMORRHAGE; if there is sudden blurring and pain in one eye, the cause may be acute IRITIS, acute GLAUCOMA, or OPTIC NEURITIS; in CHOROIDITIS there is usually sudden blurring of central vision in one eye, but no pain. Floaters and flashing lights in one eye are symptoms of a DETACHED RETINA, bleeding into the eyeball, or degeneration of the vitreous humour. Some drugs can also cause visual disturbances, but of course they affect both eyes equally. See relevant entry for homeopathic treatment.

Any damage to the choroid or retina causes scarring, which in turn causes some loss of vision; if the central part of the retina is damaged, central vision will be affected.

Lump on eyelid see also RODENT ULCER, BIRTHMARKS, STYE

Apart from styes, the lumps and bumps which most frequently develop on eyelids are chalazions, xanthelasmas, and papillomas.

A *chalazion*, also known as a meibomian cyst, is a painless lump which forms when the exit from one of the meibomian glands which lubricate the eyelids becomes blocked; a small one usually clears up of its own accord, but a large one may need to be removed via an incision in the eyelid; condition tends to recur. Traditional homeopathic remedy is *Staphisagria* 6c, taken 3 times daily for up to 2 weeks; if this does not work, take Thuja in the same dosage.

A *xanthelasma* is a yellow fatty deposit just under the outer skin of the eyelid, usually near the nose; may be a symptom of HYPERLIPIDAEMIA, but very rarely; surgical removal is not recommended as deposit tends to come back and scarring only makes appearance worse; condition is harmless in any case. Sometimes responds to *Calcarea* 6c, taken every 12 hours for up to 2 weeks; if no improvement in 1 month, repeat dosage.

Papillomas are small skin outgrowths, benign, related to WARTS, and seldom unsightly enough to warrant surgical removal; they may be dark or pink, and grow very slowly. Traditional homeopathic remedy is *Thuja* 6c, taken 3 times daily for up to 7 days; Thuja is also recommended after removal.

Macular degeneration
Deterioration of the macula, the central part of the retina where colour vision and fine resolution of detail are sharpest; with age, blood vessels in the choroid layer behind the retina constrict, and blood flow to the densely packed cones in the macula decreases; central vision becomes blurred, and reading and fine work become increasingly difficult, but outer vision remains unaffected. Not usually curable, but constitutional treatment from an experienced homeopath, who will probably recommend certain dietary changes, can prevent further degeneration.

Myopia see SHORT SIGHT

Optic neuritis
Inflammation of the optic nerve, resulting in gradual or sudden blurring of vision, and even blindness; the affected eye is painful to move. Generally affects adults between age of 20 and 40, but cause is not known. Inflammation and visual symptoms usually clear up of their own accord, though steroids are often prescribed to hasten recovery. In a small number of people, however, the condition may be an early warning of MULTIPLE SCLEROSIS; if this is the case, constitutional homeopathic treatment should be sought, and nutritional measures should be taken as for MS.

Specific remedy to be taken every hour for up to 10 doses
- At first signs of attack *Apis 30c*

Orbital cellulitis
Infection and swelling of the soft tissues lining the eye socket, pushing the eyeball outwards and causing severe pain, redness, discharge of pus, and some degree of blurred vision; offending organisms are usually bacteria which have spread from the sinuses during SINUSITIS or from BOILS near the eye. Since there is a small risk of infection spreading to the meninges of the brain and causing MENINGITIS, appropriate action is ⌷12⌷, or ②if meningitis symptoms appear. Your GP will probably prescribe an antibiotic, but if the rescue remedies listed below are given promptly they will have time to act before the antibiotic builds up sufficiently to antidote them.

Specific remedies to be taken every hour for up to 10 doses
- Lids swollen and full of fluid, eye burning and stinging, sudden piercing pains, yellow discharge *Apis 30c*
- Eye won't stop watering *Rhus tox. 6c*
- Extreme sensitivity to slightest draught or touch *Hepar sulph. 6c*

Pain in eyes
Eye pain – as distinct from soreness, tenderness, or inflammation – can be a symptom of MENINGITIS or subarachnoid BRAIN HAEMORRHAGE (pain felt behind eyes, severe headache, eye pain made worse by bright light or bending forwards, person drowsy or confused); if either condition is suspected, ⑨⑨⑨.

Can also be a symptom of TEMPORAL ARTERITIS (pain behind eyes and pain in temples, fever, a 'fluey' feeling), acute IRITIS (associated with blurred vision), or acute GLAUCOMA (blurred vision, great sensitivity to light); in all three cases, appropriate action is ②.

More commonly, eye pain is associated with SINUSITIS (pain behind eyes, pain or tenderness over one or both eyes or in cheeks) or EYESTRAIN.

Specific remedies to be given every 15 minutes until help arrives if meningitis, subarachnoid haemorrhage, or temporal arteritis suspected
- Person feverish, fearful, tense, has severe headache *Aconite 30c*
- Symptoms follow injury to head or eye *Arnica 30c*
- Great pain made worse by slightest movement, person very drowsy *Bryonia 30c*
- High fever, face red and hot, eyes wide and staring, person delirious *Belladonna 30c*
- Pain and stiffness in joints, 'fluey' feeling, person not at all thirsty *Gelsemium 6c*

Presbyopia
Deterioration in elasticity of lens due to ageing; the ciliary muscles contract in order to thicken the lens for reading and close work, but the lens responds less and less and print appears blurred unless held at arm's

length or even further away. As with long and short sight, spectacles or contact lenses can correct the immediate problem, but they do not prevent further deterioration. Constitutional homeopathic treatment or dietary changes would be well worth trying. Specific remedies are the same as those for LONG SIGHT.

Pterygium
Literally a 'wing' of tissue which grows out from the sclera and creeps across the cornea, obstructing vision; may be caused by over-exposure to ultraviolet light; very simple to remove surgically, but the remedies below should also be tried.

Specific remedies to be taken 3 times daily for up to 14 days
- *Zinc 6c*
- If Zinc produces no improvement *Ratanhia 6c*

Retinal artery occlusion
Blockage of the tiny artery which feeds the retina, or blockage of one of its branches, causing immediate total blindness or blindness in upper or lower half of visual field; blockage may be a blood clot formed locally (a thrombus), or a clot formed in a diseased artery somewhere else in the body (an embolus). This is an emergency, so ⑨⑨⑨; with drugs and/or surgery there is a chance that the clot can be moved out of the retinal artery and some sight saved.

Specific remedies to be given every 5 minutes for up to 10 doses in emergency situation
- *Aconite 30c*, followed by *Nux 6c*

Retinal vein occlusion
Blockage of the central retinal vein or one of its branches; trapped blood builds up in retina, then leaks into vitreous humour, blurring vision over the course of a few hours; often associated with GLAUCOMA or HIGH BLOOD PRESSURE. Provided any underlying condition is promptly treated, leaked blood tends to be reabsorbed over a period of months and vision improves, though the chances of this happening lessen with age. Appropriate action is ② and immediate referral to an eye specialist.

Specific remedies to be given every 15 minutes for up to 10 doses while waiting for specialist attention
- When symptoms first come on *Arnica 30c*
- If Arnica does not prevent condition worsening *Hamamelis 6c*

Once condition has stabilized, give *Lachesis 6c* every 6 hours for up to 10 days to help reabsorb blood, then seek constitutional treatment for underlying cause.

Self-help Take extra Vitamins C, E, and B$_6$, and selenium. Eat fish rather than meat.

Retinal detachment see DETACHED RETINA

Retinitis pigmentosa
Condition in which black pigment is laid down in outer areas of retina, causing gradual loss of vision to the side and at night. Your GP will refer you to an eye specialist. Constitutional treatment would also be appropriate.

Specific remedy to be taken twice daily for up to 3 weeks; if no improvement within 4 weeks, see your GP
- *Nux 6c* or *Phosphorus 6c*

Self-help Extra Vitamin A, D and calcium may be beneficial.

Scleritis
Inflammation of the sclera, the white outer tunic of the eyeball; visible as a bright red patch and felt as a dull pain in the eye; may cause loss of vision if inflammation occurs near or behind retina. Mainly affects women who suffer from RHEUMATOID ARTHRITIS, CROHN'S DISEASE, or ULCERATIVE COLITIS. Since there is a risk that the sclera will perforate, allowing the fluid contents of the eye to seep out, ⑫. Conventional treatment is by anti-inflammatory or immuno-suppressive drugs, or surgery. The homeopathic approach is constitutional, with special attention paid to diet.

Specific remedies to be taken every hour for up to 10 doses as soon as condition is suspected
- *Aconite 30c*
- If Aconite does not alleviate symptoms *Thuja 6c*

Short sight (myopia)
Usually becomes apparent during teens and early twenties, affects 1 person in 6, and tends to run in families. Distant objects are seen indistinctly because light rays from them converge not on the retina but some way in front of it; this happens either because the eyeball is too long from back to front or, more rarely, because the cornea and lens bend light too much. Focus is easily adjusted by wearing concave spectacles or contact lenses, but constitutional homeopathic treatment should also be sought.

Specific remedies to be taken 4 times daily for up to 2 weeks while constitutional treatment is being sought
- Short-sightedness becomes worse with nervous exhaustion or sexual over-indulgence *Phosphorus 6c*
- Short-sightedness seems to be getting worse *Physostigma 6c*

Squint see also SQUINT p. 332
Defined as one eye looking directly at target object while the other looks elsewhere. In adults, lack of coordination occurs either because the eye muscles themselves have been damaged, or because the motor

nerves which control the eye muscles have been damaged, usually as a consequence of DIABETES, BRAIN INJURY, BRAIN TUMOUR, HIGH BLOOD PRESSURE, or MYASTHENIA GRAVIS. The brain, used to receiving and combining two very similar pictures, cannot cope with two very different pictures, so the person sees both. In most children who squint, the brain simply ignores information from one eye and only information coming from the other is seen; if efforts are not made to correct the squint, the unused eye becomes lazy and effectively useless.

If you start seeing double, see your GP. Treatment of the underlying cause may solve the problem; if not, the options are prismatic spectacles, surgery, exercises which force the lazy eye to work, and constitutional homeopathic treatment.

Specific remedies to be taken 3 times daily for up to 2 weeks
• *Gelsemium 6c*
• If Gelsemium does not help lazy eye *Alumina 6c*

Stye
An infection which develops at the root of an eyelash; looks rather like a boil to begin with, then develops a head of pus; red and painful, but usually clears up of its own accord within 7 days. For recurrent styes, conventional treatment is antibiotics; the homeopathic approach is constitutional, intended to boost general resistance to infection.

Specific remedies to be given every hour for up to 10 doses
• *Pulsatilla 6c*
• If Pulsatilla produces no improvement *Staphisagria 6c*

Self-help To disperse a stye, try hot spoon bathing: wrap cotton wool round handle of a wooden spoon, then repeatedly dip handle in very hot water and put it against stye. You should not try to burst the stye by squeezing it. Tighten up on personal hygiene; for example, never touch or rub your eyes with dirty hands.

Tumour of the eye see also RETINOBLASTOMA, CANCER
Relatively rare but usually malignant; more cases are discovered during routine eye checks than as a result of reported symptoms; condition is usually painless, though symptoms can include visual disturbances, loss of vision, EXOPHTHALMOS, or SQUINT, depending on site and rate of growth of tumour. Tumour may be primary, affecting eye first and then other parts of the body if left untreated, or secondary, having spread from a primary cancer somewhere else. Secondary tumours, depending on their size and position in the eye, can sometimes be destroyed by radiotherapy. The usual treatment for primary tumours, however, is removal of the affected eye, unless the tumour is detected at a very early stage; *malignant melanoma*, similar to a form of skin cancer, affects either the choroid layer or the ciliary body; RETINOBLASTOMA, which affects the retina of one or both eyes, is usually seen in young children and has a strong hereditary component.

For homeopathic treatment, see CANCER.

Twitching eyelids
Brief flickering of one eyelid, with no other signs of twitching or trembling, is usually an indication of tension or tiredness, and nothing to worry about. Constitutional treatment would be appropriate.

Specific remedies to be taken every 4 hours for up to 6 doses if twitch persists
• Twitching of eyelid only *Codeinum 6c*
• Twitching of eyelid and eyeball *Agaricus 6c*
• Twitching and inflammation of eyelid *Pulsatilla 6c*

Watering eyes
Continuous watering of the eyes is fairly rare and usually the cause is blockage of the tear ducts due to infection or injury, especially injury to the bridge or side of the nose. If condition is not relieved by the remedy given below, see your GP; conventional treatment is to syringe blocked duct, give antibiotics if infection is present, or re-establish drainage from the eye into the nose by surgery. In newborn babies the tear ducts sometimes fail to open; gentle massage up the side of the nose to the inner corner of the eye may encourage them to do so, but sometimes a probe is necessary.

Specific remedy to be given 4 times daily for up to 7 days
• Tear duct infected *Silicea 6c*

EARS

THE ear performs two functions, hearing and balance, and is one of the most sensitive and delicately made structures in the whole body. It can easily be damaged, so any aches, pains, or feelings of dizziness should be investigated and treated promptly.

Vibrations in the air travel through the wax-lined outer canal of the ear and cause the eardrum to vibrate. This causes three tiny linked bones in the middle ear to vibrate too. The vibrations then pass into a fluid-filled spiral chamber called the cochlea, where they agitate the delicate endings of banks of nerve cells. These unite to form the cochlear nerve, which then becomes part of the auditory nerve, which is connected to the brain. The brain then interprets auditory nerve messages as speech, music, noise, and so on.

Two passages lead from the middle ear. One goes to the mastoid process, a cavity-filled bone which helps with resonance. The other, the eustachian tube, goes to the nose. The eustachian tube ensures that pressure inside and outside the eardrum is equal. If it is not, the eardrum will not vibrate properly. A blocked eustachian tube causes pressure in the middle ear to fall, sucking the eardrum inwards. When the tube unblocks and pressure is equalized, a sudden pop is heard. Catarrh is a frequent cause of eustachian tube blockage.

The inner ear or labyrinth, which contains all the nerve endings responsible for detecting sounds, also contains three semi-circular fluid-filled canals lined with nerve endings which detect movement and acceleration in any plane relative to gravity. The semi-circular canals are the organ of balance. As we move, the fluid in them wafts against the nerve endings, stimulating them to send messages to the brain. The brain then integrates these messages with others coming from the eye and from pressure receptors all over the body.

Barotrauma
Pressure damage to the ear caused by EUSTACHIAN TUBE BLOCKAGE. As pressure in the ear falls, the eardrum is sucked inwards, resulting in local pain, a feeling of tightness and fullness in the ear, and sometimes DEAFNESS. Most often occurs after flying in pressurized aircraft. Usually wears off within 48 hours. See remedies listed under EUSTACHIAN TUBE BLOCKAGE.

Self-help Pressure can often be relieved by trying to blow nose with nostrils pinched shut. While flying, chew gum or repeatedly swallow, and do the same on landing.

Cholesteatoma
Growth of extra tissue in middle ear due to untreated MIDDLE EAR INFECTION. Causes DEAFNESS, discharge, and occasionally damage to the eardrum, and in later stages HEADACHE, weakness of the facial muscles, and sometimes DIZZINESS. Can also cause EPIDURAL ABSCESS and MENINGITIS. If ear pain, with discharge and slight deafness, has been present for some time [48].

Deafness see also OCCUPATIONAL DEAFNESS
Conductive deafness (sound failing to reach the cochlea or auditory nerve) May be due to acute OUTER EAR INFECTION or acute MIDDLE EAR INFECTION, to EUSTACHIAN TUBE BLOCKAGE (especially after a cold), or to EAR WAX. If deafness onsets gradually, and there is a family history of OTOSCLEROSIS, see your GP.

Perceptive deafness (malfunction of cochlear nerve) May be OCCUPATIONAL DEAFNESS if work environment is noisy; may also be due to MENIERE'S DISEASE (if associated with dizziness), to side effects of prescription or recreational drugs, to ageing or to poor nutrition, and in babies to RUBELLA infection of mother during first 3 months of pregnancy. Constitutional treatment can help.

Specific remedies to be taken 4 times daily for up to 7 days
- Difficulty picking out voices from background noise *Phosphorus 6c*
- Hearing improves with background noise *Graphites 6c*
- Short periods of deafness, with ringing, humming or roaring in ears *China 6c*
- Deafness following exposure to cold *Aconite 6c*
- Deafness after a bang on the head *Arnica 6c*
- Deafness associated with nervous exhaustion, feeling weak and trembly *Gelsemium 6c*
- Old age *Chenopodium 6c*

Dizziness see MENIERE'S DISEASE, LABYRINTHITIS

Ear abscess see OUTER EAR INFECTION

Earache
Ear pain must always be investigated promptly by your GP or homeopath. Causes include OUTER EAR INFECTION (pain made worse by pulling ear lobe), BAROTRAUMA or pressure damage (a painful, blocked feeling not relieved by swallowing, especially if brought on by air travel), acute MIDDLE EAR INFECTION or EUSTACHIAN TUBE BLOCKAGE (if earache comes on suddenly), or a build up of EAR WAX (if earache comes on gradually). Earache accompanied by a discharge of pus or blood may be a sign of acute infection of the middle or outer ear. Earache after a COLD may indicate acute infection of the middle ear. Earache with pains in the jaws, teeth, face, or throat may be caused by dental infection, SINUSITIS, or throat infection. Earache after ear piercing may be due to infection of the outer ear and should be treated as for EAR ABSCESS; since both HEPATITIS and AIDS can be spread by poor sterilization procedures during ear piercing, it is extremely important to go to a reputable jeweller to have your ears pierced.

Specific remedies to be taken every ½ hour until correct diagnosis is reached, provided pain is not associated with fever, discharge, or pains elsewhere
- Throbbing pain, soothed by warmth *Hepar sulph. 6c*
- Throbbing pain made worse by warmth *Belladonna 30c*
- Severe pain in an adult, especially if he or she is irritated by trivia, or a child with ear pain who screams unless carried around *Chamomilla 6c*
- Pain as if pressure behind eardrum pushing it out, person weepy *Pulsatilla 6c.*

Self-help Hold a hot water bottle against the affected ear.

Ear infections see OUTER EAR INFECTION, MIDDLE EAR INFECTION, LABYRINTHITIS

Ear wax

Function of wax is to clean and moisten ear canal. Over-production may block canal, causing a feeling of fullness in the ear, strange noises in the ear, EARACHE, DEAFNESS, and sometimes DIZZINESS. Under-production is thought by some to be a cause of TINNITUS. There is also evidence that wax melts during ear infection, due to the heat of inflammation, so a waxy discharge and earache may indicate infection. A tendency to produce too much wax may respond to constitutional treatment.

Specific remedy to be taken 4 times daily for up to 7 days
- Copious production of wax and intermittent loss of hearing *Causticum 6c*

Self-help A few drops of pure olive or almond oil in the affected ear 5 nights running (use a dropper) will soften hardened wax and sometimes dislodge it. Lying in a warm bath with ears submerged may also be effective. If blockage persists, ask your GP to syringe the ear. Do not try to remove wax with 'Q tips', etc.

Eustachian tube blockage

Culprit is usually CATARRH associated with COLDS, MIDDLE EAR INFECTION (if blockage accompanied by discharge), TONSILLITIS (if throat is raw and sore), SINUSITIS (if cheeks and forehead are tight and tender), or infected ADENOIDS. Blockage can also be caused by swollen adenoids covering opening of eustachian tube into back of nose, and by BAROTRAUMA. Eustachian tube blockage is a stubborn condition, but responds to constitutional treatment.

Specific remedies to be taken 4 times daily for up to 7 days; if no improvement within 7 days, 48 or see your homeopath
- Constricted feeling in throat, feeling generally hot *Iodum 6c*
- Runny nose, coughing up catarrh *Kali mur. 6c*
- Catarrh and swollen adenoids *Mercurius dulc. 6c*
- Blockage tends to clear out of doors *Pulsatilla 6c*
- Blockage associated with symptoms of sinusitis *Silicea 6c*

Self-help If the blockage is caused by a small piece of catarrh at the nose end of the eustachian tube, it can sometimes be dislodged by sniffing 3 drops of pure lemon juice up each nostril 3 times a day for up to 5 days (tilt the head back and use a dropper). For children, dilute the lemon juice with an equal volume

of saline solution (made up by adding 1 teaspoon salt to 1 cup warm water). WARNING: do not use this method if the person concerned is prone to NOSE-BLEEDS.

Glue ear see also GLUE EAR p. 322

Accumulation of sticky fluid behind eardrum due to EUSTACHIAN TUBE BLOCKAGE. Use of antibiotics to treat acute ear infections may be a contributory factor. Symptoms are increasing DEAFNESS (as bones in middle ear are prevented from vibrating properly) and, in extreme cases, total deafness (if bones become fused together). Conventionally treated by making a small incision through eardrum, sucking out some of the fluid, then inserting a little tube called a grommet through the eardrum to allow the rest of the fluid to drain out. Constitutional treatment should be sought, but if there is no improvement after 6 months the risk of permanent deafness is great enough to warrant the conventional procedure.

Specific remedies to be taken 4 times daily for up to 14 days
- Thick, smelly discharge from outer ear, copious production of saliva during sleep *Mercurius 6c*
- Deafness, with a roaring noise in affected ear and eczema on ear flap *Lycopodium 6c*
- Full, stuffed up feeling in affected ear *Pulsatilla 6c*
- Snapping noises in affected ear, swollen lymph glands in neck *Kali mur. 6c*

Labyrinthitis

Infection of that part of the inner ear responsible for balance, usually caused by a virus spreading up from the eustachian tube. Symptoms are DIZZINESS (everything spinning around) and NAUSEA AND VOMITING, usually aggravated by head movements and relieved by lying down somewhere quiet. Since infection is viral, conventional medicine can only offer tranquillizers or drugs to stop the nausea and vomiting. Typically an attack lasts about 3 weeks, but homeopathic treatment can shorten this.

Specific remedies to be taken once every hour, then less frequently, for up to 12 doses
- Dizziness made worse by looking down *Phosphorus 6c*
- Dizziness made worse by lying down or turning head sideways *Conium 6c*
- Dizziness, feeling weak and trembly *Gelsemium 6c*
- Dizziness, with a feeling of fullness and congestion in affected ear, made worse by sudden movements *Belladonna 30c*
- Vomiting brought on by eye movements *Bryonia 30c*
- Dizziness made worse by looking up *Calcarea 6c*
- Dizziness made worse by downward body movements *Borax 6c*
- Dizziness accompanied by headache and constipation *Natrum mur. 6c*

For explanation of other symbols, see page 107

Meniere's disease

Increased pressure of fluid in inner ear upsets balance mechanism, causing DIZZINESS (everything spinning around), and NAUSEA AND VOMITING. Hearing may also be affected. In bad cases, muffled hearing and noises in the ear persist between attacks. If Meniere's disease is confirmed by your GP, constitutional treatment should be sought.

Specific remedies to be taken 4 times daily for up to 7 days. See also remedies listed under LABYRINTHITIS for acute attacks.
- Dizziness and muffled hearing *Salicylic ac. 6c*, followed by *Chininum sulph. 6c* in same dosage
- If attack begins on waking *Lachesis 6c*

Self-help Cut down intake of fluids and salt, and stop smoking. In acute attacks, rest quietly in bed.

Middle ear infection (otitis media)

Usually caused by germs spreading up eustachian tube from nose and throat, but occasionally by germs entering through a RUPTURED EARDRUM. May be acute (coming on suddenly and causing great pain and discharge), or chronic (slowly festering and causing only intermittent pain).

Acute infection Accumulation of pus behind eardrum causes hearing loss, a feeling of fullness in the ear, and severe stabbing pains which disturb sleep. Temperature may be higher than normal. Pressure of pus can cause the eardrum to rupture, in which case pain eases and pus drains out through eardrum. Improperly treated, acute middle ear infection can become chronic, or spread to the mastoid process, in which case surgery may be necessary. If acute infection is suspected, ⑫ or see your homeopath. Constitutional treatment can prevent recurrence.

Specific remedies to be taken every ½ hour for up to 10 doses
- Restlessness, anxiety, attack brought on by exposure to cold *Aconite 30c*
- Flushed, hot face and high temperature (particularly in children), staring eyes, excited and incoherent behaviour, unusual sensitivity to touch *Belladonna 30c*
- Pain as if pressure behind eardrum pushing it out, person weepy *Pulsatilla 6c*

Chronic infection Repeated episodes of infection, ofen as a sequel to GLUE EAR in childhood. Can cause conductive DEAFNESS, as infection progressively damages the eardrum and the tiny bones which transmit sound to the inner ear, or CHOLESTEATOMA. Requires supervision of a GP or homeopathic physician, and may take many months to clear up.

Self-help Avoid swimming. Wear a moulded earplug and shower cap when taking a bath or shower to prevent water getting into the affected ear. Take zinc and Vitamin B supplements. Dietary therapy should also be considered.

Occupational deafness

Damage to cochlea caused by prolonged exposure to noise, especially high-pitched noise, above 90 dB level. Result is perceptive deafness, especially in upper frequencies. High-risk occupations are boiler making, tractor driving, and using a pneumatic drill or power tools; also playing or listening to very loud music for hours on end, even if music is not loud enough to hurt the ears at the time. Once developed, occupational deafness is not much helped by hearing aids.

Specific remedy to be taken 4 times daily for up to 7 days
- After exposure to loud noise, as a preventive *Chenopodium 6c*

Self-help If your workplace is noisy, wear ear defenders, ear muffs, or earplugs made of rubber, foam, or plastic, have your hearing checked regularly, and report unacceptable noise levels to your trade union or direct to the Health and Safety Executive (address p. 385).

Otosclerosis

Hardening of the connections between the bones in the middle ear, particularly the connection between the stapes and the membrane leading to the inner ear, causing progressive DEAFNESS. Onset is usually slow in adults, but may be rapid in children. Hardening process may spontaneously arrest before deafness is total, in which case hearing is often better where there is background noise. Otosclerosis affects twice as many women as men, and may appear first in pregnancy or significantly deteriorate during pregnancy; it usually starts between the age of 20 and 40, and in 50 per cent of cases seems to be inherited. In severe cases, surgery may be necessary, but it is not always successful. Constitutional treatment can help.

Specific remedies to be taken 4 times daily for up to 2 weeks
- *Calcarea fluor. 6c*
- Hearing noticeably better with background noise *Graphites 6c*

Outer ear infection (otitis externa)

Infection may involve the whole outer canal of the ear or be localized as an abscess. In either case the whole outer ear is extremely sensitive to the slightest pressure or probing. Often brought on by swimming, trying to remove wax, or poking about in the ear with sharp objects. Damaged skin invites infection, resulting in inflammation, pain, discharge of pus, and sometimes DEAFNESS. Prompt treatment is necessary to prevent damage to surrounding cartilage and bone. After treatment it is important that you see your GP to make

---

⑨⑨⑨ Emergency – call GP (or dial 999) immediately. ② Consult your doctor if no improvement within 2 hours

sure there are no lingering traces of infection. Constitutional treatment is advised if infection is chronic, with dull, intermittent pain.

Specific remedies
- Acute infection, with sharp, shooting pains. First choice is *Aconite 30c* ½-hourly up to 10 doses, but if no improvement within 5 hours try *Belladonna 30c* in same dosage
- Acute infection, with discharge *Mercurius sol. 6c* hourly; if no improvement within 48 hours, [12] or see your homeopath
- Chronic inflammation, with itchiness but no infection or discharge *Graphites 6c*, 4 times daily for up to 5 days; if no improvement, see your homeopath

Oversensitive hearing (hyperacusis)
Can be extremely troublesome since it interferes with sleep, concentration, and sociability.

Specific remedies to be taken 4 times daily for up to 7 days
- Sleeplessness, with mind and body over-revving as if from too much coffee *Coffea 6c*
- Own voice sounds unusually loud *Nux 6c*
- Even a piece of paper being screwed up sounds too loud *Phosphorus 6c*
- Slightest noise (from rustling of leaves to chalk scraping on a blackboard) has almost direct effect on nervous system, producing faint nausea *Asarum 6c*
- Sounds felt as pain in ears *Silicea 6c*
- Sleeplessness, hearing so acute that a fly can be heard walking on ceiling *Opium 6c*

Protruding ears
Ears which stick out from the head at right angles. A source of embarrassment and bullying, especially among children. Can be disguised by growing hair long, but strapping the ears at night has no effect. If the condition is causing severe psychological problems, surgical correction may be appropriate. The operation is usually very successful but occasionally leaves noticeable scars.

Ringing in the ears see TINNITUS

Ruptured eardrum
Most common cause of rupture is MIDDLE EAR INFECTION. Other causes are blows on the ear, poking about in the ear with sharp objects, and blasts from loud explosions. May also be associated with a fractured skull. Surgical perforation is part of orthodox treatment of GLUE EAR. Symptoms are slight pain, slightly muffled hearing and strange noises in the ear, and sometimes a small amount of blood. Heals quite naturally within a week or two and functions perfectly normally afterwards. Be wary of infection during healing and for at least 3 months afterwards; do not go swimming during this time either. If condition is recurrent, never go swimming without moulded earplugs.

Specific remedy to be taken every hour for up to 10 doses
- Pain following rupture *Aconite 30c*

Tinnitus
Persistent ringing and other noises in the ears. Other causes of noises in the ear include insects or foreign bodies trapped in the outer ear canal (see First Aid p. 97), pressure damage or BAROTRAUMA (especially after air travel), and some drugs, especially aspirin. It is also associated with aging. If accompanied by hearing loss, see DEAFNESS for treatment. If cause cannot be pinned down, (48) or see your homeopath. Can be treated using masking noise.

Specific remedies to be taken 3 times daily for up to 2 weeks
- Roaring in ears, giddiness, deafness *Salicylic ac. 6c*
- Roaring, tingling, blocked feeling in ears *Carbon sulph. 6c*
- Buzzing, singing, or hissing in ears *China sulph. 6c*
- Longstanding ringing in ears, with no additional symptoms *Kali iod. 6c*

Self-help Put 2 drops of pure almond oil in each ear once a week (use a dropper). Take supplements of magnesium, potassium, and manganese.

Tumours of the outer ear
May be cancerous, resembling other skin tumours, in which case see SQUAMOUS CELL CARCINOMA, RODENT ULCER and CANCER for treatment, or non-cancerous. If in ear canal, may be a non-malignant outgrowth of the surrounding bone (osteoma). Any soreness or tenderness, unexplained lumps or patches of discolouration should be promptly investigated by your GP.

NOSE

LONG or short, sharp or flat, noses are designed to moisten, warm, and filter air before it is drawn into the delicate recesses of the lungs. With every breath of air, millions of foreign bodies – dust particles, spores, airborne chemicals, viruses, bacteria – gain entry to the body. Anything the nose, adenoids, and tonsils cannot deal with passes into the lungs. Strange as it may seem, quiet breathing tends to be done through one side of the nose at a time, depending on the time of day.

To function properly the inside of the nose must be moist, warm, and sensitive. The nasal cavity, divided into two by a septum of cartilage and bone and guarded at its twin entrances by hairs, is lined with millions of blood capillaries and mucus-producing cells. Projecting into the top of the nasal cavity are more hairs, microscopic in size, which trap odour molecules and stimulate the endings of the olfactory nerve.

Paired sinuses – in the frontal, sphenoid, maxillary, and ethmoid bones of the skull – lead off the nasal cavity. Their function is to add resonance to the voice. Under normal circumstances they are air-filled but if their moist linings become irritated or inflamed by infections spreading from other parts of the upper respiratory tract, they fill with fluid, causing the whole area around the nose and eyes to feel tender and congested. Allergies can also cause blocked sinuses.

According to one theory, there are seven primary odour categories, each with its own kind of receptor in the nose; the brain mixes the information coming from the 50 million or so smell receptors in the nose and forms a smell picture. Though human beings are rather poor smellers in comparison with other animals, someone with a good sense of smell can recognize several thousand distinct smells. The olfactory lobe is connected to various structures on or near the lower surface of the forebrain, specifically to areas associated with memory and emotion. Smoking and any condition which causes a runny or blocked up nose impairs sensitivity to smells.

Catarrh

Intermittent discharge of runny or viscous fluid from the nose brought on by viral or bacterial infection, ALLERGY, chemical irritants, or dry air, all of which irritate or inflame the mucous membranes lining the nasal cavity, and sometimes the sinuses as well. Result is a stuffy, blocked-up nose, and also coughing if catarrh drips down back of throat and onto vocal cords. Homeopathic medicine regards chronic catarrh – catarrh not obviously due to any of the causes mentioned above – as a symptom of general toxicity of the body; catarrh is the body's attempt to rid itself of toxins which are not being adequately dealt with by the liver or properly excreted by the kidneys, bowels, and skin.

Catarrh can be a symptom of COLDS (watery discharge which then becomes thick and yellow, mild or moderate fever), HAY FEVER AND ALLERGIC RHINITIS (clear discharge, repeated sneezing, itchy eyes and throat), a food ALLERGY, NASAL POLYPS (impaired sense of smell, sometimes facial pain), INFLUENZA (aching joints, fever, coughing, headache), or SINUSITIS (pain and tenderness in cheeks, or headache above one or both eyes). It can also be a reaction to spicy foods, dust, cigarette smoke and other chemical irritants, gas or oil fires, central heating and over-dry air, certain drugs, and cold or damp.

A large number of homeopathic remedies have catarrh as one of their symptoms, which is why very skilled prescribing is needed to clear up chronic catarrh. However, in acute cases a remedy can be chosen from the list below.

Specific remedies to be given 4 times daily for up to 14 days
- Profuse, thick, yellowish discharge, inside of nose sore and ulcerated, sneezing makes symptoms worse *Arsenicum iod. 6c*
- Sore scabs and fissures inside nose, made worse by blowing, sense of smell so abnormally acute that even the scent of flowers is unbearable *Graphites 6c*
- Nose running all the time, constant blowing, discharge from nose thin and burning but mucous dripping down back of throat thick, small ulcers on septum *Hydrastis 6c*
- Catarrh ropy, stretchy and white, feeling of pressure around bridge of nose *Kali bichrom. 6c*
- Catarrh looks like raw egg white, nose dry and sore, loss of smell and taste *Natrum mur. 6c*
- Profuse, offensive, yellow catarrh, nose feels dry and hot, frequent sneezing *Sanguinaria 6c*
- Yellow catarrh which smells offensive, person very hungry *Calcarea 6c*
- Dry scabs inside nose which bleed easily, nose stuffier indoors than out of doors, cold sores on outside of nose *Sulphur 6c*
- Yellow or green bland catarrh, worse in stuffy room, person weepy *Pulsatilla 6c*

Self-help Always blow your nose gently, one nostril at a time, keeping your mouth open; if you blow both nostrils together, catarrh may be forced up eustachian tube and cause MIDDLE EAR INFECTION, and if you keep your mouth closed air may be pushed up the eustachian tube with such force that it ruptures the eardrum. Inhaling hot steam helps to decongest the airways, but do not use Friar's balsam or other additives as these may antidote whatever homeopathic remedy you are taking; by the same token, dry air is bad for a stuffed up nose, so make an effort to humidify the rooms where you work or sleep, especially if they have central heating (see p. 30 for more information about humidifiers). If your catarrh is caused by dust or pollens, an ioniser may be helpful (see p. 30). If you smoke, try to stop, and avoid smoke-filled air. If you suffer from constant catarrh, you might gain some relief by sniffing water up the nose to prevent the inside from drying out; make sure the water is warm, sniff it half way up the nose, then blow it out; do not draw the water all the way up the nose and into the back of the throat as this may force water into the sinuses and lead to infection. Over-the-counter nasal sprays or drops should only be used if stuffiness prevents you sleeping or if you suffer from pressurization problems when flying; they can be given to babies if catarrh is causing feeding or sleeping difficulties, but make sure they are the right strength and use them very sparingly as they can damage the sensitive lining of the nose. Vitamin B complex, Vitamin C, zinc, and iron are recommended. A combination 'Q' tissue salts and Potters Antifect are of value in some people.

Colds see also COLDS p. 317, CATARRH

Virus infections which cause inflammation of the mucous membranes lining the nose, and a watery discharge which rapidly becomes thick and yellowish, and sometimes slight or moderate FEVER; if immunity is low, infection can spread to sinuses, ears, throat, larynx, trachea, or lungs, causing SINUSITIS, MIDDLE and INNER EAR INFECTIONS, PHARYNGITIS, LARYN-GITIS, TONSILLITIS, TRACHEITIS, and BRONCHITIS. Children tend to get more colds than adults (see p. 317 for specific remedies), but recurrent colds, in children or adults, are usually a sign of a weakened immune system, perhaps due to STRESS or poor nutrition, and usually require constitutional homeopathic treatment. Conventional treatment is by aspirin, antihistamines, or antibiotics; the latter cannot combat viruses, of course, but they may help to prevent bacterial infection. In acute cases, the remedies below are recommended.

Specific remedies to be taken every 2 hours for up to 4 doses
- Cold comes on suddenly, especially after exposure to cold, dry wind, sneezing, burning throat, restlessness, symptoms worse at night *Aconite 30c*
- Cold comes on suddenly, with a high temperature, skin dry, hot, and burning, light hurts eyes, sore throat worse on right side, tickly cough, person very thirsty *Belladonna 30c*
- Cold comes on more slowly, mild fever only, person prone to nosebleeds *Ferrum phos. 6c*
- Cold rather like 'flu, person feels sluggish and shivery, limbs chilly, aching, and heavy *Gelsemium 6c*
- Person more than usually irritable and critical, feels chilly, nose runs during day but becomes blocked at night *Nux 6c*
- Cold in early stages, sneezing worse in morning, catarrh like raw egg white, blocked nose, cold sores, person rejects sympathy and wants to be left alone *Natrum mur. 6c*
- Sweating, excessive salivation, sneezing, catarrh thick and yellowish-green, bad breath *Mercurius 6c*
- Person not at all thirsty but wants lot of attention and sympathy *Pulsatilla 6c*
- Catarrh thick and yellowish-green, infection spreads to ears or to throat, which feels as if it has a splinter in it, person irritable, chilly, very sensitive to draughts, breaks out in smelly sweats *Hepar sulph. 6c*
- Cough, headache made worse by coughing, dry mouth, person very thirsty, irritable, wants to be left alone, symptoms worse for slightest movement *Bryonia 30c*

- Profuse catarrh which causes burning sensation in eyes, eyes streaming, worse at night *Euphrasia 6c*
- Eyes streaming, discharge from nose burns upper lip, person feels better in fresh air *Allium 6c*

Self-help Most effective treatment is rest, plenty of fluids (hot water with fresh lemon juice and a little honey in it is good), extra Vitamin C (500 mg every 2 hours for up to 6 doses), a light diet (soups, raw fruit, vegetables), and plenty of fresh air. Some people find that regular supplements of Vitamins A and C, and zinc, help to prevent colds. A combination 'Q' tissue salts and Potters Antifect are of value in some people.

Disturbed sense of smell

Sensitivity to odours varies with air temperature and humidity, and with state of health; warm moist air carries more volatile chemicals than cold dry air, but if the nose is too dry or stuffed up with mucus the olfactory nerve endings will not be able to detect them. COLDS, HAY FEVER AND ALLERGIC RHINITIS, NASAL POLYPS, and smoking all interfere with the reception of odours; occasionally loss of sense of smell (anosmia) is due to injury of the olfactory nerves, or to a BRAIN TUMOUR or BRAIN INJURY involving the olfactory bulb at the base of the forebrain; in some cases it may be due to a deficiency of zinc. Some people suffer from exactly the opposite, an extremely acute sense of smell, and find certain smells – and not just bad smells – quite disturbing; an altered sense of smell, or suddenly experiencing strong smell sensations for no apparent reason, is sometimes a feature of pregnancy; a minority of CANCER patients report specific smell and taste changes.

Specific remedies to be taken hourly for up to 6 doses if sensitivity to certain smells becomes disturbing
- Acute sensitivity to flower scents *Graphites 6c*
- All smells overpowering and disgusting *Carbolic ac. 6c*
- Tobacco smoke intolerable, especially during acute illness *Belladonna 30c*
- Sudden smell of tarred rope, burning charcoal, soap suds, or boiled peas *Sulphur 6c*
- Sudden putrid smell *Kali bichrom. 6c*
- Sudden rotten egg smell *Belladonna 30c*
- Sudden bitter smell rather like bile *Dioscorea 6c*
- Sudden smell of fried onions *Sanguinaria 6c*
- Sudden smell rather like pigeon droppings or charred wood *Anacardium 6c*
- Sensitivity to tobacco smoke *Ignatia 6c*

Hay fever and allergic rhinitis

Both caused by allergies to airborne irritants, but whereas hay fever is mainly a summer ailment, allergic rhinitis occurs all the year round; often aggravated by some form of food ALLERGY. In both conditions there is usually a family history of ASTHMA or ECZEMA. Grass, tree, and flower pollens, and mould spores from trees, are the culprits in hayfever; in allergic rhinitis the range

---

For explanation of other symbols, see page 107

of irritants is much wider – hair, skin, fur, feathers, house dust, house dust mites, cigarette smoke, various smells. The body over-reacts to some or all of these, producing histamine which draws fluid to the site of the 'attack', causing redness, warmth, swelling, itching, and tickling. Eyes and nose are affected most, but lips, ears, throat, and lungs can also be involved. Repeated sneezing is not only very tiring, but can aggravate STRESS INCONTINENCE. Skin tests may enable your GP to pinpoint the substances you are allergic to, but skin reactions become less and less reliable the more allergies you have.

Conventional treatments include antihistamines, which block the action of histamine, but some can cause drowsiness and can increase the effects of alcohol; decongestants, which can damage the nasal membranes if used for any length of time; steroid nasal sprays, which reduce inflammation; and desensitizing injections, which eventually switch off the body's reaction to a particular allergen, but which have also been known to cause anaphylactoid SHOCK or lead to full-blown asthma; for this reason, such injections are no longer given by GPs and nowadays only rarely by allergy clinics in hospitals. In extreme cases, a helmet can be worn; this fits completely over the head and filters all the air the person breathes; it is effective, but cumbersome.

The homeopathic view of hay fever and allergic rhinitis is that they are deep-seated conditions which require, in the first instance, constitutional treatment; hay fever in particular may take two or three seasons to cure. Nosodes of pollens and other allergens can also be given as preventatives. In acute episodes, however, the following remedies are recommended.

Specific remedies to be taken as often as necessary for up to 10 doses

- Thick, honey-coloured discharge from nose following three or four days of sneezing, sore nostrils and burning sensation inside nose, warmth makes symptoms worse, burning throat, irritating cough, skin dry and scaly, person worried or anxious *Arsenicum iod. 6c*
- Temperature higher than normal, person utterly worn out but feels better for warmth, sniffing warm water up nose give some relief from sneezing, light hurts eyes, wheezing and tightness in lungs, burning throat, restlessness, worry *Arsenicum 6c*
- Early in hay fever season, tickly nose and sneezing but no discharge, roof of mouth and ears very itchy *Arundo 6c*
- Non-stop sneezing, eyes heavy, puffy, and watering, person apathetic, listless, feels dizzy and shaky *Gelsemium 6c*
- Burning discharge from nose, bland discharge from eyes, symptoms worse indoors than out of doors, light hurts eyes, larynx feels as if there are hooks sticking into it, made worse by warm food or drinks *Allium 6c*
- Thick, burning discharge from eyes, which are very swollen, bland discharge from nose, coughing up phlegm, symptoms worse indoors *Euphrasia 6c*
- Violent sneezing, watering eyes, eyelids red and swollen, headache which feels as if head is shrinking, thinking dull and slow, sore throat soothed by warm drinks, feeling generally chilly *Sabadilla 6c*
- Eyes smarting and very sensitive to light, stuffy nose and obstructed breathing, itchiness inside ears and eustachian tubes, general irritability *Nux 6c*
- Person very sensitive to cold, wants to lie down, nose streaming, nasal discharge bland or burning, breathlessness relieved by raising arms away from body *Psorinum 6c*
- Bland, yellow discharge from nose and eyes, better in open air, especially if person is of a tearful disposition *Pulsatilla 6c*
- Stuffed up nose, especially on waking in morning, sinuses feel tender, general chilliness *Silica 6c*
- Constant sneezing, stuffy or streaming nose, eyes swollen and watering, all made worse by being out of doors or in damp atmosphere, smelling new-mown hay, or becoming chilled after exertion *Dulcamara 6c*
- Chronic rhinitis, nasal membranes dry and congested, nasal polyps *Sanguinaria 6c*
- Rhinitis associated with asthma *Arsenicum iod. 6c, Kali iod. 6c, Sabadilla 6c, Iodum 6c,* or *Arsenicum 6c*
- Rhinitis made worse by warm rooms, warm clothes, or bodily exertion *Silicea 6c, Pulsatilla 6c,* or *Carbo veg. 6c*
- Stuffy nose, constant desire to blow nose although blowing does not relieve stuffiness *Lachesis 6c, Kali bichrom. 6c, Psorinum 6c, Naja 6c,* or *Sticta 6c*
- Early hay fever symptoms *Arundo 6c* or *Wyethia 6c*

Self-help Avoid known irritants if at all possible. If you suffer from hay fever, keep track of the pollen count and take preventive measures. Anyone whose hayfever is really bad at night and first thing in the morning should consider fitting air filters over open windows and fireplaces, and fitting efficient draught excluders to doors; filters can be made quite inexpensively by sandwiching a layer of cotton wool between two layers of fine-mesh gauze stretched across a wooden frame. Unfortunately very few makes of car have filtered air inlets, but filters are not difficult or expensive to fit yourself. To stop your nose becoming dry and sore, rub a little vaseline inside each nostril several times a day, or put 2 drops of pure almond oil inside each nostril once a week. Most hay fever sufferers find that direct sunlight tends to hurt their eyes, or give them a headache, or make their skin itchy, so if you must go out in the sun wear sunglasses and a hat which shades your face. Blow your nose gently – hard blowing only bursts the offending grains of pollen and increases their irritant effects. Avoid contact lenses during summer months. Try to eat a diet which is 50 per cent raw salads and fruit, and reduce the amount of sugar you eat. Some sufferers find extra Vitamin C and magnesium helpful.

Loss of sense of smell see DISTURBED SENSE OF SMELL

Nasal polyps
Chronic irritation of the mucous membrane lining the nasal cavity – the kind of irritation that occurs in HAY FEVER AND ALLERGIC RHINITIS – can cause small protrusions or polyps to develop inside the nose; lack of zinc and Vitamin B$_6$, or a sensitivity to aspirin and other salicylates, may be contributing factors. Though harmless in themselves, nasal polyps can obstruct breathing and reduce sensitivity to smells; a large polyp may block the opening to one of the sinuses and cause SINUSITIS. A polyp on one side of the nose only requires specialist investigation. Usually treated by minor surgery. Since there is a small risk of recurrence, constitutional homeopathic treatment is recommended after surgery.

Specific remedies to be given 4 times daily for up to 3 weeks
- Loss of smell, swelling around bridge of nose, nostrils dry, sore, and ulcerated, offensive yellow catarrh, extremities feel cold and clammy *Calcarea 6c*
- Polyps bleed easily *Phosphorus 6c*
- Chronic drip of catarrh down back of throat, person feels chilly and weak *Psorinum 6c*
- Yellow-green catarrh made worse by warm rooms, person weeps easily *Pulsatilla 6c*
- Large clinkers, crawling sensation in nostrils, weeping and sneezing *Teucrium 6c*
- Polyps develop as result of chronic rhinitis, profuse catarrh which smells nasty, membranes of nose dry and hot *Sanguinaria 6c*

Nosebleeds (epistaxis)
Injuries or infections which damage the moist lining of the nose can quite easily rupture tiny local blood vessels and cause bleeding; more often, bleeding occurs for no apparent reason. Contrary to popular myth, nosebleeds are not always a sign of HIGH BLOOD PRESSURE; very rarely they may be a symptom of a blood clotting disorder, in which case there will be evidence of bleeding in urine, faeces, gums, skin, etc. See First Aid p. 102 for treatment; if bleeding does not stop within 20 minutes, ②. For specific homeopathic remedies for nosebleeds, see p. 101 but constitutional treatment is recommended if they occur frequently.

Post-nasal drip see CATARRH

Runny nose see CATARRH

Septum deviation
If the septum, the cartilage which divides one nostril from the other, is crooked or is knocked crooked by a blow to the nose, the air passage on one side of the nose may become restricted or blocked; more rarely, one of the sinus openings may be obstructed, leading to SINUSITIS; not usually troublesome enough to warrant surgery to straighten septum unless exacerbating conditions such as HAY FEVER AND ALLERGIC RHINITIS are present.

Sinusitis
Inflammation of the mucous membranes of the sinuses, usually a complication of viral or bacterial infections involving some other part of the respiratory system; can also be caused by injury to nasal bones, dental treatment, swimming, inhaling foreign bodies, or SEPTUM DEVIATION; in very rare cases, infection may spread to bones of face and skull, or to brain. Symptoms are a blocked up nose, nasal-sounding speech, and generally feeling unwell; if frontal sinuses are affected, there may be a HEADACHE over one or both eyes, usually worse in the mornings and made sharper by bending forwards; if maxillary sinuses are involved, cheeks feel tender and pain may be similar to toothache in upper jaw. In susceptible individuals, condition tends to recur, especially in times of STRESS; occasionally, recurrence may be linked with a food ALLERGY, Conventionally treated with antibiotics, decongestants, or proprietary analgesics such as aspirin and paracetamol, but the remedies given below should be tried first; if these produce no improvement, 48 ; if in severe pain, 12 . Recurrent sinusitis requires constitutional treatment.

Specific remedies to be taken every 2 hours for up to 2 days
- Stringy catarrh, feeling of fullness and congestion on either side of nose *Kali bichrom. 6c*
- Throbbing, tearing pain felt deep in bones of face, tip of nose itchy *Silicea 6c*
- Yellow catarrh, face very tender and sensitive, attack brought on by cold, dry winds and accompanied by sneezing, person feels chilly and irritable *Hepar sulph. 6c*
- Pain above eyes, nose occasionally stuffed up, yellow catarrh, symptoms worse indoors, frontal and right maxillary sinuses involved, jumpy neuralgic pain on right side of face, tendency to weep *Pulsatilla 6c*
- Condition comes on suddenly, with frontal sinuses affected, temperature higher than normal, face hot and red, bleeding from nose, symptoms aggravated by slightest pressure or by lying down *Belladonna 30c*

Self-help Avoid dry atmospheres, humidify rooms, and inhale hot steam; blow nose very gently. Vitamin C and Vitaman B complex, zinc, and iron are also recommended.

For explanation of other symbols, see page 107

TEETH AND GUMS

A healthy tooth is a living structure, nourished by blood vessels and supplied by nerves; its root is sheathed in special shock-absorbing periodontal tissue, and the base of its crown is firmly held by gums which are pale pink and do not easily bleed. The enamel which covers the crown of a healthy tooth is the hardest substance in the body; the layer of dentine beneath it is also hard, but less so; inside the dentine lie blood vessels, and also nerve endings which detect heat, cold, pressure, and pain.

Permanent teeth, 32 of them, begin to replace milk teeth from the age of six onwards, with the incisors emerging first; the process usually completes itself, with the four wisdom teeth, between the age of 17 and 21.

The single most important influence on teeth at any age is, not surprisingly, food: fibrous, chewy, non-sugary, non-acidic foods keep teeth healthy; soft, acid-producing, highly refined foods packed with sugar promote decay. Good dental hygiene can help to undo the effects of sugary foods, but only up to a point. Food influences teeth in other ways too; a woman's diet before conception and during pregnancy (see pp. 23 and 282–3) can positively or adversely affect her baby's teeth, and when the child is born his or teeth will be the better for eating plenty of foods containing calcium and Vitamins A and D. Heredity influences teeth too, but there we have to abide by the luck of the draw.

When it comes to cleaning teeth, regular vigorous brushing with a small-headed, highly manoeuverable toothbrush, and occasional flossing, are far more important than the toothpaste you use; in fact most commercial toothpastes contain some form of sugar and many quite gratuitous ingredients. A 9-point plan for preventing dental decay appears on p. 23.

Fillings become necessary when part of a tooth has decayed; the dentist drills out the decayed part, shapes the cavity to receive the filling, seals the cavity with resin, then fills it with mercury amalgam or quartz and resin; the latter is sometimes used when the filling is going to be visible but is not on a biting surface. *Extraction* becomes necessary when a tooth is decayed or broken beyond repair, or loose because of gum disease, or in the way of another tooth coming through; a tooth may also be removed if it is preventing a proper bite or if teeth are overcrowded in a small jaw. *Crowns*, made of gold or porcelain, are a half-way measure between filling and extraction; if the base of the tooth is healthy but the crown is severely discoloured, decayed, or broken, just the top of the tooth is replaced. *Scaling* and *polishing* are procedures which remove plaque and calculus (hardened plaque), and help to keep both teeth and gums healthy.

All of the procedures just mentioned are minor, and can be performed by a dentist, with a local anaesthetic if appropriate. Sometimes, however, where the structure of the jaw or the arrangement of teeth is faulty, the specialist attention of an orthodontist may be required; up until the age of about 13 the jawbone is soft enough to allow teeth to be slightly repositioned, usually with the aid of a plate or brace, so that they do not recede, protrude, slope, twist, crowd each other, etc.

There is a fairly general belief among homeopaths that certain dental procedures, injections for example, can antidote homeopathic remedies. If you are receiving constitutional treatment and a dental appointment is imminent, notify your homeopath; he or she may prefer to delay prescribing until the effects of dental treatment have worn off. That said, homeopathy offers a number of specific remedies for use before and after dental treatment (see FEAR OF DENTAL TREATMENT and DISCOMFORT AFTER DENTAL TREATMENT). Cranial osteopathy also has a role to play in dental medicine.

Tooth abscess

Pus-filled cavity in root of decaying or dead tooth, formed as bacteria infect and destroy pulp and produce toxins; tooth very tender when tapped, painful to chew on, with a persistent ache or throb, and pain sometimes radiating along side of nose or across other teeth; if left untreated, pus seeps out through root, erodes a canal through adjacent bone, and causes a gumboil, a painful swelling on the gum. Up to this point, toxins are sealed off from rest of body, but if gumboil bursts, releasing foul-tasting pus into mouth and relieving pain, there may be FEVER and the lymph glands in neck and face may swell in an effort to neutralize the toxins before they get into general circulation and cause SEPTICAEMIA. Because of risk of blood poisoning, [12] if a gumboil bursts, or if abscess seems to be enlarging rapidly; antibiotics may be prescribed to prevent infection spreading.

Standard treatment of a tooth abscess is to drain pus and then disinfect and fill tooth, or remove tip of root (an apicectomy) if it cannot be disinfected, or take the tooth out.

Specific remedies to be taken every hour for up to 10 doses while waiting for dental treatment
- Copious saliva, spongy gums *Mercurius 6c*
- First hint of an abscess, tooth and surrounding gum feel hot, mouth dry *Belladonna 30c*
- Gumboil well developed and very painful, pain aggravated by both hot and cold things in mouth *Silicea 6c*
- Gumboils starts to discharge pus *Gunpowder 6c*

Self-help Wash mouth every 4 hours with a solution of Hypericum and Calendula (5 drops of mother tincture of each to 0.25 litre [½ pint] warm water).

Caries (tooth decay)

Caused by bacteria in mouth acting on sugar in food and producing acid which erodes hard enamel of teeth, allowing bacteria to enter softer dentine beneath and eventually the inner pulp; if pulp does not respond by producing secondary dentine to protect itself, bacteria will invade it, causing inflammation and the familiar pain of TOOTHACHE. Pulp may die, leaving tooth to all intents and purposes dead, or infection may spread to root of tooth, giving rise to a TOOTH ABSCESS. If decay is not too advanced, dentist will clean out pulp cavity, drain abscess if necessary, and fill cavity and root canal to seal off tooth; if this is not possible, tooth may have to be extracted.

Specific remedies to be taken twice a day for 3 weeks out of 4 for up to 3 months if tendency to decay is not solely caused by eating too many sweet things
- Teeth decayed, loose, and black, or many teeth filled, crowned, or loose, excessive salivation, bleeding gums *Mercurius 6c*
- Decay in many teeth, especially in a child who is thin and has a large head *Silicea 6c*
- Decay in many teeth, especially in a child who is overweight and prone to head sweats *Calcarea 6c*
- Teeth black *Kreosotum 6c*
- Teeth black, sensitive to slightest touch, and ache after food or drink *Sulphur 6c*

Self-help Calc. Phos. and Calc. Fluor. (see Tissue Salts p. 388) are recommended; take 3 tablets of each 3 times a day. Reduce intake of sweets, biscuits, cakes, soft drinks, etc. Make sure that your diet contains molybdenum, and check to see if your diet or environment contains excessive levels of selenium or mercury.

Denture problems

Full dentures, which rest on the ridge of the gums and are held in by suction, should be checked every 2 years, and partial dentures, usually hooked onto remaining teeth, every 6 months. With any new dentures, eat soft foods to begin with; if there is soreness, see your dentist. Always keep dentures clean, soaking them overnight in a solution of Hypericum and Calendula (5 drops of mother tincture of each to 0.25 litre [½] pint of water), and brush them daily. Enunciation problems can often be overcome by reading aloud.

In general, dentures slightly increase the risk of MOUTH ULCERS, CARIES in any remaining teeth, GINGIVITIS, and ORAL THRUSH (see individual entries for homeopathic remedies). There may also be some shrinkage of the gums and jaws, hollowing the cheeks and giving the jaw a protruding appearance, sometimes causing pain in the temporo-mandibular joints.

Specific remedies to be given every 4 hours for up to 3 days
- Tension in jaw, with difficulty opening mouth, especially after exposure to cold, dry winds *Causticum 6c*
- Cramp-like pain in temporo-mandibular joint even when resting, especially in cold, wet weather, pain relieved by firm pressure on joint, movement of jaw produces cracking sound, hot food and drinks relieve discomfort *Rhus tox. 6c*

Discolouration of the teeth

Unless due to decay – a dead tooth looks grey – discolouration usually affects all teeth. Smoking turns teeth brown; too much fluoride can cause mottling; patchy discolouration may be a side effect of WHOOPING COUGH or MEASLES; yellow teeth may be the result of taking tetracycline (an antibiotic). The most obvious course is immediately to discontinue whatever is causing discolouration – smoking, fluoride supplements – or to take the nosode (see p. 12) of the offending substance as a damage limitation measure. In the case of whooping cough and measles, the appropriate nosodes are *Pertussin 30c* and *Morbillinum 30c* respectively (3 doses only, at 12 hour intervals); if tetracycline is necessary, its after effects should be antidoted by taking the nosode of tetracycline in 30c potency (3 doses only, at 12 hour intervals). Generally speaking, once nicotine and fluoride are discontinued, teeth slowly regain their whiteness; discolouration from other causes, however, is permanent, unless one is prepared to embark on costly cosmetic treatment. Vitamin B5 is sometimes beneficial.

Discomfort after dental treatment

Homeopathy offers a number of specific remedies to aid recovery after dental procedures.

- Immediately after any kind of dental treatment *Arnica 30c* hourly for up to 10 doses
- Pain after treatment *Hypericum 6c* ½-hourly for up to 10 doses, then 4 times daily for up to 5 days
- Pain after an injection *Ledum 6c* ½-hourly for up to 3 doses
- Bleeding after an extraction *Phosphorus 6c* every 10 minutes for up to 3 doses, but if bleeding continues, contact dentist
- Infection of socket after extraction *Ruta 6c* every 3 hours for up to 24 hours, but if infection does not clear up, contact dentist

Fear of dental treatment

A very common fear, among adults as well as children. The remedies below can help to steady the nerves before a visit to the dentist.

Specific remedies to be taken once hourly as necessary

- Person very frightened *Aconite 30c*
- Person very apprehensive, shaky, legs and knees feel weak *Gelsemium 30c*
- Fear based on extreme sensitivity to pain, or a child who throws tantrums about going to dentist *Chamomilla 30c*

Fillings (problems with mercury amalgam fillings)

A controversial subject among dentists and doctors; mercury amalgam, which contains silver, tin, zinc, and copper as well as mercury, is commonly used to fill cavities where a hard biting surface is required. It has been claimed that 5 percent of mercury amalgam fillings in place for less than 5 years, and 22 percent of those in place for longer than 5 years, cause problems such as increased salivation (see SALIVARY DISORDERS), occasional blurring of vision, digestive upsets (see INDIGESTION), weakness and tingling in the limbs, chilliness, a metallic taste in the mouth, TINNITUS, irritability, SLEEP PROBLEMS, and lowered resistance to infection (mercury inhibits production of white blood cells); other researchers, studying autopsy reports, have found a positive correlation between the amount of mercury in the brain and the number of mercury amalgam fillings. Acids in the mouth, so the theory goes, cause the mercury in the amalgam to be liberated into the circulation; electric currents can also be set up in the mouth, aggravated by eating salty foods. Mercury is suspected of playing a part in ECZEMA, recurrent MOUTH ULCERS, pre-cancerous lesions in the mouth, and still births. Mercury poisoning may also mimic MULTIPLE SCLEROSIS.

Replacement of mercury amalgam fillings with mercury-free materials is not without risk as mercury may be liberated into the system in the process. If, after eliminating other possible causes, nagging symptoms continue and your own dentist is unhelpful, ask the British Dental Society for Clinical Nutrition for advice (address on p. 385).

Gingivitis see also VINCENT'S DISEASE

Infected or bleeding gums, usually caused by a build-up of plaque (a sticky mixture of bacteria and food particles) on the teeth because dental hygiene is inadequate; less often, vitamin deficiency, blood disorders, or drugs may be the cause.

Where plaque is the culprit, bacterial toxins cause the gums to become inflamed and swollen where they hug the teeth; in the pockets between the gums and teeth more decaying food gets trapped, more plaque builds up, and the inner and deeper layers of plaque harden into a substance called calculus, which begins to loosen the teeth from their sockets, with the danger of a TOOTH ABSCESS forming. Routinely treated by giving an antibacterial mouthwash, and removing offending plaque and calculus by scaling; gums usually heal satisfactorily if oral hygiene is maintained.

If gingivitis is very advanced, sensitive tissue covering root of tooth becomes exposed, causing extreme sensitivity to hot, cold, or sweet food and drinks. If gum pockets trapping food are very deep, surgery may be necessary (gingivectomy); if teeth are kept scrupulously clean, gums usually grow back again.

Specific remedies to be given every 4 hours for up to 3 days
- Gums spongy, breath smells bad *Mercurius 6c*
- Red, inflamed, swollen gums which bleed easily, with roots of teeth exposed, especially in left upper jaw *Kreosotum 6c*
- Swollen gums which bleed easily, ulcers, taste of pus in mouth, teeth very sensitive to hot and cold *Natrum mur. 6c*
- Gums which bleed easily when touched, gaps between teeth and gums *Phosphorus 6c*
- Gums which are painful, swollen, very sensitive to cold liquids, and bleed easily, tendency to gumboils *Silicea 6c*

Self-help To prevent gum disease in the first place, or to prevent recurrence, brush teeth and gums regularly, especially after sugary foods; floss between teeth every day; eat chewy foods in preference to soft foods (chewing 'massages' the gums and helps to pump blood through the teeth), but avoid foods which scratch or cut the gums; watch out for pockets of infection around ragged fillings or awkwardly spaced teeth, or around teeth next to dentures. If infection is present, rinse the mouth with Hypericum and Calendula solution (5 drops of mother tincture of each in 0.25 litre [½ pint] boiled cooled water) 4 times a day.

Grinding teeth (bruxism)

Involuntary grinding together of the teeth during FEVER or FITS; unusual but more common in children than adults; can also happen during sleep (see SLEEP PROBLEMS), possibly due to ANXIETY. If there are emotional causes, constitutional treatment may help.

Specific remedies to be given 3 times daily for up to 5 days if grinding occurs during day, or at bedtime for 5 nights running if grinding occurs during sleep
- Grinding associated with threadworms *Cina 6c*
- If Cina is not effective *Santoninum 6c*
- Intense desire to clench teeth, especially in children *Phytolacca 6c*
- Grinding causes gums to bleed and teeth to loosen *Zinc 6c*
- Grinding teeth during sleep, especially between midnight and 2 am *Arsenicum 6c*

Gum disease see GINGIVITIS, VINCENT'S DISEASE

Gumboils see TOOTH ABSCESS

Receding gums see GINGIVITIS

Sensitive teeth

May be a consequence of GINGIVITIS or over-enthusiastic brushing of teeth in one direction only. In either case, the delicate tissue covering the roots of the teeth is exposed, causing great sensitivity to hot, cold, or sweet things. Sensitivity can be reduced by applying fluoride varnish or using a special toothpaste. See GINGIVITIS for appropriate homeopathic remedies.

Teething see TEETHING p. 333

Toothache

Usually a symptom of decay (see CARIES) and a warning that prompt dental treatment is needed; paracetamol is the standard way of keeping pain at bay, but the homeopathic remedies given below should be tried first.

Continuous toothache which prevents sleep, or is associated with FEVER and swelling of face or gum, or a tooth which is loose or feels too long, may be caused by a TOOTH ABSCESS; you should see a dentist within 12 hours.

If tooth is sensitive to heat, cold, or sweet things, or gives pain lasting for more than a few minutes, nerve in tooth may be inflamed due to advanced decay; if pain is absent except when you bite, tooth or filling may be broken; in either case see your dentist within 48 hours.

Toothache after a filling is not unusual on contact with cold air or cold drinks once local anaesthetic wears off, but if pain persists and tooth becomes sensitive to heat as well, see your dentist as soon as possible. A return visit to the dentist may also be necessary if filling is not level and still hurts to bite on a week later.

Toothache can also accompany GINGIVITIS and SINUSITIS. The homeopathic remedies given below are not a substitute for prompt dental treatment, but they relieve discomfort.

Specific remedies to be given every 5 minutes for up to 10 doses
- Tooth very nervy, aggravated by cold air and slightest pressure but better for eating, teeth generally feel sensitive, as if they are somehow too long and exposed, mouth full of saliva *Plantago 6c* (mother tincture of Plantago can also be rubbed on affected tooth)
- Toothache made worse by heat and hot food, relieved by applying ice *Coffea 6c*
- Pain unbearable, made worse by cold air, by warm food and drink, and by coffee at night, person like a bear with a sore head *Chamomilla 6c*
- Tender, spongy gums which bleed easily, loose teeth, bad breath, person very thirsty, mouth full of saliva, pains shoot up to ears *Mercurius 6c*

- Severe toothache aggravated by cold air, food, and slightest pressure, drawing or tearing pain, cheek red and swollen, bad tooth black and disintegrating *Staphisagria 6c*
- Pain unbearable, especially with hot food or drink, relieved by cold water, person not at all thirsty, feels better in open air *Pulsatilla 6c*
- Pain after a filling or extraction *Arnica 30c*
- Throbbing pain and dry mouth, developing gumboil *Belladonna 30c*
- Teeth discoloured and decayed, breath smells foul, person also suffering from constipation *Kreosotum 6c*
- Gums feel tight and swollen, toothache burns and stings *Apis 30c*
- Teeth feel too long, hot food and drink and movement aggravate pain, but lying down, especially on painful side, alleviates pain, tooth less painful when pressed *Bryonia 30c*
- Toothache comes on every time person eats, cold air and cold drinks make it worse, especially during pregnancy *Calcarea 6c*
- Nervy pains like little electric shocks, soothed by warmth *Magnesia phos. 6c*

Self-help Rub oil of cloves on affected tooth, but only if three or more of the above remedies have been tried without success (oil of cloves can have an antidoting effect on homeopathic remedies).

Tooth decay see CARIES

Vincent's disease (acute ulcerative gingivitis)

Bacterial infection and ulceration of gums, often between teeth, caused by advanced tooth CARIES, poor dental hygiene, throat infection, or smoking. May cause metallic taste in mouth and BAD BREATH. In severe cases, antibiotics may be necessary, and perhaps minor surgery to prevent scarred gums from harbouring particles of food.

Specific remedies to be given every 2 hours for up to 10 doses
- Teeth loose, gums soft and spongy, bad breath *Nitric ac. 6c*
- Gums purple, spongy, and swollen, bitter salty taste in mouth *Mercurius corr. 6c*

Self-help Use Hypericum mouthwash (10 drops of mother tincture to 0.25 litre [½ pint] boiled cooled water) every 4 hours; improve dental hygiene.

Wisdom teeth problems

The four wisdom teeth, those farthest back in both the upper and lower jaw, usually erupt between the age of 17 and 21, sometimes as late as 25, and occasionally not at all. Non-emergence is not normally a problem because there are no symptoms. A wisdom tooth which emerges at an angle to its neighbour can trap food, which then causes gum infection and a nasty taste in the mouth. More seriously, a wisdom tooth may become *impacted*, unable to emerge because the tooth next to it is in the way; this causes a pocket in the gum in which food tends to accumulate, leading to pericoronitis (infection and swelling of the gum, an unpleasant taste, and pain when biting). In most cases, an impacted wisdom tooth is treated by giving paracetamol and antibiotics to reduce pain and infection, then by extraction under general anaesthetic. For appropriate homeopathic remedies, see TOOTHACHE or select a remedy from the list following.

Specific remedies to be taken every 6 hours for up to 3 days until dental appointment can be made
- Shooting, piercing pains made worse by cold air, food, or noise *Calcarea 6c*
- Where left upper molars are most affected, with warm sensation in jaw *Fluoric ac. 6c*
- Pain from erupting wisdom tooth, worse at night, forcing person to get up and walk about *Magnesia carb. 6c*

Self-help To prevent infection, rinse mouth 4 times daily with a solution of Hypericum and Calendula (5 drops of mother tincture of each to 0.25 litre [½ pint] boiled cooled water) or with salt solution (1 teaspoon salt to 0.25 litre [½ pint]).

MOUTH, TONGUE, THROAT AND VOICE

DIGESTION begins in the mouth – saliva lubricates food and adds starch-digesting enzymes to it, the teeth crush and chew it, and the muscular tongue pushes it around the mouth, then rolls it into a ball for swallowing. As the tongue pushes the ball past the soft palate, the epiglottis shuts like a lid over the entrance to the windpipe, and the ball slides into the oesophagus.

Saliva is 99.5 per cent water and is continually produced to clean the mouth – as well as digestive enzymes it contains an enzyme which destroys bacteria. Food entering the mouth stimulates taste buds on the tongue; the brain receives their messages and instructs the salivary glands to go into top gear. There are three pairs of saliva glands, the parotids just in front of the ears, which open at the back of the mouth near the molars, and the submandibulars and submaxillaries, which open beneath the tongue. Each pair of glands produces a slightly different mix of mucus and enzymes. Saliva is copiously produced in response to acids – vinegar, lemon juice, etc. Nausea also produces reflex salivation.

Some of the sensations we call 'tastes' are in fact smells. As we chew, the volatile constituents in our food are wafted up into the nasal cavity where they are sampled by the smell receptors. Altogether the tongue has about 2000 taste receptors or taste buds on its sides and upper surface. These detect four basic tastes: salt, sweet, sour, and bitter. All taste sensations – whether we interpret them as cheese, chocolate, tea, or apple pie – are blends of these primary tastes. Sweet things are tasted at the front of the tongue, salt and sour at the sides, and bitter towards the back. There are also a few taste buds on the soft palate and in the throat.

The vocal cords lie in the larynx (voice box), the short passageway between the throat (pharynx) and trachea (windpipe). When we decide to talk, muscles in the glottis contract, pulling the vocal cords (tiny elastic ligaments) taut; the outrush of air, speeded up because the glottis is narrowed, causes the cords to vibrate. The more forcefully air rushes past the cords, the louder the noise we make; the greater the tension in the cords, the higher our voice sounds. Intense emotions, infections, dry air, and irritants such as cigarette smoke can all prevent the cords from vibrating freely.

Bad breath (halitosis)
Usually smelled by others! To test your breath, breath into the cupped palm of your hand and inhale. Various mouth and upper digestive tract conditions can cause bad breath, for example CARIES, GINGIVITIS (inflamed gums), ulcer in the mouth or on the tongue (see MOUTH ULCERS), SALIVATION DISORDERS, and INDIGESTION (gases from the stomach); bad breath can also accompany infections such as COLDS, SINUSITIS, SORE THROAT, TONSILLITIS, and LARYNGITIS; metabolic disorders such as DIABETES, and smoking, drugs, and fasting can also cause the breath to smell. In such circumstances, toothpastes and mouthwashes are of little avail.

Specific remedies to be taken 3 times daily for up to 7 days
- Breath smells sour, especially after a stomach upset, after meals, or after drinking alcohol, slight nausea, worse in morning *Nux 6c*
- Breath and sweat smell offensive, whole room smells of bad breath, copious saliva, dental decay, tongue yellow and furry *Mercurius 6c*
- After eating fatty food, person not at all thirsty, mouth dry *Pulsatilla 6c*
- Breath smells putrid or bitter, especially in young people of pubertal age *Aurum 6c*
- Putrid-smelling breath, gums healthy but teeth loose, mouth ulcers *Nitric ac. 6c*
- Breath smells of onions *Petroselinum 6c*

- Breath smells of faeces *Quercus 6c*
- Bad breath due to blood in mouth, especially after injury *Arnica 6c*

Self-help The obvious course is to avoid foods and other substances which leave a strong odour behind or cause indigestion (garlic, onions, fats, alcohol, nicotine). Pay regular visits to the dentist and practice good dental hygiene. STOP SMOKING.

Burning mouth syndrome

Great soreness and smarting of the mouth, lasting for months or years, most common in women after the MENOPAUSE; cause may be decreased hormone production (see HORMONE IMBALANCES), nerve damage, STRESS; or food ALLERGY; in isolated cases, a deficiency of Vitamin B_{12} or folate has been identified. In addition to soreness and smarting, mouth may feel dry and tongue stick to palate; some sufferers also experience HEADACHES or, unjustifiably, fear that condition is due to CANCER; symptoms tend to worsen as day goes on, but mouth and tongue may look perfectly normal. Sometimes helped by Vicks lozenges, ice cubes, or cold drinks, but usually made worse by spicy or acidic foods, alcohol, nicotine, INFLUENZA, and talking. Anaesthetic and antifungal preparations, mouthwashes, and artificial saliva have no effect. Constitutional homeopathic treatment is recommended, although the remedies given below should be tried first.

Specific remedies to be taken 4 times daily for up to 14 days
- Sudden onset, mouth numb, dry, and red inside, tongue whitish and furred up *Aconite 6c*
- Mouth dry, red, and burning *Belladonna 6c*
- Symptoms made worse by cold drinks, soothed by warm ones *Arsenicum 6c*
- Person drinks lots of cold water, burning sensation extends down throat *Phosphorus 6c*
- Mouth sore, lips dry, bitter taste in mouth, centre of tongue whitish but margins and tip red *Sulphur 6c*

Self-help Suck ice cubes if pain is severe. If condition seems to be aggravated by stress, try to learn some form of relaxation or meditation. Extra Vitamin C, B_6, B_{12}, folate, and zinc, and evening primrose oil, may be beneficial.

Cold sores

Culprit is the extremely infectious *Herpes simplex* virus, which can also cause CORNEAL ULCERS and genital herpes (see SEXUALLY TRANSMITTED DISEASES), so do not touch eyes or genitals after touching cold sores. In first stage of infection, blisters and then ulcers form *inside* the mouth or on the face, accompanied by red, swollen gums, a furry tongue, mild FEVER, and feeling generally under par. Though these symptoms clear up within a few days, the virus may not be destroyed, so

whenever immunity is at a low ebb infection tends to reappear around mouth and lips, causing blisters which weep and then become encrusted; these usually clear up within 5–7 days. Though antiviral ointments are often effective, the author advises against all external applications whilst undergoing homeopathic treatment if possible. Outbreaks can be treated using the remedies given below, but constitutional treatment is the proper solution.

Specific remedies to be given 4 times daily for up to 5 days
- Many ulcers inside mouth, gums bleed easily, whole mouth very sore, worse at night *Sempervivum 6c*
- Deep crack in middle of lower lip, mouth very dry, sores puffy and burning, pearl-like blisters on lips *Natrum mur. 6c*
- Mouth and chin infected, ulcers at corner of mouth *Rhus tox. 6c*
- Cracks at corners of mouth, lips pale, red itchy rash on chin, burning blisters on tongue, breath smells nasty *Capsicum 6c*

Self-help Take extra lysine (an amino acid), Vitamin C, zinc and bioflavinoids, and avoid foods containing arginine (another amino acid, found in peanuts, chocolate, seeds, and cereals).

Glossitis see also TONGUE DISORDERS

Sore tongue caused by temporary absence of papillae, the tiny protrusions that contain the taste buds; denuded of papillae, the tongue becomes dark red and inflamed; hot, spicy, acidic, or scratchy foods should be avoided. Occasionally condition is a symptom of iron-deficient ANAEMIA, or a lack of Vitamin B_{12}, B_3, biotin, or folate. Supplying the deficiency usually re-establishes normal growth of papillae. In addition to remedies given below, those given for BURNING MOUTH SYNDROME are also appropriate.

Specific remedies to be taken 4 times daily for up to 5 days
- Sore, burning tongue with red tip and red streak in middle *Arsenicum 6c*
- Whole mouth and tongue hot, dry, and red *Belladonna 30c*

Halitosis see BAD BREATH

Hoarseness see LARYNGITIS, LARYNGEAL TUMOURS, SORE THROAT

Laryngitis

Inflammation or infection of the larynx and vocal cords, causing hoarseness or loss of voice. *Acute laryngitis* is most often caused by the same viruses and bacteria which cause COLDS, SORE THROATS, COUGHS, SINUSITIS, and BRONCHITIS; less common causes are ALLERGIES, shouting or straining the voice, continual coughing in order to bring up phlegm, vomiting, heavy smoking or drinking, inhaling toxic fumes, breathing through the mouth rather than the nose, ANXIETY, and strong emotions. If condition does not clear up within 7–10 days, see your GP; referral to an ear, nose and throat specialist may be necessary.

Chronic laryngitis is more likely to be a consequence of vocal overuse (an occupational hazard of market traders, teachers, and singers) than of infection; the vocal cords tend to swell, and in some cases develop polyps which may need to be removed surgically. However, more or less permanent hoarseness can be a symptom of HYPOTHYROIDISM, of chronic SINUSITIS or TONSILLITIS, or of food ALLERGY; progressive hoarseness may be due to a LARYNGEAL TUMOUR; paralysis of the vocal cords can occur as the result of LUNG CANCER, TUBERCULOSIS, heavy smoking or drinking, or thyroid surgery, or as part of the ageing process.

In acute cases, where infection is present, use the specific remedies given under the appropriate infection, or pick one from the list below. When laryngitis is chronic and recurrent, constitutional treatment should be sought.

Specific remedies to be taken 4 times daily for up to 7 days
- Sudden onset, made worse by cold dry winds, especially in child who has croup, fever, anxiety, restlessness *Aconite 30c*
- Throat feels worse in morning and after exposure to cold dry winds, better indoors in warm, loose cough with yellow phlegm, choking feeling *Hepar sulph. 6c*
- Dry, barking cough, especially in child with croup, loss of voice *Spongia 6c*
- Throat dry and sore, worse in evening, rasping voice, talking painful, dry, tickling cough *Phosphorus 6c*
- Throat dry and raw, mucus dripping down back of throat, person quite unable to speak, coughing causes urination *Causticum 6c*
- Person elderly, throat worse in damp, cold weather and in evening, feels chilly, comes out in sweats, has poor circulation *Carbo veg. 6c*
- Where problem is caused by an allergy and uvula (flap of skin at back of throat) is visibly swollen *Apis 30c*
- Palate and roof of mouth feel raw, corners of mouth sore and cracked, blocked-up nose and burning catarrh, hoarseness, throat feels swollen, narrowed, and burning *Arum 6c*
- Chronic laryngitis, especially if person always talks too much *Lachesis 6c*
- Sudden loss of voice due to overuse *Arnica 30c*
- Hysterical loss of voice *Ignatia 6c*
- Hoarseness worse during menstruation *Gelsemium 6c*
- Paralysis of vocal cords *Oxalic ac. 6c*
- Chronic loss of voice without obvious cause *Baryta carb. 6c*

Specific remedies for loss of voice in singers, to be taken 4 times daily for up to 3 days

- Tickle in larynx made worse by cold, voice feeble due to overuse *Alumina 6c*
- If tickle increases, voice weak, trembly, and inclined to break *Argentum 6c*
- Voice weak on starting to sing, improves after a few minutes *Rhus tox. 6c*
- Clear discharge from nose, singing feels painful, larynx tender *Phosphorus 6c*

Self-help Avoid nicotine and alcohol, and hot or smoke-filled atmospheres, rest the voice, and drink plenty of fluids. Extra Vitamin C, B complex, zinc, and iron would also be beneficial. Voice may also benefit from retraining.

Laryngeal tumours
A benign growth on the larynx is likely to cause intermittent hoarseness; if malignant, hoarseness is persistent and progressive. Benign growths, such as polyps and papillomas, seem to be related to overuse of the voice, and can be removed surgically; cancerous growths are very clearly related to heavy smoking, and if radiotherapy fails to destroy them, or if they are too far advanced, the whole larynx has to be removed. See CANCER for homeopathic treatment.

Hoarseness or other vocal changes which, in the absence of any infection, persist or get worse should always be investigated.

Leucoplakia
A whitish-grey patch of thickened or hardened skin inside the mouth or on the tongue; forms over a period of weeks as a reaction to a rough tooth, dentures, or hot cigarette smoke; feels rough and stiff, and may sting when hot, spicy food is eaten. Usually clears up within 3–4 weeks if cause is removed; if not, consult your GP as there is a very small risk of such patches turning malignant.

Specific remedies to be taken 4 times daily for up to 14 days
- Lesions in cheek, made worse by chewing and biting *Causticum 6c*
- Rough patch on palate *Phytolacca 6c*
- Tongue stiff and difficult to stick out *Hyoscyamus 6c*
- Tongue affected, mouth dry and numb, tongue sticks to roof of mouth *Nux mosch. 6c*

Lockjaw see TETANUS

Loss of voice see LARYNGITIS, LARYNGEAL TUMOURS, SORE THROAT

Mouth ulcers see also COLD SORES, ORAL THRUSH
Often a sign of being run down or under STRESS, but can also be caused by accidental damage (biting side of mouth, using toothbrush carelessly, eating food which is too hot); aggravated by acidic and spicy food, and by

cigarette smoke; in some cases, may be a symptom of food ALLERGY. Usually clear up within 10 days, or more quickly with a little self-help; if ulcers have not healed after 3 weeks, see your GP; in very rare cases, persistent ulcers may be a first sign of cancer (see TUMOURS OF THE MOUTH AND TONGUE). Constitutiomal treatment is recommended if ulcers are recurrent.

Specific remedies to be taken 4 times daily for up to 5 days
* Ulcers bleed when touched or after eating, mouth hot and tender, sometimes associated with oral thrush *Borax 6c*
* Mouth dry and burning, ulcers soothed by warm water *Arsenicum 6c*
* Ulcers mainly on tongue, where they sting and burn, especially when chewing food, tongue coated and trembly, more saliva than usual, bad breath, loose teeth *Mercurius 6c*
* Ulcers mainly on soft palate, where they feel like sharp splinters, bad breath, increased saliva *Nitric ac. 6c*

Self-help Avoid hot spicy foods and acidic foods, and stop smoking. Limit intake of sweets and refined carbohydrates. Rinse mouth with warm salt solution (1 teaspoon salt to 1 glass boiled cooled water) several times a day. If you are run down, Vitamin B complex will also help. If stress is the culprit, exercise and relaxation may be the long-term answer.

Oral thrush see also CANDIDIASIS
Fungal infection of the mouth, and sometimes the throat, most common in the young and elderly, and in people who wear dentures; communities of *Candida albicans* begin to thrive when resistance is low after illness, antibiotics, or oral corticosteroids, causing whitish, sticky patches to develop in the mouth; these are abraded by eating or cleaning teeth, leaving raw, sore areas. Your GP will probably prescribe antifungal lozenges, but if condition recurs, as it tends to, you should consider constitutional treatment to boost general immunity.

Specific remedies to be taken 4 times daily for up to 5 days
* At earliest signs of outbreak *Borax 6c*
* More saliva than usual, trembling tongue *Mercurius 6c*
* Patches hot and sore, made worse by drinking cold water *Capsicum 6c*
* Associated with cold sores on lips *Natrum mur. 6c*
* Associated with mouth ulcers and feeling worn out *Arsenicum 6c*

Self-help Aloe vera mouthwash (obtainable from most chemists and healthfood shops); this has an antifungal effect. If dentures are worn, sterilize them regularly.

Pharyngeal pouch
A rare disorder, most common in elderly men, in which a small pouch develops at back of larynx, trapping food and fluids and gradually getting bigger, making swallowing difficult. Symptoms are regurgitation of food into mouth some hours after eating, causing coughing and a metallic taste; pouch may also be visible at left side of neck after drinking. There is a slight risk of trapped food spilling into the lungs and causing PNEUMONIA, so if the above symptoms are present, you should consult your GP; surgical removal of pouch may be recommended.

Pharyngitis
Acute or chronic infection of that part of the throat between tonsils and larynx, usually less severe than TONSILLITIS; back of throat looks red and angry, swallowing may be difficult, and there may be slight FEVER. If not caused by viruses or bacteria, inflammation may be result of cigarette smoke, alcohol, or overuse of voice. See SORE THROAT for homeopathic treatment.

Salivary disorders
Most common disorder is MUMPS, a virus infection of the parotid glands and sometimes of the submaxillary glands as well (see p. 327 for description and treatment).
Bacterial infections are much rarer; these cause the affected gland to swell and discharge putrid-tasting pus into the mouth; appropriate action is 48, and Mercurius 6c every 2 hours in the meantime for up to 6 doses; an antibiotic may be necessary. Afterwards, constitutional treatment can help to boost general resistance to infection.
Salivary duct stones, hardened accumulations of various chemicals in saliva, are rare but most commonly affect the submandibular glands, which become swollen with trapped saliva; occasionally they may become infected, as above. Sucking a lemon has been known to flush out stones – the acid juice greatly stimulates the production of saliva – but if this does not work, consult your GP; stones can be removed under local anaesthetic. In the meantime, take *Calcarea 6c* every 4 hours for up to 3 days.
Excessive salivation is usually part of a wider condition, and clears up when this is treated; occasionally, it is a feature of pregnancy. Occurring in isolation, it may be due to PROBLEMS WITH MERCURY AMALGAM FILLINGS; if no other cause, or associated symptoms, can be pinpointed, try one of the remedies below.

Specific remedies to be taken 4 times daily for up to 3 days
* If associated with sore gums, saliva especially copious at night, wetting pillow *Mercurius 6c*
* If associated with mouth ulcers and splinter-like pains in ulcers *Nitric ac. 6c*

For explanation of other symbols, see page 107

- If associated with headache or migraine *Iris 6c*
- Made worse by eating *Allium 6c*
- If associated with nausea *Ipecac. 6c*

Deficiency of saliva is usually associated with a higher than normal temperature; it may also be a symptom of BURNING MOUTH SYNDROME, or a response to constantly breathing through the mouth.

Specific remedies to be taken every 2 hours for up to 10 doses
- Mouth dry, person restless and anxious *Arsenicum 6c*
- Mouth dry and hot, person feverish *Belladonna 6c*
- Lips dry and parched, great thirst, fever *Bryonia 6c*
- Mouth dry and burning *Capsicum 6c*
- Tongue sticks to roof of mouth *Nux mosch. 6c*

Sore mouth see BURNING MOUTH SYNDROME

Sore throat see also ADENOIDS, TONSILLITIS, LARYNGITIS, PHARYNGITIS, COLDS

A blanket term for inflammation or infection involving the adenoids, tonsils, pharynx, larynx and vocal cords. Infection may be generalized, involving the mucous membranes of the pharynx or larynx, or localized, affecting only the tonsils or adenoids, glands specifically designed to defend the upper respiratory tract against invading organisms. Offending microbe is usually a virus, as in COLDS, INFLUENZA, MUMPS, and GLANDULAR FEVER, but it can also be a bacterium as in streptococcal infections (RHEUMATIC FEVER usually begins with a 'strep throat'), or a fungus, as in ORAL THRUSH. Inflammation can also follow heavy smoking or drinking, abuse of gargles, general vitamin deficiency, or food ALLERGY; alternatively, inflammation can be a symptom of blood disorders such as AGRANULO-CYTOSIS, aplastic ANAEMIA, or LEUKAEMIA, or of CANCER, TUBERCULOSIS, SYPHILIS, or AIDS. If any of these conditions is suspected or diagnosed, turn to the relevant entry for description and homeopathic treatment.

If sore throat is accompanied by high FEVER and generally feeling very unwell, children ⟦12⟧, adults ⟦48⟧; depending on the diagnosis, antibiotics or analgesics may be prescribed. Antiseptic lozenges and gargles should be used with caution, as some of them contain a local anaesthetic which can trigger off an allergic reaction or simply prolong infection. A recurrent sore throat deserves constitutional treatment.

Specific remedies to be given every 2 hours for up to 10 doses
- Sudden onset, made worse by cold dry winds, throat dry, tonsils swollen, great thirst, throat looks red, rough, and dry, and also feels constricted, burning, and numb or tingly, hoarse voice *Aconite 30c*
- If person suffers from chronic nasal drip and lumbago or earache, acute sore throat comes on after exposure to cold and damp or after great exertion, throat raw and burning, saliva thick, voice

hoarse, cold sores around mouth, red itchy skin as in nettle rash, person thirsty for cold drinks and feels better moving around *Dulcamara 6c*
- Pain and soreness right-sided, throat feels as if there is a lump in it, neck glands swollen, lips dry, person thirsty but not hungry *Baryta mur 6c*
- Horrible taste in mouth, pain in neck and ears made worse by swallowing, person unwilling to drink because swallowing hurts so much, comes over hot and cold by turns, feels heavy, exhausted, weak, and shaky *Gelsemium 6c*
- Front of mouth normal, back of throat yellowish and coated, person craves fresh air, tonsil abscess threatening *Calcarea sulph. 6c*
- Sore throat due to allergy, back of throat bright red, swollen, and shiny, with uvula also swollen, pain burning and stinging, person depressed and irritable *Apis 30c*

Self-help Take plenty of Vitamin C and a course of garlic pills, and increase intake of zinc. Make up a Hypericum and Calendula gargle (5 drops of mother tincture of each to 0.25 litre [½ pint] boiled cooled water) and gargle every 4 hours.

Speech difficulties see also SPEECH

DIFFICULTIES p. 331, LOSS OF VOICE, STAMMERING
Can be due to local conditions affecting vocal cords or tongue, such as LARYNGITIS, LARYNGEAL TUMOURS, or TUMOURS OF THE MOUTH AND TONGUE, or to degeneration of those parts of the brain which coordinate thoughts and speech, as in SENILE DEMENTIA and PRE-SENILE DEMENTIA, or which control movements of mouth and larynx, as in PARKINSON'S DISEASE; can also be a consequence of a STROKE or transient ischaemic attack involving speech-related areas of the brain. Alcohol and drugs can also slow or slur a person's speech.

If speech difficulties come on suddenly, accompanied by DIZZINESS, NUMBNESS, BLURRED VISION and CONFUSION, a stroke should be suspected; appropriate action is ②.

Thrush see ORAL THRUSH

Tongue disorders see also GLOSSITIS, BURNING MOUTH SYNDROME

Condition of tongue can be a pointer to other disorders; a healthy tongue is pink and velvety, but in sickness the papillae on its surface change their colour and texture.

Enlargement of veins under the tongue may be a sign of Vitamin C deficiency.

Furring of the tongue may indicate FEVER or digestive trouble, the 'fur' being bacteria, food particles, and dead cells which accumulate when saliva flow is reduced or the tongue is less active than usual; gentle brushing with a toothbrush usually removes it. The remedies below can also be tried.

⟨999⟩ Emergency – call GP (or dial 999) immediately. ② Consult your doctor if no improvement within 2 hours

Specific remedies to be taken 3 times daily for up to 14 days
- Thick, milky, dirty furring, especially in children *Antimonium 6c*
- Thick, white coating, mouth and tongue dry, person very thirsty *Bryonia 6c*
- Tongue swollen, feels as if it has been scalded, teeth make marks in strip of yellow furring down centre of tongue *Hydrastis 6c*
- Tongue thick and swollen, teeth make marks in it, furring milky or dark, marked tremor *Mercurius 6c*
- Tongue thick, with dirty yellow furring *Sulphur 6c*

Geographical tongue is a condition in which patches of papillae fail to grow properly, sometimes due to Vitamin B deficiency; patches feel sore, and spicy foods make them sorer still.

Specific remedies to be taken 3 times daily for up to 14 days
- Tongue blistered and burning, affected areas white or yellow, rest of tongue very red *Natrum mur. 6c*
- Affected patches peeling *Taraxacum 6c*

Fissuring of the tongue occurs in people who have quite deep cracks in their tongue anyway; the cracks can turn black or brown if bacteria accumulate in them, as sometimes happens after fungal or bacterial infections, or as a result of smoking or antibiotics. Similar causes are thought to be responsible for *black hairy tongue*, in which the papillae grow extra long and become discoloured by bacteria. Both conditions are harmless, if unsightly. Recommended treatment, twice daily, is Hypericum and Calendula mouthwash (5 drops of mother tincture of each to 0.25 litre [½ pint] boiled cold water) after brushing tongue with a soft toothbrush. One of the remedies below may also be helpful.

Specific remedies to be taken 3 times daily for up to 14 days
- Tongue cracked, red, and parched *Belladonna 6c*
- Tongue moist, with blackish coating and marked tremor *Mercurius 6c*
- Tongue has inky black coating *Carbo veg. 6c*
- Tongue has black-brown coating *Phosphorus 6c*

Self-help Vitamin B₃ may help to reduce fissuring.

Tonsillitis see also TONSILLITIS p. 334, SORE THROAT
Acute infection of the tonsils, less common in adults than children; symptoms similar to those of INFLUENZA (sore throat, headache, fever, feeling hot and shivery by turns), except that tonsils at back of throat look red and swollen. Usually responds to self-help measures within 2–3 days, but if accompanied by a very high FEVER and feeling extremely ill, [12]. In susceptible individuals, tonsils tend to flare up when they are run down or overstressed; flare-ups can also be due to food ALLERGY. For recurrent tonsillitis, constitutional homeopathic treatment is recommended.

Specific remedies to be taken every 2 hours for up to 10 doses
- Throat very sore and tender to the touch, fiery pains, which shoot up into head and occur in spasms whenever person moves, pains tend to be right-sided and associated with stiff tender neck, pupils dilated, strawberry tongue with coated centre *Belladonna 30c*
- Throat feels as if there is a fishbone caught in it, pain alleviated by warm drinks, yellow pus coughed up, foul-smelling breath, person oversensitive physically and emotionally, unreasonable, feels chilly and shivery, especially in draughts, abscess developing on tonsils *Hepar sulph. 6c*
- Throat dark red, swollen, and sore, worse on right side, more painful at night and aggravated by speaking, tongue yellow and coated, breath offensive, hot sweats which make throat feel worse, excessive saliva which burns throat when swallowed *Mercurius 6c*
- Sores at corner of mouth, stringy saliva, tonsils thickly coated in slimy film, prickling sensation in throat, person not thirsty *Nitric ac. 6c*
- Throat sore on right side, associated with toothache or flatulence, tongue dry and puffy but not coated, throat feels more sore after cold drinks and food, and worse between 4 and 8 am or 4 and 8 pm *Lycopodium 6c*
- Throat sore on left side, swallowing causes pain in left ear, back of throat looks reddish purple; sleep, heat, liquids, and anything tight around neck make throat feel worse, but swallowing food seems to alleviate soreness *Lachesis 6c*
- Pain affects left and right side of throat alternately, back of throat covered in white, silvery film, saliva viscous and sticky, symptoms may coincide with a period *Lac can. 6c*
- Throat feels rough and constricted, tonsils look hot, dark red, and swollen, pain extends to ears and root of tongue, is more marked on right side, and gets worse with heat, neck glands enlarged, person exhausted, unresponsive, and feels extremely ill, also complains of cobweb sensation on face *Phytolacca 6c*

Self-help A day or two in bed, drinking plenty of fluids, usually speeds recovery. Chronic tonsillitis may be helped by taking extra Vitamin C, B complex, zinc, and iron.

Tumours of the mouth and tongue see also MOUTH ULCERS, CANCER
Both benign and malignant tumours of the mouth are very rare; however, if you notice a lump, ulcer, or colour change in your mouth, or stiffness in your

tongue, or sudden discomfort from dentures, and the problem does not clear up within 3 weeks, consult your GP. Benign tumours are usually slow-growing, pale lumps, but they should be kept under observation. A cancerous tumour of the mouth usually begins as a persistent ulcer which bleeds easily; if not detected and treated at this stage, cancerous cells from the ulcer spread to the tongue, affecting eating, speaking, and swallowing, and then to other parts of the body. A persistent ulcer on the lips may be a RODENT ULCER, a form of skin cancer. In the early stages malignancy can be removed by surgery; later, radiotherapy and chemotherapy may also be necessary.

There are a number of homeopathic remedies specifically for cancer of the tongue but, as with all forms of cancer, readers are advised to seek the care of an experienced homeopath. For homeopathic approach to CANCER, see p. 273.

LUNGS AND RESPIRATION

LUNGS developed as marine life forms began to adapt to life on dry land. With lungs it is possible to absorb oxygen directly from the air, provided their absorptive surface is kept moist. Only 21 per cent of the air we breathe is oxygen, but we do not use it all. Exhaled air is still 16 per cent oxygen. When our need for oxygen increases, blood flow through the lungs is increased by breathing faster and stepping up the heart rate. While oxygen is diffusing into the lungs, carbon dioxide diffuses out. Every cell in the body requires oxygen to liberate energy from glucose, and every cell in the body produces unwanted carbon dioxide in the process. Water is another by-product of cellular respiration; appreciable amounts are lost through the lungs, the rest is mainly disposed of in the urine.

Gaseous exchange takes place in tiny cul-de-sacs in the lungs called alveoli. These have, in the adult human lung, a combined surface area of about 70 m^2 (750 ft^2), roughly the size of a tennis court. Blood laden with carbon dioxide is pumped from the heart to the lungs through the pulmonary arteries; oxygen-rich blood returns to the heart through the pulmonary veins. Connecting these arteries and veins are many millions of alveoli, each supplied with thousands of blood capillaries constantly swopping carbon dioxide for oxygen.

The lungs are twin, conical structures, one on either side of the heart. They are enclosed in a double membrane, the pleural membrane, which is filled with fluid to allow friction-free movement inside the rib cage. The diaphragm, the dome of muscle primarily responsible for breathing movements, lies directly beneath the heart and lungs.

Each lung is a mass of branching airways which get narrower and narrower as they approach the alveoli. The walls of these airways produce mucus to keep the internal environment of the lungs moist; they are also lined with tiny hairs which beat together like wheat in the wind, trapping dust and other foreign particles and ferrying them out of the lungs so that they can be expelled by coughing or sneezing. Nicotine paralyses this extremely efficient rubbish removal system, resulting in 'smoker's cough'. Foreign particles which remain in the lungs, and of course any opportune viruses or bacteria, cause local inflammation and excessive production of mucus. If many small airways become blocked and many clusters of alveoli become flooded with mucus, respiration deteriorates. In bronchitis and pneumonia the lungs are partially suffocated by their own secretions.

We breathe in and out because the air pressure inside our lungs is constantly changing in relation to the air pressure outside. As we inhale, the diaphragm contracts and descends and the rib cage rises and expands; this decreases pressure inside the lungs, and so air rushes in. As we exhale, the diaphragm rises and the ribs fall, pulled down by gravity; this increases pressure inside the lungs, and so air rushes out. Although we can control the rate and depth of our breathing, we cannot voluntarily stop breathing.

Abscess on the lung
Most common among alcoholics and people suffering from malnutrition; also caused by inhaling foreign bodies while unconscious; more rarely, a complication of PNEUMONIA. Symptoms are chills and FEVER, CHEST PAIN, and a COUGH, with sputum containing pus and sometimes blood. Correct response is ②. Routinely treated with antibiotics. Constitutional treatment, and a change of diet and lifestyle, are recommended after antibiotic treatment, but until antibiotics take effect, or if you are unable to take antibiotics, select a remedy from the list below.

Specific remedies to be taken every ½-hour for up to 10 doses
- Skin dry and hot, restlessness, anxiety *Aconite 30c*
- In early stages of abscess development, face flushed, throbbing headache, delirium, chest pains made worse by lying on affected side *Belladonna 30c*

In later stages, once pus has formed, take *Hepar sulph. 6c* every hour for up to 6 doses; if there is no improvement within 12 hours, see your homeopath.

Asthma see also ASTHMA p. 313–4
Partial, reversible obstruction of the major and minor

---

⑨⑨⑨ Emergency – call GP (or dial 999) immediately. ② Consult your doctor if no improvement within 2 hours

airways (bronchi and bronchioles) of the lungs due to inflammation of the airways and contraction of the muscles in their walls. Asthma which onsets in childhood is usually caused by allergic reactions to house dust, house dust mite, pollens, animal fur, feathers, cigarette smoke, and other inhaled irritants (see ALLERGY), but it can also be triggered off by drugs, withdrawal from caffeine, exercise, emotional upsets, and changes in the weather. Symptoms are periodic BREATHLESSNESS, a tight feeling in the chest, WHEEZING, increased pulse rate, ANXIETY, and sometimes coughing (see COUGH). In severe cases, growth may be stunted, or sufferer may develop EMPHYSEMA; occasionally an attack proves fatal. A family history of asthma, HAY FEVER AND ALLERGIC RHINITIS, or ECZEMA seems to be a predisposing factor; asthma is also more common in affluent families with only one or two children; 1 in 10 children of school age suffers from asthma, but only 3 per cent of adults. Asthma which onsets in middle life (see case history p. 17–18) represents a more fundamental breakdown in health, and is more difficult to treat.

Once severity of condition has been assessed, GP may prescribe bronchodilator drugs to be taken during attacks, or preventive drugs such as steroids to be taken on a daily basis; such drugs are usually inhaled. Always see your GP if asthma fails to respond to orthodox or homeopathic treatment, or if inhalers or other drugs have to be used more often than prescribed (overdosage may be dangerous).

If sufferer turns bluish, or very pale and clammy during an attack, or if breathing rate climbs above 40 breaths a minute, (999); he or she may need to be put on a respirator and given drugs to relax lung and chest muscles.

Homeopathic approach to chronic asthma is constitutional (drugs such as Intal and Ventolin are compatible with homeopathic remedies). If attacks are allergen-caused, homeopathy offers allergens in homeopathic potency, i.e. Cat's hair 6c hourly before and during exposure. The remedies listed below are for use in acute attacks; however, if symptoms do not wear off within 12 hours, see your GP. If symptoms worsen, (2).

Specific remedies to be taken every 15 minutes for up to 10 doses
- Attack comes on between midnight and 2 am, person very anxious, restless, and chilly, thirsty for sips of water, feels better sitting up *Arsenicum 6c*
- Small amounts of phlegm coughed up, persistent nausea and perhaps vomiting, chest feels as if there is a heavy weight on it *Ipecac. 6c*
- Asthma bad between 2–4 am, person gets up and sits with face on knees, looks pale and tired, feels chilly *Kali carb. 6c*
- Exhaustion, weakness, mucus in lungs cannot be coughed up and causes rattly breathing, skin pale, cold, and clammy *Antimonium tart. 6c*
- Muscle spasms in lungs and in rest of body, vomiting after each spasm *Cuprum 6c*
- Asthma particularly bad after digestive upset and around 4 am *Nux 6c*
- Asthma worse in damp conditions, often associated with early morning diarrhoea *Natrum sulph. 6c*
- Attack comes on suddenly, especially after exposure to cold dry wind, anxiety and fear of dying, particularly if attack occurs at night *Aconite 30c*
- Tight, constricted feeling in throat made worse by anything worn around neck, person sits hunched forward, asthma particularly bad in morning on waking *Lachesis 6c*
- Attack comes on after grief or break-up of love affair *Ignatia 6c*
- Asthma improves in damp conditions *Hepar sulph. 6c*

Self-help During an attack, sit with elbows resting on the back of a chair – this lifts upper part of ribcage and makes it easier to exhale. Check for allergies to pollen, food, beverages, and pollutants in your home or work environment. If asthma is bad at night and early in the morning, you may be allergic to house dust mites; since these live on shed skin, they thrive in mattresses and bedclothes. Remove sheets and blankets from bed, thoroughly vacuum mattress, put an airtight plastic cover on mattress, then cover this with two or three clean blankets, clean undersheet, clean sheets, etc. Keep bedroom as dust-free as possible – this may mean removing books, soft toys, and even carpets, putting a fine screen over open windows. Invest in a humidifier – dry air only increases breathing difficulties. If you are allergic to feathers, use polyester-filled pillows and duvets. If you are allergic to pet hairs, and cannot contemplate living without pets, periodically remove pets from the house for a day or two and thoroughly clean house from top to bottom, using a Hydromist cleaner to remove hairs from carpets, curtains, cushions, and furniture. If you have a partner who smokes, try to limit his or her smoking to one room in the house; at work, agitate for smoke-free zones.

Blood in sputum

Coughing up phlegm which is bright red, pink, or rusty-brown is a proper cause for alarm. It may be a symptom of PULMONARY OEDEMA or 'water on the lung' (breathlessness even at rest, pink frothy phlegm); appropriate action is (999) and *Ammonium carb. 6c* (or, if that is not available, *Arsenicum 6c*) every 5 minutes for up to 10 doses. Alternatively, blood-tinged sputum may be a symptom of PULMONARY EMBOLISM (breathlessness, chest pain, often after prolonged bed rest); again, appropriate action is (999), plus *Aconite 30c* every 5 minutes for up to 10 doses.

If bloody sputum is associated with FEVER of more than 39°C (102°F), person may be suffering from PNEUMONIA; appropriate action is ②. Phlegm may also be blood-stained because a blood vessel in the lungs has ruptured; rupture may be due to persistent coughing, TUBERCULOSIS, or CANCER OF THE LUNG; however caused, [12].

Breathlessness see also WHEEZING
Shortness of breath, feeling of tightness in chest, difficulty drawing air into lungs and pushing it out again; usually made worse by fatigue, exercise, and lying down. In severe cases oxygen lack builds up to such a degree that lips develop bluish tinge (cyanosis); appropriate action is ⑨⑨⑨ and artificial respiration (see First Aid p. 86–7).

Sudden breathlessness, with a 'tight band around chest' feeling, or pain extending into neck and arms, may be a HEART ATTACK (see First Aid p. 101); sudden breathlessness, with chest pain and coughing up blood, may be PULMONARY EMBOLISM, or PNEUMOTHORAX. If any of these conditions is suspected, ⑨⑨⑨ and give *Aconite 30c* every 5 minutes for up to 10 doses until help arrives. PULMONARY OEDEMA (breathlessness, especially at night, with pink, frothy sputum) also requires emergency treatment; again appropriate action is ⑨⑨⑨, but give *Ammonium carb. 6c* (or, if this is not available, *Arsenicum 6c*) every 5 minutes for up to 10 doses.

Other conditions requiring prompt medical attention are PNEUMONIA and acute BRONCHITIS (difficulty breathing, temperature of 38°C (100°F) or more, greenish or rust-coloured phlegm). If either of these conditions is suspected, ②.

Other conditions associated with shortness of breath are ANGINA (sudden breathlessness, chest pain comes on with exercise or excitement), HYPERVENTILATION (light-headed feeling, tingling or numbness in hands and feet, perhaps brought on by stress), PNEUMO-CONIOSIS, chronic BRONCHITIS, EMPHYSEMA, and FARMER'S LUNG (chronic breathlessness, thick grey or yellow sputum), and congestive HEART FAILURE (puffy legs or ankles, fatigue, blood-flecked sputum, bubbling sound in lungs).

For orthodox and homeopathic treatment, see conditions mentioned above.

Bronchiectasis
Widening of one or more bronchi due to a succession of respiratory infections in childhood (SINUSITIS, MEASLES, WHOOPING COUGH), TUBERCULOSIS, or prolonged blockage by a foreign body; fluid secreted by cells lining bronchi accumulates and stagnates, increasing risk of infection and further damage to airways. Symptoms are coughing, with copious green or yellow phlegm, especially when lying down, and HALITOSIS. Orthodox treatment is to give antibiotics at earliest sign of infection. Homeopathic treatment is

constitutional, but in emergencies select a remedy from those listed under BRONCHITIS; if symptoms worsen, see your GP.

Self-help Try not to expose yourself to colds and sore throats, or to rooms full of cigarette smoke. If bronchi at base of lungs are affected, ask your GP to teach you how to drain the phlegm yourself; this is called postural drainage, and involves lying with your head over a bowl over the edge of the bed, and allowing the mucus to drain out under gravity. Supplements of the amino acids cysteine and cystine would also be of benefit.

Bronchitis see also BRONCHIOLITIS
Inflammation of mucous membranes lining airways in lungs (bronchi and bronchioles); may be acute or chronic.

Acute bronchitis is usually caused by same viruses which cause COLDS, LARYNGITIS, and INFLUENZA, and can be very serious in elderly people or people with HEART FAILURE. Symptoms include FEVER, a painful COUGH which brings up glutinous yellow sputum, difficult breathing, and WHEEZING; cold or damp air, and environmental irritants, tend to make symptoms worse. Symptoms wear off within about 10 days, but full recovery may take up to 4 weeks. If resistance is low, inflammation may become chronic (see below). Antibiotics are only given if there is secondary bacterial infection, otherwise orthodox treatment is limited to bronchodilator drugs or cough suppressants. If homeopathic remedies below do not relieve symptoms within the dose period, or if temperature rises above 39°C (102°F), or phlegm has blood in it, or breathing gets extremely difficult, ② and give *Ferrum phos. 6c* every 10 minutes for up to 10 doses.

Specific remedies to be taken every 2 hours for up to 2 days
- Dry, stabbing, painful cough, headache, chest pain relieved by supporting elbows on back of chair, great thirst *Bryonia 30c*
- Tight, dry, tickling cough, person pale, anxious, eager for reassurance, wants frequent drinks of iced water *Phosphorus 6c*
- Bronchitis comes on suddenly, dry, staccato cough, fever, symptoms aggravated by cold dry air, person chilly, restless, and anxious *Aconite 30c*
- Bronchitis in an infant or elderly person, accumulated phlegm causes rattling sound in chest, sufferer too weak to cough it up *Antimonium tart. 6c*
- Sudden onset, high temperature, pounding headache, flushed face, delirium, symptoms worse at night and when lying down *Belladonna 30c*
- Nausea, vomiting, suffocating feeling in chest *Ipecac. 6c*
- Stringy phlegm, difficulty coughing it up, person feels worse between 4 and 5 am *Kali bichrom. 6c*

---

⑨⑨⑨ Emergency – call GP (or dial 999) immediately. ② Consult your doctor if no improvement within 2 hours

- Gasping for air, skin cold and clammy, desire to be fanned, especially if sufferer is elderly *Carbo veg. 6c*
- Coughing causes involuntary passing of urine *Causticum 6c*
- Choking cough made worse by uncovering any part of body, person chilly and irritable *Hepar sulph. 6c*
- Symptoms get worse lying down or in stuffy rooms, cough is dry at night but loose in morning, lack of thirst *Pulsatilla 6c*

Chronic bronchitis, in which membranes lining airways are more or less permanently inflamed, chiefly affects people over 50, men three times as often as women; main causes are smoking and air pollution, although cold damp weather and OBESITY are aggravating factors. Over-secretion of mucus obstructs airways, mucous membranes thicken and cause airways to narrow, and muscles lining airways contract. Early symptom is coughing in morning, so-called 'smoker's cough'; gradually, amount of phlegm coughed up increases, coughing occurs throughout day, and BREATHLESSNESS and WHEEZING become more or less permanent; at this stage, even a minor cold can cause serious illness. Complications include PULMONARY HYPERTENSION, EMPHYSEMA, PNEUMONIA, and HEART FAILURE; CANCER OF THE LUNG is also a risk if bronchitis is caused by smoking. If person has been coughing up phlegm most days of the week for at least 3 months, and if this has happened for 2 years running, he or she almost certainly has chronic bronchitis and should see GP. If signs of RESPIRATORY FAILURE develop (severe shortness of breath, bluish lips) (999) and give First Aid (see p. 86–8).

Orthodox treatment is to prescribe bronchodilator drugs by inhaler or antibiotics. Homeopathic treatment is constitutional; during acute episodes the remedies given above for acute bronchitis should be tried.

Self-help Stop smoking, and avoid smoke-filled atmospheres. To raise phlegm, inhale steam (fill a bowl with boiling water, lean over the bowl with a towel over your head, and inhale). If attack is bad, stay in bed for 2 or 3 days, put a hot water bottle on your chest, and drink lots of hot drinks. If bronchitis is chronic, avoid cold, damp, dusty, or polluted air – this may mean moving house or changing your job – and keep away from people who have colds and sore throats; regular supplements of Vitamins B, C, and A, and zinc, are also advisable. You should also avoid refined carbohydrates.

Cancer of the lung see also CANCER
Most common cancer in West, causing 1 in every 18 deaths in United Kingdom; link with smoking is now irrefutable – light smokers are 10 times as likely to get lung cancer as non-smokers, and heavy smokers 25 times as likely; within 5 years of stopping smoking, provided cancer has not already developed, risks are about even, unless you are exposed to passive smoking (inhaling other people's smoke). Roughly 50 per cent of people who have chronic BRONCHITIS develop lung cancer. Symptoms are a COUGH, phlegm which may be blood-stained, difficult breathing, and perhaps CHEST PAIN; part of lung affected is usually bronchus. If you have had a cough lasting for more than 1 month, or there is blood in the sputum, see your GP.

Lung cancer develops relatively slowly, and in 12 per cent of cases is not diagnosed until secondary cancers have developed. Surgical removal of affected part of lung is feasible in about one third of cases; other cases are treated by radiotherapy or chemotherapy.

For homeopathic treatment, see CANCER.

Self-help Stop smoking now – cutting off the supply of tobacco tars which caused cancerous changes in the first place may slow down or even halt growth of cancer. See p. 273–4 for other self-care measures.

Chest pain
Can signify a range of ailments, from the minor to the life-threatening. Among the least serious are INDIGESTION (pain under breast bone after eating), PULLED MUSCLES (pain on one side of chest following injury, prolonged or severe coughing, or straining, with site of pain tender to the touch), HIATUS HERNIA (burning pain under breast bone, made worse by bending or lying down), and SHINGLES (one-sided, burning chest pain unrelated to breathing movements, followed a few days later by a blistering rash).

Other ailments which cause chest pain are PLEURISY (severe one-sided pain made worse by coughing or deep breathing, with fever and difficult breathing) and ANGINA (chest pain radiating to left arm, wearing off within 5 minutes or when exercise or excitement ceases). If either of these conditions is suspected, [12].

Chest pain can also be a symptom of PERICARDITIS (pain radiates to left shoulder blade and is made worse by moving or inhaling deeply, coughing, difficult breathing) and PNEUMONIA (breathlessness, coughing, fever). Both conditions require prompt medical attention, so (2).

Into the emergency category come HEART ATTACK (sudden constricting pain in chest, and possibly neck and arms, which does not wear off, breathlessness, collapse), PULMONARY EMBOLISM (sudden chest pain, breathlessness, perhaps coughing up blood, especially after prolonged bed rest), and PNEUMOTHORAX (sudden chest pain and breathlessness); in all cases, appropriate action is (999) and *Aconite 30c* every 5 minutes, or more often if pain is severe, for up to 10 doses.

Cough see also COUGH p. 318
Caused by irritation of mucous membranes lining trachea and airways of lungs. Coughing consists of three phases: expanding lungs to breath in, contracting

lungs to breathe out while the glottis at top of windpipe is closed, then suddenly opening the glottis and allowing air to rush out of the lungs at nearly 1000 km (600 miles) an hour! Most often associated with COLDS (in which catarrh dripping down back of nose irritates vocal cords) and a SORE THROAT (infected lining of throat), but can also be a symptom of HEART FAILURE and oesophageal reflux (see HIATUS HERNIA). Sudden bouts of coughing can also be caused by inhaling dust, fumes, or foreign bodies; if coughing does not wear off within 24–48 hours, call your GP.

A cough accompanied by a high temperature may be INFLUENZA (aches and chills, runny nose) or acute BRONCHITIS (thick yellow phlegm coughed up, wheezing); in chronic bronchitis, coughing is most marked in morning, with copious yellow sputumn, and persists for months at a time. A dry cough which has persisted for more than a month, with occasional production of blood-flecked sputum, may be a sign of TUBERCULOSIS or CANCER OF THE LUNG. Coughing, a high temperature, and difficult breathing may signify PNEUMONIA; appropriate action is ②.

If any of conditions above is suspected, see appropriate entry for description and treatment. Be very wary of cough suppressants, as overuse in young children can inhibit respiratory signals from brain, resulting in RESPIRATORY FAILURE. For specific homeopathic remedies and self-care measures, see COUGH p. 318.

Emphysema
Enlargement and rupture of air sacs (alveoli) in lungs, reducing surface area through which oxygen can be absorbed and carbon dioxide got rid of; air sacs stretch and burst if breathing out requires effort or force, as it does in ASTHMA and chronic BRONCHITIS, in heavy smokers, elderly people, and people who blow glass or play the trumpet for a living. Symptoms are increasing BREATHLESSNESS and barrel-like expansion of chest, and increased susceptibility to chest infections; complications include PNEUMOTHORAX, HEART FAILURE, and RESPIRATORY FAILURE. Condition cannot be cured, but may be slowed down by bronchodilator drugs or antibiotics, or by constitutional homeopathic treatment. When breathlessness is particularly bad, specific remedies listed under BRONCHITIS, COUGH, or ASTHMA would be appropriate.

Self-help Stop smoking, and stay away from people with coughs and colds. Take plenty of exercise in fresh air – cyling is good – and increase intake of Vitamin E.

Empyema see also PLEURISY
Accumulation of fluid in space between inner and outer membrane (pleura) around lung; usually a complication of PLEURISY, PNEUMONIA, or an abdominal infection which spreads to chest, but may also be a consequence of RHEUMATOID ARTHRITIS, HEART FAILURE, liver and kidney trouble, or CANCER of the lung, breast, or ovary.

Orthodox treatment is to give antibiotics and drain off fluid. Constitutional homeopathic treatment is recommended afterwards, but while antibiotics are being taken, author recommends *Hepar sulph. 6c*, 4 times daily for up to 3 days.

Farmer's lung
Inflammation of airways and thickening of walls of alveoli due to allergic reaction to various kinds of fungus found in mouldy grain or hay, malted cereals, mushrooms, bird droppings, laboratory animals, etc. Symptoms come on soon after exposure to fungus, and last for several hours; BREATHLESSNESS and a dry COUGH are main symptoms, sometimes accompanied by chills, HEADACHE, and FEVER, which may be mistaken for INFLUENZA. Untreated, condition may lead to HEART FAILURE or RESPIRATORY FAILURE; if detected early enough, and exposure to allergens ceases, chances of full recovery are good. See your GP if you have a persistent cough and an occupation which brings you into contact with any of the fungus sources mentioned above; steroids may be necessary. Homeopathic treatment is constitutional; for specific remedies, see COUGH p. 318.

Self-help If you cannot avoid exposure to substances which cause farmer's lung, wear a protective mask over nose and mouth.

Hiccups
Sudden contraction of diaphragm, causing sudden rush of air into lungs, which in turn causes vocal cords to snap shut with a 'hic'; probably caused by purely mechanical irritation of the diaphragm, by laughing, being tickled, or too much air in stomach, which lies directly beneath it.

Specific remedies to be taken every 15 minutes for up to 6 doses (dose may be easier to take if you crush pilule between two clean spoons, dissolve it in a little warm water, and sip)
- Hiccups accompanied by belching and retching, especially if they come on an hour or two after eating a very large or very rich meal *Nux 6c*
- Hiccups come on after eating or drinking, after smoking, or after an emotional upset *Ignatia 6c*
- Violent, noisy hiccups, with belching *Cicuta 6c*
- Obstinate hiccups, chest feels sore, retching *Magnesium phos. 6c*
- Hiccups better for drinking a little water, person has a respiratory problem *Cyclamen 6c*
- Hiccups in an infant who is feeding poorly *Aethusa 6c*
- Hiccups made worse by cold drinks, fever, feeling chilly *Arsenicum 6c*

---

⑨⑨⑨ Emergency – call GP (or dial 999) immediately. ② Consult your doctor if no improvement within 2 hours

Self-help Holding your breath, breathing rapidly, breathing into a paper bag, drinking cold water and then holding your breath, pulling your tongue forward, having someone give you a shock – all of these are effective hiccups stoppers. So is squirting lemon juice down the back of the throat. A drink of water with a little glucose in it usually stops hiccups in an infant.

Hyperventilation

Caused by rapid and irregular breathing which fails to push air deep into the lungs where gaseous exchange takes place. The stomach muscles as well as the diaphragm should be used. Excessive loss of carbon dioxide causes body fluids to become alkaline, increasing excitability of nerves, causing tingling sensations in arms and legs and sometimes tetany (muscles go into spasm, beginning with those of forearm and face). Some experts believe that this is the mechanism responsible for PALPITATIONS, ANGINA-type chest pains, DIZZINESS, ALLERGY, phobic symptoms (see PHOBIA), and ANXIETY attacks. Chronic shallow breathing is associated with a combination of fatigue and over-arousal (lack of sleep plus stress, for example); it may also stem from organic problems in the brain (after a STROKE, for example) or in the lungs themselves. Chronic hyperventilation is diagnosed by a 3-minute provocation test. Acute attacks are a reaction to emotional or physical trauma (childbirth, being in an accident, receiving bad news, etc.).

In an acute attack, breathe into a paper bag (this helps to re-establish acid-alkaline balance of blood) and take *Aconite 30c* every 5 minutes for up to 6 doses.

Chronic hyperventilation requires constitutional homeopathic treatment, attention to sleep patterns, and measures to improve breathing and reduce stress.

Interstitial fibrosis

A rare condition in which fibrous tissue progressively obstructs smaller airways of lungs and thickens walls of alveoli, reducing efficiency of gaseous exchange; cause is not known. If chronic, symptoms are slowly increasing BREATHLESSNESS, spatulate fingers with curving finger nails, and eventually RESPIRATORY FAILURE. If acute, shortness of breath is severe, even when resting, and there may also be a COUGH, with blood-flecked sputum, and CHEST PAIN; in such cases, death from respiratory failure usually occurs within a year of onset. Steroids are used to slow down progress of disease. Homeopathic treatment is constitutional.

Pleurisy

Inflammation of membranes (pleurae) surrounding lungs, caused by infections such as PNEUMONIA and TUBERCULOSIS, by injury, or by seepage of air into space between pleurae (see PNEUMOTHORAX). Inflammation causes severe CHEST PAIN, usually one-sided, and makes breathing painful; if fluid accumulates in space between pleurae (pleural effusion) pain abates because membranes are no longer rubbing together, but person may become breathless due to pressure of fluid on lung; if fluid-filled pleurae become infected, result is EMPYEMA. In addition to treating underlying condition, possibly with antibiotics, GP may prescribe painkillers. Specific homeopathic remedies should be chosen either from those listed under causes mentioned above, or from those given below.

Specific remedies to be given every hour for up to 10 doses during acute attack; if no improvement within 12 hours, see your GP
- Pleural pain aggravated by movement but soothed by lying on affected side, person thirsty and irritable *Bryonia 30c*
- Fluid pressing on affected lung, sharp cutting pains made worse by slightest movement *Sulphur 6c*
- Dry, staccato cough, sneezing, stitching pain in chest, wanting to take deep breaths *Squilla 6c*
- Sharp pain comes on suddenly after exposure to cold dry wind, breathlessness, anxiety, fear of dying *Aconite 30c*
- Fluid on lung causes breathlessness and burning pains, mild fever, heartbeat rapid and irregular, frequent dry cough *Cantharis 30c*
- Pain comes on very suddenly, face flushed and hot, great thirst, delirium *Belladonna 30c*
- If recovery from pleurisy is slow, and complicated by fluid on lung *Hepar sulph. 6c*

Pneumoconiosis

Literally 'dust in the lungs', causing breathlessness and coughing. Condition is most common among coal miners, though it may take up to 25 years to develop; inhaled particles of coal settle in lung tissue, causing patches of irritation which scar as they heal; if irritation and scarring become extensive, efficiency of lungs is drastically reduced.

Silicosis a related dust disease which affects quarry workers, metal grinders, etc., may take only 10 years to develop, and *Asbestosis* only 5 years. Silicosis brings with it increased risk of TUBERCULOSIS, and asbestosis a high risk of CANCER OF THE LUNG. Coal, silica, aluminium, iron, beryllium, talc, asbestos, and synthetic fibres can all cause lung damage if inhaled daily for long periods. Since damage is irreversible, purpose of both orthodox and homeopathic treatment is to prevent complications. If you suffer from any dust-related disease, put yourself under the care of an experienced homeopath.

Self-help Stop smoking, and avoid further exposure to dust – this may entail changing your job. If you remain exposed to dust hazards, wear a protective face mask, and make sure you have an annual chest X-ray; even if you change your job, continue to have annual check-ups.

For explanation of other symbols, see page 107

Pneumonia

Inflammation of the lungs, usually caused by same viruses which cause COLDS and INFLUENZA, or by *Pneumococcus* bacteria; other causes may be inhaled liquids or poisonous gases such as chlorine. May be mild if state of health is good, or life-threatening if person is very young or very old, immobilized or inactive, an alcoholic, or already suffering from some form of respiratory, heart, or kidney disease; people taking immuno-suppressive or anti-inflammatory drugs on a long-term basis are also likely to be very ill. If only one lobe of lung is involved, condition is known as *lobar pneumonia;* in *bronchopneumonia*, there is patchy inflammation of one or both lungs; *double pneumonia* simply means that both lungs are affected. Complications can include PLEURISY, EMPYEMA, and ABSCESS ON THE LUNG.

Symptoms usually onset within hours, but vary with virulence of microbe responsible; person may suffer from BREATHLESSNESS, even when resting, develop a FEVER and a COUGH, and feel sweaty and chilly by turns; if there is also blood in sputum or CHEST PAIN, or if lips become bluish, ②.

Most serious form of pneumonia is *viral pneumonia,* caused by influenza virus, against which antibiotics are ineffectual, although they may prevent secondary infection; *bacterial (especially staphylococcal) pneumonia* is treatable with antibiotics.

The homeopathic remedies listed below should only be used in mild cases of viral pneumonia or if, for some reason, antibiotics are contra-indicated; if there is no response within 24 hours, see your GP. Constitutional homeopathic treatment is recommended during and after recovery to boost resistance to infection.

Specific remedies to be given every 2 hours for up to 10 doses
- Sudden onset, especially if weather is cold and dry, chest pains, fever, anxiety, fear of dying *Aconite 30c*
- Cough, rust-coloured sputum, person feels weak, trembly, and nervous, numb extremities, symptoms get worse lying on left side *Phosphorus 6c*
- Sharp chest pains made worse by slightest movement but alleviated by lying on affected side *Bryonia 30c*
- Right lung affected, deep breathing causes pain which extends into right shoulder blade, exhausting, staccato cough, breathlessness, person already has a liver complaint *Chelidonium 6c*
- Pneumonia which follows on from flu, right lung affected, phlegm rust-coloured but difficult to bring up, tickly cough that seems to come from centre of chest, shortness of breath, symptoms relieved by lying on back although person has compulsion to sit up *Sanguinaria 6c*

Self-help Take extra Vitamin C and rest in bed, sitting up if possible. Dry air exacerbates pneumonia, so humidify room (see p. 30).

Pneumothorax

Trapping of air between inner and outer layer of pleural membrane around lung, exerting pressure on lung and hindering expansion; part or whole of lung may 'collapse', leading eventually to RESPIRATORY FAILURE; air gets into pleural space either from lung itself or through an injury to chest wall. For reasons which are not clear, condition is most common in otherwise healthy young men; people over 50, with lungs already damaged by ASTHMA, BRONCHITIS, etc., are also affected. Depending on severity, there may be BREATHLESSNESS, a tight feeling across the chest, or sharp pain just below collar bone on affected side. Orthodox treatment is to drain air out through a one-way catheter, and if necessary seal hole through which air is seeping into pleural space. With rest, a small pocket of air may disperse of its own accord. Removal of the pleura may be needed in recurrent cases.

Specific remedies to be taken every 5 minutes for up to 10 doses as soon as pain comes on
- Where person is afraid of dying *Aconite 30c*
- In all other cases *Bryonia 30c*

Pulmonary embolism see also EMBOLISM

Caused by a blood clot which has detached itself from the wall of a vein, travelled through the heart and into the lungs, and become stuck in an artery in the lungs, blocking flow of blood to alveoli where oxygenation takes place; result is decreased oxygen in blood returning to heart, with a very real risk of HEART FAILURE; condition is often a sequel to an operation, illness, or accident which involves prolonged bed rest or a complication of DEEP VEIN THROMBOSIS or CANCER. Symptoms are BREATHLESSNESS and feeling faint, and if blockage is severe also CHEST PAIN, COUGH (sputum may have blood in it), and blueness around lips. If these last symptoms are present, ⑨⑨⑨ and give First Aid (see p. 101). Cardiac massage, oxygen, and surgical removal of clot may be necessary; in less severe cases drugs are given to disperse blood clot or prevent clot formation. See DEEP VIEN THROMBOSIS for appropriate homeopathic remedies.

Self-help Take extra vitamin E (check with your GP first if you have high blood pressure or are taking anticoagulants). If you have to rest in bed for any length of time, get up every 2 hours and exercise feet and legs to keep circulation moving.

Pulmonary hypertension

Raised blood pressure in lungs, causing difficult breathing and OEDEMA in lower part of body, especially around ankles; skin may also develop a bluish tinge; as right side of heart works harder and harder to force blood through lungs, HEART FAILURE may develop. Of all the ailments which reduce blood flow through the lungs and so encourage blood pressure to rise, VALVULAR DISEASE

---

⑨⑨⑨ Emergency – call GP (or dial 999) immediately. ② Consult your doctor if no improvement within 2 hours

chronic BRONCHITIS and EMPHYSEMA are the most common; high altitudes produce a similar effect.

If above symptoms are present in addition to those of bronchitis or emphysema, 12. If lips turn blue and breathing becomes extremely difficult, ②. Conventional treatment is to give oxygen and diuretics; underlying condition may need to be treated with bronchodilator drugs or antibiotics.

Provided symptoms are not acute, homeopathic remedies listed under BREATHLESSNESS, PULMONARY OEDEMA, or chronic BRONCHITIS may be appropriate; if none seems entirely suitable, give *Arsenicum 6c* every 6 hours for up to 5 days.

Pulmonary oedema
Accumulation of fluid in lungs due to left-sided HEART FAILURE; because left ventricle of heart is inefficient, pressure of blood in pulmonary veins (which return oxygenated blood to heart) rises, forcing fluid out of tiny blood vessels and into air sacs in lungs, making oxygen and carbon dioxide exchange impossible. Typically, symptoms onset within a few hours, often in middle of night; person becomes increasingly breathless and hungry for air, to the point of flinging windows open or rushing out of doors; a dry, tickly COUGH may develop, which produces pink, frothy sputum; lips may also turn blue. Appropriate action is ⑨⑨⑨ and *Ammonium carb. 6c* every 5 minutes until help arrives (or, if this is not available, *Arsenicum 6c* in same dosage). Orthodox treatment for oedema is to give oxygen and drugs (morphine, diuretics, bronchodilators) to make breathing easier, or drugs to strengthen pumping action of heart.

If the above symptoms are accompanied by CHEST PAIN person may have suffered a HEART ATTACK. Again, ⑨⑨⑨, and give First Aid (see p. 101).

Self-help Persuade person to stay calm, and to sit up rather than lie down. Offer as much reassurance as you can.

Respiratory failure
Progressive or sudden loss of lung function due to destructive lung diseases such as EPHYSEMA and BRONCHIECTASIS, excessive pressure on the lungs (as in PULMONARY OEDEMA or PNEUMOTHORAX), interruption of blood supply (as in PULMONARY EMBOLISM), or disturbed nerve supply (as in drug overdose). Main symptom is increasingly severe BREATHLESSNESS. For orthodox and homeopathic treatment see conditions mentioned above; in emergencies, see First Aid pp. 86–8.

Sarcoidosis
Fleshy patches of inflammation in lungs (and occasionally other organs), not caused by infection or malignancy, and almost always diagnosed as result of routine check up; may be symptomless, or cause only mild shortness of breath; usually clears up of own accord within 2–3 years. Occasionally, healed patches become infected, causing BRONCHIECTASIS. Routinely treated with steroids. Homeopathic treatment is constitutional.

Tracheitis
Inflammation of windpipe (trachea), causing sore, burning sensation as air is taken into lungs; usually caused by viruses responsible for COLDS, INFLUENZA, and LARYNGITIS. Conventionally treated with antibiotics to prevent secondary infection.

Specific remedies to be taken every hour, then every 4 hours as symptoms subside, for up to 3 days
- Raw, scraped feeling in windpipe, tickly cough, cold air and slightest pressure on windpipe make rawness worse *Rumex 6c*
- Windpipe feels raw, frequent hacking cough, gulping ice-cold drinks to quench thirst *Phosphorus 6c*
- Soreness made worse by talking, exercise, warm rooms, and cigarette smoke, painful cough *Bryonia 30c*
- Sensation of swelling not relieved by swallowing, pain seems to invade root of tongue, symptoms worse after sleeping, person cannot stand throat being touched or wrapped up *Lachesis 6c*
- Tenacious, sticky phlegm which is difficult to bring up *Kali bichrom. 6c*
- Trachea feels as if there is a raw, sore streak down it, mucus too far down to be coughed up *Causticum 6c*
- Sweetish, yellow phlegm, sore sensation at base of trachea after coughing *Stannum 6c*

Self-help Take extra Vitamin C and humidify air if home is centrally heated.

Tuberculosis see TUBERCULOSIS p. 281

Water on the lung see PULMONARY OEDEMA

Wheezing see also BREATHLESSNESS
Laboured, noisy breathing, especially when breathing out. Chronic wheezing may be due to ASTHMA, or to chronic BRONCHITIS or EMPHYSEMA (grey or greenish phlegm coughed up frequently). If onset is fairly sudden, cause may be acute BRONCHITIS (fever, painful coughing, yellowish sputum) or PULMONARY OEDEMA (air hunger, cough which may produce pink, frothy phlegm); wheezing which onsets very suddenly may be a severe ASTHMA attack. If person is fighting to breathe, or becomes very pale and clammy, or resting respiration rate climbs above 40 breaths per minute, or lips turn blue, ⑨⑨⑨; if cause is asthma, give *Aconite 30c* every 5 minutes until help arrives; if pulmonary oedema is suspected, give *Ammonium carb. 6c* every 5 minutes until help arrives (or, if this is not available, *Arsenicum 6c* in same dosage).

For explanation of other symbols, see page 107

HEART, BLOOD, AND CIRCULATION

THE heart is really two pumps, each composed of an upper and lower chamber and two valves, one between the upper and lower chamber and one at the exit from the lower chamber. The right side of the heart is the less muscular of the two pumps; it receives oxygen-depleted blood from the venous system and sends it to the lungs for oxygenation. The other half, the left side, receives oxygen-rich blood from the lungs and sends it shooting up through the aorta and around the whole body.

Branching off the aorta are arteries and arterioles; their walls are muscular and elastic, designed to transmit the pumping force of the heart to the farthest reaches of the body. Blood is collected from every part of the body by venules and veins, which are thin-walled and have valves in them so that blood can flow one way only – back to the heart. The pumping action of muscles helps to push blood though them.

Connecting the smallest tributaries of the arterial and venous system are the capillaries, blood vessels so small that in major organs and muscles there are thousands of them per square millimetre. Oxygen-carrying red blood cells are pushed through them by the pulsing pressure of the heart. Blood pressure depends on three things: the tone of the artery walls, the pumping force of the heart, and the volume of blood in circulation. Generally speaking, blood pressure creeps up with age. This is because the kidneys become slightly less efficient at regulating the water content of the blood, and because arteries tend to become less elastic, forcing the heart to work harder.

The arch enemy of arteries is atheroma, a fatty deposit which roughens their smooth linings, reduces their elasticity, and slowly narrows their diameter. Choked or furred up arteries spell strokes, heart attacks, thrombosis, embolisms, and aneurysms.

Blood is the body's universal transport system. It carries everything the body needs – oxygen, sugars, fats, proteins, hormones, minerals, clotting factors, antibodies – as well as everything it does not need – carbon dioxide, other dissolved gases, urea, hostile micro-organisms and their toxins, general debris. A grown man has about 5 litres of blood in him, about 8 per cent of his body weight. Plasma, a straw-coloured fluid which is mostly water, accounts for 55 per cent of blood volume; red and white blood cells and platelets make up the rest. Red cells and platelets – the red cells carry oxygen bound to an iron-containing pigment called haemoglobin, and the platelets prevent blood loss by initiating the clotting process – far outnumber white blood cells, though during infections the latter multiply enormously. White blood cells are part of the immune system, protecting the body against disease organisms. At the end of their useful life, which is

seldom longer than three months even in the healthiest of us, red and white blood cells are destroyed and recycled by the liver and spleen. Destruction must of course keep pace with creation; in a healthy individual the bone marrow produces as many red blood cells as the spleen and liver destroy.

The lymph glands, the glands which swell up during infection because they are busy producing a variety of white blood cells, are part of a secondary transport network, the lymphatic system. The spleen, tonsils, bone marrow, and thymus are also part of the lymphatic system, whose vessels ramify to every part of the body. Lymph vessels have much thinner walls than veins, but like veins they have one-way valves in them and depend on the pumping action of muscles for their circulation. They transport lymphocytes to sites of injury and infection, collect emulsified fats from the small intestine, and drain fluid from the spaces between cells – this fluid contains proteins and other valuable substances which cannot be actively absorbed by the blood vessels. The contents of the lymphatic network eventually empty into the blood-stream through two ducts, one on either side of the neck at the junction of the subclavian and internal jugular veins.

Acrocyanosis see also RAYNAUD'S DISEASE

Bluish fingers and toes due to contraction of local arteries (blueness caused by reduced blood flow and build-up of toxins); reason for condition is not known, but it is painless, affects women more than men, and tends to be worse in cold weather; person may also feel cold and sweaty.

See RAYNAUD'S DISEASE for appropriate homeopathic remedies.

Agranulocytosis

Slow-down or stoppage of production of germ-destroying white blood cells (neutrophils) in bone marrow, lowering resistance to infection – most serious potential risk is PNEUMONIA; MOUTH ULCERS are often first sign, followed by depressingly frequent COLDS and other minor infections. Usually a drug side effect; in most cases, bone marrow regains neutrophil-producing capacity once drug is stopped. Orthodox treatment is to change drug responsible, and give antibiotics and perhaps drugs to stimulate bone marrow function. Homeopathic treatment is constitutional.

Anaemia

Occurs for various reasons, but essentially means that blood does not carry enough oxygen; classic symptoms are pallor, tiredness, BREATHLESSNESS, and PALPITATIONS.

Iron-deficiency anaemia is most prevalent form of anaemia, affecting mainly women; cause is lack of iron, essential for formation of oxygen-carrying pigment haemoglobin. Iron may be lacking in diet, or not absorbed properly (as in COELIAC DISEASE); or iron stores may be depleted by pregnancy or blood loss (perhaps because of injury, but also because of periods or internal bleeding from PEPTIC ULCERS, PILES, or CANCER of gastrointestinal tract); or, in conditions such as RHEUMATOID ARTHRITIS or chronic KIDNEY FAILURE, body may be unable to use its iron reserves. In addition to causing pallor and fatigue, iron deficiency lowers resistance to infection, especially to thrush (see ORAL THRUSH, VAGINAL AND VULVAL PROBLEMS, PENIS PROBLEMS). If you suspect you are anaemic, see your GP; it is important that underlying cause is diagnosed. Iron tablets or injections may solve the problem, but if iron depletion is very severe blood transfusions may be necessary.

Provided steps are being taken to remedy iron deficiency, the specific remedies below are recommended.

Specific remedies to be taken every 12 hours for up to 2 weeks
- Anaemia due to blood loss, oversensitivity, chilliness, exhaustion *China 30c*
- Face pale but flushes easily, generally robust appearance, oversensitivity *Ferrum 30c*
- Constipation, dull or muddy complexion, headache, dry mouth and lips, tendency to cold sores *Natrum mur. 30c*
- Anaemia during growth spurt (during first two years of life or during adolescence), irritability, poor digestion *Calcarea phos. 30c*
- Anaemia coupled with mental overload *Picric ac. 30*

Self-help Make sure your diet contains plenty of iron-rich foods and Vitamin C. This is especially important if you are a vegetarian since wholegrains and pulses bind iron, limiting absorption. Avoid drinking tea at mealtimes – the tannin in it makes iron absorption less efficient. Calc. Phos. and Ferrum Phos. (see Tissue Salts p. 388) are also recommended.

Vitamin B_{12} deficiency anaemia Like iron, B_{12} is essential for formation of haemoglobin, but because such small amounts are needed anaemia may take 2–3 years to develop. Diet may be deficient (vegans are particularly at risk), or small intestine may be unable to absorb vitamin (as happens in CROHN'S DISEASE and COELIAC DISEASE), or stomach may not secrete enough of special factor which enables vitamin to be absorbed – this last condition is known as *pernicious anaemia*. Symptoms of anaemia caused by B_{12} deficiency are fatigue, pallor, BREATHLESSNESS, yellowish skin, ABDOMINAL PAIN, WEIGHT LOSS, loss of appetite (see APPETITE CHANGES), and sometimes neurological impairment – poor balance, tingling extremities, CONFUSION, DEPRESSION. If poor absorption is the problem, regular injections of B_{12} will be necessary; otherwise treatment is dietary. Provided deficiency is being made up, the remedy below may be used; if there is no improvement within a month or so, see your homeopath.

Specific remedy to be taken every 12 hours for up to 2 weeks
- *Arsenicum 30c*

Self-help A varied diet, even a mainly vegetarian diet, provides adequate amounts of B_{12}, but a vegan diet does not. Healthfood shops stock many products containing B_{12} specially for vegans; yeast extract is also a good source.

Folate deficiency anaemia affects pregnant women and elderly people more than other groups, and can onset within a few weeks; again, folate is one of those nutrients vital to haemoglobin formation. Either diet is to blame (not enough green vegetables) or there is an absorption problem, as in COELIAC DISEASE. Symptoms are those of anaemia generally. Orthodox treatment is to give high doses of folate. WARNING: do not continue taking folate supplements for longer than your GP advises – they may mask a B_{12} deficiency which could lead to neurological damage.

In *sickle cell anaemia* red blood cells are misshapen because the haemoglobin in them has an abnormal structure; condition is inherited, and mainly occurs in people of African or West Indian descent. Under certain conditions – during infections, surgery, or flying, for example – sickled red blood cells tend to get stuck in small blood vessels, causing oxygen shortage in surrounding tissues; results may be life-threatening – STROKE, HEART FAILURE, KIDNEY FAILURE – depending on location of blocked blood vessels. Characteristic symptom during such crises is pain in limb bones, joints, or abdomen; at other times, all the usual symptoms of anaemia are present. Painkillers and antibiotics may be prescribed during crises, but there is no cure. Homeopathic treatment is constitutional, aimed at maximizing strengths and minimizing weaknesses so that condition puts as little strain on body as possible.

Self-help Vitamin E is recommended, but check with your GP first if you have high blood pressure or are taking anticoagulants.

Thalassaemia is also a hereditary form of anaemia, mainly affecting people of Mediterranean, Middle Eastern, or Far Eastern origin; fewer red blood cells are produced than is normal, and these contain immature haemoglobin (haemoglobin F) which is

For explanation of other symbols, see page 107

destroyed more quickly than normal haemoglobin. Symptoms are those of anaemia generally; a thalassaemic child tends not to be able to keep up with age mates. In severe cases (where defective gene is inherited from both parents), survival is not possible without regular blood transfusions and drugs to counteract resultant build-up of iron. Homeopathic treatment is constitutional, its aim being to minimize weaknesses and maximise strengths so that the condition stresses the body as little as possible.

Self-help Vitamin E is recommended, but check with your GP first if you have high blood pressure or are taking anticoagulants.

In *haemolytic anaemia* red blood cells are destroyed more quickly than they are replaced; this happens if they have been damaged by drugs, have not been manufactured properly, contain abnormal haemoglobin (as in sickle cell anaemia and thalassaemia), or are mistaken for foreign cells and destroyed by antibodies (see RHESUS INCOMPATIBILITY, AUTOIMMUNE DISEASE). In addition to the usual symptoms of anaemia, there may be mild FEVER and vomiting, JAUNDICE, and darker than normal urine. Conventionally treated by withdrawing causative drugs, or removing spleen (responsible for destroying red blood cells), or giving steroids if autoimmune system is at fault. Homeopathy offers constitutional treatment.

In *aplastic anaemia* (also called aplasia) production of blood cells (red and white) and blood platelets in bone marrow falls dramatically; certain drugs, toxic chemicals, and radiation may be the cause, or condition may develop for no obvious reason. Result is anaemia, low resistance to infection, and spontaneous bruising or bleeding; in severe cases, infection or bleeding may be fatal within a year of onset. Orthodox treatment consists of blood transfusions, antibiotics, and drugs to stimulate bone marrow; if these do not keep condition at bay or even reverse it, a bone marrow graft may be necessary. Constitutional homeopathic treatment is recommended in addition to orthodox treatment.

Aneurysm

Sac-like or cigar-shaped swelling in an artery wall due to congenital weakness of middle muscle layer, inflammation (POLYARTERITIS NODOSA and BACTERIAL ENDOCARDITIS inflame arteries), or build-up of fatty plaque inside artery (see ATHEROSCLEROSIS, HIGH BLOOD PRESSURE). Any of these conditions can cause artery to burst, resulting in loss of blood pressure and loss of blood supply to certain tissues; a burst aneurysm is potentially lethal if it happens in aorta (carrying oxygenated blood from heart) or in arteries at base of brain (aneurysms here are usually congenital 'berry' aneurysms, symptomless until they burst). Alternatively swelling may press on surrounding organs, nerves, or other blood vessels; if this occurs in upper part of aorta there may be CHEST PAIN, a persistent COUGH, and DIFFICULTY SWALLOWING. An aortic aneurysm can also stretch and damage aortic valve in heart. Another risk is that a blood clot (thrombus) may form in aneurysm; if part of it breaks away, smaller arteries may get blocked (see EMBOLISM). Sometimes blood forces its way between layers of artery wall, causing pain; this is known as a 'dissected' aneurysm.

Aneurysms mainly occur in aorta close to heart, in abdominal portion of aorta, where they are present as throbbing lumps, or in arteries at base of brain; elsewhere they are rare and may be symptomless unless they press on neighbouring nerves.

A burst aneurysm should be suspected if there is sudden, severe HEADACHE at back of head, or sudden, severe CHEST PAIN and collapse; appropriate action is (999), and *Aconite 30c* every 5 minutes until help arrives.

If any other symptoms are present (throbbing lumps in abdomen, for example), [48].

Orthodox treatment is surgery, but this is not always feasible. If your GP diagnoses a developing aneurysm or if you are awaiting surgery, constitutional homeopathic treatment should be sought; in meantime, remedies below may help; if symptoms worsen, however, see your GP.

Specific remedies to be taken every 4 hours for up 14 days
- Raised blood pressure, palpitations made worse by lying on left side, person elderly and suffering from atherosclerosis, pallor due to constriction of small arteries *Baryta carb. 6c*
- Aneurysm of aorta, person unable to lie on left side, symptoms worse between 4 and 8 pm *Lycopodium 6c*
- Bone pain, worse at night and in warm rooms, better in open air *Kali iod. 6c*

Self-help See ANGINA.

Angina

Dull, constricting pain felt in centre of chest and radiating up into neck and jaw and usually down left arm; repeated attacks can precede a full-blown HEART ATTACK; typically occurs when extra demands are made on heart already damaged by CORONARY ARTERY DISEASE, HIGH BLOOD PRESSURE, ANAEMIA, etc. Other symptoms may be DIZZINESS, nausea, sweating, and difficult breathing. Unlike pain of heart attack, angina pain wears off once exercise or excitement cease.

However, to be on safe side, (999) and give First Aid as if for a heart attack (see p. 101) if pain lasts for more than 5 minutes or does not wear off when stress or exertion ceases. If angina attacks are becoming more severe or occurring with less and less provocation, (2).

Orthodox treatment depends on condition causing angina; GP may prescribe drugs to increase blood supply to heart muscle or beta blockers to reduce heart

---

(999) Emergency – call GP (or dial 999) immediately. (2) Consult your doctor if no improvement within 2 hours

rate; if a coronary artery is badly narrowed, bypass surgery may be necessary. Homeopathic treatment for recurrent angina is constitutional; however in mild or moderate attacks the remedies below may be used.

Specific remedies to be taken every 2 minutes for up to 10 doses as soon as attack comes on

- Chest constricted, as if it has an iron band around it, difficult breathing, breaking out in cold sweat, pain down left arm, person has low blood pressure *Cactus 6c*
- Difficult breathing, relieved by lying on right side with head raised, palpitations, person thirsty for drinks of hot water *Spigelia 6c*
- Chest feels as if it is in a vice, heart feels about to burst, palpitations, pain in right arm *Lilium 6c*
- Fluttering heart, sensation of blood rushing into heart, difficult breathing, feeling faint, throbbing sensation all over body, heat makes symptoms worse *Glonoinum 6c*
- Pulse irregular, heart feels as if it has a weight on it, person anxious, afraid he or she might die, stimulants make symptoms worse *Naja 6c*
- Violent chest pains, numbness in fingers, feeble but rapid pulse *Latrodectus 6c*

Self-help Best course is to lose weight, not by crash dieting but by adopting healthier eating habits. See ATHEROSCLEROSIS for dietary and other self-help measures. Take regular gentle exercise, though not out of doors if the air is very cold, and stop immediately if you feel pain coming on. STOP SMOKING and avoid HYPERVENTILATION.

Arrhythmias

Irregular heart rhythms which develop when special group of cells (sinus node) in right atrium of heart do not function properly; these cells distribute electrical signals to other electrical relay points in heart, causing four chambers of heart to contract in correct sequence. Malfunction of sinus node can occur if brain overrides heart's own pacemaking mechanism, or if heart is damaged, by CORONARY ARTERY DISEASE or RHEUMATIC FEVER for example. It can also occur in unfit people taking unaccustomed, strenuous exercise.

Ventricular fibrillation (uncoordinated twitching of muscle fibres in ventricles) can cause CARDIAC ARREST; if person suddenly and inexplicably loses consciousness, stops breathing, and has no pulse, (999) and commence cardiac resuscitation (see First Aid pp. 88–9).

Heart block (beating of ventricles uncoordinated with beating of atria) may be mild or severe (see STOKES ADAMS ATTACK); third-degree heart block causes sudden loss of consciousness, often with FITS. Appropriate action is (999) and cardiac resuscitation (see First Aid pp. 88–9).

Atrial fibrillation (atria of heart beat much faster than ventricles) may produce symptoms such as BREATHLESSNESS, DIZZINESS, PALPITATIONS, FAINTING, and CHEST PAIN similar to ANGINA, but it is not instantly life-threatening; it may lead, however, to HEART FAILURE or to atrial EMBOLISM, so appropriate action is (2).

Paroxysmal tachycardia (sudden doubling of heart rate, lasting minutes or even days) causes a pounding feeling in chest, BREATHLESSNESS, and sometimes CHEST PAIN and FAINTING; condition slightly increases risk of congestive HEART FAILURE, but is not usually serious; however, symptoms should be reported to your GP.

Ectopic heartbeats (heart occasionally misses a beat or gains an extra beat) may be alarming, but are usually nothing to worry about; caffeine, nicotine, or alcohol may be the culprits.

For some arrythmias, GP may prescribe antiarrythmic drugs; in other cases anticoagulant drugs or beta blockers may be appropriate; sometimes normal heart rhythm can be restored by electrical shock treatment; in complete heart block, implantation of an artificial pacemaker may be necessary. Where ANXIETY is a major factor, constitutional homeopathic treatment is recommended.

Specific remedies to be taken every 2 minutes for up to 10 doses when palpitations come on, provided there is no fainting or loss of consciousness; if no improvement within 30 minutes, call GP

- Difficult breathing, relieved by lying on right side with head well raised, shuddering of whole body, person cannot bear to be touched *Spigelia 6c*
- Anginal pain and violent palpitations, made worse by lying on left side, person has atherosclerosis *Cactus 6c*
- Sensation of blood surging up into head, pulse irregular but forceful, angina pain, fear of dying *Naja 6c*
- Whole body pulsating, angina pain extending into right arm, warm room makes symptoms worse *Lilium 6c*
- Pulse loud but irregular, palpitations, feeling of heaviness and pressure in heart region, with occasional sharp, stinging pains passing from front to back, symptoms made worse by laughing, coughing, or slightest exertion *Iberis 6c*

Self-help Avoid tea, coffee, alcohol, and smoking, all of which interfere with heart rhythm. If you suffer from high anxiety levels, learn some form of meditation or relaxation (see PART 2); moderate daily exercise can also help to disperse anxiety.

If your GP has diagnosed paroxysmal tachycardia, try holding your breath, slowly drinking water, or bathing your face in cold water as soon as palpitations start; alternatively, pinch your nostrils together and try to blow through your nose – if you do this hard enough, your eardrums will pop.

Arteriosclerosis

Hardening of the arteries, a natural consequence of ageing, although age of onset seems to depend on hereditary factors; as artery walls lose their elasticity, and with it their ability to keep blood flowing vigorously, less blood reaches surrounding tissues; result may be CRAMP during exertion, especially in legs, or a transient ischaemic attack (spells of dizziness, weakness, numbness, or blurred vision – see STROKE). Rigid arteries greatly increase risk of THROMBOSIS, hence of CORONARY ARTERY DISEASE and strokes. Condition is usually complicated by some degree of ATHEROSCLEROSIS. Some nutritionists believe that silicon deficiency may be a contributing factor.

Orthodox approach is to treat any aggravating condition present (ANAEMIA or DIABETES, for example), and give drugs to widen blood vessels and prevent formation of blood clots; sometimes it may be feasible to replace a single, badly affected length of artery with an artificial tube or piece of vein. See ATHEROSCLEROSIS for homeopathic remedies.

Self-help If you suffer from pain in legs or toes at night, hang your legs over the side of the bed to speed up blood flow. Otherwise follow guidelines given under ATHEROSCLEROSIS.

Atherosclerosis

Slow clogging up and hardening of arteries due to build-up of fatty deposits (atheroma, atheromatous plaque) on smooth inner walls; as these deposits become larger and harden into plaque, artery walls lose their smoothness and elasticity, and blood flow is disrupted; plaque eats into and weakens artery walls, sometimes causing arteries to swell or burst (see ANEURYSM). Condition both contributes to and is aggravated by ARTERIOSCLEROSIS (age-related hardening of arteries). May be symptomless until arteries of heart are affected (see CORONARY ARTERY DISEASE), or arteries supplying brain and other vital organs (see STROKE, KIDNEY FAILURE); plaque-narrowed arteries are also vulnerable to blockage by blood clots and dislodged fragments of plaque.

Atherosclerosis appears to be related to high consumption of meat, eggs, butter, and cream, which contain lots of saturated fats and cholesterol, and affects nearly all Westerners to some degree, even children, though severity increases with age; women become as vulnerable as men after the MENOPAUSE. Recent American research has suggested that chlorine in the water supply may be a contributory factor; other researchers have pointed the finger at deficiencies of copper and vanadium. HIGH BLOOD PRESSURE, DIABETES, kidney trouble, OBESITY, and smoking certainly increase risk. Since furring-up process is very slow, decreased blood flow through narrowed arteries may be compensated for by extra flow through sound neighbouring arteries; in this way condition may escape diagnosis until it causes serious problems. Early warnings may be CRAMP after exertion or ANGINA.

Orthodox treatment is limited to drugs which reduce blood pressure or drugs which reduce blood cholesterol levels. The homeopathic remedies listed below are also palliative. Medication is no substitute for a change of diet and lifestyle.

Specific remedies to be taken twice a day for 1 month in addition to following self-help advice below; if there is no noticeable improvement, see your homeopath
- If person is elderly, suffers from high blood pressure and palpitations, especially if an aneurysm is present *Baryta carb. 6c*
- Frequent fainting spells, craving for salt, feeling very nervous and highly strung *Phosphorus 6c*
- Fainting spells, dizziness, confusion, and general mental deterioration, liver problems, heart feels compressed within chest *Vanadium 6c*
- Tight, congested headache, pounding sensation in arteries *Glonoinum 6c*

Self-help The suggestions which follow are mainly preventive; they are unlikely to undo the effects of decades of unhealthy eating, overeating, or inadequate exercise, but they may prevent further damage to your arteries and your heart. If there is a history of artery disease in your family, you should regard yourself as particularly at risk.

First of all, cut down on full-fat milk and cheese, cream, butter, eggs, fatty meat, lard, dripping, and hydrogenated vegetable fats; look for margarines and oils high in polyunsaturates (those based on sunflower, safflower, and corn oil are best), and don't heat them above 120°C (250°F). Eat oily fish (herring, mackerel) twice a week. Add garlic to your food and take brewer's yeast (containing B vitamins and chromium); these will help to reduce cholesterol levels. Add fresh ginger to your cooking; this will help to reduce stickiness of blood platelets and prevent clotting. Cut down on refined carbohydrates, at their most concentrated in sugar, sweets, chocolate, biscuits, cakes, and soft drinks. Other items to be wary of are shellfish and salt; avoid salty foods and don't add salt to your food. If you cannot wean yourself off caffeine and alcohol entirely, make them a twice-a-week treat only. Make sure you eat plenty of unrefined, high-fibre foods – principally that means wholegrain cereals, leafy vegetables, and pulses. Take extra Vitamin B_6, C, and E (if you have high blood pressure or are taking anticoagulants, check with your GP before taking extra Vitamin E). Take fish oils, e.g. Max EPA, evening primrose oil and recommended daily amounts of manganese, calcium, selenium, magnesium, iodine, lecithin, and rutin.

Stop smoking. Some form of relaxation or meditation (see PART 2) would also be beneficial. Both relaxation and exercise dissipate stress, and lower stress levels generally mean lower blood cholesterol levels.

Oral contraceptives and hormone replacements should be avoided if at all possible; if you are taking them and want to stop, consult your GP.

Bacterial endocarditis
Infection primarily affecting heart valves (tissue covering these is continuous with tissue lining chambers of heart); valves already damaged in some way – by RHEUMATIC FEVER, SYPHILIS, congenital heart defects (see CONGENITAL DISORDERS), or possibly by surgical repair or replacement – are most susceptible to bacteria (and occasionally fungi), which are transmitted through bloodstream. Untreated, bacteria may eat into heart valves, weakening them and eventually causing HEART FAILURE, or break away in clumps and lodge in small arteries (see EMBOLISM). Symptoms include mild FEVER, aching joints, chills, HEADACHE, fatigue, loss of appetite (see APPETITE CHANGES), and possibly mild ANAEMIA. Routinely treated with antibiotics, and iron tablets if anaemia is present. Homeopathic treatment is constitutional, designed to boost immunity to infection.

Blood poisoning see SEPTICAEMIA p. 273

Blood pressure see HIGH BLOOD PRESSURE, LOW BLOOD PRESSURE

Bruising
Accumulation of blood in tissues around a ruptured blood vessel; as soon as rupture occurs, blood platelets pour into the breach, causing blood vessel to contract so that further blood loss is minimized, then strands of protein in blood serum mat together, trapping more platelets, and breach is sealed. Bruising occurs very easily if one component in complex blood-clotting mechanism is absent, as in HAEMOPHILIA; if blood platelet count is low because bone marrow has been damaged by drugs or radiation; or if antibodies are destroying platelets faster than they can be produced in the bone marrow, as in thrombocytopenia (see PLATELET DISORDERS). Lack of Vitamin C, essential for formation of collagen in walls of blood vessels, also leads to easy bleeding and bruising.

Specific remedies to be taken 4 times daily for up to 3 days; if no improvement, see your homeopath
- Bruising due to injury *Arnica 30c*
- Bruising with broken skin, or bruising due to poor return of blood to heart, as in varicose veins *Hamamelis 6c*
- Where bruising involves many nerve endings, as in fingers or toes *Hypericum 30c*
- Bruises on breast *Bellis 6c*
- Where bruising feels as if it is in a bone *Ruta 6c*

Self-help Apply a cold compress or Arnica ointment. Step up intake of Vitamin C.

Buerger's disease
Inflammation of arteries (occasionally of veins), causing formation of blood clots (see THROMBOSIS), most commonly occurring in legs; cause is not known, but most sufferers are cigarette smokers aged 25–45; quite often condition remits of its own accord within a few years. Shortage of oxygen in surrounding tissues causes legs to feel cold and painful, particularly after exertion; complications include ARTERIOSCLEROSIS, dry GANGRENE, VARICOSE ULCERS, and RAYNAUD'S DISEASE. If veins are affected, legs may tingle and become painfully swollen and hot; in bad cases, THROMBOPHLEBITIS may develop. Orthodox approach is to give drugs to dilate blood vessels, or sever nerves which cause arteries to constrict; in cases of gangrene, amputation may be unavoidable. For homeopathic treatment see conditions mentioned above.

Cardiac arrest
Heart stops beating, either because coronary arteries are diseased (see CORONARY ARTERY DISEASE) or because ventricles have gone into fibrillation (see ARRHYTHMIAS); person suddenly loses consciousness, stops breathing, and has no pulse. Give artificial respiration immediately, followed by cardiac resuscitation (see First Aid pp. 86–9), and ⑨⑨⑨. Some ambulance crews carry a machine called a defibrillator which sends a surge of electric current through heart via two metal plates held against chest; this may or may not restart heart. After cardiac arrest, person will be kept in hospital in intensive care for several days. Constitutional homeopathic treatment is advisable after discharge.

Cardiac infarction see HEART ATTACK

Chilblains
An extreme reaction to cold, in which superficial blood vessels contract excessively causing skin to go pale and numb, then red, swollen, and itchy; eventually skin may break; most common on hands and feet. Problems gets worse with repeated exposure to cold and damp. If the remedies given below do not seem to be effective, see your homeopath.

Specific remedies to be taken every ½-hour for up to 6 doses
- Chilblains which burn and itch, skin red and swollen, and not relieved by cold applications *Agaricus 6c*
- Chilblains get worse in cold weather, person feels chilly, is prone to head sweats, and puts on weight easily *Calcarea 6c*
- Chilblains most painful when limbs hang downwards, veins swollen, warmth makes discomfort worse *Pulsatilla 6c*
- Chilblains itch and burn, skin weepy and watery, damp makes problem worse, person prone to rough skin *Petroleum 6c*

Self-help Keep affected parts as warm and as dry as possible during cold or damp weather. If skin is broken, apply Calendula ointment; if not, apply Tamus ointment. Try not to scratch.

Circulation problems see CHILBLAINS, RAYNAUD'S DISEASE, BUERGER'S DISEASE, VARICOSE VEINS, VARICOSE ULCERS, ARTERIOSCLEROSIS, ATHEROSCLEROSIS

Symptoms which point to circulatory problems are fingers and toes which go numb or dead-looking in cold weather, cuts and bruises which seem slow to heal, and cramping pains or aching in calves. If any of these symptoms are persistent, see your GP.

Congenital heart defects see CONGENITAL DISORDERS

Coronary artery disease

Narrowing or blockage of the arteries (the two coronary arteries and their branches) which deliver oxygen to heart muscle; cause is ATHEROSCLEROSIS, which not only narrows and hardens arteries but also encourages formation of blood clots. During exercise, and at times of great stress, heart needs extra oxygen; if this is not available, starved heart muscle produces CHEST PAIN. This may be the dull, constricting pain known as ANGINA (pain is focused in centre of chest but may also radiate up to neck and jaw, down left arm, or to back), which ceases when exercise or stress ceases, or it may be the more agonizing, bursting pain of coronary thrombosis (see HEART ATTACK), which may be associated with collapse and loss of consciousness and does not go away when stress or exercise ceases. Starvation of heart muscle can also cause difficult breathing, sweating, DIZZINESS, and nausea. For preventive measures, see ATHEROSCLEROSIS.

Coronary thrombosis see HEART ATTACK

Deep vein thrombosis see also THROMBOSIS

Presence of blood clot in a deep vein, usually in leg or lower abdomen, obstructing return of blood to heart; pressure in veins and capillaries below clot rises, causing pain, swelling (see OEDEMA), and sometimes dark red discolouration of skin. If you have these symptoms, 12. Danger is that fragments of blood clot will be swept into lungs (see PULMONARY EMBOLISM). Prolonged immobility, POLYCYTHAEMIA, OBESITY, and oestrogens (in oral contraceptives and post-menopausal hormone preparations) encourage development of deep vein thrombosis. Orthodox treatment options are painkillers, anticoagulant drugs, drugs to dissolve, or surgical removal of clot.

Specific remedies to be taken every 2 hours for up to 6 doses while waiting to see GP

- Purplish-blue extremities, pain and swelling relieved by warmth, especially if left side of body is affected *Lachesis 6c*
- Limb extremely swollen and sensitive, causing unbearable bursting sensation, allowing limb to hang makes symptoms worse *Vipera 6c*
- Deep vein thrombosis accompanied by varicose veins, great pain, fatigue *Hamamelis 6c*
- Right side of body most affected, limbs swollen and cold, condition follows bad bruising *Bothrops 6c*

Self-help If you are on the pill, discuss alternatives with your GP. Losing weight, giving up cigarettes, adding garlic and fresh ginger in cooking, and taking regular exercise all decrease risk of thrombosis. See ATHEROSCLEROSIS for other sensible precautions.

Embolism see also PULMONARY EMBOLISM

Blockage of an artery by an embolus, a largish piece of debris temporarily in general circulation (normally, provided they do not obstruct blood flow, such pieces of debris are removed by scavenging white blood cells called macrophages). Embolus may be a blood clot or fragment from a blood clot formed in a vein (see DEEP VEIN THROMBOSIS) or in an artery, a fragment of atheromatous plaque (as in ATHEROSCLEROSIS), a clump of bacteria (as in BACTERIAL ENDOCARDITIS), or even a foreign body which has entered through a wound. Most at risk are people suffering from ATHEROSCLEROSIS, ARTERIOSCLEROSIS, or THROMBOSIS, and people over 50.

An embolus which lodges in an artery in the brain will cause a STROKE, or at the least a transient ischaemic attack. If pulmonary vein is blocked (see PULMONARY EMBOLISM), blood returning to heart will be inadequately oxygenated and circulation will be unbalanced; this is likely to cause BREATHLESSNESS, CHEST PAIN, a dry COUGH, FAINTING, and cyanosis (bluish lips); in severe cases, person may collapse and die within minutes unless emergency help is available. An embolism in an intestinal artery may cause ILEUS (paralysis of intestines); symptoms of an embolism in a limb artery include NUMBNESS or tingling, weakness, dead white or blue-tinged skin, and in severe cases GANGRENE. Orthodox treatment options depend on cause of embolism, but may include painkillers, drugs to dilate blood vessels, prevent further clotting, or disperse clots, or surgery to remove embolism. After an acute episode, constitutional homeopathic treatment is recommended.

Self-help Take extra Vitamin E, but if you have high blood pressure or are taking anticoagulants, consult your GP before doing so. If embolism affects a limb, keep the limb cool.

Enlarged spleen

One of the symptoms of MALARIA, CIRRHOSIS OF THE LIVER, LEUKAEMIA, LYMPHOMA, HODGKIN'S DISEASE,

---

POLYCYTHEMIA, etc. Spleen enlarges when called on to remove massive numbers of red blood cells, defective cells, or bacteria from circulation. Enlargement produces a dull, heavy sensation just under left ribs. Though this may not be only symptom, 12 .

In adults, spleen may have to be removed if it has been ruptured by injury or if it is destroying too many red blood cells (as in HAEMOLYTIC ANAEMIA); its functions are taken over by rest of reticulo-endothelial system. In small children, splenectomy is usually avoided because organ plays a larger role in dealing with hostile bacteria.

While awaiting investigation, give one of the remedies listed below. If enlargement is related to any of conditions mentioned above, consult relevant entry for homeopathic remedies.

Specific remedies to be taken 4 times daily for up to 2 weeks
- Spleen greatly enlarged, discomfort increased by movement and by lying on left side, or where enlargement is a result of leukaemia, with pain deep under left ribs *Ceanothus 6c*
- Enlarged spleen associated with alcoholic cirrhosis of liver, ankles swollen *Quercus 6c*
- Stitch-like pains under left ribs, short, dry cough, sneezing, involuntary passage of urine *Squilla 6c*
- Swollen spleen accompanied by constipation and craving for salt, especially if person is oversensitive and gets even more upset when consolation is offered *Natrum mur. 6c*

Gangrene

Flesh which has died from oxygen starvation; causes include EMBOLISM, poor circulation (see DIABETES, ARTERIOSCLEROSIS), FROSTBITE, or a major wound which has been poorly disinfected. Dying tissue causes pain, then becomes numb and turns black, with clear line between dead and living tissue. *Dry gangrene* is dead tissue which has not been infected; *wet gangrene* develops when dead tissue becomes infected by bacteria which thrive in absence of oxygen; some strains of bacteria are very virulent and produce a type of wet gangrene known as *gas gangrene*, so called because of the putrid-smelling gas they give off. Wet gangrene can cause BLOOD POISONING if not promptly treated, and gas gangrene can swiftly lead to SHOCK and death.

Orthodox treatment consists of drugs to improve circulation or surgery to bypass blocked arteries, but if tissue is already dead, affected area will have to be removed surgically; if underlying muscle and bone are also dead, amputation will be necessary; any remaining bacteria are destroyed by antibiotics, antiserum, or hyperbaric oxygen treatment.

If gangrene is suspected, 12 and choose a remedy from the list below.

Specific remedies to be taken every hour for up to 10 doses
- Affected area bluish-purple and on left side of body, pain worse after sleep *Lachesis 6c*
- Burning sensation in affected area, lessened by cold applications, increased by covering or applying heat *Secale 6c*
- Ulceration of surrounding skin, cold makes pain worse, person feels chilly and restless *Arsenicum 6c*
- Affected area cold, bluish, and bruised-looking, symptoms begin in toes, especially if person is elderly *Carbo veg. 6c*
- Wound which turns septic, or wet gangrene with foul smell *Echinacea 6c*
- Long-standing ulcer which develops wet gangrene, especially if person is elderly *Euphorbia 6c*

Glandular enlargement see also ENLARGED SPLEEN

Occurs when lymph glands – most numerous in neck, armpits, and groin – step up production of white blood cells (lymphocytes) to fight infection; generally speaking, glands nearest site of infection become tender and swollen, but in GLANDULAR FEVER all lymph glands are more or less affected. LYMPHOMA and HODGKIN'S DISEASE also cause lymph glands to swell; both conditions are forms of cancer which affect lymphocyte production; if left untreated, cancerous lymphocytes quickly spread to other lymph glands and to spleen. For homeopathic treatment, see conditions mentioned above.

Haemophilia

Inherited sex-linked condition in which body fails to manufacture or does not manufacture enough Factor VIII, one of many chemicals essential for staunching bleeding. Symptoms are prolonged or uncontrollable bleeding, and easy BRUISING which causes swelling and pain; repeated bruising around joints eventually restricts movement. Defective blood clotting gene is part of X chromosome, not of Y chromosome (XX codes for a girl, XY for a boy), so a girl whose mother carries the gene and whose father is a haemophiliac may suffer from haemophilia, but this is extremely rare; defective gene almost always expresses itself in a boy whose mother carries the gene but whose father is quite normal. It follows that haemophiliac fathers cannot pass haemophilia on to their sons, though they may produce daughters who carry the faulty gene. In 25 per cent of cases, there is no family history of haemophilia; in such cases, disease is usually attributed to spontaneous mutation in one of mother's X chromosomes. Fatal consequences of disease can now be prevented by regular transfusions or injections of Factor VIII; all diagnosed haemophiliacs wear or carry some form of identification in case of emergencies. Suitable homeopathic remedies are given under BRUISING, and under BLEEDING and WOUNDS in First Aid.

Self-help Keep fit by swimming, running, cycling, etc., but avoid sports which are likely to cause injury (football, rugby, judo, skiing, etc.). Do not take any drugs, not even aspirin, without first consulting your GP. Carefully clean any wounds and apply firm pressure to staunch bleeding; if bleeding continues, contact local or nearest hospital. If you have bruised a joint, apply an ice pack, firmly bandage the joint, and go to hospital.

Haemorrhage see BRAIN HAEMORRHAGE, ANTE-PARTUM HAEMORRHAGE, POST-PARTUM HAEMORRHAGE, SHOCK

Heart attack (coronary thrombosis, cardiac or myocardial infarction)

Heart attacks occur when the heart muscle becomes damaged through lack of oxygen. This usually happens when a coronary artery or one of its branches becomes blocked by a blood clot; the technical name for this is *coronary thrombosis*. The result of coronary thrombosis is *cardiac or myocardial infarction*, death of part of the heart muscle.

Symptoms are CHEST PAIN in centre of chest, radiating up into neck and into both arms; person may also collapse and lose consciousness; other symptoms may be BREATHLESSNESS, DIZZINESS, sweats and chills, and nausea – sometimes these symptoms occur without chest pain, in which case episode is called a 'silent infarct'. Severity of chest pain varies, depending on proportion of heart muscle starved of oxygen; some sufferers describe pain as 'crushing', 'agonizing', or 'vice-like', or as a bursting sensation; others merely complain of tightness or constriction. Attack may be quite unexpected or preceded by episodes of ANGINA, which produces very similar symptoms.

If a heart attack is suspected and person collapses and loses consciousness, ⑨⑨⑨ and give First Aid (see pp. 88–90). Action taken in first 3 minutes may mean difference between life and death. One in three heart attacks is fatal, usually within 2 hours, either because electrical pacemaker mechanism or heart muscle is irretrievably damaged, or because person goes into SHOCK. Later complications may include HEART FAILURE, ANEURYSM, EMBOLISM, and THROMBOSIS. Statistically, however, anyone who survives a first heart attack has a 70 per cent chance of recovering fully and living for at least another 5 years, provided he or she makes certain changes in diet and lifestyle.

Heart attacks occur for different reasons in different people, and for different combinations of reasons. Conditions such as ATHEROSCLEROSIS, ARTERIO-SCLEROSIS, HIGH BLOOD PRESSURE, and DIABETES increase risk; so does STRESS and SMOKING, being male (though women are equally at risk after the MENOPAUSE), smoking, eating lots of refined carbohydrates and saturated fats, being overweight, doing a sedentary job, driving everywhere rather than walking, taking oral contraceptives (particularly over age of 35) if smokers,

and living in areas where water is soft. Heredity also plays a part.

Recent evidence has shown that stress – whether one interprets this as free-floating anxiety, excitement, strong emotions, or as mental or physical exhaustion – over-stimulates nerves which control coronary arteries, causing them to go into spasm, slowing blood flow, and creating conditions in which a blood clot is likely to form and cut off blood flow.

Specific remedy to be taken every 3 hours for up to 1 week during recovery from heart attack
• Left arm still feels numb and weak *Rhus tox. 6c*

Self-help Immediately after a heart attack, get plenty of sleep, rest whenever you feel tired, and try to avoid situations which arouse anger, moral indignation, helplessness, or anxiety. After 4–5 weeks your heart will have recovered sufficiently for you to be able to resume most activities, including sexual intercourse, but go gently to begin with. Moderate, regular exercise is something to be aimed for, not feared; try to walk, swim, or cycle at least 20 minutes a day, use the stairs rather than the lift, leave the car keys at home occasionally. . . STOP SMOKING. Learn some form of relaxation or meditation to relieve stress (see PART 2). Avoid HYPERVENTILATION.

For dietary self-help measures see ATHEROS-CLEROSIS.

Heart block see ARRYTHMIAS

Heart failure

A rather drastic name for a condition which may not be immediately threatening; what is meant is that pumping action of one or both sides of heart is inefficient due to faulty valves, HIGH BLOOD PRESSURE, CORONARY ARTERY DISEASE, congenital heart defects (see CONGENITAL DISORDERS), etc.

In *right-sided heart failure*, pressure of blood in main veins returning blood to heart rises, forcing fluid into organs and tissues (see OEDEMA); typical symptoms are tiredness, weakness, puffiness around ankles, legs, or abdomen (skin pits when pressed), and sometimes ABDOMINAL PAIN caused by a swollen liver.

In *left-sided heart failure*, pressure of blood in the veins returning blood from lungs to heart rises because left side of heart is pumping inefficiently; fluid forced out of blood vessels accumulates in lungs (see PULMONARY OEDEMA), causing BREATHLESSNESS and WHEEZING, and sometimes CHEST PAIN and expectoration of frothy, blood-tinged phlegm. These are symptoms which deserve immediate medical attention, so ⑨⑨⑨, keep person in sitting position, and give *Ammonium carb. 6c* (or *Arsenicum 6c* if this is not available) every 15 minutes for up to 6 doses.

Congestive heart failure is a combination of both left- and right-sided heart failure; in addition to symptoms mentioned above, person may lose appetite (see

---

⑨⑨⑨ Emergency – call GP (or dial 999) immediately. ② Consult your doctor if no improvement within 2 hours

APPETITE CHANGES) and suffer from CONFUSION; muscles may also begin to waste, though at first this may be masked by fluid retention. PNEUMONIA is a very real risk once lungs become waterlogged.

Depending on cause of heart failure, orthodox treatment options include diuretics to deal with fluid retention, and drugs to strengthen heart beat and discourage formation of blood clots; if these fail, only solution may be a heart transplant, but demand far exceeds availability.

Sufferers are advised to seek constitutional treatment from an experienced homeopath. In meantime, remedies given below, and also under OEDEMA, PULMONARY OEDEMA, HIGH BLOOD PRESSURE, or ATHEROSCLEROSIS may be appropriate.

Specific remedies to be taken 4 times daily for up to 3 days
- Palpitations brought on by slightest exertion, swollen ankles, slow irregular pulse, occasional blueing of lips, sudden feeling that heart has stopped *Digitalis 6c*
- Symptoms of heart failure and also of angina, with pain in left arm *Cactus 6c*
- Symptoms of heart failure and also of angina, strong irregular pulse, anxiety, fear of dying *Naja 6c*
- Symptoms alleviated by lying on left side with head raised and drinking hot water *Spigelia 6c*
- Symptoms of failure accompanied by general chilliness, extremities blue and mottled, desire to be fanned *Carbo veg. 6c*
- Heart disease well advanced, arteriosclerosis, fluid in membranes around lungs *Arsenicum iod. 6c*

Self-help Plenty of rest is important – sitting is probably better than lying down – but keep the legs moving. If breathing is difficult at night, use more pillows for support. Cut down on salt. See HIGH BLOOD PRESSURE for more dietary suggestions.

High blood pressure (hypertension)

Pressure of blood within circulatory system depends on elasticity of artery walls and also on volume of blood in circulation, which in turn depends on how well kidneys regulate salt and water content of blood. Since both arteries and kidneys slowly deteriorate with age, blood pressure steadily increases with age. The greater the pressure of blood within the system, the harder the heart has to work, the greater the strain on the arteries, and the greater the risk of ATHEROSCLEROSIS, HEART FAILURE, ANGINA and HEART ATTACKS, STROKE, and KIDNEY FAILURE. Even mild hypertension can decrease life expectancy.

Current medical opinion is that diastolic pressure of 90–100 or over, recorded on three separate occasions, or systolic pressure of more than 160 in a young person, requires treatment. Blood pressure is given as two figures e.g. 130/80. The top figure is the systolic, the lower the diastolic. (Diastolic pressure represents the reflux or recoil pressure due to the elasticity of the aorta, systolic pressure the pumping force ex-

erted by the left side of the heart). Often condition goes unnoticed because there are no symptoms; symptoms only set in when high blood pressure has taken its toll of heart and kidneys.

Most cases of high blood pressure are described as *essential hypertension*, which means that there is no underlying ailment, unlike cases of *secondary hypertension*, which arise because of kidney problems, or renal artery narrowing (which is the most treatable surgically), because person is suffering from ALDERO-STONISM or CUSHING'S SYNDROME, or because oral contraceptives or non-steroidal anti-inflammatory drugs are being taken; secondary hypertension can also develop during pregnancy. There is a hereditary element in essential hypertension, but staying slim, not adding salt to food, not eating too much saturated fat or drinking too much alcohol, and walking for at least half an hour a day seem to have a protective effect; so does breast-feeding. High blood pressure which develops very suddenly, is described as *malignant hypertension*; it is most common in heavy smokers, quickly damages kidneys, and can be fatal within 6 months if left untreated.

Drugs used to treat high blood pressure include beta blockers, which reduce force of heartbeat, diuretics, which encourage kidneys to excrete more water, calcium antagonists, wich regulate the amount of calcium going into the cells, and ACE inhibitors which block the conversion of a substance which causes narrowing of the arteries. The latter two lead to lowering of arterial resistance and therefore of blood pressure. However, once you are put on these drugs, you may have to take them for the rest of your life; if your blood pressure is raised but not dangerously so, see what the self-help measures below will achieve first, and seek constitutional treatment from an experienced homeopath.

Self-help Have your blood pressure checked every 3 to 5 years, especially if you are on the pill, take moderate and regular exercise, keep your weight within the limits appropriate for your height and build (see charts p. 261), stick to the 'twice a week rule' for alcohol and for the animal products mentioned on p. 24, and cut down on salt. If you often feel angry, resentful, depressed, or helpless, some form of meditation or relaxation (see PART 2) would be a good insurance policy.

If your GP has already diagnosed high blood pressure, both your blood pressure and your general health would be improved by changing to a diet low in animal protein and high in raw vegetables and fruit, a mainly lacto-vegetarian diet in fact. The occasional short fast would also be beneficial (see p. 350), but if you have any doubts on this score consult your GP first. Other measures you might like to consider, because of their detoxifying, vitality-boosting effects, are dry skin brushing, sunbathing, warm baths, gradually in-creasing exercise periods, and deep breathing, all of

For explanation of other symbols, see page 107

which are discussed in PART 2 – Prevention is better than cure.

Hodgkin's disease see also LYMPHOMA

Cancer of lymph glands, especially those in neck; lymphocyte production accelerates, causing pain, swelling, and ITCHING, but lymphocytes may be defective, unable to produce antibodies which fight infection; 90 per cent of early cases are curable by chemotherapy and radiotherapy; outlook is less good once cancer spreads to other lymph glands. Condition affects three times as many men as women. See pp. 273–4 for homeopathic approach to CANCER.

Hypertrophic cardiomyopathy

Thickening of heart muscle to compensate for defective muscle fibres; eventually heart wall may become so thick that blood flow into and out of heart is impeded, causing CHEST PAIN, PALPITATIONS, BREATHLESSNESS, and fatigue. Orthodox medicine offers symptom relief in the form of beta blockers and diuretics; in isolated cases, a heart transplant may be recommended. For specific homeopathic remedies, see ANGINA and PALPITATIONS; if selected remedy produces no improvement, see your GP or homeopath.

Hypertension see HIGH BLOOD PRESSURE

Hypotension see LOW BLOOD PRESSURE

Immunodeficiency diseases see LEUKAEMIA, LYMPHOMA, MYELOMA, HODGKIN'S DISEASE, AIDS

Leukaemia see also LEUKAEMIA p. 325, CANCER

Cancer of white blood cells, causing massive over-production of both normal and abnormal cells; may be acute or chronic, involving either lymphatic system (lymphocytes produced in lymph glands and elsewhere) or myeloid system (neutrophils produced in bone marrow), but all forms are very rare.

Chronic lymphatic leukaemia causes enlargement of lymph glands, an ENLARGED SPLEEN (felt as a dragging sensation in upper left abdomen), ANAEMIA, WEIGHT LOSS, loss of appetite (see APPETITE CHANGES), slight FEVER, night sweats, and recurrent infections such as PNEUMONIA; as condition worsens, BRUISING and bleeding occur with less and less provocation. Condition may take 5 years or more to develop. Problem is that defective lymphocytes, which are unable to fight infection, invade all parts of lymphatic system, then interfere with production of red cells, white cells, and platelets in bone marrow. Treatment options are chemotherapy, steroids, and radiotherapy, and antibiotics if necessary, but eventually disease becomes resistant to treatment.

Acute lymphatic leukaemia is most common in children – see LEUKAEMIA p. 325 – and onsets within a matter of weeks.

Chronic myeloid leukaemia leads to a massive increase in neutrophil production in bone marrow; this inhibits production of red blood cells, causing symptoms of ANAEMIA (pallor, tiredness, shortness of breath, palpitations), but resistance to infection remains good; lymph glands, spleen, and liver begin to enlarge as neutrophils invade bloodstream, causing WEIGHT LOSS and loss of appetite (see APPETITE CHANGES), night sweats, and general ill health. Usually occurs in people over 50, and onsets over a few months; blood transfusions and chemotherapy may keep disease at bay for 2–3 years.

In *acute myeloid leukaemia*, neutrophils also multiply exponentially and take over bone marrow and invade other organs, but they are abnormal, so drastically reduce resistance to infection as well as producing symptoms of ANAEMIA; onset is extremely rapid. Steroids, antibiotics, blood transfusions, and chemotherapy may check disease for a year or so.

For homeopathic treatment, see CANCER pp. 273–4.

Low blood pressure (hypotension)

Chronic low blood pressure is almost never serious; problems occur when blood pressure drops suddenly, and arteries do not constrict quickly enough to maintain blood supply to brain; this is most likely to happen when one stands up suddenly from a sitting or lying position and feels dizzy and faint. This phenomenon is known as *postural hypotension*, occurring most frequently in people who are taking drugs to control HIGH BLOOD PRESSURE; it can also be a feature of pregnancy, a symptom of ARTERIOSCLEROSIS or DIABETES, or a consequence of strong emotion, lack of food, prolonged standing in the heat, or being generally run down.

If you faint frequently, and especially if you are on drugs for high blood pressure, see your GP. Homeopathic treatment is constitutional.

Lymphangitis

Inflammation of lymph vessels, visible as thin red lines under skin; these radiate from site of infection – broken skin infected with *Streptococcus* bacteria, for example, as in ERYSIPELAS – to nearest lymph gland. To be on safe side, 12 as there is a risk of SEPTICAEMIA. If inflammation is severe and FEVER has set in, ②; GP will probably prescribe antibiotics. While waiting for medical attention, try one of the remedies below.

Specific remedy to be taken every 10 minutes for up to 10 doses if inflammation is severe
- Skin swollen and discoloured, discomfort relieved by pressure, temperature starting to rise, worse on right side of body *Crotalus 6c*

Specific remedies to be taken every hour for up to 10 doses
- At first signs of inflammation, skin dry, hot, and tender, neighbouring lymph glands swollen *Belladonna 6c*
- Left side of body most affected, blue discolouration of skin, symptoms worse after sleep *Lachesis 6c*
- Thin red line threading up arms or legs from a septic lesion *Hepar sulph. 6c*

---

999 Emergency – call GP (or dial 999) immediately. ② Consult your doctor if no improvement within 2 hours

Lymphoma see also CANCER

A form of cancer which attacks lymphocytes in lymph glands, similar to HODGKIN'S DISEASE but more malignant; affected lymphocytes divide and multiply unchecked, then spread to rest of lymphatic system, and to spleen, where process is repeated; since many of these cancerous lymphocytes are abnormal, the body's ability to fight infection deteriorates. First sign may be a single swollen gland, usually in neck, accompanied by WEIGHT LOSS, poor appetite (see APPETITE CHANGES), mild FEVER, night sweats, and a series of minor infections. Discomfort in upper left abdomen usually indicates an ENLARGED SPLEEN. Most lymphomas develop slowly, and eventually become resistant to steroids, radiotherapy, and chemotherapy; fast-growing lymphomas, however, stand a good chance of being cured. For homeopathic treatment, see CANCER.

Myeloma see also CANCER

A form of cancer which speeds up growth of plasma cells in bone marrow, disrupting production of other kinds of blood cell, interfering with infection-fighting activities of normal plasma cells, and causing pressure to build up within marrow cavity and weaken surrounding bone. Person succumbs to repeated infections, becomes anaemic, and suffers from bone pain, typically in vertebrae; weakened vertebrae tend to split causing permanent stooping, and weakened limbs fracture easily. Condition is rare, mainly affecting people over 50, men twice as often as women; chances of cure are slim, but steroids, blood transfusions, radiotherapy, and chemotherapy may keep disease under control for several years. For homeopathic treatment, see CANCER pp. 273–4.

Myocardial infarction see HEART ATTACK

Myocarditis

Inflammation of heart muscle, a rare complication of MUMPS, DIPTHERIA, TOXOPLASMOSIS, and viral respiratory infections; if any of these ailments is accompanied by CHEST PAIN and BREATHLESSNESS, 12; GP will probably arrange for hospital admission for observation and prescription of steroids to make heart heal quickly, antibiotics, and rest. Untreated, condition may lead to HEART FAILURE. If breathing difficulties become acute, or if lips turn bluish, ②.

Specific remedy to be given every 15 minutes for up to 6 doses in acute attack
- Fainting, anxiety, irregular pulse, bluish lips and tongue *Lachesis 6c*

Specific remedies to be given every 2 hours for up to 6 doses
- Palpitations made worse by slightest exertion, rapid pulse, shortness of breath, heart feels as if it has stopped, puffiness around ankles *Digitalis 6c*

- Swollen ankles which feel as if they are about to burst, especially if legs are allowed to hang down, area over liver feels tender *Vipera 6c*

Nutritional cardiomyopathy

Damage to heart muscle caused by insufficient amounts of Vitamin B_1 in diet or loss of potassium as result of persistent DIARRHOEA or long-term use of diuretics; condition is most common in alcoholics, whose diet is notably lacking in B_1, though some specialists believe damage is directly due to alcohol poisoning; symptoms include swelling of hands and feet, PALPITATIONS, and disturbed heart rhythm (see ARRYTHMIAS); eventually HEART FAILURE may set in. Chances of recovery are good in non-alcoholics, if missing nutrients are supplied; in alcoholics, only total abstinence can halt damage. See PALPITATIONS, ARRYTHMIAS, and HEART FAILURE for appropriate homeopathic remedies.

Palpitations

Sensation that heart is beating irregularly, or faster or more forcefully than it should, given the level of activity demanded of it; may be a symptom of heart disease (see ARRHYTHMIAS, ATHEROSCLEROSIS), of an overactive thyroid gland (see THYROID PROBLEMS), or of food ALLERGY; a high FEVER can also disturb heart-beat. Palpitations brought on by ANXIETY or over-consumption of caffeine and nicotine are nothing to worry about unless a heart condition already exists.

If palpitations are accompanied by CHEST PAIN, difficult breathing, DIZZINESS, sweating, or FAINTING, ② and select a remedy from the list below. GP may prescribe beta blockers or anti-arrhythmia drugs, depending on underlying problem. Where anxiety is a major factor, constitutional treatment is recommended.

Specific remedies to be taken every 5 minutes for up to 6 doses as soon as palpitations come on
- Palpitations after overindulgence in food or alcohol, or after prolonged expenditure of nervous energy, feeling chilly and irritable *Nux 6c*
- Violent palpitations, made worse by lying on left side, and distinctly worse just before a period, dizziness, shortness of breath, flatulence *Cactus 6c*
- Fainting, constricted feeling in chest, anxiety, especially during menopause *Lachesis 6c*
- Palpitations brought on by hysteria or exposure to cold, trembling heart, weak pulse, fainting *Moschus 6c*
- Palpitations seem to shake entire body, constricted feeling in chest, heat and sympathy make discomfort worse *Natrum mur. 6c*
- Palpitations brought on by heat or rich, fatty foods, general weakness *Pulsatilla 6c*
- Breath smells foul, person thirsty for drinks of hot water, which seem to have a calming effect on heart *Spigelia 6c*

- Palpitations begin with feeling that heart has stopped, then person feels that slightest movement might make heart stop *Digitalis 6c*
- Palpitations come on suddenly, especially after a shock, fear of dying *Aconite 6c*

Self-help See general advice given under ATHEROS-CLEROSIS. STOP SMOKING; reduce or stop caffeine-containing drinks.

Pericarditis

Inflammation of membrane around heart (pericardium), sometimes with accumulation of fluid between membrane and heart. *Acute pericarditis* comes on suddenly as result of viral infection, RHEUMATIC FEVER, SYSTEMIC LUPUS ERYTHEMATOSUS, KIDNEY FAILURE, chronic HEART FAILURE, or a HEART ATTACK. Person experiences pain in centre of chest, perhaps radiating to left shoulder, and usually finds that coughing, twisting or turning, or taking deep breaths makes pain worse; BREATHLESSNESS may also be a symptom. Since underlying condition is often serious, ② and select a remedy from the list below. Fluid around heart may need to be drawn off by syringe; steroids may also be given.

Long-standing inflammation of pericardium can cause a condition known as *constrictive pericarditis*; after each inflammatory episode pericardium scars, thickens, and shrinks, progressively restricting beating of heart; this causes sluggish blood flow and OEDEMA in lower part of body, and eventually HEART FAILURE. Surgery to remove thickened tissue is the only solution.

Specific remedies to be taken every 15 minutes for up to 10 doses

- Dry cough, exhaustion, pericardium full of fluid *Arsenicum iod. 6c*
- Sharp, stitch-like pains in centre of chest made worse by warmth and slightest movement, alleviated by cold drinks and by lying on left side, person thirsty *Bryonia 30c*
- Pain comes on suddenly, and is made worse by cold or sudden emotional shock, person afraid of dying *Aconite 30c*
- Stitch-like pain in chest, pain subsides when lying on right side with head raised *Spigelia 6c*
- Fluid around heart, difficulty breathing, dry cough, ankles swollen *Arsenicum 6c*
- Sudden onset of pain, with severe breathlessness, especially after midnight, person looks flushed and hot, fears for his or her life, and feels as if heart is about to force itself upwards out of chest *Spongia 6c*
- Severe pain, heavy, tight feeling in chest, shortness of breath, thin pulse; symptoms relieved by stooping forwards but made markedly worse by loss of sleep *Colchicum 6c*

Phlebitis see THROMBOPHLEBITIS

Platelet disorders

Platelets are formed in bone marrow and are vital to the blood clotting process which follows rupture of blood vessels (see BRUISING).

Abnormal stickiness Oral contraceptives and oestrogens, HIGH BLOOD PRESSURE, DIABETES, and high levels of fat in blood increase stickiness of platelets, encouraging them to clump together and form blood clots (see THROMBOSIS, CORONARY THROMBOSIS, STROKE); also, clumps of platelets readily combine with cholesterol to form atheroma inside arteries (see ATHEROSCLEROSIS). Vitamin B_6, C, and E, and also evening primrose oil, fish oils, garlic, and ginger are effective counter-measures. See THROMBOSIS for homeopathic remedies.

Thrombocytopenia Condition in which there are too few platelets in circulation, causing easy BRUISING and prolonged bleeding. Most common cause is AUTO-IMMUNE DISEASE, in which antibodies are produced which destroy platelets faster than they can be manu-factured by bone marrow; this condition, known as idiopathic thrombocytopaenia purpura, usually begins between age of two and six, manifesting as a rash of small, reddish-purple dots (really tiny bruises) which persist when pressed. Other causes include antibiotics, diuretics, and non-specific anti-inflammatory drugs, all of which can damage bone marrow. Can also be a symptom of LEUKAEMIA. If condition is suspected, 48 as there is a risk of internal bleeding.

If drug-induced, most cases clear up within 6 months if drug is stopped; steroids may also be given to control bleeding. Other orthodox treatment is removal of spleen, which plays leading role in destruction of platelets. Homeopathic treatment is constitutional. While treatment is being sought, one of the remedies below should be tried.

Specific remedies to be taken 4 times daily for up to 7 days
- *Crotalus 6c*
- *Phosphorus 6c*

Polyarteritis nodosa (PAN)

An AUTOIMMUNE DISEASE affecting connective tissue in walls of arteries; this causes local inflammation and swelling, and weakens artery walls; affected arteries develop multiple small swellings (see ANEURYSM) and offer ideal conditions for formation of blood clots (see THROMBOSIS). Symptoms vary according to organs or part of body affected, but are likely to include persistent low FEVER, WEIGHT LOSS, poor appetite (see APPETITE CHANGES), sweating, and general aches and pains; if heart is affected, symptoms may be those of ANGINA, PERICARDITIS, or HEART FAILURE; if peripheral nervous system is involved, person will probably suffer from NEURALGIA AND NEURITIS; if kidneys are damaged, there may be BLOOD IN URINE; if lungs are damaged, symptoms may mimic those of ASTHMA.

Disorder is notoriously difficult to diagnose, but is most common in men aged 20–50; in some cases onset is triggered by a bad reaction to immunization, blood transfusions, penicillin, or sulphonamides. Routinely controlled by means of steroids or immuno-suppressive drugs. For homeopathic treatment, see AUTOIMMUNE DISEASE.

Polycythemia

Too high a concentration of red blood cells in the blood. In *primary polycythemia* bone marrow produces red blood cells at a faster rate than they are destroyed, though reason for this is not known; this produces congested feeling in head (see HEADACHE), DIZZINESS, flushed skin which becomes very itchy after a hot bath (see ITCHING), and an ENLARGED SPLEEN, felt as a swelling under left ribs. Condition may take years to develop, and is seldom seen in people under 40; left untreated, it can lead to DEEP VEIN THROMBOSIS, STROKE, HEART ATTACK, GOUT, and kidney damage. Orthodox treatment consists of regular removal of blood, and drugs or injections of radioactive phosphorus to depress red cell production. Constitutional homeopathic treatment is recommended in addition to orthodox treatment.

Secondary polycythemia is usually a complication of chronic BRONCHITIS; because lungs are congested, existing red blood cells are unable to pick up all the oxygen the body needs, so bone marrow responds by producing more. If bronchitis can be treated, size of red cell population returns to normal. In *pseudopoly-cythemia*, blood contains less plasma than it should and therefore more red blood cells; disorder is associated with STRESS, overeating, and high alcohol consumption, but poses no direct risk to health.

Pulmonary hypertension see PULMONARY HYPERTENSION p. 182

Raynaud's disease see also ACROCYANOSIS

Sudden contraction of small arteries in fingers and toes, causing skin to turn very pale, then bluish; an occasional, short-lived phenomenon at first, with affected digits feeling weak and numb; returning circulation is accompanied by pins-and-needles sensation. In severe cases, blood-starved tissues may cause VARICOSE ULCERS or dry GANGRENE. Condition may be brought on by cold, STRESS, abnormal reactions to drugs such as beta blockers, or repeated use of a pneumatic drill or chain saw; sometimes it is a feature of BUERGER'S DISEASE, SCLERODERMA, ARTERIOS-CLEROSIS, PULMONARY HYPERTENSION, DIABETES, or NEURALGIA AND NEURITIS. If fingers or toes frequently become numb and bluish, see your GP. Orthodox treatment consists of drugs to dilate arteries and improve circulation; cutting nerve supply to affected arteries may also produce improvement. Homeopathic treatment is constitutional, although the remedies below should be tried first.

Specific remedies to be taken every ½ hour for up to 10 doses
- Burning sensation in fingers or toes, made worse by heat, rest of body feels cold *Secale 6c*
- Skin icy cold and mottled, natural colour returns with fanning *Carbo veg. 6c*
- Skin bluish-purple, especially after sleep *Lachesis 6c*
- Applying heat or letting limb hang down makes symptoms worse *Pulsatilla 6c*
- Skin very pale, flushes easily, cold applications relieve symptoms *Ferrum phos. 6c*
- Swelling, burning, and itching, cold makes symptoms worse *Arsenicum 6c*
- Hands icy cold and swollen, swollen feet, restless legs *Cactus 6c*

Self-help To restore circulation to hands and feet, whirl your arms about in the air and swing your legs. Make sure your hands and feet are thoroughly warm before you go out in cold weather; toast gloves and socks on a radiator before you put them on, and don't wear them too tight. Stop smoking – nicotine makes blood vessels contract – and take the occasional nip of alcohol – that does the opposite!

Rheumatic heart disease

A consequence of one or more attacks of RHEUMATIC FEVER in childhood or young adulthood; today, joints are more often attacked than heart tissue, but if heart alone is affected, person may look tired and wan, or develop definite symptoms of heart trouble – BREATH-LESSNESS when exercising or lying down, for example, or OEDEMA in legs or back. Majority of victims suffer some degree of damage to heart valves (see VALVULAR DISEASE; in severe cases, HEART FAILURE may develop. In short term, orthodox treatment consists of steroids to reduce inflammation, and antibiotics to reduce chances of rheumatic fever recurring. If valves are affected, beta blockers and anticoagulants may be sufficient; if not, valve replacement may be necessary. For homeopathic treatment see OEDEMA, HEART FAILURE.

Shock

Sets in when flow of blood through body suddenly becomes inadequate, either because a HEART ATTACK has occurred (cardiogenic shock), person has lost a lot of blood (hypovolaemic shock), or blood vessels have suddenly dilated in response to an allergen or an infection (anaphylactic or septic shock). As blood pressure plummets, brain no longer receives enough oxygen, so nervous control of blood vessels is lost, which causes them to dilate further, lowering blood pressure even more; heart and kidneys then begin to fail, and brain and other organs begin to die.

First symptoms are sweating, faintness, nausea, rapid breathing and pulse, pallor, and cold, clammy skin; as brain runs out of oxygen, person becomes confused and drowsy, then loses consciousness.

Immediate action is necessary, so ⑨⑨⑨. Put person in recovery position (see First Aid pp. 91–1), with legs raised above level of hips to encourage blood flow to brain, and loosen tight clothing; cover with one blanket or coat only; if possible, give *Aconite 30c* every 5 minutes until help arrives. In hospital, blood pressure will be restored by means of blood or plasma transfusions; even so, damage to brain or kidneys may be irreversible.

Stokes Adams attack
Severest form of heart block (see ARRHYTHMIAS), in which ventricles contract independently of electrical signals from pacemaker cells in right atrium; fault may occur spontaneously or be result of damage done by a HEART ATTACK; if ventricles slow down drastically or stop pumping altogether for a few seconds, blood supply to brain starts to fail and person faints, or may go into convulsions (see FITS). If this happens, ⑨⑨⑨ and give artificial respiration and cardiac resuscitation if necessary (see First Aid pp. 86–9). Installation of an artificial pacemaker will prevent heart block recurring.

Temporal arteritis
An AUTOIMMUNE DISEASE in which lining of temporal arteries (those which supply scalp and branch just behind temples above the ears) become inflamed and thickened, reducing blood flow and causing dull, throbbing HEADACHE in one or both temples; affected arteries may feel swollen and painful if touched; other symptoms may be slight FEVER, aching muscles, poor appetite (see APPETITE CHANGES), and WEIGHT LOSS. Condition is increasingly common after age 55, and affects twice as many women as men. Complications include eye trouble, and some loss of vision, and STROKE. If you suffer from persistent, throbbing headaches and deteriorating vision, see your GP; steroids are essential in temporal arteritis, both to control inflammation and save eyesight. Constitutional homeopathic treatment is recommended.

Thrombocytopenia see PLATELET DISORDERS

Thrombophlebitis
Inflammation of a vein, usually due to injury or infection; roughening of wall of affected vein encourages development of blood clots (see THROMBOSIS). Condition is most common in superficial veins of legs, and in people who suffer from VARICOSE VEINS. Symptoms are pain, redness, tenderness, ITCHING, and hard swelling along length of affected vein. If infection is present, person may also have FEVER; if this is the case, ⑤⑧. Main risks are SEPTICAEMIA and fragmenting of blood clots (see EMBOLISM). Orthodox medicine offers antibiotics and compression bandaging. Homeopathic treatment is constitutional, aimed at increasing resistance to infection and promoting natural resorption of

blood clots. In the meantime, the following remedies will ease pain and promote healing.

Specific remedies to be taken 4 times daily for up to 7 days
- If condition follows injury *Arnica 30c*
- After taking Arnica, if bruising and soreness persist *Hamamelis 6c*
- Swollen veins, pain made worse by heat and letting affected limb hang down *Pulsatilla 6c*
- Skin has purplish appearance *Lachesis 6c*

Self-help Take moderate exercise, and apply hot and cold compresses alternately. Zinc and a multivitamin and mineral supplement are also recommended.

Thrombosis see also DEEP VEIN THROMBOSIS, PLATELET DISORDERS
In normal circumstances blood only clots when blood vessels have been ruptured (see BRUISING for brief description of clotting process). A thrombus is a blood clot which forms on the roughened or inflamed wall of a vein or artery; sluggish circulation and high blood lipid levels (see ATHEROSCLEROSIS) encourage this to happen. As thrombus enlarges, blood flow through affected channel decreases and may be blocked altogether; if an artery in the heart or brain is affected, result will be CORONARY THROMBOSIS or a STROKE. A blood clot, or fragments of a blood clot, can also be swept into general circulation and lodge in a distant blood vessel (see EMBOLISM); if heart, brain, or lungs are affected the result will be a HEART ATTACK, a STROKE, or PULMONARY EMBOLISM.

Thrombosis is conventionally treated with anticoagulants, which dissolve clots. Homeopathic treatment is constitutional; while seeking constitutional treatment the following remedies are recommended.

Specific remedies to be taken 4 times daily for up to 7 days
- Sluggish circulation, family or personal history of strokes or transient ischaemic attacks *Bothrops 6c*
- Where site of thrombosis has purplish appearance *Lachesis 6c*

Self-help Take extra Vitamin B_6 and C. Vitamin E is also recommended, but should be avoided if you are already taking anticoagulants. Eat oily fish (herring, mackerel) twice a week, and add garlic and fresh ginger to your cooking. Evening primrose oil is also beneficial.

Valvular disease
Heart valve disorders may be congenital (see CONGENITAL DISORDERS) or acquired through infections such as RHEUMATIC FEVER or BACTERIAL ENDOCARDITIS. Inflammation of heart valves can lead to stenosis or incompetence; in stenosis, valve is thickened by scar tissue so cannot open very wide, which forces heart to work harder to push blood through it; an incompetent valve is one that is so

---

⑨⑨⑨ Emergency – call GP (or dial 999) immediately. ② Consult your doctor if no improvement within 2 hours

distorted that it cannot close properly, so blood leaks back after it has been pumped through, again forcing the heart to work harder.

Valve disorders commonly cause weakness and BREATHLESSNESS; they can also cause ARRYTHMIAS, HEART FAILURE, ANGINA, or HEART ATTACK depending on nature of damage and valve affected. In some cases, heart valve replacement is recommended; otherwise treatment is palliative. See conditions mentioned above for suitable homeopathic remedies.

Varicose veins

A sign that valves in affected veins are weak and unable to prevent backflow of blood; veins become lumpy and distended with blood, and smaller veins and capillaries show as twisted, purplish lines on skin; poorly drained tissues may develop brown staining. Condition mainly affects legs, but also testicles (see VARICOCELE), and rectum and anus (see PILES); legs tend to ache or swell, and become tender and itchy. Valves may be naturally weak, or become so as result of prolonged sitting or standing, DEEP VEIN THROMBOSIS, CONSTIPATION, OBESITY, or pregnancy; complications include VARICOSE ULCERS and THROMBOPHLEBITIS. Orthodox treatment is to 'strip' or remove varicosed sections of veins, or give injections to close them; surrounding smaller veins rapidly enlarge to compensate. Support stockings are also prescribed.

Homeopathy offers the remedies below; if there is no improvement within 3 weeks, or if condition becomes dramatically worse, see your GP.

Specific remedies to be taken every 12 hours for up to 7 days
- Varicose veins feel bruised and sore, person may also suffer from piles *Hamamelis 30c*
- Warmth and allowing legs to hang down make varicose veins worse, especially during pregnancy, person feels chilly *Pulsatilla 30c*
- Legs look very pale but redden easily, walking slowly makes weak, achy feeling wear off *Ferrum 30c*
- Skin mottled and marbled *Carbo veg. 30c*

Self-help Sit with feet raised above hip level whenever you can, and spend as little time standing as possible. Always wear support stockings. If a vein bursts and bleeds, apply a pad and bandage it on tightly, and keep leg raised until bleeding stops; if it doesn't, see your GP as soon as possible. Guard against constipation by eating more fibre, and increase your intake of Vitamins E and C, and bioflavinoids.

MUSCLES, BONES AND JOINTS

THE body is a wonderful system of bony levers and casings, bound together by ligaments, and moved, supported and protected by muscles. Where bones meet there are joints. Most joints are enclosed in a sleeve or capsule of tough, fibrous tissue lined with cells which secrete a special lubricating fluid, synovial fluid. The ends of the bones themselves are covered in a special kind of cartilage, hyaline cartilage, which is smooth and tough, and nourished by the synovial fluid. The fluid and the smooth articulating surfaces of the bones ensure friction-free movement. The largest synovial joints in the body occur at the shoulder, elbow, hip, and knee, and between the pelvis and sacrum.

There are other kinds of joints too, though these occur in lesser numbers. The weight-bearing surfaces of the vertebrae, for example, are separated by discs of fibrous cartilage with a tough outside and a softer inside; the vertebrae stack up on each other separated by these shock-absorbing discs. The knee, because it is both load-bearing and freely movable, has a fluid-filled joint capsule with two partial discs of cartilage (menisci) inside it.

Where muscle tendons cross joints, there are special anti-fraying structures called bursae, small fluid-filled sacs of connective tissue; there are bursae above and behind the knee, at the top of the femur and humerus, at the back and front of the elbow, and so on. The knee is unique in having a small shield of bone, the patella, in front of the joint; without it, kneeling would be impossible and the tendon of the quadriceps at the front of the thigh would soon wear through or get nipped in the joint as the knee straightened.

Every joint in the body has its own range of movement – the shoulder has the greatest, followed by the wrist, the head and neck, and the hip. Healthy ligaments check joint movement, keeping it within stable limits. Healthy muscles, whose inelastic tendons insert into bone close to the joints they move, also keep joints within stable limits. An extra-mobile joint, therefore, is not necessarily a healthy one. A hyper-mobile joint in the spine, for example, usually means that other vertebral joints are not as mobile as they should be.

If muscles are weak, giving little stability or protection to a joint, the task of stabilizing and protecting falls entirely on the ligaments and the joint capsule itself. Unlike muscles, ligaments and joint capsules have no contractile powers; they can only stretch. With traumatic or habitual strain the joint becomes inflamed, causing stiffness, pain, swelling, and loss of mobility. It may even dislocate, becoming useless because the fulcrum against which the muscles exert their leverage has fallen apart. If trauma is sudden and severe, ligaments tear, tendons rupture or rip away from their bony moorings, muscle fibres break, and bones fracture. However, most of the muscular aches and pains which take people to their GP, osteopath, chiropractor, physiotherapist or acupuncturist do not have such spectacular causes. They are the result of poor posture, depression, anxiety, occupational demands, lack of exercise, and the slow process of ageing.

Pain and stiffness in joints can be dramatically relieved by steroid (hydrocortisone) injections. The procedure is not particularly pleasant, and repeated injections can actually damage joints, but if all other treatments fail, a single injection should be considered. After an injection, or if a joint has not felt right since an injection, take *Ledum 6c* every 8 hours for up to 6 doses.

Bone, contrary to popular conception, is one of the most active tissues in the body. It is well supplied with blood vessels, and is continuously repairing and remodelling itself in response to stress and load. Exercise, and sufficient calcium and Vitamin D in the diet, encourage growth, maintenance, and repair. In fact calcium is continually swopped between the bones and the blood in order to keep sufficient calcium in the blood for nerves and muscles to function properly. In an adult, the manufacture of blood components – red and white blood cells, and platelets – is carried out in the marrow inside the vertebrae, breastbone, ribs, pelvis, and heads of the humerus and femur.

Ankle problems

If an ankle has been injured, is causing severe pain, and cannot be moved, (999) and give *Arnica 30c* every 5 minutes until help arrives; likely cause is a FRACTURE (see First Aid p. 99). A SPRAIN (see First Aid pp. 104–5) causes pain and swelling, but usually the ankle remains mobile. Tissues around ankle joint remain prone to swelling for several months after such injuries.

Other conditions affecting the ankles and requiring prompt treatment are TENDONITIS (partial or complete rupture of Achilles tendon, causing pain and inflammation), DEEP VEIN THROMBOSIS (swelling of one ankle and tenderness in corresponding calf), RHEUMATIC FEVER (fever, and redness and swelling which affect other joints too), and INFECTIVE ARTHRITIS (fever, and redness and swelling of one ankle only); appropriate action in such cases is 12 .

Swollen ankles can also be a sign of PRE-ECLAMPSIA in later stages of pregnancy or, more prosaically, of sitting or standing for long periods; if puffiness persists for longer than 48 hours, see your GP.

Chronic conditions sometimes accompanied by ankle problems are RHEUMATOID ARTHRITIS or OSTEO-ARTHRITIS (ankles red, hot, swollen, and painful), PYELONEPHRITIS and KIDNEY FAILURE (puffy ankles – see OEDEMA), HEART FAILURE (ankles swollen, breath-

lessness, wheezing, tiredness), and VARICOSE VEINS (swollen veins in legs, feet and ankles swell after standing for short time). Hot weather can also cause ankles to swell and shoes to feel tight; in some women swollen ankles are a side-effect of oral contraceptives or part of PRE-MENSTRUAL SYNDROME.

See conditions mentioned above for homeopathic remedies; if none seems suitable, choose one of the remedies below. If cause of ankle pain cannot be pinpointed, constitutional treatment should be considered.

Specific remedy following injury
- *Arnica 30c* every hour for up to 48 hours, then in 6c 4 times daily for up to 5 days

Other remedies to be taken 4 times daily for up to 5 days
- If Arnica does not produce improvement after 48 hours *Bellis 6c*
- Ankle injury, bruising kind of pain in ankle bones *Ruta 6c*
- Ankle injury, pain in ankle feels like rheumatism and becomes more insistent with rest but wears off with gentle movement *Rhus tox. 6c*
- Swollen ankles with varicose veins *Hamamelis 6c*
- Ankles swell up in hot weather *Apis 6c*

Specific remedies to be taken every 12 hours for up to 1 week
- Drawing or tearing pains in ankle, aggravated by cold, dry weather *Causticum 30c*
- Ankles weak and turn easily, also painful, especially in heat, person prone to constipation and headaches *Natrum mur. 30c*
- Tearing pains in ankles, warm glow from feet to head, body feels as if it is on fire *Viscum 30c*

Self-help If you suffer from swollen ankles in hot weather, take *Natrum Mur.* 3 times daily while weather remains hot. For weak ankles, *Calcium Phos.* tissue salt, taken 3 times daily for 1 month, may be beneficial.

Ankylosing spondylitis

An AUTOIMMUNE DISEASE affecting facet joints between vertebrae; joints become inflamed, then stiff, effectively fusing vertebrae together, causing spine to become increasingly rigid. Condition usually starts in sacroiliac joint (joint between sacrum and ilium of pelvis) with low backache and morning stiffness; if stiffness progresses up spine, joints between ribs and spine may be affected, causing CHEST PAIN or breathing difficulties; if upper spine is affected, jaw and movement and even eyes may be affected. Orthodox treatment is physiotherapy, steroids or other anti-inflammatory drugs, and in severe cases surgery. Homeopathy offers constitutional treatment and, in the early stages, the remedy below.

Specific remedy to be taken 3 times daily for up to 5 days
● Pain around sacroiliac joint, aggravated by walking and stooping *Aesculus 6c*

Self-help Take *Calcium Fluor.* 3 times daily, and do some form of daily exercise – swimming is especially good. Deep breathing for several minutes each day will help to keep the joints between your spine and ribs mobile. Use a hard mattress, and sleep on your front without a pillow, rather than on your back or side; that way your spine can relax into its natural curve. Avoid prolonged sitting, especially driving; if you have a sedentary job, get up and walk about every 30 minutes or so. You should also do as little bending and lifting as possible. If you smoke, try to stop.

Arm problems see also ELBOW PROBLEMS, SHOULDER PROBLEMS

If there is severe pain in or misalignment of upper or lower arm bones after some kind of injury, ⑨⑨⑨ and give *Arnica 30c* every 5 minutes until help arrives; likely cause is a FRACTURE (see First Aid p. 99). A wrist SPRAIN (see First Aid pp. 104–5) will be painful, but joint retains some of its function.

Pain extending from chest into left arm, with sweating, DIZZINESS, and nausea, may be a sign of ANGINA (typically pain increases with activity or excitement, but wears off after 5 minutes); if pain extends from chest into both or either arms, with collapse and loss of consciousness, person may be having a HEART ATTACK, in which case ⑨⑨⑨ and give First Aid (see p. 101).

Pain, redness, and swelling around the wrists may be a symptom of RHEUMATIC FEVER (both wrists affected) or INFECTIVE ARTHRITIS (great tenderness over bone in one wrist); if either of these conditions is suspected, ⑫.

Numbness and tingling in the hands may be a symptom of CARPAL TUNNEL SYNDROME (thumb side of hand affected, pains shoot up arm from wrist) or CERVICAL SPONDYLOSIS (stiff painful neck, dizziness on turning head, one or both hands affected). Knuckle and elbow joints can be affected by GOUT (joint suddenly becomes red, shiny, and extremely tender); injury, overuse, or pressure can cause TENDONITIS or BURSITIS in an elbow or shoulder; if all the joints in both arms are more or less swollen and painful, the cause is probably RHEUMATOID ARTHRITIS.

See individual entries for description and treatment.

Arthritis see INFECTIVE ARTHRITIS, OSTEOARTHRITIS, RHEUMATOID ARTHRITIS

Back problems

The single largest cause of lost working hours, often caused by lifting, twisting, poor posture, and in-adequate back support when sitting or lying down; pain is felt when back muscles are over-tense or pulled (see FIBROSITIS, PULLED MUSCLES) or go into spasm to prevent further damage to overstrained ligaments (see SPRAINS), or when discs between vertebrae rupture, pressing on adjacent nerves (see PROLAPSED DISC). Anything which puts sustained extra strain on the back – pregnancy, OBESITY, having one leg shorter than the other, habitually carrying one shoulder higher than the other – can cause backache; mental and emotional over-load can aggravate and sometimes cause a bad back.

Back pain may be localized, as in LUMBAGO (pain in middle of the back just below waist), SCIATICA (pain radiates from lower back into buttock, then shoots down leg), COCCYDYNIA (pain around coccyx, right at base of spine) or CERVICAL SPONDYLOSIS (pain and stiffness in neck), or more general, as in INFLUENZA (with fever, sore throat, headache) or OSTEOARTHRITIS, especially in an older person. Where chief symptom is general stiffness or pain around sacroiliac joint (which links sacrum to pelvis) cause may be ANKYLOSING SPONDYLITIS. Other ailments which can affect the spine are TUBERCULOSIS, SHINGLES (knife-like pains stabbing out from one side of spine at chest level), and PAGET'S DISEASE (spine tender when pressed, perhaps developing sideways curve). Extremely rarely, back pain may be due to a SPINAL CORD TUMOUR.

If a back injury causes loss of control of bowel or bladder, or loss of movement, NUMBNESS, or tingling, ⑨⑨⑨ and give *Arnica 30c* every 5 minutes for up to 10 doses until help arrives; likely cause is SPINAL CORD INJURY.

If back pain onsets suddenly after a period of immobility, especially in someone over 60, ⑫; cause may be a FRACTURE brought on by OSTEOPOROSIS. Back pain accompanied by FEVER may be a sign of acute PYELONEPHIRITIS (back pain one-sided and radiating into groin, nausea and vomiting); again, appropriate action is ⑫.

Homeopathic treatment of back trouble caused by tension and stress is mainly constitutional; for specific remedies, see LUMBAGO, SCIATICA, COCCYDYNIA, FIBROSITIS. Other remedies appear under other con-ditions mentioned above. Osteopathy, chiropractic, physiotherapy and acupuncture are also recommended – they bring swift relief to many thousands of back sufferers each year.

Orthodox treatment options, depending on severity of problem, include muscle relaxants, painkillers, steroid injections, traction, wearing a collar or surgical corset, physiotherapy; surgery is usually a last resort.

Self-help Local heat – a hot water bottle held against the small of the back, for example – can help to relax knotted muscles. Rest your back as much as possible; if you can, lie flat on your back on a fairly hard mattress with a foam pad about the thickness of two paperbacks under your head; if lying on your back is uncomfortable because you cannot let your legs go flat, lie on your side with your knees pulled up and a foam pad in the hollow of your waist.

To prevent back pain in the first place, never lift things with a bent or twisted back; bend your knees instead and keep your back straight. Don't try to lift and twist at the same time. Wear low-heeled shoes. Sit as upright as possible; if you spend a lot of time sitting down, have a stretch and a walk around every half hour or so, and use a chair which supports the small of your back or a back support cushion. Special back chairs, which have a seat which tilts forward (see Posture p. 19) oblige one to sit up straight, allowing the back to assume its natural inward curve at the waist. Make sure your mattress is fairly hard, but not uncomfortably so; if it has a dip in the middle, put a board or a door underneath it. Losing weight also takes some of the strain off the spine.

Shoulder bags, especially if worn on the same shoulder all the time, do untold damage to backs. Wherever possible, split the loads you carry – carry a bag in each hand rather than one heavy bag in one hand. Make a habit of carrying things in alternate hands.

Your GP or physiotherapist may recommend special exercises to strength your back. If not, try the following exercises twice a day. Do not try 2 until you can do 1, or 3 until you can do 2, and go very gently to start with.
1 Lie on the floor, on your back with your knees bent; tighten the muscles around the anus and raise your hips an inch or so off the floor, then relax. Repeat 10 times.
2 Lie on the floor, on your back with your knees bent; breathe in and arch your back as strongly as possible, then breath out and flatten your back against the floor. Repeat 10 times.
3 Kneel on all fours, supporting yourself on straight arms, with your hands flat; arch your back upwards as far as possible and tuck your chin as close to your chest as you can; now let your back sink slowly down and raise your face to the ceiling; now arch your back up again, and so on. Repeat 10 times, holding each posture for a few seconds. Try to breathe out as you arch up and in as you sink down. This is a a yoga exercise known as The Cat.

Swimming is also beneficial.

Bone pain

A well known symptom of ailments such as INFLUENZA and MALARIA but a persistant aching or pain in any bone should be investigated by your GP in order to rule out hairline FRACTURES, OSTEOMYELITIS, BONE TUMOURS, secondary CANCER, etc. Occasionally bone pain is due to potassium deficiency. For treatment of GROWING PAINS in children, see p. 323.

Specific remedies to be taken 4 times daily for up to 3 days while waiting to see GP
- Bone feels 'bruised', especially after a bad knock *Ruta 6c*
- Pains at night, mainly involving skull, nose, or palate, made worse by cold *Aurum 6c*

- Pains associated with flu or malaria *Eupatorium 6c*
- Rheumatic pains, aggravated by cold, pressure, or movement, and worse at night *Mezereum 6c*
- Limbs feel achy, numb, and chilly, feeling of great weariness when climbing stairs *Calcarea phos. 6c*
- Pains stab like lightning *Fluoric ac. 6c*

Bone tumours see also CANCER

Usually appear as hard, painless lumps on bone, causing weakening and susceptibility to FRACTURE at slightest strain. Most bone tumours are secondary, offshoots of well established tumours of the lungs, breast, prostate, kidney, or thyroid gland, so treatment can only be palliative. Tumours which start in bones are rare and usually benign.

Bunions

Caused by weakness of joint at base of big toe and made worse by pointed and high-heeled shoes or collapsed arches; big toe twists inwards over or under first toe (hallux valgus), forcing joint at base of big toe to stick out sideways; with continued friction and pressure, a CALLUS may develop on side of joint, or joint may be affected by BURSITIS, causing pain and swelling and even more difficulty getting shoes to fit; eventually OSTEOARTHRITIS may set in. In most people, both feet are more or less equally affected. If bunions are causing unbearable discomfort, your GP may recommend surgery to straighten big toes. Calluses can be dealt with by a chiropodist. For homeopathic remedies, see BURSITIS and CORNS AND CALLUSES.

Self-help If bunions are inflamed by bursitis, sort out your oldest, softest pair of shoes, cut holes in the uppers over the bunions, and wear only that pair of shoes until the bursitis clears up.

If bunions run in the family there are various preventive measures you can take. First of all, wear roomy comfortable shoes, and whenever possible go without shoes or socks. Keep the arches of your feet strong by picking up squash balls with your toes. Do exercises to strengthen the weak muscles down the side of each big toe: standing with feet together at heels and toes, try to move your big toes towards each other, hold for 10 seconds, then relax. Don't cheat by moving your heels apart. Difficult at first, but persevere!

Bursitis

Inflammation of the little pads (bursae) around joints which allow bones and tendons to move over or under each other without friction, usually brought on by injury or constant pressure; inflamed bursae fill with fluid, causing swelling and tenderness. Best known example of condition is *housemaid's knee*. Condition usually clears up of its own accord within a week or two, provided pressure is kept off joint, but if it persists, see your GP; he or she may drain off fluid, then bandage joint, or prescribe steroid injections. If condition

---

recurs, removal of offending bursa is a minor surgical procedure.

Specific remedies to be taken 4 times daily for up to 7 days
- Burning, stinging pain made worse by heat *Apis 30c*
- Tearing pain, joint stiff and swollen, made worse by rest and cold damp weather, alleviated by heat and gentle exercise *Rhus tox. 6c*
- Dragging pain and tightness over bursa, discomfort worse when affected limb is allowed to hang, general chilliness *Pulsatilla 6c*
- Shooting pains *Sticta 6c*
- Pains much worse at night *Kali iod. 6c*
- Pain made worse by heat or slightest movement *Bryonia 30c*
- Pain made worse by slightest jarring, joint red, hot, swollen, and throbbing *Belladonna 30c*
- Housemaid's knee, pain in thigh when knee is straightened, or a joint which feels bruised and weak *Ruta 6c*

Self-help Rest the affected joint as much as possible and avoid putting pressure on it. Hot or cold compresses can help to disperse swelling.

Carpal tunnel syndrome see CARPAL TUNNEL SYNDROME p. 126

Cervical spondylosis
A form of arthritis in which the vertebrae of the neck grow extra bone and start to press upon adjacent nerves, causing a stiff and painful neck, and tingling sensations, NUMBNESS, pins and needles, or pain in the hands and legs of one or both sides of the body, and sometimes HEADACHE, DOUBLE VISION, and DIZZINESS or unsteadiness when neck is turned in certain directions.

Homeopathic treatment is the same as that for OSTEOARTHRITIS, but the remedies listed below are also helpful.

Specific remedies to be taken 4 times daily for up to 14 days
- Headache behind forehead, limbs numb, flatulence *Argentum nit. 6c*
- Tenderness at back of neck (over backward-pointing spines of neck vertebrae), chest feels constricted, person weak and shaky *Agaricus 6c*
- Shooting pains up spine and into head, burning sensation in spine *Picric ac. 6c*

Coccydynia
Continuous, aching pain in area of coccyx (small fused bones at base of spine), caused by injury or a heavy fall on rear end; can also occur after childbirth.

If the remedies below produce no improvement, see your homeopath.

Specific remedies to be taken 3 times daily for up to 7 days

- Brought on by a fall *Hypericum 6c*
- Coccyx feels bruised and aching, improves in damp, wet weather *Causticum 6c*
- Pressure and draughts increase pain, constipation *Silicea 6c*
- Coccyx feels as if it has a heavy, dragging weight attached to it *Antimonium tart. 6c*
- Recurrent tearing or jerking pain *Cicuta 6c*
- Pain gets worse when sitting down or walking *Kali bichrom. 6c*

Self-help Rest as much as possible, lying down on your front to take pressure off coccyx. Pressure can also be alleviated by sitting on a rubber ring. Local heat may also help. Chiropractic or osteopathy would also help if problem was caused by a bad fall.

Cramp
Acute discomfort caused by muscles going into spasm (violent, uncontrollable contraction) because of shortage of oxygen and build up of lactic acid; prolonged sitting or standing, lying in an awkward position, strenuous or unaccustomed exercise and pregnancy are the most common causes of cramp; less often, cramp may be a symptom of ATHEROSCLEROSIS or BUERGER'S DISEASE. Occasionally cramp can be a symptom of sodium deficiency caused by excessive sweating while exercising, working in extreme heat, or taking a sauna (SEE HEAT EXHAUSTION).

If cramp occurs frequently for no obvious reason, constitutional homeopathic treatment may help. The remedies given below are for emergency use.

Specific remedies to be taken every 5 minutes for up to 6 doses
- Severe cramps mainly in feet or legs, cramp begins with twitching of muscles *Cuprum 6c*
- Cramps accompanied by headache, loss of appetite, nausea, and constipation, often worse at night *Nux 6c*
- Cramp which comes on as a result of fatigue *Arnica 30c*
- Cramp in someone who is overweight, flabby, pale, chilly, and prone to head sweats *Calcarea 6c*
- Cramp in calves, feet feel icy cold *Camphora 6c*
- Cramp in calves, alleviated by massage but made worse by walking about, recent diarrhoea and vomiting *Veratrum 6c*
- Cramp in thighs or legs *Chamomilla 6c*

As a preventive against cramp at night, take *Cuprum ars. 6c* at bedtime for 14 nights running.

Self-help When cramp comes on, try to stretch muscles involved, and massage them to increase blood supply. If cramp comes on at night, raise the foot of your bed by about 10 cm (4 in). Extra magnesium might also help.

Dermatomyositis and polymyositis

Rare forms of AUTOIMMUNE DISEASE mainly affecting voluntary muscles. Dermatomyositis usually occurs in children, and in its acute form causes swollen ankles, weakness of muscles in thighs and upper arms, FEVER, lesions on skin, and in some cases death from RESPIRATORY FAILURE. In its chronic form it affects muscles in lower arms and legs, and is sometimes associated with CANCER, especially of the stomach or intestines; if there are no skin lesions, this form is known as polymyositis. Conventionally treated by steroids. Homeopathic treatment is constitutional and dietary.

Dislocations see also First Aid p. 97

Joints are held together by ligaments, but shearing blows or falls can knock their articulating surfaces apart, tearing or permanently overstretching the ligaments, damaging the joint capsule, and perhaps surrounding blood vessels and nerves as well. Joint may go back into place when first dislocated, or have to be manipulated back (reduced); since joint is permanently weakened, dislocation is likely to recur, with an increased risk of OSTEOARTHRITIS. Shoulders and jaws dislocate most easily; dislocation of the vertebrae can cause SPINAL CORD INJURY. If a joint is congenitally weak, dislocation may occur spontaneously, without injury. Congenital dislocation of the hip (see CONGENITAL DISORDERS) is seen in about 1 in 60 newborn babies. Joints badly deformed by RHEUMATOID ARTHRITIS can also dislocate.

If dislocation keeps recurring, surgery may be necessary to tighten ligaments or reconstruct joint socket, followed by physiotherapy. After a first dislocation, joint is immobilized for 2 to 3 weeks to allow tissues to heal; subsequent dislocations are usually less painful.

Specific remedy to be taken every 4 hours for up to 3 doses
● To promote healing after dislocation *Ruta 30c*

Dupuytrens contracture

Thickening and shrinking of sheet of fibrous tissue under skin of palm, usually pulling third and fourth fingers towards palm; may be hereditary, but mainly affects alcoholics, epileptics, and men over 40. Can be corrected by surgery and physiotherapy in early stages. However, before consulting your GP, try the remedies given below.

Specific remedies to be taken every 12 hours for up to 2 weeks
● Condition has come on recently *Gelsemium 30c*
● Condition well established *Thiosinaminum 30c* or *Calcarea fluor. 30c*

Self-help Vitamin E is known to help this condition.

Elbow problems

Structure of elbow joint makes it vulnerable to TENDONITIS – in *tennis elbow* the outer elbow tendon is torn, in *golfer's elbow* the inner tendon is injured – and also to BURSITIS. Elbows are sometimes affected by GOUT (extreme tenderness, fever, sudden onset), and more frequently by RHEUMATOID ARTHRITIS and OSTEOARTHRITIS. Like all other joints, elbows are subject to FRACTURES (see First Aid p. 99), SPRAINS (see First Aid pp. 104–5), and DISLOCATIONS (see First Aid p. 96); a fractured or dislocated elbow gives severe pain at slightest attempt to move it, and may look misshapen; appropriate action is (999) and *Arnica 30c* every 5 minutes until help arrives.

Fibrositis

Small adhesions between individual muscle fibres, causing pain and stiffness; commonly caused by habitual strain due to occupational or postural habits, by unaccustomed strain, or by emotional tension; one of the commonest causes of backache (see LUMBAGO). Usually clears up in 3–4 days, provided muscles have not been torn (see PULLED MUSCLES).

Specific remedies to be taken 3-hourly for up to 2 days
● Pain comes on suddenly in cold dry weather and seems to be aggravated by movement, person restless and apprehensive *Aconite 30c*
● Muscles feel bruised, as if from sleeping on a bed that is too hard, movement makes pain worse, physical restlessness, irritability *Arnica 30c*
● Fibrositis in neck, back, and limbs, made worse by movement and by dry, cold, east winds, soothed by pressure *Bryonia 30c*
● Aching, tearing pains in limb muscles, with stiffness or weakness, pain wears off in warm, wet weather, but gets worse in cold *Causticum 6c*
● Pain and stiffness, having to get up in night because of pain, feeling bad tempered, as if nothing is going right *Chamomilla 6c*
● Affected muscles feel cold but pain and stiffness relieved by cold applications *Ledum 6c*
● Pain and stiffness worse in damp weather, in cold dry weather, after exercise, and around 4 am, turning over in bed hurts, pressure brings some relief, feeling very irritable *Nux 6c*
● Muscles stiff after overuse, stiffness improves with gentle movement, restlessness *Rhus tox. 6c*

Self-help Take hot baths, and apply hot and cold compresses alternately to stimulate circulation. Soft tissue treatment from a physiotherapist or osteopath would also help. Also, you could try the Liver Diet (see p. 352) for 1 month.

Foot problems see also BURNING FEET

Less serious problems include verrucas (small, thickened patches of skin on soles of feet causing pain on walking – see WARTS), ATHLETE'S FOOT (itchy, peeling skin between toes), CORNS OR CALLUSES (lumps or pads of hard skin on toes or side of feet), and BUNIONS (big toe beginning to cross over or under others, swollen joints at base of big toes). General pain and tiredness in both feet, made worse by prolonged standing, may be the result of fallen arches or being overweight. Pain, redness, and swelling in a toe joint may be GOUT, RHEUMATOID ARTHRITIS, or OSTEOARTHRITIS. Arterial diseases such as ARTERIOSCLEROSIS or BUERGER'S DISEASE are more likely to cause pain in one foot, especially on walking.

Feet are also subject to injuries which cause FRACTURES (see First Aid p. 99), and SPRAINS (see First Aid pp. 104–5). A fracture should be suspected if there is severe pain, loss of movement, and deformity; appropriate action is ⑨⑨⑨ and *Arnica 30c* every 5 minutes until help arrives. A stress fracture of the foot (a hairline crack in a bone, typically after prolonged exercise, particularly marching) declares itself as increasing pain on walking; prompt attention is necessary, so ②. If foot is merely sprained, it is painful, but can be walked on, and shows no deformity.

Joints which suddenly become painful and swollen, accompanied by FEVER, suggest RHEUMATIC FEVER; appropriate action is [12].

If a cut or bite on a foot turns septic, see First Aid pp. 90–2 and 106, and [48].

Specific remedies to be given every 4 hours for up to 3 doses; if no improvement within 48 hours, see your GP
- Feet ache after too much walking or standing *Arnica 30c*
- Feet feel burning, stiff, and swollen *Apis 30c*
- Soles of feet burning, made worse by walking *Graphites 30c*
- Feet very hot, smelly, and sweaty, with tearing pain in heel or gimlet-like pain in big toe, especially at night *Silicea 30c*
- Feet more painful when resting, pain wears off with movement, wrenched or sprained feeling *Rhus tox. 30c*
- Rheumatic, drawing kind of pain in ankles and toes *Caulophyllum 30c*
- Soles of feet painful to step on, tightness and pain in one or both Achilles tendons *Muriatic ac. 30c*
- Soles of feet burning and itchy, made worse by hot baths and worse in bed *Sulphur 30c*
- Soles of feet hurt, especially when walking on hard pavements, tenderness, swelling, and heat worse towards balls of feet *Petroleum 30c*
- Soles of feet sweaty and painful, as if walking on pins *Nitric ac. 30c*

Fractures see also First Aid p. 99
Bones break if they are put under sufficient stress, and may break with little or no provocation if they are weakened by OSTEOPOROSIS, BONE TUMOURS, or old age. A *simple fracture* involves just the bone – the skin is not broken. In a *compound fracture*, skin is broken and other tissues may be damaged as well; if fracture is bad, splinters of bone may sever nerves or blood vessels, or bone may become infected (see OSTEOMYELITIS, INFECTIVE ARTHRITIS). In a *complete fracture* the bone is broken clean through, but in an *incomplete fracture*, also known as a 'green stick' fracture, the break is more like a crack. Most serious of all are fractures of the skull and spine, which can injure the brain and spinal cord (see BRAIN INJURY, SPINAL CORD INJURY).

Even if skin is not broken, most fractures cause severe pain, especially if you try to move, and some swelling and BRUISING; however, broken bones do not always look obviously crooked or deformed. Fractures in small bones of wrist or ankle are sometimes mistaken for SPRAINS.

Routine treatment of broken bones is to put the broken ends back together (reduction); give antibiotics to combat infection if skin is broken or if surgery is necessary to reduce the break; hold the realigned limb in place by means of a plaster cast, pinning with metal screws or plates, strapping, or traction; and finally re-establish full range of movement with physiotherapy. Even while break is healing it is important to keep nearby joints as active as possible to prevent muscles wasting; the longer a joint is immobile, the greater the risk of OSTEOARTHRITIS at a later date. If break does not reunite, a bone graft may be necessary. Pulsed electromagnetic therapy, not yet widely available in Britain, can also help resistant breaks to heal; small electrical coils worn around the fracture induce tiny currents in the bone, stimulating the repair process.

Specific remedy to be taken twice a day for up to 3 weeks
- If a fracture is slow to heal *Symphytum 6c*

Frozen shoulder see also SHOULDER PROBLEMS
May be a consequence of minor injury, or a sequel to BURSITIS or TENDONITIS; pain provokes disuse, which provokes stiffness and pain, which provokes more disuse, until range of movement is minimal and pain is severe enough to disrupt sleep; although joint may gradually heal and pain disappear, mobility may be permanently restricted. If you suspect you have this condition, see your GP as soon as possible. Pain-killers, antirheumatic drugs, or steroid injections into shoulder joint may be prescribed, and possibly physiotherapy or manipulation under anaesthetic. See SHOULDER PROBLEMS for homeopathic remedies.

Ganglion
A small swelling in a joint capsule or in a sheath around a tendon; swelling is filled with a jelly-like substance which may be soft or quite firm; harmless and usually painless, and most common on wrist or upper surface of foot. If such a swelling develops, see your GP to make sure it is nothing serious. Surgery is seldom

advised as ganglia tend to recur and sometimes disappear of their own accord; instead, GP may try to disperse swelling with percussion.

Specific remedies to be taken 4 times daily for up to 7 days
- Ganglia in tendons on inside of arm or wrist *Ruta 6c*
- Ganglia associated with strong-smelling urine *Benzoic ac. 6c*

Gout see GOUT p. 259

Hand and wrist problems
Like other joints, those of hand and wrist can be affected by GOUT, BURSITIS, RHEUMATOID ARTHRITIS, and OSTEOARTHRITIS. A problem peculiar to the wrist is CARPAL TUNNEL SYNDROME (tenderness over inner aspect of wrist, numbness and tingling in thumb side of hand, pains shooting up the arm). Numbness or tingling in one or both hands, if combined with a chronically stiff neck and DIZZINESS on turning the head in certain directions, suggests CERVICAL SPONDYLOSIS. FEVER and pain in one wrist might indicate RHEUMATIC FEVER; if both wrists are involved INFECTIVE ARTHRITIS would be the likelier cause. Sudden pain extending from chest down into one or both arms and wrists is usually a symptom of ANGINA or a HEART ATTACK; if a heart attack is suspected, (999) and give First Aid (see p. 101). Wrists and hands are also subject to FRACTURES (see First Aid p. 99) and SPRAINS (see First Aid pp. 104–5). A fracture does not necessarily cause obvious deformity, but may nevertheless be painful and immobilizing; with a sprain, movement is still possible. In either case give *Arnica 30c* every 5 minutes for up to 10 doses.

Hernia see also HIATUS HERNIA
Bulging of soft tissue through a weak point in a sheet of muscle or between muscles – muscles may be congenitally weak, or weakened by overstrain or lack of use; most common in abdominal wall, occurring just above or below navel, or in fold between abdomen and thigh. Some hernias develop gradually, others suddenly, after strenuous lifting, for example; some produce a noticeable bulge, others merely a feeling of heaviness and tenderness. If a small portion of intestine protrudes through a weak point, there is a danger that it will become obstructed or, if blood supply is cut off, strangulated; if this happens, (999). A strangulated hernia looks very red and swollen and is extremely painful; an obstructed hernia causes ABDOMINAL PAIN, and NAUSEA AND VOMITING.

If you suspect that a bulge or area of tenderness may be a hernia, see your GP. Even if soft tissue can be pushed back inside hernia, muscle wall remains weak and hernia is likely to recur. Routine treatment is surgical repair of muscle wall, but until surgery can be arranged, you may have to wear a corset or truss.

Specific remedies to be taken 4 times daily for up to 14 days while waiting for surgery
- Remedy of first resort *Nux 6c*
- Hernia on right side of groin, cutting pain *Aesculus 6c*

Self-help Avoid lifting all but the lightest objects. After surgery, you should not attempt to lift anything heavy for at least 3 or 4 months.

Hip problems
The hip joint is the commonest site for OSTEOARTHRITIS; in severe cases, a hip replacement (replacing head and neck of femur with a steel prosthesis) is the only way to relieve pain and restore mobility; in chronic cases and after hip replacement constitutional homeopathic treatment is recommended; see OSTEOARTHRITIS for self-help measures.

Bursae over the greater trochanter of the femur can also become inflamed (see BURSITIS); ligaments and muscles holding head of femur in its socket can be over-stretched or torn (see SPRAINS, PULLED MUSCLES). Falls and other accidents can dislocate the joint or fracture femur or pelvis – see FRACTURES and DISLOCATIONS under First Aid; in either case the joint will be useless and painful. Congenital dislocation of the hip (see CONGENITAL DISORDERS) is evident at birth and is corrected by splinting the legs so that the head of the femur is kept pressed into the hip socket.

Housemaid's knee see KNEE PROBLEMS

Infective arthritis
A rare form of bacterial infection causing swelling, pain, and redness in a single joint, and FEVER; bacteria may invade joint through a wound or from an infection nearby, or be carried to joint through bloodstream. Prompt medical attention is necessary to prevent joint becoming permanently stiff, so (12); fluid may have to be drained off, and antibiotics will be prescribed.

Specific remedies to be taken every hour for up to 10 doses while medical help is being sought
- Infection comes on suddenly, high fever, pain, person very apprehensive *Aconite 30c*
- Joint swollen and painful, aggravated by slightest movement, sensitive to slightest touch *Bryonia 30c*
- High fever and delirium, slightest jarring to joint causes unbearable pain, person has red face and staring eyes *Belladonna 30c*
- Joint swollen with pus (at this late stage antibiotics are essential) and extremely sensitive to draughts or slightest pressure *Hepar sulph. 6c*

Knee problems
Like other important joints, knees can be affected by RHEUMATOID ARTHRITIS (loss of weight and appetite, muscular pains, then red, swollen, painful joints, with

stiffness most noticeable first thing in morning) and OSTEOARTHRITIS (episodes of pain, swelling, and stiffness, eventually knee may lock or give way); osteoarthritis of the hip may give pain in the corresponding knee. Knees can also be affected by GOUT (only one knee affected, pain and swelling come on in matter of hours, fever, joint unbearably tender) and by BURSITIS – *housemaid's knee* and 'water on the knee' are forms of bursitis, caused by injury or pressure.

Infections such as RHEUMATIC FEVER, OSTEO-MYELITIS, and INFECTIVE ARTHRITIS can involve knee joints. If any of these is suspected, [12]. All are of sudden onset, and involve fever, heat, swelling, and pain.

Knee injuries can take the form of FRACTURES (see First Aid p. 99), DISLOCATIONS (see First Aid p. 96), or damage to cartilages and ligaments (see SPRAINS and First Aid pp. 104–5). Unfortunately, all such injuries increase risk of OSTEOARTHRITIS at a later date. If knee is fractured or dislocated, there is severe pain, loss of movement, and deformity; appropriate action is (999), and *Arnica 30c* every 5 minutes until help arrives. If a ligament is torn, or if a cartilage is crushed or torn, as frequently happens in violent twisting injuries on the sports field, there will be escalating pain, stiffness, and swelling; appropriate action is (2). Joint will probably be put in plaster; while it is healing, it is important to do exercises to prevent thigh muscles wasting.

With its two extra pads of cartilage (menisci) between the articulating surfaces of the upper and lower leg bones, the knee is well adapted for load bearing, but with age the cartilage may start to disintegrate, causing the joint to jam or give way unexpectedly. If this happens, both pads of cartilage may have to be removed; the knee is left weaker but remains perfectly serviceable if used sensibly. Quadriceps exercises (tendon of quadriceps muscle keeps kneecap firmly in place) are important in post-operative period.

Specific remedies to be taken every 2 hours for up to 3 days
- Knee painful and swollen, skin over joint very dry, joint gives a cracking sound *Benzoic ac. 6c*
- Knees crack when walking *Causticum 6c*
- Knees feel stiff and sore, as if from a beating *Berberis 6c*
- Knees feel cold *Agnus 6c*

Leg problems
Pain in thigh or calf muscles may be PULLED MUSCLES (especially after unaccustomed exercise or exercising without warming up properly) or it may signal a vascular problem such as VARICOSE VEINS (legs ache, especially after prolonged standing), inflammation of a vein as in THROMBOPHLEBITIS (hard swelling, tenderness, or itchiness along length of vein), ARTERIOS-CLEROSIS or BUERGER'S DISEASE (pain worse with exercise, better for rest), CRAMP (comes on after strenuous or unaccustomed exercise, but quickly wears off), or DEEP VEIN THROMBOSIS (calf pain, with swelling and tenderness). Deep vein thrombosis requires prompt attention, so [12].

FRACTURES (see First Aid p. 99) can be caused by injury, OSTEOPOROSIS, or BONE TUMOURS; a fractured leg causes pain, loss of movement, and sometimes visible deformity; appropriate action is (999) and *Arnica 30c* every 5 minutes until help arrives.

Localized pain and FEVER, and feeling generally unwell, may indicate OSTEOMYELITIS. Pain which shoots down one leg when you sneeze or cough may be SCIATICA.

For homeopathic remedies, see conditions above as appropriate. If none of the remedies listed seems entirely suitable, choose one from the list below; if there is no improvement within 48 hours, see your GP.

Specific remedies to be taken every 2 hours for up to 2 days
- Shooting pains which shift around, or aching, rheumatic pains, causing limping and sudden muscle contractions *Belladonna 30c*
- Pains between calf and ankle, causing limping, or 'growing pains' in lower leg *Guaiacum 6c*
- Pains which shift around, noticeably worse in warm rooms *Kali sulph. 6c*
- Tearing pain worse in right leg, especially in hot thundery weather *Rhododendron 6c*
- Tearing pains and stiffness, made worse by cold wet weather and by not moving around, alleviated by gentle exercise *Rhus Tox. 6c*

Lumbago see also BACK PROBLEMS
Pain in small of back brought on by lifting or over-strenuous exercise; muscles may be strained or torn (see FIBROSITIS, PULLED MUSCLES) and go into spasm, or ligaments between vertebrae may be torn (see SPRAINS). Pain may be severe and immobilizing, and come on suddenly or develop overnight; chronic lumbago tends to be worse in cold or damp weather.

If rest and one of the remedies listed below do not produce some improvement within the dose period, see your GP or refer yourself to an osteopath or chiropractor.

Specific remedies to be taken every hour for up to 10 doses if back pain comes on suddenly
- Sharp pain made worse by exposure to cold dry weather and draughts *Aconite 30c*
- Severe pain comes on after injury *Arnica 30c*

Specific remedies to be taken 4 times daily for up to 10 days
- Lower back feels stiff and bruised, especially after resting and in damp cold weather, moving around reduces pain and stiffness *Rhus tox. 6c*

- Pain comes on in cold dry weather and is made worse by slightest movement, back feels bruised and sensitive to slightest touch *Bryonia 6c*
- Continuous pain, with nausea and vomiting, cold makes pain worse and causes cold sweats and fatigue, pain less insistent when standing up and moving around, eating aggravates pain *Antimonium tart. 6c*
- Violent stitching pain on stooping, aggravated by movement and especially bad at night in heat of bed *Sulphur 6c*
  Lumbago causes restlessness and prevents sleep *Cimicifuga 6c*
- Pain aggravated by stooping and by exertion followed by exposure to cold and damp *Dulcamara 6c*
- Lumbago worse before a thunderstorm or in dry cold weather *Rhododendron 6c*
- Lumbago aggravated by movement or a chill *Nux 6c*
- Lower back pain aggravated by walking and stooping *Aesculus 6c*

Self-help See BACK PROBLEMS for various self-help measures.

Lupus see SYSTEMIC LUPUS ERYTHEMATOSUS

Myasthenia gravis

An AUTOIMMUNE DISEASE in which muscles weaken because transmission of nerve impulses across nerve-muscle junctions is faulty; muscles of face and throat are usually affected first, causing DROOPING EYELIDS and DOUBLE VISION, and perhaps DIFFICULTY SWALLOWING or talking; arms and legs can also be affected. Condition is rare, mainly affects women, and is sometimes associated with a growth in the thymus gland, one of whose jobs is to destroy any lymphocytes which might attack the body's own cells. Degree of weakness can vary from day to day, but drug treatment or removal of thymus growth usually produces improvement. Constitutional homeopathic treatment might help.

Neck problems

A stiff neck accompanied by a severe HEADACHE, NAUSEA AND VOMITING, intolerance of light, ABNORMAL SLEEPINESS OR DROWSINESS, or CONFUSION, may be MENINGITIS or a subarachnoid haemorrhage (see BRAIN HAEMORRHAGE); immediate action is required, so ⑨⑨⑨ and give *Arnica 30c* every 5 minutes until help arrives.

'Whiplash' neck injuries (where the neck is flung violently backwards or forwards) are common in motor accidents. A PROLAPSED DISC in the neck makes any movement to straighten the neck extremely painful, sends shooting pains into shoulders and arms whenever you move your head, and may even cause hands and arms to feel tingly; if you suspect a disc injury, [12];

your GP will probably recommend that you wear a support collar for a while. Strained neck muscles and ligaments (see PULLED MUSCLES, SPRAINS) cause rapid stiffening and pain; if rest and appropriate homeopathic remedies do not relieve stiffness within 7 days, see your GP.

At worst, whiplash may cause SPINAL CORD INJURY (see First Aid p. 104) and some loss of sensation and movement below the neck; immediate help is vital, so ⑨⑨⑨ and if possible give *Arnica 30c* every 5 minutes until help arrives, and then *Hypericum 30c* every 8 hours for up to 5 days if possible.

Slow onset of pain and stiffness in the neck, with tingling in the hands, may denote CERVICAL SPONDYLOSIS. More prosaically, a stiff neck can be the result of sitting in a draught or lying in an awkward position; if the stiffness is not relieved within 24 hours by 6 doses of *Aconite 30c* taken at 2-hourly intervals, see your GP.

For other homeopathic remedies, see conditions mentioned above; if none seems particularly suitable, select a remedy from the list below. The author strongly recommends physiotherapy, osteopathy, and chiropractic as complementary treatments for neck problems.

Specific remedies to be taken 4-hourly for up to 3 days
- Neck stiff, with chin fixed in raised position, whole cervical and upper thoracic spine very sensitive *Cimicifuga 6c*
- Pain down right side of neck, with pain in upper arm and elbow, made worse by movement, more perspiration than usual *Lacnanthes 6c*
- Pain at top of nape of neck, as if from lying in awkward position, alleviated by heat, aggravated by becoming chilled in hot weather *Dulcamara 6c*
- Pain worse for slightest touch or movement *Bryonia 6c*
- Dull pain at top of nape of neck, with stiffness between shoulder blades, ache less insistent in wet weather *Causticum 6c*

Self-help Local heat can help to relax tense muscles. Use a firm, low pillow so that you lie with your neck as straight as possible.

Osteoarthritis (osteoarthrosis)

With age, injury, or overuse, cartilage covering articulating surfaces of bones breaks down; underlying bone becomes thickened and distorted, restricting joint movement and sometimes causing episodes of inflammation, pain, and swelling; joints most commonly affected are the load-bearing ones – hips, knees, and spine; 90 per cent of people over 40 have some degree of osteoarthritis in one or more joints. Condition can be aggravated by being overweight, by an over-acid diet, and by laxative abuse. Conventional treatments include painkillers, anti-inflammatory drugs, steroid injections into joints, physiotherapy to prevent muscles wasting, and replacement of worn joints, especially hips, with artificial ones; hip replacements have a high success rate, but may themselves have to be replaced within about 20–30 years.

Homeopathy offers constitutional treatment if osteoarthritis is chronic, but for isolated flare-ups the remedies below should be tried; if they do not improve matters, consult your GP or homeopath. Many sufferers get great benefit from osteopathy, chiropractic and physiotherapy, naturopathy and acupuncture.

Specific remedies to be taken 4 times daily for up to 2 weeks

- Pain relieved by heat but aggravated by cold and damp, more insistent when resting but wears off with continued movement, stiffness worse in morning *Rhus tox. 6c*
- Severe pain, made worse by heat and movement, relieved by cold applications *Bryonia 30c*
- Heat and warm rooms make joint pains worse, feeling weepy *Pulsatilla 6c*
- Affected joints feel cold and numb, pain and stiffness increase when weather changes, weakness on climbing stairs *Calcarea phos. 6c*
- For after effects of steroid injections, or for small joints, especially toes, which give pain and make cracking noises, joint pains seem to progress up the body, pain relieved by cold applications *Ledum 6c*
- Joints pains a consequence of, or made worse by, injury *Arnica 30c*
- Severe flare-up in cold dry weather *Aconite 30c*

Self-help Two-thirds of osteoarthritis sufferers find the Alkalinizing Diet (see p. 350) beneficial; stick strictly to the diet for 1 month, and see if it helps you. Take some of the weight off your joints by using a stick or by losing weight. Sleep on a firm bed and take several short rest periods during the day. Don't give up on exercise – your muscles need regular exercise to keep them strong. If you are severely disabled, contact the Disabled Living Foundation (address p. 358) for information on special equipment – long-handled dustpans, retrieving sticks, electrical plugs with handles on them, etc. Some sufferers say that green lipped mussel extract, devil's claw, and extra Vitamin B_5 help. Vitamins A, B, C and E, and also iron, zinc, copper, selenium, and manganese would certainly be beneficial.

Osteomalacia

Loss of bone tissue due to deficiency of Vitamin D (essential for absorbing calcium from food); deficiency may be caused by poor diet, lack of sunlight, chronic KIDNEY FAILURE, COELIAC DISEASE, or by drugs used to treat EPILEPSY. Symptoms are tender, painful bones which fracture easily, tiredness, and CRAMP; hip muscles may also become weak, making climbing stairs and getting out of chairs difficult, and causing a waddling gait. Unlike RICKETS, which at one time affected many children in Britain, osteomalacia is generally reversible, given regular amounts of Vitamin D.

Osteoporosis

Loss of bone mass due to ageing, prolonged inactivity, hormone changes, drugs (excess oral steroids as in CUSHING'S SYNDROME, and also drugs given for ASTHMA and RHEUMATOID ARTHRITIS), or calcium deficiency; bones remain same size and shape, but their honeycomb structure becomes less dense because bone is broken down faster than it is replaced; lighter bones fracture easily and heal slowly. Condition is more common in women than men because after the menopause the parathyroid glands produce less calcitonin, the hormone which stimulates bones to absorb calcium; in three-quarters of women bone loss is fairly slow, but by the age of 80 most women have lost between half and a quarter of their bone mass. Scientists returning from prolonged periods of weightlessness in Spacelab were found to have lost bone mass.

Though bone loss is not reversible, constitutional homeopathic treatment may help to slow the process down. For bone and joint pains, see remedies listed under BONE PAIN.

Self-help Increase intake of calcium and magnesium, and increase exercise to at least 3 hours a week. Try a more vegetarian diet. If the menopause is imminent, consult your GP about hormone replacement therapy; however, HRT should probably be discontinued after age 55 as there may be costs as well as benefits in the long term.

Paget's disease

Disease in which new bone is produced faster than old bone is destroyed; initially old bone is replaced by blood vessels and fibrous tissue; these then calcify, but never become as hard or as strong as healthy bone; cause is not known. Affected bones – usually pelvis and tibia, but also femur, collar bone, spine, and skull – are weakened and become more vulnerable to FRACTURES; they also ache all the time, especially at night, and may become misshapen. Complications include DEAFNESS (if auditory nerve is compressed), HEART FAILURE (extra vascular tissue in bones puts extra demands on heart), and BONE TUMOURS. Orthodox treatment is to relieve pain with analgesics or give regular injections of the hormone calcitonin to encourage bones to absorb more calcium. Homeopathic treatment is constitutional; as a temporary measure, one of the remedies given under BONE PAIN may be appropriate.

Self-help Extra Vitamin D, which has a similar action to calcitonin, may be beneficial in mild cases.

Paralysis see PARALYSIS p. 133

Polymyositis see DERMATOMYOSITIS AND
POLYMYOSITIS

Poliomyelitis see POLIO p. 134

Polymyalgia rheumatica

Inflammatory condition affecting connective tissue in
and around muscles, especially those of the shoulder
and pelvis, causing pain, tenderness, early morning
stiffness, and in some cases mild FEVER, WEIGHT LOSS,
and ANAEMIA; most common in women over age 50,
and often associated with TEMPORAL ARTERITIS;
eventually clears up of its own accord, though this may
take months or years. Routinely treated with steroids;
plenty of rest is also recommended. Homeopathic
treatment is constitutional, and may include nutritional
supplements and diet recommendations, investigation
of allergies, and bowel cleansing routines.

Prolapsed disc see also BACK PROBLEMS

Rupture of tough outer casing of an intervertebral disc,
allowing soft nucleus of disc to protrude and rupture
adjacent ligaments or press on a spinal nerve. Discs do
not really 'slip'; some 'slipped discs' are in fact
herniated discs (only partly ruptured) or prolapsed
discs (badly ruptured), but many are FIBROSITIS,
PULLED MUSCLES, or SPRAINS. Discs in lower back are
most vulnerable to prolapse since they bear the brunt of
injudicious lifting and twisting; unfortunately, unless
one is extremely careful, middle and lower back disc
injuries tend to recur; discs in the neck (see NECK
PROBLEMS) usually heal completely. Pain may come on
suddenly, when twisting or lifting, or build up
gradually; attempts to straighten back usually increase
pain; pains which shoot into the leg, described as
SCIATICA, indicate that injured disc is lumbar spine at
point of entry of sciatic nerve. If there is any weakness,
NUMBNESS, or tingling in arms or legs, or loss of
bladder or bowel control, ⑫. Orthodox treatment
includes rest and painkillers, and in bad cases
injections of local anaesthetic to numb affected nerves
or enzyme injections into injured disc; surgery to
remove pressure of disc on nerve is risky, and only
undertaken as a last resort.

Gentle manipulation, by a physiotherapist, osteopath, or chiropractor, can help to take pressure off
nerves and speed healing. For specific homeopathic
remedies, see BACK PROBLEMS, SCIATICA, NECK PROB-
LEMS. For self-help measures, see BACK PROBLEMS.

Pulled muscles

Overstrenuous or unaccustomed exercise can tear
individual muscle fibres, causing internal bleeding and
swelling, and immediate pain and stiffness as muscle
contracts. Conventionally treated with painkillers or
muscle relaxants; a crutch or a sling may be necessary,
followed by physiotherapy once muscle fibres have
healed. For ruptured muscles (muscles which have

been torn right through), only possible treatment may
be surgery.

Specific remedies
- Immediately after injury *Arnica 30c* every hour
  for up to 6 doses, then 4 times daily for up to 3
  days
- If pain persists after course of Arnica *Rhus tox. 6c*, 4
  times daily for up to 7 days

Self-help Rest until pain eases, then gently exercise
muscle to prevent stiffness; if exercise causes pain, stop
immediately.

Reiter's syndrome see SEXUALLY
TRANSMITTED DISEASES

Restless legs

Tickling, burning, or pricking sensation in lower legs,
causing involuntary twitching or jerking; condition
affects between 5 and 10 people in 100, seems to be
nervous in origin, partly hereditary, and is often
associated with DIABETES, iron or Vitamin B deficiency,
drug withdrawal, or over-consumption of caffeine.
Orthodox treatment consists of painkillers or tranquillizers.

Specific remedies to be taken 4 times daily for up to 14
days
- Legs twitching and jerking, irresistible urge to move
  them all the time, yawning *Tarentula 6c*
- Legs always on the move, general restlessness,
  anxiety, feeling chilly *Arsenicum 6c*
- Twitching worse when lying on right side, especially
  in elderly person with limb tremor, catnaps seem to
  steady limbs *Phosphorus 6c*
- Trembling, twitching feet and restless legs, even
  when asleep *Zinc 6c*
- Legs jerk, twitch, and tremble, and feel itchy and
  tingly, becoming even more uncomfortable in cold
  weather or in early sleep, causing person to wake
  with a start *Agaricus 6c*
- Legs jerk and go into spasm, person feels generally
  hot but has cold extremities, slightest jarring makes
  jerking worse, discomfort increases when trying to
  go to sleep *Belladonna 6c*
- Problem comes on after grief or broken love affair,
  legs jerk in sleep causing person to wake and despair
  of ever sleeping again *Ignatia 6c*
- Jerking worse between 2 and 4 am *Kali carb. 6c*
- Twitching and jerking worse during day but helped
  by exercise *Sepia 6c*

Self-help Warmth – warm socks or a hot water bottle –
is the best treatment for jumpy muscles. Make sure diet
contains plenty of folate and Vitamin E.

Rheumatic fever see RHEUMATIC FEVER p. 329

Rheumatism

Though muscular aches and pains in cold or damp weather are real enough to many elderly people, 'rheumatism' has no precise medical meaning. Vague muscular pains may be early warnings of RHEUMATOID ARTHRITIS, which only later affects the joints, or they may be the result of a virus infection such as INFLUENZA, a FOOD ALLERGY, or CANDIDIASIS, all of which can cause mild inflammation in muscle tissue. Muscular pains in the limbs are not part of the symptomology of OSTEOARTHRITIS, which affects joints only. While conventional medicine prescribes anti-inflammatory drugs and painkillers, homeopathic treatment is constitutional, although the remedies given below should be tried first.

Specific remedies to be taken 4 times daily for up to 14 days
- Aches and pains worse in cold dry weather, aggravated by movement, relieved by pressure *Bryonia 6c*
- Pains flit from one part of body to another, warm rooms make pains worse, feeling weepy, digestion upset by fatty foods *Pulsatilla 6c*
- Pains mainly in jaw and neck, with muscle spasms, pains tend to wear off in warm or wet weather *Causticum 6c*
- Aching and stiffness, especially in cold damp weather, in morning, or after rest, stiffness tends to wear off once person starts to move around, causing restlessness *Rhus tox. 6c*
- Pain and stiffness worse at night and during winter *Colchicum 6c*
- Pain and stiffness worse in cold damp weather, especially after becoming overheated *Dulcamara 6c*
- Aches and pains worse at night, with offensive sweats, discomfort made worse by both heat and cold *Mercurius 6c*
- Pain affects joints, especially larger joints, and tendinous insertions of muscles rather than muscles themselves *Ruta 6c*
- Aches and pains in muscles and ligaments, discomfort more insistent in sultry, thundery weather, and in cold weather *Rhododendron 6c*
- Sharp pains in wrists and hands *Calcarea hypophos. 6c*
- Sharp pains which onset suddenly, especially in cold dry weather, general feeling of anxiety and restlessness *Aconite 6c*

Self-help Follow the Alkalinizing Diet (p. 350) for 1 month. If aches and pains subside, continue to eat a moderate amount of alkalinizing foods. Also, take extra Vitamin B$_6$, magnesium, and calcium.

Rheumatoid arthritis

An AUTOIMMUNE disease in which the linings (synovial membranes) of joint capsules become inflamed and swollen; inflammation spreads to other joint tissues and, in severe cases, to the bones themselves, causing deformity, DISLOCATION, and disability. Joint symptoms may onset suddenly or be preceded by vague muscular pains, WEIGHT LOSS, loss of appetite (see APPETITE CHANGES), and feeling generally unwell; in many sufferers, inflammation affects tissues of heart and blood vessels as well as joints; some sufferers also develop ANAEMIA. Condition mainly affects smaller joints, chiefly knuckles and toe joints, but also wrists, neck, ankles, and knees; pain and stiffness are worst in morning, but tend to wear off as day progresses. Nearly half of all sufferers recover completely after one or more attacks. Routinely treated with painkillers, steroids and other anti-inflammatory drugs, and physiotherapy; surgery is considered risky, but may be advised in special cases. Homeopathic treatment is constitutional, with special attention to diet and nutrition; for specific remedies see ARM PROBLEMS, ANKLE PROBLEMS, BACK PROBLEMS, ELBOW PROBLEMS, FOOT PROBLEMS, HAND AND WRIST PROBLEMS, HIP PROBLEMS, KNEE PROBLEMS, LEG PROGLEMS, NECK PROBLEMS, SHOULDER PROBLEMS.

Self-help Take regular, moderate exercise – swimming is excellent for keeping joints mobile, especially if pool is heated. Plenty of rest is also important – if you can, take a nap or two during the day. If you are severely disabled and need special aids or appliances, contact the Disabled Living Foundation (address p. 385). Extra Vitamin B$_6$, B$_3$, B$_5$, C, and E, and also zinc are recommended, as are evening primrose oil and green lipped mussel extract. Wearing a copper bracelet might also be beneficial.

Sacroiliac pain see BACK PROBLEMS

Sciatica

Nerve pain caused by compression of, or presssure on, sciatic nerve supplying leg; can be caused by a PROLAPSED DISC or disc degeneration, by OSTEOARTHRITIS (distorted or thickened vertebrae), or by ANKYLOSING SPONDYLITIS (fusion of facet joints between vertebrae); pains shoot into buttock and leg, especially when bending, sneezing, or coughing; standing may be more comfortable than sitting. Orthodox treatment depends on cause of pain, but options include painkillers, muscle relaxants, steroid injections, and physiotherapy. Osteopathy, chiropractic and acupuncture also offer relief from the pain of trapped nerves. Homeopathy offers the remedies listed below; if these do not produce some improvement, see your GP or homeopath.

Specific remedies to be taken every hour for up to 10 doses, or every 30 minutes if pain is acute
- Pain shoots down right leg to foot, causing occasional numbness and weakness, pain seems worse in cold or damp weather *Colocynth 6c*

- Pain worse when sitting, difficulty straightening knee of affected leg because hamstring has shortened, pain wears off when walking, lying down, or sleeping *Ammonium mur. 6c*
- Severe pain, numbness, and cramps in affected leg, made worse by movement, alleviated by rest and sitting down *Gnaphalium 6c*
- Tearing pain, relieved by heat and movement, but aggravated by inactivity, cold, and damp *Rhus tox. 6c*
- Sciatic pain in invalid or elderly person, worse at night and aggravated by cold, improves with gentle exercise *Arsenicum 6c*
- Pain in right leg, aggravated by pressure and lying on right side, most severe between 4 and 8 pm *Lycopodium 6c*
- Tearing pains, especially in right leg, bending backwards relieves pain but most other movements, including sitting up, make pain worse *Dioscorea 6c*
- Pain in left leg, aggravated by both heat and cold, increasing stiffness and difficulty walking *Carbon sulph. 6c*
- Burning pains shooting into knee and foot, aggravated by coughing, leg feels itchy, pain especially bad around 3 am *Kali carb. 6c*
- Lightning-like pains in right leg, soothed by heat, aggravated by coughing *Magnesia phos. 6c*
- Burning pains especially bad at night, preventing sleep, also bad after rest or as you start to walk *Gelsemium 6c*

Self-help See BACK PROBLEMS.

Scleroderma

A very rare AUTOIMMUNE DISEASE in which connective tissue in and around smallest blood vessels (capillaries) becomes inflamed, then shrinks and hardens; if this happens to capillaries in heart, lungs, or kidneys, result may be HEART FAILURE, RESPIRATORY FAILURE, or KIDNEY FAILURE; more commonly, skin and oesophagus are affected, the skin becoming unbearably tight and the oesophagus stiff and resistant to swallowing (see DIFFICULTY SWALLOWING). Conventionally treated with steroids and penicillamine (an anti-rheumatic). Homeopathic treatment is constitutional.

Self-help If scleroderma is diagnosed, avoid all forms of heat.

Severed tendon

If you are unable to move fingers or toes properly after a bad cut or injury to the corresponding hand, forearm, foot, or calf, you may have severed a tendon; appropriate action is (999) and *Arnica 30c* every 5 minutes for up to 6 doses. Surgery may be needed to locate severed, retracted ends of tendon and sew them together; repairs to foot tendons are generally more successful than repairs to hand tendons.

Specific remedy to be taken 4 times daily for up to 1 week
- After Arnica, to assist healing *Ruta 6c*

Shoulder problems see also FROZEN SHOULDER FRACTURES (see First Aid p. 99) and DISLOCATIONS (see First Aid p.96) are most serious kinds of injury to shoulder, causing pain, loss of movement, and visible deformity; appropriate action is (999) and *Arnica 30c* every 5 minutes for up to 10 doses. Strenuous exercise or overuse can also result in PULLED MUSCLES, SPRAINS, and BURSITIS, though shoulder will still be movable. Standard treatment is to put arm in sling to rest shoulder joint until it heals, then physiotherapy.If shoulder dislocates repeatedly, an operation to tighten ligaments or build up rim of shoulder socket may be necessary. OSTEOARTHRITIS may develop in a shoulder joint which has been injured and immobilized for any length of time; another consequence of injury may be FROZEN SHOULDER (stiffness, pain, loss of mobility).

RHEUMATOID ARTHRITIS (swelling, stiffness, and pain) is uncommon in shoulder joints and GOUT even less common.

Choose appropriate homeopathic remedy from those listed under conditions mentioned above; if none seems particularly suitable, choose one of the remedies below. If shoulder pain persists, see your GP or homeopath.

Specific remedies to be given 4 times daily for up to 14 days
- Rheumatic pain in right shoulder, wears off during sleep but is made worse by movement or pressure *Sanguinaria 6c*
- Pain in right shoulder, especially around lower angle of shoulder blade, headache *Chelidonium 6c*
- Rheumatic pain in shoulder, relieved by walking, cold makes pain worse, as does sitting still or getting overheated, pain most intense around midnight *Ferrum 6c*
- Burning pain in shoulder, worse in cold damp weather and after sleep or rest, pains wear off with gentle exercise *Rhus tox. 6c*
- Rheumatic pain in left shoulder, which feels dead and heavy, tendency to bring shoulder forward as if protecting chest *Sulphur 6c*

Self-help Rest is the best medicine. Hot or cold applications may help to ease pain.

Sjogrens syndrome

A fairly rare AUTOIMMUNE DISEASE characterized by dry eyes, dry mouth, and painful joints, sometimes accompanied by an increase in respiratory tract infections, HAIR LOSS, and damage to nails (see NAIL PROBLEMS). See RHEUMATOID ARTHRITIS for conventional and homeopathic treatment.

Slipped disc see PROLAPSED DISC

Sprains see also FIRST AID p. 105

Partial or complete rupture of ligaments which hold joints together; most vulnerable joints are ankles, wrists, knees, and fingers. A mild sprain causes some pain and swelling, but joint remains functional; rest, a support bandage, ice packs to reduce swelling, and then very careful resumption of use is all that is required. A severe sprain, in which most of the ligaments around a joint are torn, may be mistaken for a FRACTURE; joint quickly swells, stiffens, and becomes too painful to move, and may need to be immobilized in plaster for several weeks; very badly torn ligaments may need to be repaired surgically; in either case, physiotherapy will be necessary to restore range of movement.

Specific remedy to be taken every 12 hours for up to 1 week
- Recurrent sprained ankle *Natrum carb. 30c*

Systemic lupus erythematosus (SLE)

An AUTOIMMUNE DISEASE which causes inflammation of connective tissue, in particular of membranes around joints (with symptoms similar to those of RHEUMATOID ARTHRITIS) and around lungs, kidneys, heart, and other organs; red rash also develops on cheeks and may involve entire upper body. Condition is rare, but mostly affects women aged 30–50; may be triggered off by an infection, by exposure to strong sunlight, by certain drugs, including oral contraceptives, and by excessive consumption of alfalfa sprouts, seeds, or juice. First signs may be mild but persistent FEVER, flitting joint pains, characteristic butterfly-shaped rash on cheeks, HAIR LOSS, WEIGHT LOSS, and poor appetite (see APPETITE CHANGES); later, there may be circulation problems, leading to RAYNAUD'S DISEASE and VARICOSE ULCERS; in some cases, persistent inflammation of the kidneys leads to KIDNEY FAILURE.

Orthodox treatment is to give steroids and immuno-suppressive drugs to slow down progress of disease, and regularly check for protein in urine to assess state of kidneys.

The author's approach to this and other auto-immune diseases is multi-pronged, a combination of constitutional homeopathic treatment, attention to diet, vitamin and mineral supplements, allergy identification, perhaps a bowel cleansing routine, and rest.

Tendonitis

Tearing of fibres in tendons (which connect muscles to bones), causing inflammation, soreness, and pain; usually caused by injury or overuse; Achilles tendon in heel is particularly vulnerable, as are tendons in elbows, causing *tennis elbow* and *golfer's elbow* (see ELBOW PROBLEMS), although hitting balls is not a prerequisite! If the specific remedies and self-help measures mentioned below do not improve matters within 7 days, see your GP; steroid injections may be given in bad cases.

Specific remedies to be taken 4 times daily for up to 7 days
- Tearing pain aggravated by rest, movement, or damp weather, wears off with continued movement *Rhus tox. 6c*
- Tearing pain, lameness, affected ankle feels bruised and broken *Ruta 6c*

Self-help Rest and support are important for the first few days after injury – bandage affected ankle and calf, or put arm in a sling, and use limb as little as possible. Then start exercising very gently, avoiding movements which caused tendon to tear in first place; tendon may take two or three months to heal properly.

Tennis elbow see ELBOW PROBLEMS, TENDONITIS

Tenosynovitis

Inflammation of membrane sheath around certain tendons, notably those attached to bones of fingers and thumb; as membrane heals it may shrink, restricting movement or causing jerky movements known as *trigger finger*. Often occupational in origin, affecting people who do repetitive work with their hands, but occasionally caused by infection. Affected fingers hurt and make a soft cracking sound on bending or straightening. Orthodox treatment is non-steroidal, anti-inflammatory drugs.

Specific remedies to be taken every 2 hours for up to 10 doses in acute cases
- Affected finger hot and swollen, with stinging pains *Apis 30c*
- Condition caused by injury *Arnica 30c* followed by *Ruta 6c*
- Slightest movement makes fingers hurt *Bryonia 30c*
- Affected finger swollen, movement more painful after rest and in cold damp weather, eased by warmth and gentle movement *Rhus tox. 6c*

Specific remedy to be taken 4 times daily for up to 14 days if condition is chronic; if no improvement within 14 days, see your GP or homeopath
- *Causticum 6c*

Self-help Use the affected hand as little as possible; hot or cold applications will help to reduce pain.

Wrist problems see HAND AND WRIST PROBLEMS

OESOPHAGUS, STOMACH, AND DUODENUM

THE digestive processes begun in the mouth continue in the stomach and duodenum. Food is rhythmically squeezed down the oesophagus, a muscular tube about 24 cm (10 in) long, past a one-way sphincter or valve, and into the stomach. Usually food stays in the stomach for 3 or 4 hours, then enters the duodenum through another one-way sphincter, but a fatty meal can slow the process down, just as great stress can speed it up.

When we see or smell food, or anticipate a good meal, the brain not only tells certain cells in the stomach lining to start secreting digestive chemicals but also tells others to secrete the hormone gastrin, which sets full-scale production of digestive juices in train. The most important chemicals produced by the stomach are hydrochloric acid and the enzymes pepsin and lipase. The acid produced by the stomach is of sufficient strength to liquefy meat and to kill the bacteria in food, efficiently protecting the rest of the digestive system from infection caused by putrefaction; it is also necessary for the absorption of calcium, iron, and other nutrients. Pepsin breaks down proteins into smaller units and lipase has a similar effect on fats; both enzymes require an acid environment. However, if the stomach did not also have millions of mucus-producing cells in its walls, it would start to digest itself; ulcers are, in effect, areas where the mucous lining has been destroyed.

Although the stomach mostly secretes substances which break food down, it also absorbs small molecules such as water, salts, Vitamin B_{12}, and alcohol, and feeds them into the bloodstream.

Once in the duodenum, semi-digested food is made alkaline and further broken down by secretions from the pancreas, and any untreated fat in it is emulsified or broken down into very small droplets by bile from the gall bladder. Both the pancreas and gall bladder have ducts which open into the duodenum, and the flow of digestive juices through them is controlled by a series of hormones secreted as soon as food mixed with acid enters the duodenum.

Achalasia

Loss of nervous coordination of rhythmic squeezing movements (peristalsis) at lower end of oesophagus, causing build-up of swallowed food, pain on swallowing, CHEST PAIN, bad breath, a nasty taste in the mouth, and eventually WEIGHT LOSS and malnutrition. Cause is not known, though Vitamin E deficiency may be a contributory factor. At first fluids are difficult to swallow, then solids too; if food is regurgitated, it may spill into the lungs and cause PNEUMONIA. Condition is diagnosed by barium swallow and/or endoscopy, then treated by antispasmodic drugs, by stretching the muscles at the base of the oesophagus with water-filled

bags or special dilator rods (bougies), or by cutting through some of the muscles at the entrance to the stomach (cardiomyotomy).

ACHALASIA IS BEST TREATED BY AN EXPERIENCED HOMEOPATH, but the remedies below may help to relieve discomfort while treatment is being sought.

Specific remedies to be taken 4 times daily for up to 3 weeks
- Remedy of first choice *Cimicifuga 6c*
- Symptoms accompanied by a dry throat which feels plugged up, and by chronic constipation and straining even when stools are soft, only small amounts can be swallowed at a time *Alumina 6c*
- Heartburn, craving for ice-cold water which is vomited up as soon as it becomes warm in stomach, food regurgitated shortly after swallowing, sour taste in mouth, sour belching *Phosphorus 6c*

Self-help Vitamin E is recommended.

Acid secretion problems

The acid-producing cells in stomach can produce too much or too little hydrochloric acid; either condition can cause INDIGESTION.

Over-acidity is one of the causes of PEPTIC ULCER and GASTRITIS. Coffee, especially decaffeinated coffee, increases acid production. Under-acidity allows food to ferment in the stomach, causing BAD BREATH, BELCHING, and flatulence. Marijuana, pollutants such as DDT, and FEVER seem to depress acid production. Among the conditions associated with under-production of acid are PERNICIOUS ANAEMIA, ASTHMA, OSTEOPOROSIS, DIABETES (diabetes mellitus), food ALLERGY, RHEUMATOID ARTHRITIS, THYROID PROBLEMS, COELIAC DISEASE, and ECZEMA.

For homeopathic remedies, see INDIGESTION or PEPTIC ULCER, or read whichever of the above entries seems appropriate. Normalizing acid secretion by making dietary or lifestyle changes is infinitely preferable to taking antacids, drugs, or supplements of hydrochloric acid on a long-term basis.

Appetite changes see also ANOREXIA, BULIMIA

Loss of appetite is quite common in acute or chronic illness, can be aggravated by drugs, and can be directly caused by gross over-consumption of Vitamins A and D, and fluoride, or by a deficiency of iron, zinc, Vitamin B_1, folate, or biotin. Appetite usually returns to normal once the offending substance is withdrawn or the deficiency made up, but if there is no improvement within 3 or 4 weeks, consult your GP or homeopath. In rare cases continuing loss of appetite is an early sign of CANCER OF THE STOMACH.

Specific remedies to be taken every 8 hours for up to 2 weeks, provided appetite loss is not due to excess or deficiency, drugs, or a diagnosed illness

- Loss of appetite caused by grief, complete loss of interest in food (solids and fluid), cigarettes, etc., but no aversion to them *Ignatia 30c*
- Person not at all thirsty, has a particular aversion to fat and eggs *Pulsatilla 30c*
- Person put off food by bitter taste in mouth, yellow tongue, and feeling generally 'hung over' *Nux 30c*
- Person hungry but feels full up after just a few mouthfuls, a lot of wind in stomach *Lycopodium 30c*

Specific remedy to be taken after acute illness, when person has no appetite but feels in need of a tonic

- *Gentiana 3x*, 5 drops to be taken ½ hour before meals for up to 10 days

Increased appetite may be a symptom of hyperthyroidism (general speeding up of all body processes – see THYROID PROBLEMS), HYPOGLYCAEMIA, and sometimes DEPRESSION; in BULIMIA, sudden craving for huge amounts of food is followed by guilt, self-induced vomiting, and abuse of laxatives.

Specific remedies to be given 3 times daily for up to 2 weeks

- Increased appetite but no corresponding weight gain, feeling hot and faint, with gnawing pains in stomach if food is not eaten at regular intervals, person increasingly forgetful so checks everything twice *Iodum 6c*
- Increased appetite accompanied by weight loss, especially around neck, and craving for salt *Natrum mur 6c*
- Increased appetite associated with worms *Cina 6c*
- Non-stop craving for food *Psorinum 6c*
- Increased appetite, but a feeling of fullness after just a few mouthfuls *Lycopodium 6c*

Cravings and aversions are well known in pregnancy, and in some cases are an indication of deficiency or food ALLERGY. Homeopaths take special note of food likes and dislikes when prescribing constitutionally. Remedies for specific cravings and aversions will be found in the Food and Drink section of the General Remedy Finder (see pp. 68–71).

Belching (eructation) see also INDIGESTION, WIND

Usually caused by swallowing air when nervous or by eating too fast; to relieve discomfort in the stomach, the air is regurgitated as wind. Belching may also be a symptom of INDIGESTION, especially after rich food, HIATUS HERNIA (if bending or lying down makes wind worse), PYLORIC STENOSIS, or GALLSTONES (wind after eating fatty food); wind is also common in babies, and in the later stages of pregnancy, as the uterus presses on the stomach.

Specific remedies to be taken every ½ hour for up to 10 doses

- If belching relieves discomfort *Carbo veg. 6c*
- If belching does not relieve discomfort *China 6c*
- Craving for sweet things, abdomen distended, diarrhoea, wind made worse by worrying about some future event *Argentum nit. 6c*
- Person very hungry, feels full after a few mouthfuls of food, produces a lot of wind *Lycopodium 6c*
- Belching accompanied by nausea, person feels worse in hot rooms *Pulsatilla 6c*.

Self-help See INDIGESTION.

Blood in vomit see also NAUSEA AND VOMITING

May look red or, if partially digested by stomach, like coffee grounds. If caused by violent or repeated vomiting, 48. Can also be caused by a bleeding PEPTIC ULCER, CANCER OF THE STOMACH, or bleeding from swollen oesophageal veins associated with CIRRHOSIS OF THE LIVER; if person is known to have any of these conditions, (999) and give *Phosphorus 30c* every 5 minutes for up to 6 doses until help arrives.

Cancer of the oesophagus see also CANCER

A rare form of cancer thought to be associated with heavy smoking and drinking, and perhaps molybdenum deficiency. First symptom is difficulty or pain on swallowing solids and then liquids; tumour grows fairly swiftly, increasing swallowing difficulties and causing rapid WEIGHT LOSS. Prompt surgery and radiotherapy are usually necessary. See CANCER for homeopathic treatment.

Cancer of the stomach see also CANCER

Much more common than oesophageal cancer and twice as common in men as in women. May be due to heavy smoking and drinking, nutritional deficiencies, or excessive amounts of nitrite in diet. Usually starts as a PEPTIC ULCER, though very few peptic ulcers become malignant: symptoms are pain in upper abdomen, WEIGHT LOSS, NAUSEA AND VOMITING, and sometimes BLOOD IN VOMIT or BLOOD IN FAECES. In the early stages surgery may be successful; later, if surgery is not feasible, radiotherapy is given to retard growth of tumour.

There are specific homeopathic remedies for stomach cancer, Ornithogallum for example, but THEY SHOULD ONLY BE TAKEN UNDER THE GUIDANCE OF AN EXPERIENCED HOMEOPATH.

Difficulty swallowing (dysphagia)

May be brought on by ANXIETY, which interferes with nervous control of peristalsis and usually feels like a ball or lump in the throat; a fishbone lodged in the throat can cause coughing and pain on swallowing (see p. 95 for First Aid treatment); some narrowing of the throat is quite normal with a SORE THROAT or

TONSILLITIS; if food feels stuck high up in chest and pain worsens when you bend or lie down, cause may be HIATUS HERNIA or reflux oesophagitis (see under HIATUS HERNIA) or STRICTURE OF THE OESOPHAGUS; pain on swallowing, accompanied by inexplicable WEIGHT LOSS of more than 0.5 kg (1 lb) per week, may be CANCER OF THE OESOPHAGUS, in which case 48.

See remedies under conditions above; if none diagnosed try these specific remedies to be given every 4 hours for up to 2 days

- Throat feels as if there is a lump in it, but swallowing otherwise normal *Ignatia 30c*
- Person can't stand scarves or tight clothes around neck *Lachesis 30c*
- Throat feels as if fishbone stuck in it, but no fishbone swallowed *Nitric ac. 30c*
- Muscles go into spasm on swallowing *Stramonium 30c*

Duodenal ulcer see PEPTIC ULCER

Dysphagia see DIFFICULTY SWALLOWING

Food poisoning see FOOD POISONING p. 276, SALMONELLOSIS

Foreign bodies, swallowed

Though extremely worrying, swallowed objects are not necessarily a cause for alarm, provided they are smooth. If a child has just swallowed a marble, for example, holding him or her upside down will probably expel it; if it has travelled further along the digestive tract, 12; it may be passed in the faeces in 2–3 days, provided child does not suffer from constipation; if the object is not excreted, or if the child has difficulty swallowing, or stomach pain, or FEVER, endoscopy may be necessary to remove it. Sharp objects such as needles and fishbones, however, can cause a lot of damage and should be removed as soon as possible, so ②.

Gastric erosion and gastritis

Localized inflammation of and damage to the stomach lining is known as gastric erosion, and general inflammation of the stomach lining as gastritis; repeated bouts of gastritis can lead to gastric erosion. In both cases the culprit may be aspirin, steroids and other antiflammatory drugs, nicotine, or alcohol; occasionally, gastritis is caused by a virus infection. Symptoms of gastritis are those of INDIGESTION or, if virally caused, of GASTROENTERITIS. Gastric erosion causes bleeding, which can go on for some time without the sufferer being aware of it; first signs may be dark or black streaks in stools, or vomiting, with 'coffee grounds' (partially digested blood) in vomit; if bleeding continues, symptoms of ANAEMIA develop.

If person is vomiting blood, ⑨⑨⑨ and give *Phosphorus 30c* every 5 minutes for up to 10 doses; a blood transfusion may be necessary if a lot of blood has been lost. If persistent indigestion develops while taking drugs mentioned above, 48; alternative drugs may have to be prescribed.

If symptoms are those of gastritis, homeopathic treatment is the same as that for INDIGESTION and GASTROENTERITIS; if symptoms are those of gastric erosion, remedies for ANAEMIA would be appropriate.

Self-help To allow stomach to heal, fast for 24 hours, taking nothing but boiled cooled water. Then, for the next 24 hours, take only arrowroot, tapioca, or semolina, and water. On the third and fourth day, eat lightly and often – bland foods such as potatoes, brown rice (well chewed), and mashed apples are good, but avoid acid foods. On the fifth day, resume normal diet, and follow self-help suggestions given under INDIGESTION. If you smoke or drink . . . stop. Extra Vitamin C and Zinc would also be beneficial.

Gastritis see GASTRIC EROSION AND GASTRITIS

Gastroenteritis (gastric flu) see GASTROENTERITIS p. 276

Hiatus hernia see also INDIGESTION

Caused by a weakening of the tissue around the hole (hiatus) in the diaphragm through which the oesophagus descends to the stomach; this allows the top of the stomach to protrude up through the diaphragm, exerting back pressure on the valve between it and the oesophagus; this gradually weakens the valve, allowing acid from the stomach to well up into the oesophagus (reflux oesophagitis). This backflow of acid is felt as heartburn, a burning pain in the chest; pain sometimes extends to the neck and arms, and may be mistaken for ANGINA; bending or lying down encourages backflow and so makes discomfort worse. If condition is not treated, oesophagus may become ulcerated – in rare cases the ulcers bleed and lead to ANAEMIA – or very scarred, leading to STRICTURE OF THE OESOPHAGUS. Conventionally treated by giving antacids, taken after meals, to neutralize the acid floating on top of the stomach contents (however, antacids may not be appropriate if person has HIGH BLOOD PRESSURE, kidney disease, KIDNEY STONES, or intestinal bleeding); also by giving drugs which increase rate at which stomach empties; surgery is a last resort.

Homeopathic remedies are the same as those given for INDIGESTION.

Self-help If you are overweight, try to lose weight (hiatus hernia is seldom helped or cured in people who remain overweight). Eat slowly, so that you do not swallow air, and never have a meal late at night. Avoid stooping, especially after meals. Raise the head of your bed by 10 cm (4 in) or so – if you cannot do this because you have swollen ankles, see your GP. Wear loose clothing. Avoid alcohol and smoking. Slippery Elm Food, taken last thing at night, is often beneficial.

Hiccups see HICCUPS pp. 180–1

Indigestion

A blanket term for hiccups, belching, vague discomfort after eating, heartburn, CHEST PAIN, stomach ache, acidity (see ACID SECRETION PROBLEMS), and wind. The mechanisms of digestion – the automatic muscle contractions of the gut, and the secretion and flow of various digestive fluids, enzymes, and hormones – can be upset by emotions such as ANXIETY, rage, fear, resentment, and impatience; they also become less efficient as we get older; and they can be aided or hindered by the kind of food we eat. Citrus fruits, fruit skins, cooked cabbage, tomatoes, onions, cucumbers, beans and pulses, nuts, bread, pork, spices, wine, neat spirits, fizzy drinks, and rich fatty foods are all quite difficult to digest and cause flatulence unless eaten in small quantities; tea, coffee, and refined carbohydrates also interfere with stomach function. Eating too much at once, eating too quickly, or swallowing air while eating also cause indigestion. Pregnancy, smoking, CONSTIPATION, and OBESITY also reduce digestive efficiency.

Most minor indigestion problems are amenable to the self-help measures outlined below. However, if indigestion is long-standing and chronic, constitutional homeopathic treatment is recommended. Over-the-counter antacid preparations may give temporary relief, but they should not be taken on a regular basis, nor if you suffer from HIGH BLOOD PRESSURE, kidney disease, KIDNEY STONES, or any form of intestinal bleeding.

If digestive problems do not seem to be related to any of the factors mentioned above, or if digestive patterns change over a period of 1–2 months without obvious reason, see your GP; other possible causes of 'indigestion' are food ALLERGY, HYPO-GLYCAEMIA, CANDIDIASIS, HIATUS HERNIA, STRICTURE OF THE OESOPHAGUS, reflux oesophagitis (see HIATUS HERNIA) GALL STONES, CHOLECYSTITIS, PANCREATITIS, CANCER OF THE PANCREAS, PEPTIC ULCER, and CANCER OF THE STOMACH.

If indigestion is accompanied by vomiting, with blood in vomit, (999) and give *Phosphorus 30c* every 5 minutes for up to 10 doses. If there is agonizing pain radiating towards back, with or without vomiting, (2).

Specific remedies to be given every 10–15 minutes for up to 7 doses during acute attacks
- Stomach feels full of wind even after eating plainest food, belching gives some relief, digestion seems slower than usual, faint burning sensation in stomach goes through to back, craving for fresh air *Carbo veg. 30c*

- Heartburn ½ hour after eating, painful retching leaves putrid taste in mouth, attack brought on by too much food, too much alcohol, or too much work, person irritable *Nux 6c*
- Attack brought on by rich food, beginning 2 hours after eating, attacks worse in evening, feeling of pressure under breastbone, pounding heart, bad taste in mouth, headache around eyes, nausea with or without vomiting, weepiness *Pulsatilla 6c*
- Heartburn after food, worse in small hours of morning, stomach feels as if there is a stone weight in it, person retches and vomits until exhausted, then feels chilly and restless, but better for warmth and small sips of water, peptic ulcer suspected *Arsenicum 6c*
- 'Heavy stone in the stomach' feeling comes on soon after food, with heartburn, nausea, and faintness, mouth fills with bitter tasting fluid (waterbrash) person gulps down cold drinks, feels worse for pressure or slightest movement, but better for lying on back *Bryonia 6c*
- Stomach full of wind, bloated feeling not relieved by belching, recent loss of body fluids (sweat, blood, semen), person sluggish and apathetic, feels worse at night, stools have 'chopped egg' appearance *China 6c*
- Indigestion comes on 1 to 2 hours after meals, though can be delayed by eating again, foul taste in mouth, stomach feels blocked up, cold drinks make things worse, urge to pass stool ineffectual, person tends to be forgetful, peptic ulcer suspected *Anacardium 6c*
- A lot of belching, especially after sweet foods, alternating constipation and diarrhoea, fluttery feeling in stomach, suspected peptic ulcer *Argentum nit. 6c*
- Sudden empty feeling in stomach, especially in evening, relieved by eating, craving for pickles and acid foods, tongue white-coated, sour taste in mouth, a lot of flatulence, tenderness over liver, person nauseated by smell of food, feels better lying on right side *Sepia 6c*
- Heartburn, stomach bloated and full of gas, person quickly feels full up even when hungry, mainly because food causes almost instant indigestion, discomfort not relieved by belching, constipation, suspected peptic ulcer *Lycopodium 6c*
- Burning sensation in chest, craving for ice-cold water, which is vomited up as soon as it becomes warm in stomach, likely peptic ulcer *Phosphorus 6c*
- Burning hunger pangs relieved by food or hot drinks (especially milk) but soon followed by indigestion, person nauseated by sweet things, suspected peptic ulcer *Graphites 6c*
- Nausea and vomiting after drinking beer, a feeling that all digestive processes have stopped, stomach distended and painful in a particular spot, likely peptic ulcer *Kali bichrom. 6c*

Self-help Relax or meditate for a few minutes (see pp. 27–9 for hints on stress reduction) before you eat; eat calmly, sitting down; and try to relax for at least 30 minutes after eating. Avoid late-night eating and foods which particularly upset you. Reduce coffee, tea, and alcohol consumption and try to stop smoking. If flatulence is the main problem, steer clear of pulses, onions, cabbage, etc. and try cooking your food with cumin, aniseed, or ginger.

If stomach is not producing sufficient hydrochloric acid, there are acid-containing supplements available; however these should only be taken under direction of your GP.

Loss of appetite see APPETITE CHANGES

Nausea and vomiting see also TRAVEL SICKNESS, BLOOD IN VOMIT

Bouts of nausea, with or without vomiting, which last less than 24 hours are often associated with MIGRAINE (one-sided headache, visual disturbances), GASTRO-ENTERITIS (diarrhoea), acute GASTRITIS (after fatty foods or bingeing on alcohol), FOOD POISONING (after eating contaminated food), LABYRINTHITIS and MENIERE'S DISEASE (disturbed balance), JAUNDICE (whites of eyes turn yellow), WHOOPING COUGH (repeated spasms of coughing), and urinary tract infections (pain or frequently passing water). If nausea, with or without vomiting, occurs frequently or lasts, on and off, for more than a day or two, the cause is more likely to be a drug, HIATUS HERNIA (heartburn, worse bending or lying down), chronic GASTRITIS (especially if nausea follows alcohol), CHOLECYSTITIS (fever and pain under right ribs), GALLSTONES, or PYLORIC STENOSIS (stomach very distended, foul belching).

Nausea and vomiting can also be indicators of more serious conditions such as a PEPTIC ULCER (especially if it bleeds or perforates), severe GASTRIC EROSION, APPENDICITIS, a BRAIN INJURY, a subarachnoid or subdural BRAIN HAEMORRHAGE, a BRAIN TUMOUR, acute GLAUCOMA, MENINGITIS, and CANCER OF THE STOMACH, all of which require prompt medical attention.

If nausea and vomiting are accompanied by severe abdominal pain lasting for more than 1 hour, or if they follow a head injury, or if vomit is blood-stained or contains 'coffee grounds', (999).

Specific remedies for use in (999) emergencies, to be taken every 5 minutes for up to 10 doses
- Vomiting and severe abdominal pain lasting for 1 hour or more, pain not relieved by vomiting, burst ulcer or appendicitis suspected *Aconite 30c*
- Vomiting of dark red blood or 'coffee grounds', bleeding peptic ulcer suspected *Phosphorus 6c*
- Vomiting follows head injury *Arnica 30c*

If, in addition to feeling nauseous and vomiting, person is suffering from ABNORMAL SLEEPINESS OR DROWSINESS, CONFUSION, intolerance of light, and HEADACHE made worse by bending forwards, (2) and give *Belladonna 30c* every 5 minutes until help arrives. If person is nauseous and vomiting, and has a severe pain in one eye and blurred vision, appropriate action is also (2). If there is recurrent vomiting *without* nausea, and a headache in the morning, 12. If there is recurrent vomiting and constant pain in stomach, or frequent vomiting and weight loss of more than 0.5 kg (1 lb) per week, 48.

Other causes of nausea and vomiting include intense emotion, radiation, food ALLERGY, deficiencies of zinc and Vitamin B_6 (especially in pregnancy), and also of sodium, magnesium, and biotin, and sometimes an excess of Vitamin D, calcium, or lithium.

Specific remedies to be taken ¼-hourly, or less frequently depending on severity, for up to 10 doses
- Persistent nausea, griping pains in abdomen, vomit may contain greenish mucus, symptoms worse when in a car or looking at moving objects, headache, perspiration *Ipecac. 6c*
- Nausea and vomiting accompanied by diarrhoea, perhaps as result of eating spoiled food (especially overripe fruit) or because person has peptic ulcer, pain in stomach alleviated by warm drinks, person feels worn out, restless, and chilly, symptoms worse between midnight and 2 am *Arsenicum 6c*
- Vomiting occurs 2–3 hours after eating, with painful retching, tendency to wake around 4 am and not be able to get back to sleep for 2–3 hours, person feels 'hung over', especially after reckless eating or if he or she has a peptic ulcer *Nux 6c*
- Craving for cold water, which is vomited up as soon as it becomes warm in stomach, blood in vomit and burning pains in pit of stomach, suspected peptic ulcer *Phosphorus 6c*
- Vomiting after rich fatty food, yellow-green discharge from nose, person feels better in open air, but generally tearful *Pulsatilla 6c*
- Vomiting occurs very soon after meals, especially after very large meals, lack of hunger after vomiting, tongue white and furred, weighed-down sensation in stomach, person feels worse in hot stuffy rooms *Antimonium 6c*

Self-help Repeated vomiting can be very dehydrating, so drink plenty of fluids (especially boiled cooled water), a little and often to begin with; avoiding solids for a day or two will also give your stomach a rest. If you smoke, try to stop. If you are taking prescription drugs of any kind, and suspect that they are having side effects, consult your GP.

Oesophageal cancer see CANCER OF THE OESOPHAGUS

Peptic ulcer

Both stomach (gastric) ulcers and duodenal ulcers are referred to as peptic ulcers. Whereas duodenal ulcers affect four times as many men as women, stomach ulcers are more or less equally distributed; for women, however, the risk of ulcers increases after the MENOPAUSE, perhaps because high levels of oestrogen have a protective effect.

Stomach ulcers are coin-sized raw areas on the walls of the stomach where the protective mucus coating has been eroded. May be due to over-production of acid (see ACID SECRETION PROBLEMS), failure to produce enough mucus, or regurgitation of bile from the duodenum, which may in turn be due to heavy smoking or drinking, irregular eating habits, ALLERGY to foods such as wheat and milk, STRESS, recurrent GASTRITIS, or drugs, especially aspirin, steroids, and non-steroidal anti-inflammatory drugs.

The symptoms of a stomach ulcer are a gnawing or burning pain in the chest or upper abdomen, sometimes lasting for 2–3 hours, INDIGESTION, and NAUSEA AND VOMITING; pain may or may not coincide with eating. Groups most at risk are older people, people on low incomes, and blood group A. With time, if ulcers are left untreated, there may be loss of appetite (see APPETITE CHANGES) and WEIGHT LOSS. PERITONITIS (if ulcer perforates stomach wall), PYLORIC STENOSIS (if ulcer blocks exit from stomach), and CANCER OF THE STOMACH (if ulcer turns malignant) are also slight risks. A bleeding stomach ulcer is fairly rare, but can cause rapid blood loss and SHOCK, especially in an elderly person, or ANAEMIA.

Conventional treatment of stomach ulcers includes bed rest, antacids, and H$_2$ Receptor antagonists (such as Ranitidine and Cimetidine); only if ulcers refuse to heal is surgery (partial gastrectomy) recommended.

Duodenal ulcers are raw spots in the lining of the duodenum eroded by acid from the stomach; somewhat smaller than stomach ulcers, they usually cause gnawing upper abdominal pain 3–4 hours after eating. As with stomach ulcers, heavy smoking, aspirin, steroids, and anti-inflammatory drugs, and over-production of stomach acid (see ACID SECRETION PROBLEMS) are the culprits; condition is more common in blood group O and among people with EMPHYSEMA or alcoholic CIRRHOSIS OF THE LIVER. Possible complications include bleeding, leading to ANAEMIA, PYLORIC STENOSIS (narrowing of exit from stomach), and PERITONITIS (infection of abdominal cavity if ulcers perforate duodenal wall).

Conventionally treated by giving antacids to neutralize acid produced by stomach or drugs to reduce the amount of acid produced; surgery is seldom necessary.

A *perforated ulcer* is an ulcer which has eroded through the wall of the stomach or duodenum; symptoms are severe abdominal pain lasting for 1 hour or more, with or without vomiting, and sometimes BLOOD IN VOMIT; appropriate action is (999).

See INDIGESTION and NAUSEA AND VOMITING for specific homeopathic remedies; many of these include 'peptic ulcer' as one of their symptoms.

Self-help Ulcers can be helped to heal by eating only small quantities of food at a time; Slippery Elm Food, taken every 2 hours, is especially recommended. Rich fatty foods, acid foods, highly concentrated carbohydrates, tea, coffee, and alcohol should all be avoided. Cut out smoking. If you are particularly prone to stomach ulcers, try the Liver Diet on p. 352. Make sure your diet contains plenty of Vitamins A, C, and E, and zinc.

Pyloric stenosis see also PYLORIC STENOSIS p. 302

Narrowing (stenosis) or total blockage of the duodenum (pylorus) caused by a PEPTIC ULCER or CANCER OF THE STOMACH; symptoms are a distended stomach, BELCHING of gas from trapped stomach contents, heavy vomiting, DEHYDRATION, and eventually WEIGHT LOSS and malnutrition. If condition is suspected, |48|; endoscopy will almost certainly be necessary to establish diagnosis. In the meantime, specific remedies given under INDIGESTION and NAUSEA and VOMITING may be appropriate.

Stomach ache see ABDOMINAL PAIN p. 220, INDIGESTION

Stomach cancer see CANCER OF THE STOMACH

Stricture of the oesophagus

A rare condition in which repeated scarring of the inner walls of the lower part of oesophagus narrows it, making swallowing difficult; mainly affects elderly HIATUS HERNIA sufferers, scarring being due to persistent backflow of acid from the stomach. If you suffer from heartburn and experience increasing difficulty swallowing, consult your GP. Can be treated by mechanically dilating the oesophagus or by surgical removal of scar tissue. For suitable homeopathic remedies, see ACHALASIA.

Travel sickness see also NAUSEA AND VOMITING

Motion, especially motion while reading or trying to focus on something stationary, can upset the balance mechanism of the inner ear; children are especially susceptible. Symptoms are pallor, feeling cold and clammy, and NAUSEA AND VOMITING; hot, stuffy, enclosed conditions, and the smell of food or tobacco, do not help.

Specific remedies to be given ¼-hourly to hourly, depending on severity beginning 1 hour before starting journey
- Person afraid of death and disaster *Aconite 30c*
- Person nauseous, giddy, faint, pale, cold and sweaty, with 'tight band around head' feeling, finds cigarette smoke especially nauseating *Tabacum 6c*

- Person fidgety, but feels better lying down *Rhus tox. 6c*
- Sight of food causes nausea and sudden increase in saliva, person feels giddy and worn out, and wants to lie down *Cocculus 6c*
- Feeling hungry, hunger satiated by small amounts of food, sudden increase in saliva, giddy feeling made worse by loud noise or by sitting up, pain in back of head and neck *Petroleum 6c*
- Fear of sudden downward motion (hitting an air pocket, for example) when travelling by air *Borax 6c*
- Feeling queasy, with headache at back of head or over one eye, food, tobacco, or coffee make queasiness worse, painful gagging and retching, feeling chilly, constipated *Nux 6c*

Ulcers see PEPTIC ULCER

Vomiting see NAUSEA AND VOMITING

SMALL AND LARGE INTESTINE, LIVER, GALL BLADDER AND PANCREAS

FROM the stomach food enters the duodenum and small intestine, squeezes into the caecum through a small valve, then passes into the ascending, transverse, and descending parts of the colon or large intestine, and finally to the rectum and anus. The total distance between the stomach and the anus is about 8 m (26 ft), the whole journey taking 18–30 hours from the time food leaves the stomach.

Liver and pancreas empty their digestive secretions into the duodenum through a common duct, the bile duct. Bile produced by the liver emulsifies fats, and enzymes produced by the pancreas get to work on proteins, starch, and fat.

The liver does many things besides aiding digestion. It stores glycogen (a compact form of glucose) and also vitamins (A, B, D, E, and K); it removes toxins, for example alcohol, from circulation; it manufactures blood proteins and blood clotting agents; it synthesizes cholesterol, a vital component of all cell membranes and the precursor of many hormones; it converts saturated fats to unsaturated fats when the body is obliged to use fat rather than glucose for energy; it breaks down and recycles the iron-rich, oxygen-carrying pigment haemoglobin; it dismantles excess amino acids and excretes their nitrogen-containing components into the blood as urea (urea is one of the constituents of urine); it also produces a great amount of heat because of all the chemical reactions going on inside it.

The pancreas, a gland about 15 cm (6 in) long lying beneath and behind the stomach, produces large amounts of sodium bicarbonate as well as digestive enzymes, sodium bicarbonate is alkaline, and therefore neutralizes the hydrochloric acid produced by the stomach. It also produces two important hormones, insulin and glucagon, which control sugar uptake by every cell in the body.

The gall bladder has no secretory function. It merely stores and concentrates bile sent to it by the liver and empties it into the duodenum in response to a hormone called cholecystokinin, secreted whenever fatty food leaves the stomach.

The small intestine has two functions, to complete the food breakdown process, and to absorb nutrients into the bloodstream. Although it is only 6.4 m (21 ft) long, it has a total absorptive area of about 18.5 m^2 (200 ft^2). This is because its inner walls are lined with millions of finger-like projections called villi, each containing blood capillaries and tiny tributaries of the lymphatic system called lacteals. Amino acids, glucose, small fat droplets, vitamins, and minerals pass into the capillaries, and larger fat droplets into the lacteals.

Whatever remains unabsorbed by the small intestine – about 5 per cent of fats, 10 per cent of amino acids, fibre, some vitamins, bacteria, intestinal secretions, salts, water – passes into the colon where it is gradually compacted into semi-solid faeces. The bacterial populations of the colon manufacture vitamin K, B$_{12}$, B$_1$ and B$_5$, and certain amino acids; these are absorbed by the walls of the colon, together with salts, water, and other valuable substances. Transit time through the colon depends mainly on the amount of roughage in the diet. Too little roughage causes constipation, and related ailments such as haemorrhoids and diverticulitis.

Abdominal pain see also ABDOMINAL PAIN pp. 312–3
Strictly speaking, the term abdominal pain covers all forms of pain (aches, cramps, colic, etc.) felt between diaphragm and groin; it therefore includes 'stomach ache', although pain due to ailments of the upper parts of the digestive tract – stomach, duodenum, pancreas, gall bladder, and liver – is likely to be felt in the upper abdomen, behind the lower ribs or between the ribs and the navel.

Acute abdominal pain, pain so severe that the slightest movement is agony, may be due to APPENDICITIS (if appendix ruptures, there is severe pain in lower right abdomen, with vomiting and fever), OBSTRUCTION of part of the intestine or bowel (abdomen distended, vomiting, constipation or diarrhoea, inability to pass wind), acute PANCREATITIS (severe pain in upper abdomen, radiating to back, with vomiting), a perforated PEPTIC ULCER (sudden intense pain, followed by shock), diverticulitis (pain in lower left abdomen, fever, nausea – see DIVERTICULAR DISEASE), or internal injury, all of which can very swiftly lead to PERITONITIS. All are emergency situations, so ⑨⑨⑨; once in hospital, it may be necessary to open up the abdomen to find out what is wrong.

Self-help If pain is severe, do not drink or eat until you have seen your GP, and do not take painkillers or drink alcohol. A hot water bottle or an ice pack applied to the site of the pain may help.

Specific remedies to be given, for up to 10 doses only, until medical help arrives
- Suspected burst appendix *Lachesis 6c* every 5 minutes
- Suspected obstruction *China 6c* every 5 minutes
- Person in state of fear and shock *Aconite 30c* every 10 minutes
- If pain follows injury *Arnica 30c* every 10 minutes

Acute abdominal pain can also be due to GASTRO-ENTERITIS or FOOD POISONING (diarrhoea, vomiting, fever), RENAL COLIC (pain extends from small of back to groin), acute PYELONEPHRITIS (fever as well as pain), GALLSTONES or CHOLECYSTITIS (pain under right ribs), CYSTITIS (painful or frequent urination), SHINGLES (burning pain localized to strip down one side of abdomen, tenderness), INDIGESTION (especially after alcohol or heavy meals), diverticulosis or diverticulitis (cramps and tenderness in lower left abdomen – see DIVERTICULAR DISEASE), CONSTIPATION, disruption to blood flow in the area of bowel and intestines (possibly caused by THROMBOSIS, a haemorrhage, or an aortic ANEURYSM), or even a sudden change of diet (constipation, lots of wind). In pregnancy, acute lower abdominal pain, especially if associated with vaginal bleeding, may signal an ECTOPIC PREGNANCY or a MISCARRIAGE.

If pain is severe and continues unabated for more than 1 hour, or occurs during first 3 months of pregnancy, ②.

Among the many causes of chronic or recurrent abdominal pain are PELVIC INFECTION (smelly vaginal discharge), HIATUS HERNIA (heartburn made worse by bending or lying down), INDIGESTION and PEPTIC ULCER (pain relieved by antacids), PANCREATITIS (pain in upper abdomen), GALLSTONES (pain in upper right abdomen), CROHN'S DISEASE (cramps after eating, diarrhoea), HERNIAS in the abdominal wall in the area of the navel or groin, IRRITABLE BOWEL SYNDROME (often one-sided abdominal cramps), and ULCERATIVE COLITIS (left-side abdominal pain relieved by passing stools).

If pain is localized between navel and breastbone and person is losing weight at rate of 0.5 kg (1 lb) or more per week, cause may be CANCER OF THE STOMACH; if there is persistent pain in the lower abdomen, with fever, and alternate bouts of constipation and diarrhoea, cause may be CANCER OF THE COLON. In either case, appropriate action is ⁴⁸.

If abdominal pain can be traced to any of the causes mentioned above, see relevant entry for homeopathic treatment. Where pain is recurrent but the cause cannot be found, constitutional treatment would be a sensible course.

Specific remedies to be given ½-hourly for up to 10 doses when pain comes on
- Pain onsets and stops with equal suddenness, as if abdomen has been gripped by a hand and then released, face red and hot, abdomen tender and sensitive to slightest jarring *Belladonna 30c*
- Pain like a stitch, abdomen feels as if it is about to burst, pressure makes pain worse, pain so severe that person cannot move, think, or talk, breathing shallow *Bryonia 30c*
- Cutting pain causes person to double up and cry out, abdomen distended with wind, attack may follow anger outburst *Chamomilla 6c*
- Violent, cutting, twisting pain just below navel, relieved by passing wind, bending forwards, or pressing on abdomen *Colocynth 6c*
- Pain so violent that person cries out, relieved by warmth, friction, and pressure on abdomen *Magnesia phos. 6c*

Anal fissure
An elongated split in the rectum close to the anal sphincter, often associated with internal PILES; though rare, condition is most common in middle age, but affects some children. When a stool is passed, split is irritated, causing sphincter muscles to go into painful spasm; split may also bleed. CONSTIPATION is the root cause.

Orthodox treatment is to soften stools with liquid paraffin, or to use a local anaesthetic or KY jelly to make stooling less painful; in some cases, stretching of the anus (dilatation) or surgery may be necessary.

Specific remedy to be taken 4 times daily for up to 14 days
- Sore, burning pain from fissure, ache in lower back, stools large, dry, hard, and knobbly *Aesculus 6c*
- Sore, smarting pain on passing stools, which are lumpy and covered in mucus *Graphites 6c*
- Sharp, spiky pains during and after passing stools, constipation, chilliness, irritability *Nitric ac. 6c*
- Burning or stabbing sensation in rectum, worse after passing stools, bowels loose or constipated *Ratanhia 6c*

Self-help Increase amount of roughage in diet, especially raw vegetables. Add natural laxatives (see p. 354) to diet for a while, until regular bowel habits are established.

For explanation of other symbols, see page 107

Anal fistula

A rare condition in which an abscess in the rectum erodes a tiny canal (fistula) through to the skin somewhere near the anus, and discharges watery pus through it; abscess may or may not be painful, and may be associated with CROHN'S DISEASE or CANCER OF THE RECTUM. Standard procedure is to clean out abscess under local anaesthetic so that fistula heals.

Specific remedies to be taken every 4 hours for up to 14 days
- Abscess painful *Calcarea sulph. 6c*
- If there is still discharge after abscess has been cleansed *Silicea 6c*
- Stitching pains darting up rectum, made worse by coughing or sneezing *Lachesis 6c*

Self-help Bathe anal area with Hypericum and Calendula solution (5 drops of mother tincture of each to 0.25 litre [½ pint] boiled cooled water).

Appendicitis

Infection and swelling of appendix due to increased activity of harmful bacteria inside it; seems to happen when appendix is partially or totally blocked off from colon by hard faecal matter, a swollen lymph gland, a tumour, or even a tapeworm; appendix either bursts, releasing pus into abdominal cavity and causing PERITONITIS, or surrounding tissues envelop it in an abscess, effectively sealing if off from the rest of the abdomen. Classic symptoms are vague pain around navel, followed by loss of appetite, CONSTIPATION or DIARRHOEA, then NAUSEA AND VOMITING; then person develops FEVER, and pain becomes sharp and moves to lower right abdomen, which feels very tender. A burst appendix causes severe pain, not relieved by vomiting, and a DISTENDED ABDOMEN.

If appendicitis is suspected, 12. If appendix bursts, 999. The cure is usually swift surgical removal (appendicectomy), but if abscess has formed, removal may be delayed until infection in surrounding tissues can be cleared up by antibiotics.

Specific remedies to be given every 15 minutes for up to 10 doses while waiting for help
- Face red and hot, slightest movement makes pain worse *Belladonna 30c*
- Even slightest touch of hand on skin over appendix area causes intense pain *Bryonia 30c*
- Cutting, tearing pains, abdomen distended, skin over appendix area acutely sensitive, person extremely tetchy and irritable *Lachesis 6c*
- Pain most intense over appendix area *Iris ten. 6c*

Self-help Go to bed, eat nothing, and drink only water (a full stomach and surgery do not go together). Even if you are constipated, do not take laxatives. A high-fibre diet, with plenty of green vegetables, is the best preventive.

Blood in faeces

Not an ailment as such, but bright red, dark red, or tarry blood in stools should never be ignored. If stools are bloody, and person has a FEVER and feels very ill, 2; he or she may have DYSENTERY or ULCERATIVE COLITIS. In children under 12 months, red jelly-like stools may be a sign of INTUSSUSCEPTION, which also causes severe pain; appropriate action is again 2. Other conditions causing bloody stools are PILES, ANAL FISSURE, DIVERTICULAR DISEASE, and CANCER OF THE COLON OR RECTUM; if a person has a bleeding PEPTIC ULCER, stools may be black and tarry. If any of these conditions is suspected, 12. See appropriate entry for orthodox and homeopathic treatment.

Cancer of the colon or rectum see also CANCER pp. 273–4

May take the form of an ulcer, a constriction, or a growth containing cancerous cells liable to spread to other parts of the abdomen or, via the blood, to more distant sites in the body. Symptoms may be marked change in bowel movements, either increased CONSTIPATION or DIARRHOEA, ABDOMINAL PAIN, and BLOOD IN FAECES. In later stages, ulcer may erode through wall of bowel and cause PERITONITIS; a constriction or growth may block the bowel and cause OBSTRUCTION. Most at risk, it seems, are people who eat a highly refined, low-fibre diet, and people over 40 and between 60 and 70; plenty of calcium and adequate Vitamin A in the diet may be a preventive. In a few cases, cancer of the colon follows ULCERATIVE COLITIS.

Treatment is surgical removal of part of the colon or rectum (colectomy or proctocolectomy), or radiotherapy and drugs if surgery is not feasible. If healthy parts of the colon or rectum cannot be rejoined, a hole is made in the abdominal wall to allow solid wastes to be discharged into a bag. Constitutional homeopathic treatment is recommended after surgery.

Cancer of the liver see also CANCER pp. 273–4

Occasionally primary, but more often secondary to CANCER OF THE COLON OR RECTUM; most at risk are heavy drinkers. Because the liver performs so many vital metabolic functions, general health is fairly rapidly affected; specific symptoms are WEIGHT LOSS, loss of appetite, INDIGESTION, and JAUNDICE; as a rule, once jaundice has appeared, treatment of this form of cancer can only be palliative. Chemotherapy can buy time, but the side-effects of cytotoxic drugs are often more unpleasant than the effects of the cancer. Constitutional treatment from an EXPERIENCED HOMEOPATH would almost certainly improve the quality of life.

Cancer of the pancreas see also CANCER

Apart from a possible link with over-consumption of coffee, the cause of pancreatic cancer is not known. Symptoms are WEIGHT LOSS, loss of appetite, NAUSEA

---

999 Emergency – call GP (or dial 999) immediately. 2 Consult your doctor if no improvement within 2 hours

AND VOMITING, JAUNDICE, and ABDOMINAL PAIN (felt in upper abdomen, often extending to the back); sitting up and leaning forwards usually reduces pain. If detected early enough, surgery may be possible; the whole pancreas is removed, although this results in DIABETES; at a later stage, radiotherapy and chemotherapy are used, their effects being palliative rather than curative. For homeopathic approach, see CANCER.

Cholecystitis see also GALLSTONES

An acute condition in which the gall bladder becomes inflamed and swollen because flow of bile into duodenum is blocked by GALLSTONES; result is biliary colic – intense pain in upper right abdomen or between shoulders, INDIGESTION, especially after fatty food, and NAUSEA with or without vomiting; untreated, condition can lead to JAUNDICE and occasionally, if gall bladder bursts, to PERITONITIS. If site of pain is as described above, and pain persists for more than 3 hours, ②; painkillers and antibiotics will probably be prescribed, and then surgery recommended to remove the gall bladder; only in exceptional cases are gallstones dissolved *in situ*.

Occasionally, infection elsewhere in the intestines can spread to the gall bladder; treatment is by antibiotics and painkillers.

Specific remedies to be given ½-hourly for up to 6 doses while waiting for medical treatment
- Obstructed bile duct, radiating, tearing pains made worse by jarring, pale stools, signs of jaundice *Berberis 30c*
- Pains extend from under right ribs to right shoulder blade, especially after eating fatty food *Chelidonium 30c*
- Great flatulence which is not relieved by belching, person feels chilly, especially in draughts, prefers to move around rather than sit still, bending double reduces discomfort *China 30c*
- Cutting pains relieved by bending double, intestines feel as if they are being pinched between two stones, diarrhoea *Colocynth 30c*
- Griping, drawing, bursting, or cutting pains made worse by pressure on abdomen, relieved by bending backwards *Dioscorea 30c*
- Pain markedly better if a hot water bottle is held to abdomen *Magnesia phos. 30c*

Cirrhosis of the liver

Damage to intricate architecture of liver caused by alcohol, malnutrition, HEPATITIS, HEART FAILURE, and certain drugs and toxins; magnesium deficiency may also be a factor. Damaged tissue is replaced by hard lumps of scar tissue, yellowish (*cirrhos* means tawny) in appearance, which cut off hard-working liver cells from the vessels and ducts which enable them to function. As liver function deteriorates, there is WEIGHT LOSS, loss of appetite, NAUSEA AND VOMITING,

INDIGESTION, general weakness, and a tendency to bleed and bruise easily; in later stages, JAUNDICE develops and periods cease (see MENSTRUAL PROBLEMS), followed by fluid retention (see OEDEMA) and liver failure. Sufferers are always advised to stop drinking alcohol, and to cut down intake of salt and fat; diuretics, steroids, cytotoxic drugs, and vitamin and mineral supplements may also be prescribed.

A number of specific homeopathic remedies are given below, but sufferers are advised to seek the care of an EXPERIENCED HOMEOPATH.

Specific remedies to be taken 4 times daily for up to 7 days while seeking homeopathic treatment
- Jaundice, empty or gnawing sensation in pit of stomach, craving for ice-cold water, which makes sensation worse and which is vomited up as soon as it becomes warm in stomach, tendency to bleed easily *Phosphorus 30c*
- Liver swollen, with pain under right ribs, pain aggravated by slightest touch, person chilly and sensitive to draughts, stomach full of wind but not relieved by belching *China 30c*
- Fluid retention, especially around ankles and abdomen, person feels worn out, chilly, restless, and markedly worse between midnight and 2 am *Arsenicum 30c*

Self-help Cut out alcohol (fatal liver failure is almost inevitable if the liver is given no respite from alcohol), and cut down on salt and fat. Stop taking any non-prescription drugs. Extra Vitamin A, zinc, magnesium, nickel, and selenium are recommended.

Colic see ABDOMINAL PAIN

Any fairly sharp, spasmodic pain in the upper or lower abdomen is popularly called 'colic'; most common cause is INDIGESTION and GALLSTONES.

Constipation see also CONSTIPATION pp. 317–8

Delayed transit of solid wastes through colon, resulting in irregular, infrequent, or difficult bowel movements; the longer faeces stay in the colon, the more water is absorbed from them, the harder they become, and the more straining is required to pass them; the risk of faecal toxins passing into the bloodstream and adversely affecting the metabolism of the rest of the body is also increased (see OBESITY).

Though conditions such as CANCER OF THE COLON OR RECTUM, IRRITABLE BOWEL SYNDROME, DIVERTICULAR DISEASE, ANAL FISSURE, and PILES may contribute to difficult or painful bowel movements, the root cause of constipation is usually dietary – not enough fibre, not enough fluids, a lack of Vitamin B_1, B_5, B_6, potassium, magnesium, and zinc, too much animal protein (meat, eggs), too many dairy products, too much Vitamin D, too much aluminium, and too much vinegar, pepper, salt, and spices.

If diet is not at fault, cause may be eating meals too fast, not taking enough exercise, tension, ANXIETY, DEPRESSION, delaying or not regularly obeying the urge to open the bowels, taking antibiotics or abusing laxatives (both of which upset balance of micro-organisms in gut), abuse of certain over-the-counter drugs, especially cough mixtures, hypothyroidism (see THYROID PROBLEMS), liver malfunction leading to inadequate bile production, impairment of nerves supplying colon due to spinal abnormality or injury. . .

The list of disorders for which constipation is blamed, or in which constipation is thought to play a part, is even longer, ranging from vague symptoms such as 'liverishness' and sluggishness to heart disease and CANCER. The roll call includes HEADACHE, INSOMNIA, various skin complaints, eye problems, dental problems, EPILEPSY, STROKE, ATHEROSCLEROSIS, premature ageing, ASTHMA, TUBERCULOSIS, DIABETES, GALLSTONES, liver trouble, ULCERATIVE COLITIS, PILES, GLOMERULONEPHRITIS, RHEUMATISM, OBESITY. . .

If there is bleeding from the anus, or blood in stools, 12. If there is a marked change in bowel function accompanied by inexplicable weight loss of more than 0.5 kg (1 lb) per week, 48. Also, if no motion has been passed for several days despite self-help measures, and abdomen is painful, see your GP. Orthodox treatment is by laxatives, suppositories and, if necessary, enemas. In osteopathy or chiropractic, constipation is treated by manipulation; in naturopathy, the colon is flushed out.

In homeopathy, constipation is regarded as a constitutional problem, and is therefore treated constitutionally; bowel nosodes may be given (see p. 12 for definition of nosode). The remedies given below are for use on an occasional basis only, for example when travel or holidays disrupt normal diet and exercise habits.

Specific remedies to be taken 2 hourly for up to 10 doses
- Great urge to pass stool, but nothing passed, or passing stools and feeling that there is more to come, especially if person is sedentary, elderly, or studying hard, chronic use of laxatives, chilliness, irritability *Nux 6c*
- Stools large, dry, hard, and burnt-looking, especially in elderly person, dry mouth, head aches and feels congested, abdomen distended, burning feeling in rectum after passing stool, great thirst and irritability *Bryonia 30c*
- No desire to open bowels until rectum is completely full, even soft stools are difficult to pass, and may be mucous-covered or soft and clayey, sensation of stools getting caught up in splenic flexure (under left ribs, where colon starts to descend) *Alumina 6c*
- Rectum feels dry and painful when straining, stools hard and crumbly, and only passed every second day, or at longer intervals during periods, stools feel like wind and vice versa *Natrum mur. 6c*

- Ineffectual urging accompanied by painful burning sensation, when passed stools are dark, large, hard, and dry, always feeling that there is more to come, person suffers from piles or anal fissure, constipation alternates with bouts of diarrhoea, stools are passed every 2–4 days when constipated *Sulphur 6c*
- Contraction of anal sphincter not strong enough to expel stool, so stool slides back in again, anus feels sore, stools scanty, hard, and mucous-covered, person chilly and prone to head sweats *Silicea 6c*
- No desire to open bowels for days on end, then stools are hard and pill-like, bowels lazy, appetite poor, person drowsy during day but wakeful at night, alert to the slightest sound *Opium 6c*
- No desire to open bowels for several days, then griping, colicky pain followed by passage of large stool covered in white mucus, bowels ache afterwards, person may have piles or an anal fissure and be overweight *Graphites 6c*
- Rectum feels dry and hot, as if full of sticks or spikes, sensation of knife being jabbed upwards on attempting to open bowels, sensation of fullness in rectum, pain in lower back, crawling sensation in anus, symptoms worse after sleep, person elderly *Aesculus 6c*
- Boiling sensation in bowels, splinter-like pains last for hours after passing stools as if something has been torn, also burning and itching *Nitric ac. 6c*
- Sharp griping pains, straining produces little pills which are hard, black, and dry, and at the same time bowels feel as if they are being drawn up towards the spine on a piece of string, person habitually constipated *Plumbum 6c*
- Great flatulence, no desire to open bowels for days on end, hard incomplete stools passed with pain and difficulty, patches of wind in intestines relieved by rubbing, person craves sweet things and feels worse between 4 and 8 pm *Lycopodium 6c*

Self-help Pay more attention to diet, and in particular eat plenty of raw vegetables. Also take extra Vitamin C and magnesium. For information on natural laxatives – linseed, blackstrap molasses, and dried fruit – see p. 354; senna pods and proprietary laxatives based on senna should be avoided as they irritate the lining of the colon. Take some form of brisk outdoor exercise every day, or try the slant board exercises on pp. 19–21, 22. The occasional cold bath is also beneficial. As a general rule, suppositories should be avoided; however, if dietary or physical measures fail or are not practical, the occasional glycerine suppository (obtainable from chemist) may be used.

Crohn's disease (terminal ileitis)
Recurrent inflammation of the ileum as it nears the large intestine, often with months or years between episodes; cause is not known. Between attacks, inflamed tissue heals and scars over, narrowing lumen

of ileum and reducing absorption of nutrients (see MALABSORPTION); during flare-ups, symptoms are cramping pains after eating, DIARRHOEA, general malaise, and sometimes slight FEVER; if condition is very bad, there may be a risk of OBSTRUCTION, severe bleeding leading to ANAEMIA, or, if the wall of the ileum perforates, PERITONITIS; in rare cases, inflamed tissue may become malignant (see CANCER). In some people, condition is associated with joint, liver, skin, or eye problems.

Orthodox treatment includes painkillers, anti-inflammatory and anti-diarrhoeal drugs, and steroids; an ileostomy, in which affected section of ileum is removed, is a last resort.

For specific homeopathic remedies, see ABDOMINAL PAIN and DIARRHOEA. Constitutional treatment from an EXPERIENCED HOMEOPATH is advised.

Self-help Conventional wisdom is to increase intake of milky foods. However, many people with bowel problems are allergic to milk. If you have any suspicions on this score, consult a dietary therapist first. Sugar and other refined carbohydrates should be avoided. You may also need to take extra Vitamin A, B, and D, and zinc.

Diarrhoea

Failure of the large intestine to absorb water from faeces; this can happen with IRRITABLE BOWEL SYNDROME (diarrhoea alternates with constipation), GASTROENTERITIS (diarrhoea and vomiting), ULCERATIVE COLITIS (blood in faeces), FOOD POISONING (diarrhoea and vomiting), worms and other intestinal parasites (see THREADWORMS, TAPEWORMS), LACTOSE INTOLERANCE and other food intolerances, and even ANXIETY. Certain drugs, especially antibiotics cause diarrhoea; also antacids because of their magnesium content, and so does a lack of Vitamin B_3 or folate; too much Vitamin D can cause constipation as well as diarrhoea. Liquid stools can also be the price of eating too many pulses or prunes. Chronic diarrhoea can cause potassium deficiency.

If diarrhoea continues for more than 48 hours, or is accompanied by FEVER or BLOOD IN FAECES, ②; regardless of the cause, person may be seriously dehydrated. Orthodox treatment onsists of rehydration with electrolyte solutions for 12–24 hours, followed by investigation and, if persistent, antidiarrhoeal agents such as kaolin and morphine or drugs which inhibit peristalsis or cause constipation.

A tendency towards diarrhoea is best treated constitutionally, although in acute attacks the remedies below may be used.

Specific remedies to be taken every ½ hour for up to 10 doses
- Diarrhoea comes on suddenly after shock or exposure to cold wind, or overheating in summer, abdomen distended, person feels better after passing stool *Aconite 30c*

- Diarrhoea after a summer chill, after food which disagrees, or after anger outburst, tip of tongue very red, symptoms worse in morning and made worse by eating, painful urination, yellowish-green stools, a lot of wind, difficult to distinguish between wanting to pass stool and wanting to pass wind *Aloe 6c*
- Anxiety and apprehension, belching, craving for salt and sweet things *Argentum nit. 6c*
- Scanty, odourless, brown stools which seem to burn skin around anus, especially after cold drinks, ice creams, ice lollies, or over-ripe fruit, person finds small sips of hot drinks soothing *Arsenicum 6c*
- Copious and offensive stools the colour of pea soup and the consistency of batter, with a lot of wind and colic, urgency early in morning, empty feeling afterwards *Podophyllum 6c*
- Profuse, watery stools with bits of food in them, person feels better after passing them *Phosphoric ac. 6c*
- Need to pass stool propels person out of bed at 5 am, anus feels hot, piles may be present *Sulphur 6c*
- Profuse stools, vomiting, forehead breaks out in cold sweat, craving for iced water *Veratrum 6c*
- Stools like chopped egg, a lot of wind, made worse by summer chills or fruit, person very irritable *China 6c*
- Diarrhoea accompanied by spasmodic, griping pains, doubling up or pressing on abdomen lessens pain, stools copious, thin, frothy, and yellowish, attack possibly brought on by anger *Colocynth 6c*
- Diarrhoea comes on in damp weather or as a result of getting chilled after exertion, stools are slimy, green or yellow, and may have blood in them *Dulcamara 6c*
- Diarrhoea worse at night, also made worse by cold drinks, onions, and rich, fatty foods, no two stools alike *Pulsatilla 6c*

Self-help To combat dehydration, drink plenty of boiled cooled water, with a little honey in it, or rice water, or barley water (water in which rice or barley has been cooked). Once diarrhoea settles down, eat arrowroot, tapioca, semolina, or Slippery Elm Food for a day or two, then gradually revert to your normal diet. If diarrhoea has been caused by antibiotics, take Acidophilus capsules or Acidophilus yoghurt. Take extra folate and Vitamin B for 1 month, and cut down intake of Vitamin D. Avoid analgesics.

Distended abdomen see also ABDOMINAL PAIN
Usually due to retention of wind, faeces, or body fluids, as in IRRITABLE BOWEL SYNDROME (wind and pain, relieved by passing wind or stool), CONSTIPATION, or PREMENSTRUAL TENSION, or after eating too many pulses; can also be due to MALABSORPTION (pale, greasy stools, weight loss), swallowing air (see BELCHING), under-production of stomach acid (see

ACID SECRETION PROBLEMS), food intolerance, intestinal CANDIDIASIS, etc.

Perhaps the most serious conditions signalled by abdominal distention are OBSTRUCTION (severe pain with or without vomiting, inability to pass wind, fever) and APPENDICITIS (if appendix has burst); if obstruction or a burst appendix is suspected, (999).

Other distension-related conditions requiring prompt medical attention are RETENTION OF URINE (relieved by passing urine), CIRRHOSIS OF THE LIVER (with jaundicing), congestive HEART FAILURE (with puffy ankles which pit when pressed, breathlessness which gets worse at night and during exercise) and GLOMERULONEPHRITIS (swollen ankles which pit when pressed, small amounts of urine); if any of these conditions is suspected, [12].

Give specific homeopathic remedies appropriate to the cause; if none of the remedies listed elsewhere seems to answer the case, the remedies given below may be used.

Specific remedies to be given every ½ hour for up to 10 doses
- Marked constipation, passing of wind *Lycopodium 6c*
- Passing wind, abdominal pain relieved by bending backwards, bowels loose *Dioscorea 6c*
- Hysterical distention of abdomen, particularly after grief *Ignatia 6c*
- Bowels feel as if there is a live animal in them, lots of wind and rumbling, abdomen distended, chronic diarrhoea *Thuja 6c*

Self-help If wind is the problem avoid gas-producing foods such as pulses, nuts, onions, and cabbage.

Diverticular disease see also MECKEL'S DIVERTICULUM
Diverticula (plural of the Latin word *diverticulum*, meaning a wayside house of ill repute!) are small pouches which extrude through the walls of the colon and into the abdominal cavity; they may be congenital, or the result of not eating enough fibre.

The presence of diverticula – signalled in some people by occasional cramps and tenderness in lower left abdomen, relieved by passing wind or stools, bouts of DIARRHOEA and CONSTIPATION, and occasional bleeding – is known as *diverticulosis*. The symptoms of *diverticulitis*, in which the diverticula become infected and inflamed, are generally more severe; as well as intense ABDOMINAL PAIN, FEVER, and NAUSEA, there is a risk of abscess formation and PERITONITIS. If symptoms are those of diverticulosis, especially if there is blood in faeces, [12]; if symptoms include severe pain and fever, (2). Endoscopic examination of the lower colon or a barium enema (which should not be given while infection is in acute phase) may be necessary in order to rule out CANCER OF THE COLON, which has similar symptoms. Painkillers and/or antibiotics will

probably be prescribed, and a high-fibre diet. If diverticulitis is recurrent, surgery may be advised.

For specific homeopathic remedies, see ABDOMINAL PAIN, DIARRHOEA.

Self-help Diverticulosis can be helped or forestalled by a high-fibre diet. Bran is only a temporary solution, because although it increases bulk and brings extra calcium and magnesium to the bowels, it also carries calcium, magnesium, and zinc away with it. Fibre-rich foods, such as raw vegetables and fruit, are more nourishing and more appetizing.

Dysentery see DYSENTERY p. 275

Gallstones see also CHOLECYSTITIS
Solid accretions of various substances present in bile, including calcium and cholesterol; may be few and large, or many and small, and cause few symptoms while they remain in gall bladder; in fact, many gallstones are discovered during routine scans or X-rays. However, if a stone blocks exit from gall bladder or becomes stuck in duct leading to duodenum, gall bladder becomes swollen with trapped bile and fats in duodenum pass into small intestine undigested, causing pain and tenderness under right rib cage, NAUSEA with or without vomiting, and discomfort after eating fatty food – all the symptoms in fact of acute CHOLECYSTITIS.

Women are more at risk than men, especially women who take or have taken oral contraceptives, and risk increases with age and being overweight; gallstones also seem to increase risk of acute PANCREATITIS. Cause may be under-production of bile by the liver, excessive elimination of toxins through the liver, food ALLERGY, or abnormally high blood cholesterol levels.

Conventional treatment for gallstones is removal of the gall bladder, even if symptoms are not those of full-blown cholecystitis, on the principle of 'better safe than sorry'; occasionally, it may be feasible to dissolve chemically stones *in situ* or remove them using an endoscope but there is a risk of recurrence. If stones are present but causing no symptoms, consult your homeopath.

Specific remedies to be taken 4 times daily for up to 14 days while seeking homeopathic treatment
- *Berberis 6c*
- If Berberis is not effective, or if person is nervy, chilly, and oversensitive *China 6c*

Self-help Both as a preventive and after removal of the gall bladder, cut rich fatty foods, fried foods, and refined carbohydrates down to a minimum, and eat plenty of vegetables, fruit, and fibre. The possibility of a food allergy would also be worth investigating.

If gallstones have been diagnosed, and PROVIDED NO SYMPTOMS OF CHOLECYSTITIS ARE PRESENT, it is possible to flush out the stones yourself using the

---

following method, called a *liver and gall bladder flush*: in the five days leading up to the flush, eat a normal diet but drink as much fresh-pressed apple juice as possible; on the day of the flush, eat a normal lunch but for supper have only citrus fruit or juice; at bedtime, blend ½ cup pure warm olive oil with ½ cup freshly squeezed lemon juice, and drink it; go to bed and lie on your right side, with your knees pulled up to your chest for the first 30 minutes. When you open your bowels the next day, the gallstones will appear as irregular, gelatinous, green objects in the stools. If you are constipated, take 2 dessertspoons Epsom salts in warm water 4 hours before taking the oil/lemon mixture, and repeat the Epsom salts the next morning.

There is a theoretical risk that flushing may cause stones to lodge in the bile duct rather than pass into the duodenum, but in the author's experience this has never happened; if the oil/lemon mixture can be kept down, and not vomited up, flushing can be extremely effective.

Gastroenteritis see GASTROENTERITIS p. 276

Haemorrhoids see PILES

Hepatitis

An infected liver; infection may be chronic and grumble on for months or years, or it may be sudden and acute, caused by hepatitis A or B virus, or by the viruses which cause GLANDULAR FEVER and YELLOW FEVER, or by alcohol and certain drugs. In some cases acute episodes may lead on to chronic infection.

Hepatitis A onsets suddenly, although incubation time is up to 3 months; virus is spread by faecal-oral route, through contaminated food or sewage. At first, symptoms resemble those of INFLUENZA (aching, FEVER, weakness), often with NAUSEA and loss of appetite; as these subside, JAUNDICE appears and lasts for 2–3 weeks, until the liver is sufficiently recovered to remove yellow pigment (bilirubin) from blood. Person feels weak, run down, sometimes depressed, for a month or two afterwards, and may suffer further attacks, but no lasting damage is sustained by the liver.

Hepatitis B produces similar symptoms to hepatitis A, has a longer incubation time (3–6 months), and is potentially more serious as it can lead to acute liver failure or chronic hepatitis (see below) or CIRRHOSIS OF THE LIVER. Virus is transmitted by blood (unsterilized needles used in tatooing, acupuncture, ear piercing, or drug-taking, transfusions in countries where blood screening is poor) or by body fluids (saliva, semen, vaginal secretions); a few people are carriers of the virus, though they may not know it until they donate blood.

Chronic hepatitis is rare, causing fatigue, INDIGESTION, loss of appetite, some degree of JAUNDICE, and eventually CIRRHOSIS OF THE LIVER. It may develop insidiously, or set in after an attack of hepatitis B, or occur in conjunction with ULCERATIVE COLITIS or

CROHN'S DISEASE. Though the root cause is thought to be an autoimmune reaction (see AUTOIMMUNE DISEASE), the culprit may also be large quantities of alcohol or paracetamol.

If flu-like symptoms develop after suspected exposure to hepatitis A or B, or if jaundice appears after 'flu, 48 .

Since acute hepatitis is virally caused, antibiotics are of no use; the liver has to be helped to heal itself, by rest, abstention from alcohol, fatty foods, and other causative or aggravating agents, and by taking plenty of fluids. In the case of chronic hepatitis, steroids may be prescribed to retard further damage to the liver. Injections of gammaglobulin, which boost resistance to hepatitis A for about 6 months, are a sensible precaution if you live with a hepatitis A sufferer or travel to countries where the disease is endemic.

Homeopathic treatment of chronic hepatitis is constitutional. In cases of acute hepatitis, or while waiting for a diagnosis, the remedies below may be beneficial.

Specific remedies to be taken 4 times daily for 7 days; if symptoms do not abate, see your GP or homeopath
- Symptoms come on after exposure to cold, sharp pain and tenderness in liver region, made worse by movement but alleviated by applying pressure *Bryonia 30c*
- Tongue dirty and yellow, breath smells bad, jaundice, smelly perspiration, great sensitivity to heat and cold, liver feels tender, especially when lying on right side *Mercurius 30c*
- Weak, empty, cold feeling in abdomen, craving for cold water followed by vomiting as water warms up in stomach *Phosphorus 30c*
- Jaundice, abdomen feels distended and constricted at same time, as if there is a string round it, pain in liver area extends to right shoulder blade *Chelidonium 30c*
- Liver feels swollen and tender, anything tight around waist is unbearable, abdomen distended, sensitive, and painful, and distinctly worse for heat or after sleep *Lachesis 30c*
- Liver feels swollen and tender, nose and throat discharging yellow, ropy catarrh *Hydrastis 30c*

Self-help If hepatitis B is diagnosed, person may remain infectious for several months, so meticulous hygiene in the bathroom and kitchen is essential; lavatory, bath, and washbasin should be thoroughly disinfected after each use, and separate crockery and cutlery used. Bed rest should continue for as long as person feels weak. Plenty of fluids, especially rice water or barley water with added sugar, will help to cleanse the system. Extra Vitamin C is also recommended.

Ileus

Paralysis of the intestines, a serious condition because digestion depends on food being squeezed through the gut by muscular contraction. Cause may be OBSTRUCTION or a perforated PEPTIC ULCER, an EMBOLISM (a blood clot blocking a vital artery), or abdominal surgery. Trapped, half-digested food stagnates, producing gas which distends abdomen; CONSTIPATION, FEVER, and vomiting of foul-smelling fluid follow, accompanied by dull ABDOMINAL PAIN which gradually wears off.

If ileus is suspected, *even if pain subsides*, ⑨⑨⑨. Give nothing to eat or drink.

Specific remedies to be given every 5 minutes for up to 10 doses while waiting for help
- Gas in abdomen cannot be expelled through mouth or anus, abdomen hard and swollen, griping pains around navel, vomit looks like stools *Raphanus 6c*
- Symptoms accompanied by drowsiness and a heavy, stupid appearance *Opium 6c*

Incontinence see INCONTINENCE OF URINE pp. 340–1, INCONTINENCE OF FAECES p. 341, STRESS INCONTINENCE

Intussusception see INTUSSUSCEPTION pp. 306–7

Irritable bowel syndrome (spastic colon)

Also known as functional or nervous diarrhoea, colon or vegetative neurosis, or mucous colitis; main symptoms are CONSTIPATION and DIARRHOEA, turn and turn about, occasional cramping pains in lower abdomen, and sometimes pain on defecating. Muscular contraction in the colon or ileum is uncoordinated and spasmodic, though not for any reason which can be detected by X-rays or endoscopy; causes are as likely to be psychological – family, marital, or work problems, cancer PHOBIA, in fact STRESS in general – as dietary. However, a low-fibre diet, or intolerance to wheat, corn, dairy products, citrus fruit, tea, coffee, apples, pears, and salads – in that order – is sometimes the culprit (see food ALLERGY). Less often, spasms can be triggered off by a bowel infection, bowel parasites (THREADWORMS, TAPEWORMS, amoebae, etc.), overgrowth of bowel flora, CANDIDIASIS, spinal maladjustment, or excessive use of laxatives. Twice as many women are affected as men.

The diagnosis is mainly made by excluding other conditions, but if the symptoms mentioned above are accompanied by persistent WEIGHT LOSS, 48; if there is also FEVER or BLOOD IN FAECES, 12. Prompt investigation is especially important in people over 50, if only to rule out CANCER. Anti-spasmodic drugs may be prescribed, and also a high-fibre diet (although bran may aggravate problems if there is intolerance to wheat).

The homeopathic approach to irritable bowel syndrome is constitutional, although the remedies given below may be tried first. The remedies listed under ABDOMINAL PAIN and DIARRHOEA would also be appropriate.

Specific remedies to be given 4 times daily for up to 14 days
- Great flatulence, constipation alternating with diarrhoea, pain in upper left abdomen, mucus in stools, fluttery, tense feeling in stomach *Argentum nit. 6c*
- Burning pains in abdomen, great thirst, nausea and vomiting, person also has cystitis *Cantharis 6c*
- Watery stools, tearing pains, and nausea made worse by smell of food *Colchicum 6c*
- Griping pains relieved by doubling up or pressing on abdomen, attack associated with or brought on by anger *Colocynth 6c*

Self-help If a particular food is suspect, eliminate it from your diet for 4 days, then reintroduce it and see if problems recur. If the results are inconclusive, consult a dietary therapist. If problem is due to a trapped spinal nerve, consult a physiotherapist, chiropractor, or osteopath.

Jaundice

Yellowing of the whites of the eyes and the skin, usually due to poor liver function (see CIRRHOSIS OF THE LIVER, HEPATITIS, and CANCER OF THE LIVER); normally the liver removes the yellow-brown pigment bilirubin (formed as ageing red blood cells are dismantled) from the blood and sends it, via the gall bladder and bile duct, to the intestines, where it colours the faeces brown; in a person with jaundice the faeces are grey and chalky, while the urine is darker than normal. GALLSTONES and CHOLECYSTITIS, which prevent bile from entering the duodenum, can also cause jaundice, and so can drugs such as paracetamol, anabolic steroids, Valium, Largactil, monoamine oxidase inhibitors, and some oral contraceptives. Haemolytic ANAEMIA, in which red blood cells are broken down more quickly than they can be replaced, also causes jaundice.

Jaundice fades once the underlying cause has been treated. See causative ailments for specific homeopathic remedies.

Specific remedy to be given every 4 hours for up to 3 days
- Jaundice caused by haemolytic anaemia *Crotalus 6c*

Malabsorption see also COELIAC DISEASE

Failure of the small intestine to absorb nutrients contained in food; this happens either because the absorptive suface of the small intestine is in some way defective, or because food has not been sufficiently broken down. Symptoms are WEIGHT LOSS, lack of energy, DISTENDED ABDOMEN, DIARRHOEA (with very soft, pale, bulky stools which float and smell offensive), and deficiency ailments such as ANAEMIA (iron, B_{12}, folate), RICKETS AND OSTEOMALACIA (calcium and Vitamin D), a general tendency to bleed easily (Vitamin K), a sore tongue and cracked lips (Vitamin B), dry skin (Vitamin A), and OEDEMA (protein). Children who have

---

⑨⑨⑨ Emergency – call GP (or dial 999) immediately. ② Consult your doctor if no improvement within 2 hours

absorption problems fail to grow and thrive (see FAILURE TO THRIVE).

Among the many ailments which cause malabsorption are CROHN'S DISEASE, COELIAC DISEASE, CYSTIC FIBROSIS, ANAEMIA (iron-deficient and pernicious), DIABETES (diabetes mellitus), THYROID PROBLEMS, chronic PANCREATITIS, LACTOSE INTOLERANCE, chronic DIARRHOEA, SCLERODERMA, LYMPHOMA and bowel infections such as giardiasis and tropical sprue. Absorption problems are fairly common after laxative abuse and during recovery from digestive tract surgery. Excessive amounts of Vitamin B₃, C, E, zinc, choline, fructose, lecithin, ginseng, spirulina, and starch blockers can also interfere with absorption.

For orthodox and homeopathic treatment, see conditions mentioned above.

Meckel's diverticulum

A small pouch protruding from small intestine near its junction with colon; congenital and usually symptomless unless it becomes infected and inflamed; symptoms are BLOOD IN FAECES, vomiting, and ABDOMINAL PAIN, and are sometimes mistaken for those of APPENDICITIS or a PEPTIC ULCER. If pain is severe, possibly indicating that diverticulum has perforated, ②; if there is bleeding from rectum, ⑿. Routine treatment is to open abdomen and remove diverticulum. For specific homeopathic remedies, see APPENDICITIS.

Obstruction of the intestine

A serious turn of events, causing severe ABDOMINAL PAIN and a DISTENDED ABDOMEN, vomiting, CONSTIPATION, and total inability to pass wind. Appropriate action is ⑨⑨⑨ and *China 6c* every 5 minutes for up to 10 doses while waiting for help.

A strangulated HERNIA, a foreign body in the gut, volvulus (twisting of the gut), and CANCER OF THE COLON can all cause obstruction; complications include DEHYDRATION, ILEUS, SHOCK, and PERITONITIS.

Pancreatitis

Acute or chronic inflammation of the pancreas, often associated with GALLSTONES; occurs when powerful enzymes secreted by pancreas, destined for the gut, leak into pancreatic tissue instead.

Acute pancreatitis can be precipitated by blockage of the pancreatic duct by a gallstone, PARATHYROID PROBLEMS, excessive amounts of food or alcohol, abdominal injury, or in rare cases MUMPS; symptoms come on 12–24 hours after excessive eating or drinking, with agonising pain in the upper abdomen, radiating to the back and chest, and vomiting; person may even go into SHOCK. Appropriate action is ⑨⑨⑨ and *Aconite 30c* every 15 minutes for up to 6 doses until help arrives. In hospital, painkillers will be given, and an intravenous drip to enable digestive system to rest; surgery to remove gall bladder may also be necessary.

Chronic pancreatitis develops slowly, sometimes as a sequel to acute pancreatitis, causing dull upper abdominal pain, usually relieved by bending forwards; most sufferers are heavy drinkers or have gallstones. As enzyme and hormone manufacturing functions of pancreas deteriorate, chronic INDIGESTION, mild JAUNDICE, or DIABETES may set in. Orthodox treatment is to prescribe painkillers and replacement enzymes, or, in severe cases, to remove damaged part of pancreas.

For chronic pancreatitis, constitutional homeopathic treatment is recommended, although the following remedies may be taken while expert help is being sought.

Specific remedies to be taken ½-hourly for up to 10 doses
- All food being vomited up, everything appears larger than usual, dry throat, difficulty swallowing *Atropine 6c*
- Empty, gnawing feeling in upper abdomen, made worse by cold, and by food and drink (especially milk), person thirsty, stomach full of wind, with painful burning sensation in navel region *Kali iod. 6c*
- Stabbing pains in upper abdomen, feeling chilly, sweat smells offensive, signs of jaundice *Mercurius 6c*
- Cutting pains in upper abdomen, watery stools, burning sensation in bowels and rectum *Iris 6c*
- Cutting pains in upper abdomen which intensify in warm, quiet surroundings, especially when lying on right side *Iodum 6c*
- Fiery, burning pains in upper abdomen which get worse between midnight and 2 am, person chilly and restless *Arsenicum iod. 6c*
- Jaundice, with large yellow patches on abdomen, empty sensation in stomach, sharp cutting pains in upper abdomen, craving for cold drinks, although these are vomited up as soon as they become warm in stomach *Phosphorus 6c*

Self-help Give up alcohol altogether – chances of recovery are minimal if pancreas continues to be poisoned by alcohol. Eat a low-fat diet.

Peritonitis

Inflammation of the membrane (peritoneum) which lines the abdominal cavity and covers the abdominal organs; usually a complication of conditions such as a perforated PEPTIC ULCER, DIVERTICULAR DISEASE, a ruptured appendix (see APPENDICITIS), or PELVIC INFLAMMATORY DISEASE, but occasionally a result of injury or abdominal surgery. Symptoms are severe ABDOMINAL PAIN, a rigid DISTENDED ABDOMEN, NAUSEA AND VOMITING, and FEVER; there is also a danger of DEHYDRATION (from vomiting) and ILEUS. Appropriate action is ⑨⑨⑨ *even if pain decreases.*

Specific remedies to be given every 5 minutes for up to 10 doses until help arrives

- Sudden onset of severe abdominal pain, person chilly and fearful *Aconite 30c*
- Pain feels as if intestine is being gripped by nails, transverse colon above navel swollen and clearly outlined *Belladonna 30c*
- Griping, cutting pains, great tenderness over painful area, great urge to pass stool *Mercurius corr. 6c*
- Cramping pains relieved by bending double or pressing on abdomen *Colocynth 6c*
- Fever, sharp pain made worse by slightest movement *Bryonia 30c*

Piles (haemorrhoids)

Swollen or strangulated veins in lower rectum and around anus; straining to pass faeces, usually as a result of CONSTIPATION, raises pressure in veins, causing them to bulge and protrude into the anal canal or through the anal opening; as stools are passed, there may be pain and bleeding. Occasionally, blood inside a haemorrhoid clots. Apart from constipation, piles can be caused by persistent coughing, pregnancy and childbirth, standing for long periods, laxatives, sitting on cold surfaces, and travelling long distances sitting on heated car seats, all of which raise pressure in rectal veins.

Anal bleeding should never be ignored; it may be due to piles, but can also be a sign of ULCERATIVE COLITIS or CANCER OF THE COLON OR RECTUM. If pain and bleeding last for more than 12 hours, [12]. Conventionally treated by painkilling ointments and/ or steroid suppositories, and also bulking and laxative agents; if piles persist, anal opening can be stretched to reduce straining, or piles can be shrunk by injection, or removed by ligation or surgery.

Homeopathy regards piles as a constitutional problem, and treats them accordingly. However, in the short term, the remedies and self-help measures given below should be tried.

Specific remedies to be taken 4 times daily for up to 5 days
- Piles internal, associated with constipation and pain in lower back, dry spiky sensation in rectum, lumpy stools which cause stabbing, tearing, or splinter-like pains when passed, anus hot, dry, and itchy *Aesculus 6c*
- Piles protrude like a small cluster of grapes, frequent bleeding reduced by cold applications, burning sensation in rectum and anus, spattery diarrhoea, stool feels like wind and vice versa *Aloe 6c*
- Great itching, constant bleeding, constipation, desire to pass stool *Collinsonia 6c*
- Bleeding, anus feels sore and bruised *Hamamelis 6c*
- Burning, cutting pains before, during, and after passing stool, presence of anal fissure *Nitric ac. 6c*
- Where person is sedentary, has frequent urge to pass stool but never feels that bowels empty properly, wakes very early then falls into heavy sleep just as it is time to get up, feels chilly and irritable, has large piles which burn and sting *Nux 6c*
- Painful piles which bleed easily and cause more discomfort when lying down, person not at all thirsty *Pulsatilla 6c*
- Piles do not bleed but are aggravated by warmth, skin around anus red and sore *Sulphur 6c*
- Piles extremely painful, pain worse when lying down or during menstruation *Ammonium carb. 6c*
- Protruding piles, burning sensation *Capsicum 6c*
- Piles feel sore, inability to strain to pass stool *Causticum 6c*

Self-help Change to the Liver Diet (p. 352) for at least 1 month and avoid tea, coffee, milk, eggs, gelatine, jellies, white bread, arrowroot, tapioca, semolina, etc. Increase the amount of exercise you take, and do the slant board exercises shown on pp. 19–21, 22. Try to open the bowels regularly, and avoid overstuffed or heated seats.

For external piles, Paeonia ointment can be applied; for internal piles, Peony suppositories or lint soaked in Hamamelis solution (5 drops of mother tincture to a small cup of boiled cooled water) can offer relief; gently push lint or suppositories into the rectum and leave in place overnight. Hamamelis solution can also be applied externally. Mother tinctures of Paeonia and Hamamelis, and also Paeonia ointment, can be obtained from homeopathic pharmacies (addresses p. 361).

For piles which are thrombosed or strangulated and protrude through the anus as small blood-filled pouches, raise the foot of the bed, lie down, and apply an ice pack or a Hamamelis compress to the anal opening. Do not try to push the pouches back inside. Warm salt water baths may also give relief. Alternatively, make up a potato poultice (a layer of hot mashed potato between two layers of muslin) and sit on it as soon as the heat is bearable; this encourages the piles to shrink back in. *Aconite 6c* taken at ½-hourly intervals for up to 10 doses would also be beneficial.

Polyps see TUMOUR OF THE INTESTINE

Pruritis ani

Intractable itching around the opening of the anus. External causes include excessive sweating due to wearing woollen or nylon knickers or tights, lack of cleanliness, irritants in washing powders and possibly in coloured toilet paper, and liquid paraffin used to relieve constipation; discharge from PILES, an ANAL FISSURE or ANAL FISTULA, or from the vagina can also cause it, and so can DIABETES (diabetes mellitus), THRUSH, THREADWORMS, and DIARRHOEA (particularly in children with alactasia, in which milk sugars cannot be digested). In some cases, itching may have a psychological component.

Specific remedies to be taken 4 times daily for up to 14 days

---

- Itchiness of vulva or scrotum which seems to get worse in company *Ambra 6c*
- Violent itching and a crawling sensation around anus, made worse by warmth *Ignatia 6c*
- Itching worse when walking outdoors or after passing stool *Nitric ac. 6c*
- Itching feels like lots of pin pricks, burning sensation in anus, stools soft but passed with difficulty *Alumina 6c*
- Itching due to threadworms, continous irritation, especially on going to bed, restlessness, crawling sensation in rectum after passing stool *Teucrium 6c*
- Where sufferer is a child who takes unreasonable hatreds to people, itching worse at night, grinding of teeth in sleep *Cina 6c*
- Itchiness and smarting worse at night, alternate constipation and diarrhoea, especially if person is elderly, mucous discharge from anus, heat, wine, acid foods, and water make itching worse *Antimonium 6c*
- Anal area red and sore, burning diarrhoea worse in morning *Sulphur 6c*

Self-help Try not to scratch – this only damages the skin and makes it easier for particles of faeces to cause further irritation – and wear cotton underwear. Do not use toilet paper. First thing in the morning and last thing at night, and after passing stool, wash anal area with warm soapy water, rinse with clean warm water, and pat dry with a towel reserved for the purpose. Then rinse your hands and apply Hamamelis ointment.

Tumour of the intestine
The majority of growths in the lower part of the digestive tract are benign, not cancerous; most are small, about the size of a cherry, and are called polyps; very few become large enough to cause OBSTRUCTION. Once detected by endoscopy, or by a barium meal or enema, a small tissue sample (biopsy) is taken for analysis. Surgical removal is usually recommended as there is a small risk of such growths becoming malignant.

Ulcerative colitis
A fairly rare condition in which lining of rectum and colon become progressively ulcerated, causing periodic attacks of left-sided ABDOMINAL PAIN, DIARRHOEA, mucus and BLOOD IN FAECES, and in severe cases FEVER and NAUSEA. Complications include ANAEMIA, as ulcers bleed, and SEPTICAEMIA, as toxins from ulcers get into bloodstream; risk of developing CANCER OF THE RECTUM OR COLON is slight. Cause is not known, but condition can be aggravated by broad spectrum antibiotics. Diagnosis is by barium enema and endoscopy of the rectum and lower colon. Conventionally treated by steroids; in severe cases steroids and nutrients may have to be given intravenously to rest colon and allow it to heal; colostomy, or surgical removal of affected part of colon, is a last resort.

After a first attack, constitutional homeopathic treatment is recommended.

Specific remedies to be given every 2 hours for up to 10 doses during acute attack while constitutional treatment is being sought
- Hot stools which smell offensive and have blood and mucus in them, cutting pains on passing them, abdominal pain not relieved by passing stools *Mercurius corr. 6c*
- Person chilly, restless, and anxious, burning pain in abdomen accompanied by vomiting, symptoms worse after midnight, wanting warm drinks and sipping them at frequent intervals *Arsenicum 6c*
- Blood in stools, passing stools relieves pain but anus feels wide open afterwards *Phosphorus 6c*

Self-help Further attacks may be prevented by changing to a high-fibre diet and reducing intake of milk and dairy products. Be very wary of antibiotics; if you have a bacterial infection and consult your GP, remind him or her that you have a history of ulcerative colitis. Stop smoking.

KIDNEYS AND BLADDER

IN the average adult the kidneys filter the total volume of the blood nearly 300 times a day, producing about 1 litre (2 pints) of urine, passed on four to six occasions. As urine is produced it filters into collecting ducts in the neck of the kidneys and trickles down the ureters into the bladder. As soon as the bladder is half full – its total capacity is about 0.5 litre (1 pint) – stretch receptors in its wall signal the urge to urinate. After the age of about four the sphincter between the bladder and urethra is under voluntary control.

The male urethra, which acts as a passageway for semen as well as urine, is nearly four times as long as the female; this, and the fact that its opening at the tip of the penis is well removed from the anus, explains why men are less susceptible to urinary infections than women. Unfortunately, the short female urethra provides bacteria with a relatively swift invasion route to the bladder.

Urine, the sterile product of the non-stop filtering activities of the kidneys, is 96 per cent water and 4 per cent organic and inorganic solids, and its colour can be a valuable guide not only to the function of the kidneys,

For explanation of other symbols, see page 107

but also to the state of the liver and gall bladder. The kidneys regulate the amount of water and also the balance of acid and alkaline constituents in the blood, and on those two things all the chemical functions of the body intimately depend.

Inside each kidney the branches of the renal artery subdivide into a million or so tiny tufts of blood vessels called glomeruli; small molecules – water, salt, various minerals, glucose, and wastes such as urea, a by-product of protein breakdown – squeeze through their walls under pressure and enter a million adjacent tubules called nephrons which selectively reabsorb them; in a healthy kidney, 99 per cent of the water and all the glucose are reabsorbed. This reabsorption process is controlled by hormones made in the pituitary gland at the base of the brain and in the adrenal glands which sit on top of the kidneys. The kidneys themselves produce a number of hormones which help to control blood pressure, stimulate production of red blood cells in the bone marrow, and activate Vitamin D.

Abnormal-looking urine

Under normal circumstances, urine is straw-coloured, but if the kidneys, urinary tract, or liver are not functioning as well as they should, the colour may change.

Blood in the urine should never be ignored. If urine has a pink, red, or smoky tinge, or if it appears to have tea-leaves or clots of blood in it, 12. Source of bleeding may be kidneys, bladder, urethra, or prostate gland – see KIDNEY STONES, BLADDER STONES, KIDNEY TUMOURS, BLADDER TUMOURS, PYELONEPHRITIS, GLOMERULONEPHRITIS, CYSTITIS, PROSTATE PROBLEMS; injury to the kidneys, impaired renal blood supply, and certain drugs can also present as blood in the urine. Some foods – beetroot, blackberries – and food colourings can also turn the urine reddish or smoky. Blood can also enter the urine from the vagina or the anus (see PILES, ANAL FISSURE, ULCERATIVE COLITIS, etc), or it may be present in semen.

Orange/dark yellow urine usually means that it is more concentrated than usual; concentration happens quite naturally in hot weather or when perspiration rate is high; is also happens with FEVER, DIARRHOEA, and VOMITING, all of which cause water loss. Rhubarb, Vitamin B complex (riboflavin or B$_2$), and laxatives containing senna also intensify orange colour.

Dark brown urine, associated with pale faeces and yellowing of the whites of the eyes, is usually a sign of JAUNDICE.

Cloudy urine suggests infection.

Greenish/bluish urine is usually due to artificial food colourings.

Bladder control problems see also
BEDWETTING
Loss of bladder control can occur after a fright or extreme psychological shock, or as the result of injury, especially SPINAL CORD INJURY, or as the result of progressive nerve damage, as in MULTIPLE SCLEROSIS; more commonly, it is a feature of STRESS INCONTINENCE or PROSTATE PROBLEMS. Stress incontinence occurs in women, usually because the muscles of the pelvic floor have been weakened by childbirth; urine is involuntarily passed when coughing, sneezing, running, lifting, or laughing. In men, an enlarged prostate leads to a frequent urge to urinate, difficulty starting the flow of urine, weak flow, and dribbling after urination. IRRITABLE BLADDER (bladder suddenly contracts, making it imperative to pass urine immediately, though only a small amount is passed) and BLADDER STONES can also cause control problems.

If involuntary urination follows a back injury, and is accompanied by weakness or numbness in the legs, (999).

Bladder stones (vesical calculi)
Nodules of calcium and other salts, which tend to collect at urethral exit of bladder, causing frequent urge to urinate, pain as urine is passed, and blood in urine due to irritation of bladder lining; if all these symptoms are present, 12. Stones can be fragmented *in situ* using ultrasound or an instrument called a cytoscope; the pieces are then washed out. Alternatively, the bladder is opened surgically and the stones sucked out.

For reasons which are not clear, both bladder and kidney stones are much less common now than 40 years ago; they are slightly commoner in men who have had a vasectomy; however, both conditions are related to concentration of urine by high rates of perspiration. To prevent recurrence, constitutional homeopathic treatment is recommended.

Specific remedies to be given 4 times daily for up to 14 days until surgery or fragmentation can be carried out
- Red sediment in urine, frequent urge to urinate, especially at night, especially if there is constipation and a lot of wind in the bowels *Lycopodium 6c*
- Stones interrupt or stop flow of urine, which contains blood and mucus and scalds urethra, all-over bruised feeling *Uva ursi 6c*
- Urine slimy, with sandy sediment and particles of mucus in it, severe pain felt around urethral exit as flow stops, causing person to cry out, frequent urge to urinate *Sarsaparilla 6c*
- Urine has stony particles in it, cold sweats, especially on feet, person overweight and in poor physical shape, craves eggs *Calcarea 6c*
- Fluttering sensation in region of kidneys (around waist at back), mucus in urine, distinct sensation of sitting on a ball *Chimaphila 6c*
- After an operation to remove bladder stones *Staphysagria 6c*

Self-help Drink plenty of water (this reduces concentration of urine). When pain is bad apply heat or cold (hot water bottle or ice pack) to bladder area.

Bladder tumours see also CANCER

Warty or cauliflower-like growths in bladder lining, benign or malignant; thought to be associated with protein-rich Western diet, which leads to high level of L-leucine (an amino acid) in blood. If tumour blocks ureter, urine may be forced back into kidney, causing a condition known as hydronephrosis, or acute PYELONEPHRITIS; because of tumour, bladder may also be more vulnerable to CYSTITIS. Symptoms are BLOOD IN URINE, PAINFUL URINATION, FREQUENT URINATION, and perhaps pain in kidney area. In early stages, tumours can usually be successfully destroyed; if a large area of bladder lining is affected, whole bladder may have to be removed and an external bladder fitted.

Constitutional homeopathic treatment is compatible with surgery.

Specific remedies
- When symptoms are most painful and while waiting for surgery *Thuja 30c* every 12 hours for up to 3 days
- Immediately after operation *Staphysagria 6c*, 3 times daily for up to 5 days

Bright's disease see GLOMERULONEPHRITIS

Cystitis

Mainly affects women, principally because the female urethra is short and easily invaded by bacteria and other microbes present in bowel, vagina, and vulval area. In men, cystitis is usually secondary to PROSTATE PROBLEMS, BLADDER TUMOURS, BLADDER STONES, or congenital abnormality of the bladder or urethra.

The term 'cystitis' is often used, rather loosely, to describe three different conditions which have similar symptoms: a frequent urge to urinate, and scanty urine which smells strongly and stings or scalds as it is passed, and may have blood in it; sometimes there may be a dull ache in the lower abdomen.

Cystitis proper is inflammation of the bladder due to infection, usually by *E. coli* bacteria transferred from the bowel; it is particularly common in the early stages of pregnancy, and attacks tend to recur. *Urethral syndrome* is chronic irritation of the bladder and urethra due to causes other than bacterial infection; antibiotics, certain contraceptives, hormone imbalances caused by STRESS or fear, diet, food ALLERGY, hygiene, clothing, urination patterns, intercourse, and bruising of the urethra during intercourse have all been cited as possible causes. *Urethritis* is inflammation of the urethra only, occasionally due to infection (see *non-specific urethritis* in SEXUALLY TRANSMITTED DISEASES) but more often to bruising during intercourse; it lasts for 2 or 3 days at most, and is common in women who have just started to have intercourse.

Though it poses little risk to general health, cystitis should be treated. If an attacks lasts for more than 48 hours, see your GP. The standard weapon of orthodox medicine is antibiotics, and urine analysis if the condition recurs; some of the self-help methods given below may also be recommended. The homeopathic approach to recurrent attacks is constitutional, although the remedies given below will relieve symptoms in isolated flare-ups.

Specific remedies to be taken every ½ hour for up to 10 doses
- Burning, cutting pains in lower abdomen too severe to ignore, non-stop urge to urinate, ache in small of back tends to get worse in afternoon, merest trickle of urine with blood in it, inability to empty bladder properly *Cantharis 30c*
- Frequent and painful urging with little result *Nux 6c*
- Sharp, stinging pains in lower abdomen, frequent urge to urinate, urine scanty, hot, and bloody, symptoms seem worse for heat and better for cold *Apis 30c*
- Burning sensation along urethra, bladder sensitive to jarring, urine bright red with little clots of blood in it, urging persists even after urine has been passed *Belladonna 30c*
- High fever, excruciating pain in bladder area, bladder swollen and hard, feeling extremely restless, great sense of hurry *Tarentula 6c*
- Urine slimy, with fine mucus in it, burning, radiating pains which get worse during and after passing urine, and during rest *Berberis 6c*
- Frequent urge to pass urine, made worse by coughing and sneezing, acute sensitivity to cold, obeying urge produces nothing but is followed, 15 minutes later, by involuntary passage of urine, itching around urethral opening, perhaps with vaginal discharge *Causticum 6c*
- Attack comes on after getting damp and cold after exertion, especially in autumn, urine bloody and frequent *Dulcamara 6c*
- Pains come on as urination ceases, urine thick and milky-looking, urgency and pressure to pass urine, feeling thirsty *Sarsaparilla 6c*
- Frequency and burning sensation as urine is passed, with pain in small of back, blood in urine, drowsiness, tingling in ears, tongue red and shiny, rest makes symptoms worse but walking in open air alleviates them *Terebinth 6c*
- Attack comes on after sexual intercourse or after catheterization for an operation, urethra feels as if a drop of urine is continuously trickling along it, burning sensation almost constant, even when not passing water *Staphisagria 6c*
- Stream of urine slow and intermittent *Clematis 6c*
- Burning pains in lower abdomen, feeling restless, chilly, and anxious *Arsenicum 6c*
- Pain worse at start of urination, no urine passed despite intense and urgent straining, muscles at base of bladder in spasm, cold makes symptoms worse *Camphora 6c*

For explanation of other symbols, see page 107

If an attack has been brought on by fear or stress, the Bach Flower Remedies Mimulus and Aspen (see p. 388 for suppliers) may be helpful.

Self-help There is a lot you can do for yourself in an acute attack of cystitis. To reduce acidity of urine – responsible for the stinging and scalding – and to flush infected urine out of the bladder as quickly as possible, drink 0.25 litre (½ pint) cold water, barley water, or water with bicarbonate of soda in it every 20 minutes. Don't overdo the bicarbonate – 1 teaspoon per hour for up to 3 hours only is the maximum you should take; if you have a heart condition, stick to plain water or barley water. Curling up with a hot water bottle or ice pack clasped to the lower abdomen also offers relief.

There are also a number of preventive measures you can take, whether you suffer from cystitis, urethral syndrome, or urethritis.

Urinary habits Never suppress the urge to urinate; try to develop the habit of emptying the bladder every 4 hours, and do it twice each time to make sure the bladder is completely empty.

Fluid intake and diet Increase fluid intake to 3 litres (5 pints) per day, or until urine is a normal colour and there is no discomfort on passing urine. Tea, coffee, and alcohol are not a good idea, except perhaps twice a week. The more alkaline your urine the better; a daily bowl of vegetable broth, or a teaspoon of bicarbonate of soda taken in water twice a day, or a daily glass of Mist. Pot. Cit., obtainable from the chemist, will achieve this. Alkaline urine turns pink litmus paper blue, so buy some litmus from the chemist and test it.

Foods known to aggravate cystitis and related conditions are asparagus, spinach, beetroot, raw carrots, potatoes and tomatoes, citrus fruits and strawberries, red meat, milk and ice cream, condiments, junk food in general; chlorinated water and alcohol are also aggravating. Aduki beans are said to be beneficial.

Hygiene In her invaluable book on cystitis (see Books for Further Reading p. 364), Angela Kilmartin recommends the following cleansing routine after every bowel movement.
1 Wipe bottom from front to back with soft white toilet paper
2 Wash hands
3 Soap hands with non-perfumed soap and wash anal area (not vaginal area) with fingers
4 Rinse hands
5 Fill a small bottle with warm water, sit back on lavatory, and pour water down past urethral opening and vagina, using free hand to wash out nooks and crannies
6 When all traces of soap have been washed away, pat dry with a soft towel kept only for that purpose.

This method uses only hands, unscented soap, and the flow of clean warm water to clean anal and vulval area; using flannels, cloths, or cotton wool is not recommended – they only harbour germs. Nor are bidets or squatting in the bath and douching with the shower – that way germs may spread or be forced up the urethra. Nor are vaginal deodorants, vaginal douches, medicated creams, bath oils, bath salts, bubble baths, talcum powder, or antiseptics like Dettol – all of which can irritate the skin. If possible, tampons should be avoided too.

Sexual intercourse If possible have a drink of water and empty the bladder before intercourse. Be as relaxed as possible and spin out time spent in foreplay. Use KY jelly as a lubricant, and don't be afraid to experiment with different positions to see if these relieve pressure on bladder or urethra. After intercourse, empty bladder and wash away semen using the bottle-of-warm-water technique described above. The man should wash his hands and penis before intercourse. Since long finger nails harbour germs, both partners should keep nails short.

Clothing Swap nylon underwear for cotton, and nylon tights for those with a cotton gusset, and change them every day. Wash them in pure soap – never with biological washing powders or bleach – and rinse them thoroughly.

Antibiotics These should be avoided in cystitis unless absolutely necessary, as they tend to promote thrush (SEE VAGINAL AND VULVAL PROBLEMS). If a course of antibiotics is necessary – for example, if other measures have failed or if there is FEVER, indicating that infection may be spreading – eat a small carton of natural yoghurt every day for 5 days as soon as the course finishes. This helps to re-populate the body with the healthy bacteria which the antibiotics destroyed along with the undesirables.

Frequent urination

Urinating more frequently than usual is quite normal in cold weather, in the first and last trimester of pregnancy, and in moments of anxiety or excitement; frequency of urination also tends to increase in old age. Tea, coffee, alcohol, excessive Vitamin D, and certain drugs, especially diuretics prescribed for high blood pressure and heart disease, also make visits to the toilet more frequent.

The disorders most commonly associated with frequent urination are DIABETES (wanting to pass urine at night, feeling thirsty, losing weight, tiredness, itchy genitals), IRRITABLE BLADDER (uncontrollable urgency, involuntary leaking of urine), PROSTATE PROBLEMS (if prostate is enlarged, flow of urine may be weak and difficult to start, with dribbling afterwards), urethral stricture (stream of urine weak and reluctant to start, only small amounts passed – SEE PENIS PROBLEMS), and CYSTITIS (overwhelming urge to urinate, urine passed in trickles which burn or sting, dull pain in lower abdomen). See individual entries for specific homeopathic remedies. If none seems suitable, try the remedies below; however, if frequency continues, see your GP.

Specific remedies to be taken every 4 hours for up to 3 days
- Person elderly and suffers from frequency all the time, day and night *Causticum 6c*
- Urge to pass urine strongest around 4 am, difficulty starting stream *Kali carb. 6c*
- Frequent urging, associated with constipation and irritability *Nux 6c*
- Intense urging, dragging pains in lower abdomen *Lilium 6c*

Glomerulonephritis (Bright's disease)

Inflammation of the tiny filtering units (glomeruli) in the kidneys, causing red blood cells and proteins to leak into the urine. If blood and protein loss is severe, as it tends to be in children, NEPHROTIC SYNDROME may develop, and some degree of ANAEMIA; if many filtering units are affected, preventing kidneys from effectively regulating composition of blood, HIGH BLOOD PRESSURE may develop, and as waste products accumulate in blood KIDNEY FAILURE becomes a possibility. Symptoms are smoky or red urine passed in small amounts, puffy ankles (due to fluid retention), NAUSEA AND VOMITING, ABNORMAL SLEEPINESS OR DROWSINESS, and generally feeling unwell, and may onset fairly suddenly or insidiously over months or years. Since condition affects every aspect of metabolism, ⏍12⏍ if above symptoms are present. Orthodox approach is to treat inflammation, fluid retention, high blood pressure, and anaemia with steroids, diuretics, anti-hypertensive drugs, and iron respectively; in severe cases, a blood transfusion may be necessary.

Constitutional homeopathic treatment is recommended in chronic cases; as a temporary measure, until treatment can be arranged, take *Arsenicum 6c* 4 times daily for up to 7 days.

Specific remedies to be given every ½ hour for up to 10 doses in acute cases while waiting to see GP
- In early stages, symptoms mild but include fluid retention *Apis 30c*
- Burning pains in region of kidneys, pain passing urine or inability to pass it at all, especially after scarlet fever *Cantharis 30c*
- Fluid retention all over body due to loss of protein through urine, person thirsty for sips of cold water, chilly, restless *Arsenicum 6c*

Incontinence of urine see also INCONTINENCE OF URINE pp. 340–1

Involuntary urination can be due to weakness of the pelvic floor or prolapse of the uterus (leakage of urine when sneezing, coughing, laughing, running, lifting things, etc., with dragging pain between legs – see STRESS INCONTINENCE, UTERUS PROBLEMS), IRRITABLE BLADDER (sudden uncontrollable urge to urinate), PROSTATE PROBLEMS (urgency and frequency, drib-

bling after flow has stopped), bladder and urethral infections (urgency, frequency, scalding pain on passing urine, having to get up in night – see CYSTITIS), or the result of injury (INJURY TO KIDNEYS, BLADDER, OR URETHRA). Lower abdominal surgery can also cause temporary loss of control. Urinary incontinence can also be a part of SENILE DEMENTIA. It may also occur during an epileptic fit (see EPILEPSY). Suitable homeopathic remedies are listed under each of the conditions mentioned above.

If loss of control is accompanied by sudden weakness, confusion, dizziness, numbness, paralysis or great heaviness in any part of the body, blurred vision, slurred or difficult speech, or loss of consciousness, ② since a STROKE may have occurred. If, after an accident of some kind, there is weakness, numbness, paralysis, and loss of bowel as well as bladder control, SPINAL CORD INJURY should be suspected; ⑲⑲⑲ and give *Arnica 30c* every 5 minutes for up to 10 doses until help arrives; *Hypericum 30c*, given 4 times daily for up to 7 days, will aid recovery.

Self-help The best way of toning up weak pelvic floor muscles, especially after childbirth, is to practice stopping and starting the flow of urine several times while urinating. Standing, tucking the coccyx in, and tightening the muscles around the anus has a similar toning effect.

In elderly people, problems can be minimized by establishing a regular pattern of urination; use an alarm clock if necessary, and set it to go off every 2 or 3 hours. Bedtime drinks should be kept to a minimum. If there is a problem getting to the toilet quickly, use a chamber pot or commode.

Injury to kidneys, bladder, or urethra

Kidney injuries Usually caused by a blow under the ribs, or a crushing injury to the ribcage or upper abdomen; injury may merely bruise kidneys and ureters; more seriously, it may rupture them, releasing urine into the abdominal cavity and causing PERITONITIS. Most kidney injuries declare themselves by BLOOD IN URINE. Rupture causes severe back pain in kidney area, made worse by pressure and movement, plus the symptoms of peritonitis (nausea, vomiting, distended abdomen, fever); appropriate action is ⑲⑲⑲, and *Aconite 30c* every 5 minutes until help arrives. If kidney is damaged beyond repair, it may need to be removed. If kidney is merely bruised, recovery takes 7–10 days.

Specific remedy to be given every 2 hours for up to 2 days during recovery from injury
- *Arnica 30c*

Bladder and urethra injuries Most bladder injuries are caused by blows which fracture the pelvis and cause splinters of bone to puncture the bladder; in addition to severe pain in the lower abdomen, BLOOD IN URINE, and inability to urinate, urine may seep into the abdominal cavity and cause PERITONITIS or person may go into SHOCK. In men, the urethra can be ruptured by a straddling fall or a blow to the groin; as well as agonising pain, there may be subsequent difficulty urinating, and narrowing of the urethra as the injury heals (see urethral stricture – PENIS PROBLEMS); urethral injuries in women are rare.

If rupture of either urethra or bladder is suspected, (999), and give *Aconite 30c* every 5 minutes until help arrives. If urination is still possible, even if scanty or painful, give one or other of the remedies below, but if blood appears in urine or RETENTION OF URINE sets in, (2).

Specific remedies to be given ½-hourly for up to 10 doses immediately after injury
- Injury involves bruising only *Arnica 30c*
- Very scanty amounts of urine passed *Opium 6c*

If injury leads on to CYSTITIS, take *Staphisagria 6c* every 2 hours for up to 10 doses.

Irritable bladder (urge incontinence)

Sudden contraction of the bladder causing instant urge to pass urine regardless of time or place, often associated with STRESS INCONTINENCE or prolapse of the uterus (see UTERUS PROBLEMS), in which the pelvic floor muscles are weak, or with urinary tract infections such as CYSTITIS (frequency, burning sensation on passing urine). Orthodox treatment depends on cause, but if nervous control is faulty drugs may be prescibed to suppress nervous impulses to bladder or relax bladder muscles.

For homeopathic treatment, look up whichever of the above conditions is most appropriate; if none of the remedies mentioned seems suitable, select one from the list below.

Specific remedies to be taken every 4 hours for up to 7 days
- Great urge to pass urine but nothing comes, chilliness, irritability *Nux 6c*
- Non-stop urge to pass urine, straining produces only a few drops at a time, burning pain at neck of bladder and in urethra, especially in older women *Copaiva 6c*
- Involuntary passage of urine when coughing or sneezing *Causticum 6c*
- Involuntary passage of urine on sitting down, walking, coughing, or passing wind *Pulsatilla 6c*

Self-help See STRESS INCONTINENCE for exercises to strengthen pelvic floor muscles; nervous control of bladder muscles may also be improved by not instantly answering the urge to urinate, but holding on for as long as possible.

Kidney failure (renal failure)

May be acute or chronic, involving a sudden or gradual build-up of water and waste products in the blood.

Acute kidney failure means that the kidneys stop working within the space of several hours or days. Cause may be SHOCK (usually due to heavy blood loss or a heart attack), sudden blockage of the ureters, bladder, or urethra (by KIDNEY STONES, for example), or, more rarely, GLOMERULONEPHRITIS (widespread damage to filtering units in kidneys). Symptoms may be secondary to those of immediate cause, but include scanty urine, loss of appetite (see APPETITE CHANGES), NAUSEA AND VOMITING, and eventually CONFUSION, ABNORMAL SLEEPINESS OR DROWSINESS, and coma. Orthodox treatment depends on underlying cause; to restore kidney function, person may need intravenous drip of blood or plasma, and diuretic drugs; in more severe cases, several weeks of dialysis (machine-assisted elimination of water and wastes) may be necessary, or even a kidney transplant; to assist recovery, a high calorie/low protein/low fluid regime is prescribed, together with careful monitoring of potassium and sodium levels.

If failure symptoms follow severe blood loss or heart attack, (999) and give *Aconite 30c* every 5 minutes for up to 6 doses until help arrives; if failure sets in for other reasons, appropriate action is [12], plus one of the remedies below.

Specific remedies to be given every hour for up to 10 doses while waiting for help
- In early stages of failure, person feverish, anxious, and afraid of dying *Aconite 30c*
- In early stages of failure, person feverish, with flushed face and staring eyes *Belladonna 30c*
- No urine passed, or blood only *Terebinth 6x*
- Face and feet look puffy with retained fluid, burning, stinging pains in kidney region *Apis 30c*
- Person drowsy, especially after stroke or heart attack *Opium 6c*
- Symptoms worse for exposure to cold *Camphora 6c*

In *chronic kidney failure*, brought about by mild but recurrent attacks of inflammation (see chronic PYELONEPHRITIS, GLOMERULONEPHRITIS, KIDNEY STONES, HIGH BLOOD PRESSURE), kidney efficiency slowly decreases as more and more tissue becomes scarred; certain drugs, notably aspirin, paracetamol, and phenacetin, and the toxic element cadmium can also cause inflammation. Symptoms are insidious – tiredness, feeling lethargic, passing urine more often than usual, and a gradual increase in blood pressure. As time goes on, person may begin to suffer from ANAEMIA, OSTEOMALACIA, and hyperparathyroidism (see PARATHYROID PROBLEMS) as metabolism of iron and calcium fails, or may develop the symptoms of end-stage kidney failure (see below). Since kidney damage is irreversible, treatment is directed towards

---

slowing down the failure process. Homeopathic treatment is constitutional and dietary, although the specific remedies given above for acute kidney failure may be used while treatment is being sought. Orthodox treatment is also dietary, with drugs to control blood pressure and to prevent bones losing calcium. Iron, vitamins, and a low protein/high fluid diet are usually recommended.

End-stage kidney failure occurs in three out of four people already suffering from chronic kidney failure, the last straw often being a minor urinary infection. Symptoms are many and varied – HEADACHES, NAUSEA AND VOMITING, ORAL THRUSH, HALITOSIS, a furred tongue (see TONGUE DISORDERS), DIARRHOEA, retention of fluid in the lungs and under the skin (see OEDEMA), itchy skin (see ITCHING), cessation of periods (see MENSTRUAL PROBLEMS). . .

Orthodox treatment is to alleviate as many symptoms as possible by drugs; in suitable cases, dialysis (long-term use of a kidney machine) or a kidney transplant may be offered. Homeopathic treatment is constitutional, though until dialysis or a transplant is possible it can only be palliative.

Kidney stones (renal calculi)

Hard accretions of calcium and other salts which form in the larger urine-collecting ducts in one or both kidneys; sometimes associated with GOUT, PARATHYROID PROBLEMS, or kidney disease. If very small, stones may pass into ureters and out of the body unnoticed; if too large to pass into the ureters, they remain in the kidneys, perhaps giving mild pain whenever fragments break off. If a medium-sized stone enters a ureter, then becomes stuck or only gradually works its way down to the bladder, the result is *renal colic*, waves of severe stabbing or cramping pain which abate when the stone stops moving; pain follows the route of the ureter. Once in the bladder, kidney stones are removed in the same way as BLADDER STONES. If a stone is stuck in a ureter, blocking the flow of urine, surgery may be necessary. To prevent recurrence, constitutional homeopathic treatment should be sought. A kidney with a stone in it is vulnerable to infection (see PYELONEPHRITIS); in a few cases, scarring from large stones leads to KIDNEY FAILURE.

If symptoms are those of renal colic, ②, and select an emergency remedy from the list below; the appropriate remedy should relax the circular fibres in the ureter wall, allowing the stone to descend to the bladder.

Specific remedies to be given as often as necessary for up to 10 doses while waiting for help
- Stitching pain felt between lower ribs and hip bone when urinating, pain radiates from a specific point and is made worse by slightest movement but is relieved by lying on painful side *Berberis 6c*
- Right-sided pain which stabs towards genitals and down right leg, causing nausea and vomiting, or right-sided pain which shoots into rectum, causing urge to stool, weak urine flow which stops altogether on straining to increase flow, person chilly and irritable *Nux 6c*
- Pain in right side, which stops at bladder and does not go down into the leg, also pain in the back relieved by urinating, urine clear with red sediment in it, symptoms worse between 4 pm and 8 pm *Lycopodium 6c*
- Pain darts down ureter, causing nausea and cold sweat *Tabacum 6c*
- Pain feels like knives stabbing in all directions, burning sensation in bladder and intolerable urge to urinate, person thirsty but sickened by thought of food *Cantharis 6c*

Specific remedy to be given 4 times daily for 5 days immediately after removal of a kidney stone
- *Staphisagria 6c*

Self-help A hot water bottle or an ice pack held over the site of the pain usually offers some relief.

Recurrence can be avoided by taking some or all of the following measures.
1 Avoid high-dose long-term supplementation with Vitamin C.
2 Avoid calcium and Vitamin D supplements.
3 Avoid foods containing sucrose and lactose.
4 Reduce intake of animal protein.
5 Reduce intake of salt and alcohol.
6 If previous stones contained oxalates, reduce intake of tea, coffee, chocolate, peanuts, spinach, rhubarb, and beetroot.
7 Increase fluid intake (not tea), but if you live in a hard water area do not drink more than 2 litres (3 ½ pints) a day.
8 Eat a high fibre diet.
9 Take supplements of magnesium and B_6.
10 Lose any excess weight.

Kidney tumours see also WILM'S TUMOUR, CANCER

One kind of tumour, known as a hypernephroma, affects the kidneys in adults; it is malignant, and causes general symptoms such as FEVER, WEIGHT LOSS, blood in urine (see ABNORMAL LOOKING URINE) and loss of appetite (see APPETITE CHANGES), and also VOMITING, ABDOMINAL PAIN, and reddish or cloudy urine; it can spread to the lungs or bones. Smaller cauliflower-like tumours may grow in the kidney. Orthodox treatment is removal of the affected kidney, leaving the job of cleansing the blood to the remaining healthy kidney.

Painful urination

In men, painful urination accompanied by a dull ache in the groin, and sometimes FEVER, may be due to prostatis (see PROSTATE PROBLEMS). Other conditions causing painful urination include urethritis (see CYSTITIS), SEXUALLY TRANSMITTED DISEASES such as non-specific urethritis (discharge from urethral opening – see SEXUALLY TRANSMITTED DISEASES) and gonorrhea (discharge from penis or vagina, anal infection causing discharge and irritation, and in women fever, chills, and pains in abdomen and joints), genital infections such as thrush, trichomoniasis, and pruritis vulvae (see VAGINAL AND VULVAL PROBLEMS, PENIS PROBLEMS), CYSTITIS (frequent urge to urinate, stinging or burning sensation when urine is passed), and acute PYELONEPHRITIS (high fever, intense pain in kidney area extending down to groin, nausea and vomiting, shivering, pink or cloudy urine). If pyelonephritis is suspected, 12 .

See CYSTITIS and PYELONEPHRITIS for specific remedies.

Pyelonephritis

Acute or chronic infection of the kidneys, usually following bacterial infection of the urethra or bladder (see CYSTITIS), especially in women.

In *acute pyelonephritis* inflammation results in sudden intense pain in the back, just above the waist, usually worse on one side; pain then extends down to groin, accompanied by high FEVER, NAUSEA AND VOMITING, rigours (intense shivering) PAINFUL URINATION, and frequent urge to pass urine; urine also turns pink or cloudy, and person feels generally cold and shivery. KIDNEY STONES, BLADDER TUMOURS, an enlarged prostate (see PROSTATE PROBLEMS), or blockage of a ureter during pregnancy – all of which make transit of urine through urinary system slower – tend to increase risk of acute infection. If above symptoms are present, 12 ; antibiotics and bed rest will probably be prescribed, and x-ray investigation of the kidneys once attack has subsided.

Specific remedies to be taken every hour for up to 10 doses while waiting to see GP
- Scanty urine, burning sensation as urine is passed, person exhausted and restless *Arsenicum 6c*
- Sudden onset, person fearful, feverish, and thirsty, painful urination and anxiety at start of urination, urine hot, red, and scanty, kidney area tender, symptoms come on after exposure to cold dry air *Aconite 30c*
- Frequent urge to pass urine, burning or tearing pains in kidney area, blood and mucus in urine, vomiting *Uva ursi 6c*
- Constant desire to pass urine, cutting, burning pains in kidney area *Cantharis 30c*

In *chronic pyelonephritis* there are repeated infections, sometimes from childhood onwards, but no clear symptoms until kidney function is considerably impaired; then early signs of KIDNEY FAILURE – tiredness, increased urination, itchy skin, nausea – set in; in most cases, condition is detected as the result of tests for other ailments. Repeated infection is often due to weakness of valves between ureters and bladder, allowing urine and any bacteria present in bladder to spurt back into ureters as bladder is emptied. Surgical repair of valves may be possible in children, but in adults usual treatment is to give low-dose antibiotics for long periods.

Homeopathic treatment is constitutional; however, while treatment is being sought, one of the remedies given for chronic kidney failure (p. 236) may be suitable.

Self-help Increase fluid intake to at least 5 pints per day, and cut down protein and salt in diet. In acute attacks, eat only light, bland foods until infection abates.

Renal colic see KIDNEY STONES

Retention of urine

Acute failure to pass urine, causing great pain as bladder is stretched by accumulating urine; not unusual after abdominal surgery and catheterization (passage of a small tube into bladder to drain urine), or after injury to bladder or urethra (see INJURY TO KIDNEY, BLADDER, OR URETHRA); more commonly, it may be due to enlargement of the prostate gland (see enlarged prostate and prostatitis under PROSTATE PROBLEMS). Prompt action is necessary, so ②; a catheter will have to be inserted into the bladder to drain it.

Increasing difficulty in passing urine – less and less urine passed over a period of months or years – results in gradual expansion of the bladder; in severe cases the bladder pushes up to just below the navel! Sneezing, coughing, laughing, straining, etc. cause leakage of urine, and there is great vulnerability to infections such as PYELONEPHRITIS and CYSTITIS. Sooner or later retention becomes acute.

Specific remedies to be given ½-hourly for up to 10 doses where retention is acute
- Problem follows injury to groin or lower abdomen *Arnica 30c*
- Problem brought on by surgery *Causticum 6c*
- Inability to pass urine in presence of others *Natrum mur. 6c*
- Pain but no urge to urinate *Opium 6c*
- Person too hyped up and restless to relax urethral muscles and let urine out *Tarentula 6c*
- If retention is a hysterical reaction to grief *Ignatia 6c*

Stress incontinence see also IRRITABLE BLADDER

A very common and embarrassing complaint, almost unique to women, in which small quantities of urine are involuntarily passed when coughing, sneezing, laughing, lifting things, etc. Because the muscles of the pelvic floor are weak – often as the result of childbirth, being overweight, or general loss of muscle tone after the menopause – the urethral sphincter does not close properly. If the problem only occurs once in a while, the self-help measures below will almost certainly improve matters. If incontinence occurs more often, ask your GP to refer you to a specialist for assessment; the options, depending on the severity of the problem, are pelvic floor exercises, wearing special briefs, or an operation to tighten the pelvic floor muscles.

Specific remedies to be taken 4 times daily for up to 3 weeks while waiting for specialist treatment
- Problem made worse by coughing, laughing, sneezing, excitement, person unaware that leakage is occurring *Causticum 6c*
- Problem made worse by sitting down, walking, passing wind, desire to pass urine increases when lying down *Pulsatilla 6c*
- Problem worse during day, with tickling sensation in urethra and bladder, especially if sufferer has pale complexion *Ferrum 6c*
- Incontinence associated with 'bearing down' sensation, as if abdominal contents are escaping through vagina, stream of urine slow to start *Sepia 6c*

Self-help The pelvic floor muscles can be strengthened by alternately tightening and relaxing them as you urinate, so that stream of urine stops and starts, and stops and starts, or by tightening the muscles around the anus, as if controlling the passage of a stool; this last exercise can be done sitting or standing, reading the paper or waiting for a bus! If you are overweight, try to lose weight; this will relieve some of the downward pressure of the abdominal organs on the bladder and pelvic floor.

Urethritis see CYSTITIS

Urethral syndrome see CYSTITIS

SPECIAL PROBLEMS IN WOMEN

BETWEEN puberty and the menopause, a span of some 35 years, a woman ovulates about 400 times, normally at intervals of 28 days. If an egg is fertilized, pregnancy follows; if not, menstruation occurs as the vascular lining of the womb is shed. This remarkable cycle of fertility is maintained by three hormone-producing glands, the hypothalamus, pituitary, and ovaries. The ovaries produce two hormones, oestrogen and progesterone, in response to two hormones produced by the pituitary, follicle stimulating hormone (FSH) and luteinizing hormone (LH). Oestrogen levels, responding to FSH levels, rise dramatically in the 12 days leading up to ovulation, and are at their lowest during menstruation. Levels of progesterone, secreted in response to LH, are highest after ovulation, preparing the lining of the uterus (endometrium) for implantation of the egg. Menstrual bleeding begins approximately 2 days after oestrogen and progesterone secretion reach their lowest level. About 35 ml (1½ fl oz) of blood are then lost over 3–7 days.

The uterus or womb is a thick-walled, pear-shaped organ about 7.5 cm (3 in) long, with a narrow neck or cervix at its lower end; the mouth of the cervix juts into the top of the vagina. Opening into the bulbous, upper end of the uterus are two tubes about 10 cm long (4 in), the Fallopian tubes. These are lined with tiny waving hairs which transport eggs from the ovaries to the uterus. It is in one or other Fallopian tube that fertilization usually occurs. There is no direct connection between the ovaries and the Fallopian tubes, however; eggs are simply released into the fluid-filled peritoneal cavity and wafted towards their fringed entrances.

The ovaries themselves are almond-shaped and about 3.5 cm (1 ½ in) long. At birth they contain many millions of immature eggs and follicles, but as already mentioned only about 400 reach maturity. Although several eggs may begin to mature each month under the influence of FSH, only one matures. Once it has been released from its follicle, the follicle turns into a 'corpus luteum' (literally 'yellow body') and proceeds to secrete large amounts of progesterone.

The external female genitals, referred to as the vulva, consist of the fleshy inner and outer labia or lips which conceal the entrance to the vagina, and the clitoris, which lies just above the urethral opening where the inner labia meet. The clitoris is very sensitive and a focus for many of the sensations which trigger orgasm. The vagina is about 10 cm (4 in) long, expands and lubricates during sexual arousal, and is most sensitive near its entrance. It is protected from infection by populations of acid-producing bacteria.

Breast development is one of the first signs of puberty. The breasts move with the pectoral muscles underneath and their hang is greatly influenced by posture and the tone of the muscles which brace the shoulders back. Embedded in the fatty tissue of each breast are 15–20 clusters of milk-producing glands whose ducts converge on the nipple. The pigmented area around the nipple, the areola, contains glands which keep the nipple supple.

Amenorrhea see MENSTRUAL PROBLEMS

Bartholinitis, Bartholin's cyst see VAGINAL AND VULVAL PROBLEMS

For explanation of other symbols, see page 107

Breast problems see also CANCER OF THE BREAST

The best insurance against breast cancer and other problems is regular self-examination of breasts; this should be done just after every period or, if periods have ceased, on same date each month; just before a period breasts can be misleadingly lumpy or tender due to activation of milk-producing tissue; it is also quite normal for one breast to be slightly larger than the other. If you detect anything suspicious, see your GP. You are not wasting his or her time.

Undress to waist and stand in front of mirror. Can you see any differences between breasts when you lean forwards, lift breasts upwards, stretch arms above head, press hands on hips? Things to watch for are different 'hang' and 'swing', and areas of dimpling or flattening.

Lie in bath or on bed and feel each breast with flattened fingers. Does one breast feel different from the other? Are there any lumps or areas of thickening or tenderness in breast or armpit? Has one nipple begun to retract or stick out in an odd direction? Is there any discharge from it? Is there any new or persistent pain?

Breast abscess (mastitis) Due to milk stasis in the breast glands post-natally. If breast-feeding, continue to do so unless symptoms are very severe; symptoms are red, painful swelling in breast, some tenderness in armpit glands, and possibly mild FEVER. Homeopathic remedies below are recommended as first resort; if they do not work, see your GP; if antibiotics do not subdue infection, abscess may have to be drained. However, antibiotics are best avoided if you are breast-feeding; tell your GP you are breast-feeding if he or she proposes antibiotics, for whatever reason.

Specific remedies to be taken every hour for up to 10 doses
- Abscess brewing, with hardening of breast tissue and pain on slightest movement *Bryonia 6c*
- Symptoms as above, with red streaks on affected breast *Belladonna 6c*
- Pain very localized, area extremely tender, irritability *Hepar sulph. 6c*
- Armpit glands swollen, looking generally pale, feeling shivery *Phytolacca 6c*
- Nipple cracked and discharging pus, general exhaustion *Silicea 6c*

Self-help At first sign of pain bathe breast in hot water. Use gravity to help drain the affected area of milk by positioning breast and baby so that abscess is uppermost. Apply Calendula ointment to nipple. For other self-help measures see BREAST-FEEDING PROBLEMS.

Galactorrhea Abnormal production of small quantities of breast milk, usually from both breasts, unrelated to childbirth or breast-feeding; discharge is whitish or greenish; causes include excessive production of milk-stimulating hormone prolactin by pituitary (see PITUITARY PROBLEMS), malfunction of hypothalamus, CANCER OF THE BREAST, drugs such as oral contraceptives, tranquillizers, and diuretics, and more rarely injury, burns, or surgery, nervous disorders such as SHINGLES, and problems with cervical part of spine. Problem affects very few women, notably women who suffer from amenorrhea (see MENSTRUAL PROBLEMS), and can occur in men. Milk production ceases once underlying cause is found and treated.

Specific remedies to be taken 4 times daily for up to 7 days
- Discharge of milk follows injury to breast *Arnica 30c*
- If breast remains swollen after taking Arnica *Bellis 6c*
- Where breast is hard and painful to touch *Conium 6c*

Lumps in breasts May be due to a cyst (fluid-filled sac of tissue), to fibroadenosis (thickening of milk-producing tissue), to a benign growth, or to cancer (see CANCER OF THE BREAST); pain is rare in such cases, so regular self-examination of breasts is important. Only a breast infection or abscess (see above) can be relied on to cause pain; it is also of sudden onset. If you notice *any* changes in nipple shape, skin colour, skin texture, or 'hang' of breasts, or any hard or tender areas you have not felt before, see your GP as soon as possible. Breasts may feel slightly tender before a period, but this is perfectly normal and due to changing hormone levels.

Cysts are conventionally treated by draining off fluid, provided diagnosis has been determined; otherwise they need surgical removal. Benign tumours are also treated by surgical removal; after such treatments, check-ups are carried out every 2 years. In homeopathic medicine, all of these conditions are treated constitutionally, although the remedies listed below may be used while constitutional treatment is being sought. For conventional and homeopathic treatment of malignant tumours, see CANCER OF THE BREAST.

Specific remedies to be taken 4 times daily for up to 14 days
- Cyst diagnosed, affected area hard and painful, stitching pains in nipple, and itching inside the breast, discomfort worse just before and during period, wanting to press breast hard with hand *Conium 6c*
- Cysts present, breasts have purplish tinge and feel extra tender before and during period, chill, damp weather and emotional strain make discomfort worse *Phytolacca 6c*
- Pain comes and goes suddenly, reducing you to tears *Pulsatilla 6c*
- Breasts swollen, hard, and thickened, nipples sore, cracked, and blistered *Graphites 6c*

---

(999) Emergency – call GP (or dial 999) immediately. (2) Consult your doctor if no improvement within 2 hours

- Breasts painful and engorged with milk at time of period *Mercurius 6c*
- Breasts red, throbbing, and heavy, lying down makes discomfort worse *Belladonna 30c*
- Breast feels hard, slightest movement makes pain worse *Bryonia 30c*

Self-help Reduce intake of animal fats and of tea, coffee, and other beverages containing caffeine. Occasionally substitute oily fish (herring, mackerel, sardines) for meat or dairy products. An 8-week course of Vitamin E is also recommended, gradually increasing daily dosage from 100 to 600 units; however, if you have HIGH BLOOD PRESSURE, check with your GP first as extra Vitamin E can temporarily raise blood pressure. Extra Vitamin B$_6$, magnesium, and zinc, and also evening primrose oil and kelp, would also be beneficial.

Nipple problems Dark red discharge from one nipple may indicate a benign tumour called a duct papilloma, which requires surgical removal, or CANCER OF THE BREAST; white or greenish discharge from both breasts, unrelated to childbirth, may be galactorrhea (see above). Brown area around nipple (areola) can be affected by cysts (see SEBACEOUS CYSTS) or BOILS. Eczema only affecting the nipple area may be Bowen's disease, which may lead to cancer. Nipples which do not protrude are said to be retracted or indented; in some women this is quite normal, but may make breast-feeding difficult; recent indentation, however, may be a sign of cancer and requires prompt investigation by GP. For other nipple problems see POST-NATAL BREAST PROBLEMS.

Specific remedy to be taken every 12 hours for up to 7 days
- Long-standing indentation of nipples, provided cancer has been ruled out *Silicea 30c*

Painful breasts General tenderness is quite common before period (see PREMENSTRUAL SYNDROME); localized pain may be an abscess (see above) or a lump (see above for possible causes).

Size problems Except post-natally, when milk glands are working hard, breast tissue is largely fat, laid down and maintained by action of female sex hormone oestrogen; since fat distribution is determined genetically, losing or putting on weight is not an infallible way of reducing or increasing breast size; however, if you are over-weight and suffer from pain in neck and shoulders because your breasts are too heavy for the muscles which support them, do try to lose weight; if you are underweight, extra calories will enable you to lay down more fat, which will encourage oestrogen production. Breast reduction is occasionally necessary on medical grounds, breast augmentation almost never.

Homeopathy offers a number of remedies for enlarged or shrunken breasts and associated symp-toms; if there is no improvement within 1 month, see your homeopath.

Specific remedies to be taken every 12 hours for up to 7 days
- Breasts large because of fluid retention *Natrum mur. 30c*
- Breasts heavy and pendulous, especially if woman is obese, pale, and prone to sweats and chills *Calcarea 30c*
- Enlargement associated with pain and tenderness *Conium 30c*
- Enlargement associated with darting pains *Carbo an. 30c*
- Small, flaccid breasts which enlarge and harden before period *Conium 30c*
- Gradual loss of fatty tissue, bluish-red lumps in skin of breasts, tendency to feel hot all the time *Iodum 30c*
- Breasts poorly developed or wrinkled and shrunken *Sabal 30c*

Cancer of the breast see also BREAST PROBLEMS
Most common form of cancer in women, affecting 1 woman in 20, usually between age of 40 and 50; risk is slightly higher if MENOPAUSE is late, if breast cancer runs in family, and in women who have not had children and in smokers. Warning signs are a lump, usually in outer or upper part of breast, which may or may not be painful, dimpling or creasing of skin in region of lump, discharge from nipple, and recent indentation or reorientation of nipple (see self-examination routine p. 240); usually only one breast is affected. Not all lumps are malignant (see BREAST PROBLEMS) but immediate investigation is essential as even small tumours can quickly spread. Orthodox treat is to remove lump ('lumpectomy'), affected breast (simple mastectomy), or affected breast plus adjacent lymph nodes (radical mastectomy), with radiotherapy or chemotherapy as necessary; however, with new radioactive implant techniques, removal of whole breast is likely to become a less common procedure. In some cases diseased tissue can be replaced by a silicon implant, preserving shape of breast. For some women the psychological effects of losing a breast can be devastating; this is why counselling before and after mastectomy is important; spouses can give enormous reasssurance too.

See HYSTERECTOMY for post-operative remedies and pp. 273–4 for general homeopathic approach to CANCER.

Cancer of the cervix see also CERVICAL PROBLEMS
Affects 1 women in 80, especially after age of 40; usually a late consequence of untreated cervical erosion which has developed into cervical dysplasia (see CERVICAL PROBLEMS); incidence is higher in women who have had many sexual partners or who start having inter-course very young and in smokers; genital warts (see

VULVAL WARTS, PENILE WARTS) and a deficiency of Vitamin B$_6$ may also be contributory factors. Symptoms are offensive, watery bleeding between periods, after intercourse, or after MENOPAUSE; cervical polyps (see CERVICAL PROBLEMS) cause similar symptoms. See your GP immediately if you have any suspicions; a cervical smear will rule out or confirm malignancy. Routine treatment, provided cancer has not spread beyond uterus, depends on grading of cancer by cervical smear and biopsy. It may range from laser treatment or local surgery through to HYSTERECTOMY (usually removal of ovaries and fallopian tubes along with uterus and cervix), backed up by radiotherapy. See CANCER for homeopathic approach.

Cancer of the ovary

Rare and difficult to detect in early stages because ovaries are deep-lying; once symptoms develop – lower ABDOMINAL PAIN and swelling, general malaise, perhaps WEIGHT LOSS – cancer may be well established and already have spread; occasionally, an untreated OVARIAN CYST becomes cancerous. Routine treatment is to remove ovary, or ovary and uterus (see HYSTERECTOMY); if cancer has spread, its progress can be kept at bay for several years with radiotherapy and chemotherapy. For homeopathic treatment, see CANCER.

Cancer of the uterus see also UTERUS PROBLEMS

Most common in women aged 50–60 who have not had children; warning signals are period-type pains at abnormal times, spotting of blood between periods, or reappearance of blood after MENOPAUSE, sometimes accompanied by watery pink or brown discharge which smells unpleasant; a cervical smear and a D and C (removal of tissue from inside uterus) are necessary to confirm or rule out presence of cancer; malignant change in lining of uterus is fairly slow, although eventually muscular walls of uterus, fallopian tubes, ovaries, and other abdominal organs may be affected. If detected early enough, chances of HYSTERECTOMY and radiotherapy effecting a complete cure are very good. For homeopathic treatment, see CANCER.

Cancer of the vulva see also VAGINAL AND VULVAL PROBLEMS

A very rare, slow-growing form of cancer, most common in women over 60; begins as hard lump on labia or at entrance to vagina, often on site of persistent irritation or infection, and develops into an ulcer with a thick rim and a moist centre; almost always curable, if detected early enough, by surgical removal and radiotherapy; in some cases lymph glands in groin may have to be removed. For homeopathic treatment, see CANCER.

Cervical problems see also CANCER OF THE CERVIX

Often discovered during a routine check-up rather than as a result of obvious symptoms. Check-up involves manual and visual examination of vagina, and a cervical smear or 'Pap' test, which involves taking a few cells from mouth of cervix for analysis.

Current medical opinion is that all women should have a smear test within 1 year of becoming sexually active, and then at 3–5 year intervals until age of 65–70. More frequent, even yearly, tests are recommended if woman (or her partner) has many sexual partners, has vulval warts (or if partner has penile or anal warts), smokes heavily, or has had a previously abnormal smear.

Cervical dysplasia Just occasionally, when delicate tissue around tip of eroded cervix (see cervical erosion below) reverts to tougher tissue typical of lining of vagina, certain cells become abnormal and may eventually cause CANCER OF THE CERVIX; to minimize risk of malignant change, suspect tissue is surgically removed or destroyed by laser or cauterization; in some cases, and certainly if cancer is already present, HYSTERECTOMY is advised. Dysplasia is likely to be symptomless, although its precursor, cervical erosion, may not. Homeopathic treatment is constitutional.

Cervical erosion Signalled by watery bleeding after intercourse or between periods (see unusual discharge – MENSTRUAL PROBLEMS); cause is extension of delicate, mucus-secreting lining of cervical canal to outer part of cervix during or after pregnancy or as result of taking oral contraceptives; in itself, condition is harmless, although it makes mouth of cervix more vulnerable to infection; if discharge is heavy, cauterization of affected tissue may be recommended. Constitutional homeopathic treatment is advised, but in the meantime the following remedies may lessen discharge and clear up any infection.

Specific remedies to be taken 4 times daily for up to 14 days
- Burning discharge, worse during day, especially in afternoon *Alumina 6c*
- Profuse, smarting discharge, with bleeding after intercourse *Phosphorus 6c*
- Bloody discharge, lower abdomen feels heavy and sore, intercourse painful *China 6c*
- Copious discharge between periods, feeling drained and weak *Cocculus 6c*
- Brown watery discharge with strands of mucus in it *Nitric ac. 6c*
- Discharge milky and itchy *Calcarea 6c*

Cervical polyps Grape-like outpouchings of lining of cervical canal which occasionally bleed after intercourse, between periods, or after MENOPAUSE, or increase menstrual bleeding; discharge is usually heavy and watery. Since CANCER OF THE CERVIX produces similar symptoms, ask your GP to investigate; surgical removal of polyps is a quick, painless procedure, but a D and C (dilatation of cervix and curettage or scraping of lining of uterus under general anaesthetic) may also be necessary to exclude possibility of more serious causes of bleeding (see UTERUS PROBLEMS).

Specific remedy to be taken 4 times daily for up to 14 days
• Before or after surgical removal of polyps *Calcarea 6c*

Endometriosis see UTERUS PROBLEMS

Fibroids see UTERUS PROBLEMS

Galactorrhea see BREAST PROBLEMS

Hormone imbalances
Hypothalamus, pituitary, and ovaries carry out a delicate balancing act in order to maintain fertility, nourish new life, and ensure that body chemistry is biased towards femaleness; if balance is upset, ovulation and periods are the first processes to go awry (see MENSTRUAL PROBLEMS). Function of hypothalamus can be disturbed by severe illness, by drastic weight changes, by STRESS and very strong emotions, and by coming off the pill; these in turn affect function of pituitary, although most common cause of pituitary malfunction is a tumour (see PITUITARY PROBLEMS); underproduction of FSH (follicle stimulating hormone) or LH (luteinizing hormone) by pituitary can affect oestrogen- and progestogen-producing activities of ovaries, although OVARIAN CYSTS and CANCER OF THE OVARY can have similar effects; low oestrogen levels means that testosterone (male hormone) produced by adrenal glands exerts greater influence, perhaps resulting in spotty skin, more facial and body hair, a deeper voice, and WEIGHT GAIN. If you have any of these symptoms, and also have period problems or are approaching the MENOPAUSE, see your GP. Homeopathic treatment is constitutional.

Hysterectomy
Surgical removal of uterus and cervix, and sometimes fallopian tubes and ovaries as well, through horizontal incision ('bikini incision') in lower abdomen or through the vagina; convalescence can take up to 2 months, depending on age and general state of health. After the operation, some women experience temporary DEPRESSION associated with imagined 'loss of femininity'; once vaginal and lower abdominal scars have healed, intercourse can be resumed; sexual enjoyment and ability to have orgasm are not usually impaired.

Unfortunately, for CANCER OF THE UTERUS or CANCER OF THE OVARY, for fibroids (see UTERUS PROBLEMS) which occupy space equivalent to that occupied by a 12-week-old foetus, and in cases where there is great pain and persistent bleeding, hysterectomy is the only effective treatment; in all other cases, hysterectomy should be a last resort. Homeopathic remedies below alleviate post-operative pain and promote healing.

Specific remedies to be taken after operation
• Immediately after operation as soon as anaesthetic wears off *Arnica 30c* hourly for up to 3 doses, then every 12 hours for up to 5 days
• If healing is slow or there are complications *Staphisagria 6c* every 4 hours for up to 5 days

Mastitis see BREAST PROBLEMS

Menopause
Not a disorder as such but, like puberty, a period of physical and emotional change to which some women adjust better than others. First sign is disruption of the menstrual cycle, an early warning that the delicate balance between ovaries, hypothalamus, and pituitary which ensures fertility is beginning to change; most women have their last period (strictly speaking 'menopause' means cessation of periods) around age of 50, but for some women periods cease as early as 40 or as late as 58. Symptoms of diminishing hormone production by ovaries can include hot flushes and sweating, joint pains, HEADACHE, dryness of vagina, irritability, DEPRESSION, SLEEP PROBLEMS, etc., but only 1 in 4 women experiences these symptoms to a distressing or inconvenient degree.

Homeopathic view of menopausal problems is that they represent imbalances which have been present for a long time; treatment is therefore constitutional, although the remedies and self-help measures given below should be tried first.

Orthodox approach used to be suppress distressing emotional and mental symptoms with tranquillizers, anti-depressants, and sleeping tablets, but now the first line treatment is to prescribe hormone preparations, a form of treatment known as hormone replacement therapy (HRT). HRT lessens physical symptoms by temporarily restoring hormone levels, but many gynaecologists are uneasy about long-term effects of HRT, despite its usefulness in preventing postmenopausal conditions such as OSTEOPOROSIS, and recommend that it be discontinued after age of 55. HRT should not be prescribed if you suffer from circulatory problems.

If periods are prolonged, or if spots of blood appear between periods, or if 'last' period is followed, 6 months or more later, by another period, see your GP; source of bleeding may be fibroids (see UTERUS PROBLEMS), which are benign, or a malignant growth (see CANCER OF THE UTERUS, CANCER OF THE CERVIX).

Specific remedies to be taken every 12 hours for up to 7 days

- Hot flushes, sweating, constricted feeling around abdomen, headache on waking, dizziness, flooding during periods, great talkativeness *Lachesis 30c*
- Flooding during periods, sweating, backache, sinking feeling in pit of stomach, chilliness, tearfulness, irritability *Sepia 30c*
- Hot flushes, piles, varicose veins, especially if woman is fair-haired, weeps easily, often feels chilly, and prefers open air to stuffy rooms *Pulsatilla 30c*
- Dryness and thinning of walls of vagina, constipation, stools which look blackish and burnt *Bryonia 30c*
- Hot flushes which come on very suddenly *Amyl nit. 30c*
- Hot flushes, loss of appetite, backache, feeling very taut and nervous, palpitations, symptoms worse around 3 am *Kali carb. 30c*
- Hot flushes, especially on face, nosebleeds, weight gain, scanty periods, cutting pains in lower abdomen *Graphites 30c*
- Hot flushes worse in evening and after exercise, great weariness *Sulphuric ac. 30c*

Self-help Avoid tea, coffee, alcohol, and spicy foods. Guard against constipation by eating plenty of fibre-rich foods, and avoid rich, heavy foods; several light meals a day will be much better for you than one big blow out. You may also find the Liver Diet on p. 352 beneficial. Supplements of calcium, zinc, Vitamin E, and Vitamin B complex, and also cod liver oil and evening primrose oil are recommended.

If you suffer from hot sweats, wear cotton underwear and light clothes, and avoid hot baths. Practise regular deep breathing (see pp. 18–19) and take moderate exercise.

If vulva is dry and sore, apply Calendula ointment; if vagina is dry and sore, apply Aci-gel (available from chemist) or douche vagina with yoghurt solution (1 small pot live natural yoghurt to 1.75 litres [3 pints] boiled cooled water).

Menstrual problems see also PREMENSTRUAL SYNDROME

Amenorrhea Temporary or permanent absence of periods; may be primary if periods have not started by age of 16 (see DELAYED PUBERTY for specific homeopathic remedies), or secondary if periods have started and then stopped because of ANOREXIA or excessive WEIGHT LOSS, excessive exercise (especially on vegetarian diet), or STRESS; an established menstrual cycle can also be disrupted by HORMONE IMBALANCES (as MENOPAUSE approaches, for example) or by coming off the pill; after childbirth, periods may be absent or irregular for 6 weeks to several months. In rare cases, amenorrhea may be due to a gross displacement of the uterus (see UTERUS PROBLEMS), although this can be corrected by special exercises.

If periods have been absent for more than 9 months and woman wishes to get pregnant, GP may prescribe a fertility drug; however, absence of periods cannot be relied on as a method of contraception since ovulation may restart (or start) at any time. Homeopathy offers constitutional treatment in appropriate cases; provided secondary amenorrhea is not due to pregnancy, childbirth, or anatomical problems, remedies below may be of benefit; if periods do not restart within 2 months, see your homeopath.

Specific remedies to be taken every 12 hours for up to 14 days
- Periods stop suddenly due to great emotional shock or exposure to dry cold *Aconite 30c*
- Periods stop after becoming extremely chilled after strenuous exercise *Dulcamara 30c*
- Feeling tired, giddy, and chilly, with legs as heavy as lead, breasts swollen and painful, nerviness and jumpiness *Calcarea 30c*
- Thinning hair, headaches, constipation, irritability, recent emotional shock *Natrum mur. 30c*
- Periods cease because of grief or loss *Ignatia 30c*
- Dryness of vagina, lower abdominal pain, headache, slightest emotional upset disrupts periods, feeling faint and shivery, weepy and sad *Lycopodium 30c*
- Abnormal vaginal discharge, sallow patches on face, feeling weak, tearful, and irritable *Sepia 30c*
- Weariness, weakness, wanting to sit down all the time, face usually pale, occasional hot flushes *Ferrum 30c*

Self-help Take a multivitamin and mineral supplement.

'Breakthrough' bleeding or *abnormal bleeding* Always consult your GP. Spotting of blood between periods can be due to STRESS, or may be a side effect of intrauterine devices, certain oral contraceptives, and other drugs. Profuse discharge of watery blood between periods, possibly made worse by intercourse, suggests cervical erosion (see CERVICAL PROBLEMS) or cancer (see CANCER OF THE CERVIX, CANCER OF THE UTERUS); early diagnosis is important, so see your GP as soon as possible. Cancer is also a possibility if bleeding restarts more than 6 months after the MENOPAUSE.

If you are pregnant, bleeding accompanied by pain in lower abdomen may signal an ECTOPIC PREGNANCY or impending MISCARRIAGE; prompt medical attention is vital, so ②. In an ectopic pregnancy (most often associated with IUD failure, or with infection or abnormality of fallopian tubes), embryo starts to develop outside womb, causing severe pain and internal bleeding; risk of SHOCK setting in is very real.

Heavy periods (menorrhagia) Defined as profuse bleeding ('flooding') which quickly soaks through sanitary protection, discharge of large clots of blood, or bleeding which continues for more than 7 days. Causes

---

include HORMONE IMBALANCES, fibroids or endometriosis (see UTERUS PROBLEMS), and PELVIC IN-
FECTION; in a minority of women, IUDs increase
monthly flow. Consistently heavy periods can lead to
iron deficiency ANAEMIA. If cycle is regular but periods
are getting heavier and heavier, see your GP. If you
have had intercourse recently and your period is late
and heavier than usual, you may have lost a pregnancy
(see MISCARRIAGE); appropriate action is 12 just in
case there is an ECTOPIC PREGNANCY.

Heavy periods caused by hormonal imbalance are
conventionally treated by prescribing oral contraceptives or drugs to lessen bleeding; in other cases,
antibiotics or surgery may be appropriate; iron tablets
may also be given.

Homeopathy offers constitutional treatment, and
also the specific remedies given below and under the
causative conditions mentioned above.

Specific remedies to be taken every 8 hours for up to 10
doses starting just before period is due
- Intermittent bleeding, dark clots of blood, abdominal cramp, headache, giddiness, faintness, face
very pale *China 30c*
- Blood dark or red, with or without clots in it, labour-
like pains in small of back, emotional upsets
increase blood loss, difficulty controlling weight
Sabina 30c
- Blood bright red, dragging pains, face hot and
flushed, throbbing headache *Belladonna 30c*
- Profuse bleeding, blood bright red, nausea *Ipecac.
30c*
- Cramping pains in abdomen, pain in small of back,
head feels congested, chilliness, general pallor,
weight problem *Calcarea 30c*
- Flooding, blood dark and watery, face pale,
occasional flushes, walking around seems to improve things *Ferrum 30c*
- Clots of blackish blood, sensation of movement
inside uterus, feeling weak, sick, and worried *Crocus
30c*
- Blood thin and watery, without clots, cold extremities, general exhaustion, fear of dying, warmth
makes you feel worse *Kali carb. 30c*
- Profuse bleeding, with abdominal cramps and
nausea, especially in first day or two of period, pain
and bleeding worse at night *Borax 30c*

Self-help Try the following: cut out tea, coffee, and
alcohol, reduce consumption of milk and dairy foods,
eat lots of raw vegetables, increase intake of calcium,
zinc, iron, Vitamins A and B$_6$, and bioflavinoids (see
nutritional supplements pp. 343–9), take 30 minutes
of moderate exercise a day but avoid over-straining
yourself, and in between periods take several short
cold baths. If these measures fail, try the Liver Diet on
p. 352 for 1 month.

Infrequent periods (oligomenorrhea) Periods of normal
duration occurring less frequently than once every
26–28 days; very common as MENOPAUSE approaches,
although for a few women infrequent periods are the
norm due to their particular hormone cycle. Only
problem is reduction of chances of getting pregnant; if
checks reveal that INFERTILITY is due to irregular
egg production, hormone injections or fertility drugs
may be prescribed; homeopathic treatment is constitutional.

Painful periods (dysmenorrhea) Most women experience some discomfort during first 2 or 3 days of
period; this is quite normal. Depending on the
individual, 'discomfort' may be a dull ache in lower
back or abdomen, or cramping pains severe enough to
cause NAUSEA AND VOMITING; STRESS and ANXIETY can
make pain considerably worse. In general, women who
have painful periods can expect some respite after
childbirth and as they reach their 30s.

However, if periods suddenly become painful after
several years of relative freedom from pain, underlying
cause may be fibroids (prolonged or heavy periods –
see UTERUS PROBLEMS), endometriosis (pain worsens
towards end of period – see UTERUS PROBLEMS), or
PELVIC INFECTION (early or heavy periods, mild fever,
smelly vaginal discharge); if any of these conditions is
suspected, see your GP. An intrauterine device or
coming off the pill can also make periods more painful.

Where there is no obvious organic cause, homeopathy offers constitutional treatment, but the specific
remedies below are effective relievers of pain and
tension and should be tried in preference to over-the-
counter analgesics.

Specific remedies to be taken every hour for up to 10
doses as soon as period pains come on
- Pain worse just before period, aching, dragging
sensation made worse by lying down, skin hot and
flushed, bright red blood *Belladonna 30c*
- Severe cramping pains, especially if associated with
anger, great restlessness *Chamomilla 30c*
- Pain comes in spasms, soothed by heat, pressure,
and movement, membranes present in blood flow
Magnesia phos. 30c
- Periods late and scanty, pain extends into thighs
Viburnum 30c
- Scanty periods, nausea and vomiting, weepiness
Pulsatilla 30c
- Periods late and scanty, sharp pains which are
soothed by heat, uterus feels heavy *Gelsemium 30c*
- Prolonged periods which arrive early, chilliness,
exhaustion, constipation, irritability *Nux 30c*
- Strong contractions of uterus, rather like labour
pains, headaches in days leading up to period
Cimicifuga 30c
- Pain extends down into thighs, nausea, muffled
buzzing in ears *Borax 30c*

Self-help A general toning up and rebalancing of all the body systems is the best route to pain-free periods. Eat more raw fruit and vegetables, take extra Vitamin E, C, B complex, and magnesium, calcium, zinc, and evening primrose oil, perhaps go on the Liver Diet (p. 352) for 1 month, step up the amount of exercise you take, and if you are heavier than you should be, try to do something about it. In the week before your period, take a long hot bath every other night; in between periods take the occasional short cold bath. Osteopathic or chiropractic manipulation sometimes achieves excellent results; slant-board exercises (see pp. 19–22), which gently shift the contents of the abdomen, can also be beneficial.

Unusual discharge see VAGINAL AND VULVAL PROBLEMS, PELVIC INFECTION

Nipple problems see BREAST PROBLEMS

Ovarian cysts see also CANCER OF THE OVARY
Fluid-filled outgrowths of tissue which develop on or near ovaries; often symptomless unless large enough to press on bladder or cause visible swelling in lower abdomen or pain on intercourse; if production of ovarian hormones is affected (see HORMONE IMBALANCES), menstrual cycle may become irregular, but this is rare; risk of cancerous change is small, the greater risk being PERITONITIS (sudden, severe abdominal pain, nausea, fever, abdominal distention) if cyst bursts. Where possible, especially in younger women, cyst is removed without damaging ovary; in other cases removal of ovary and fallopian tube may be advised. Constitutional homeopathic treatment is usually required, but the remedies given below may be of some benefit.

Specific remedies to be taken 4 times daily for up to 14 days
- Left ovary affected, local pain which is worse in morning but wears off during period *Lachesis 6c*
- Lower abdominal pain which feels like a wedge being driven through ovary and womb *Iodum 6c*
- Right ovary affected, sore, stinging pains locally, painful periods with tenderness in lower abdomen *Apis 6c*
- Small, round cysts which cause pain which seems to bore through lower abdomen, bending double and pressing fists into abdomen gives some relief *Colocynth 6c*

Ovulation pain
Ovulation occurs, on average, 12–14 days before onset of menstruation, but it is an event of which many women are unaware, unless they practise natural contraception; some women, however, experience what is called 'mittelschmerz', lower ABDOMINAL PAIN which is more localized and qualitatively different from period pain. If the homeopathic remedies below prove ineffective, see your homeopath; if pain is part of a wider picture, constitutional treatment may be recommended.

Specific remedies to be taken every hour for up to 10 doses
- Nervy pains, relieved by warmth, by bending double, or by pressing fists into lower abdomen, often worse on left side, and often associated with anger *Colocynth 6c*
- Violent, cramping pains, worse on left side, ovary feels as if it is being dragged up towards heart *Naja 6c*
- Right-sided pain, worse between 4 and 8 am, constipation and wind, apprehensiveness *Lycopodium 6c*
- Right-sided pain which shoots up to breast, alleviated by pressure, abdomen feels bloated *Palladium 6c*

Pain in lower abdomen
Menstrual pain occurs just before and during first 2 or 3 days of period, with lower abdominal pain often accompanied by dull, aching pain in small of back (see painful periods – MENSTRUAL PROBLEMS). Pain due to PELVIC INFECTION is accompanied by heavy, unpleasant discharge from vagina. Burning or scalding pain while urinating suggests CYSTITIS. OVARIAN CYSTS and CANCER OF THE OVARY can also cause lower abdominal pain. If pain occurs during sexual intercourse, possible cause may be fibroids, endometriosis, or retroversion of the uterus (see UTERUS PROBLEMS). Severe pain and abnormal bleeding from vagina suggests ECTOPIC PREGNANCY. For other causes, see ABDOMINAL PAIN pp. 220–1.

Period problems see MENSTRUAL PROBLEMS

Pelvic infection (salpingitis, pelvic inflammatory disease or PID)
Acute or chronic infection of uterus, fallopian tubes, ovaries, or surrounding tissue by germs which enter through vagina, especially during intercourse, although sometimes infection follows ABORTION, MISCARRIAGE, or fitting of an IUD. For unknown reasons, the pill appears to protect against PID. Condition is related to frequency of intercourse, and is most common in younger women. Symptoms include early or heavy periods (see MENSTRUAL PROBLEMS), profuse and smelly vaginal discharge between periods (see VAGINAL AND VULVAL PROBLEMS), PAINFUL INTERCOURSE, and PAIN IN LOWER ABDOMEN; if infection is acute, pain is likely to be severe and persistent, and temperature higher than normal. Early treatment is essential, since infection can lead to ABSCESS formation, PERITONITIS, and even BLOOD POISONING; INFERTILITY is also a risk if delicate membranes of reproductive tract become scarred. Routinely treated with antibiotics and, if necessary, painkillers. Homeopathic

treatment is constitutional, designed to boost general resistance to infection; in acute cases, specific remedies given below should relieve pain and inflammation, but if there is no improvement within 24 hours or if temperature suddenly rises, see your GP.

Specific remedies to be taken every 2 hours for up to 10 doses in acute cases
- Sudden onset, mild fever, anxiety, symptoms aggravated by emotional shock or exposure to cold *Aconite 30c*
- Stinging, burning pains, mainly on right side of abdomen, lack of thirst *Apis 30c*
- Sudden onset, severe abdominal pain made worse by slightest jarring, face bright red and burning hot *Belladonna 30c*
- Cramping pains, relieved by doubling up and pressing fists hard into abdomen *Colocynth 6c*
- Alternate chills and sweats, sweat smells unpleasant, rest makes you feel better *Mercurius corr. 6c*

Self-help Rest in bed until symptoms wear off, and refrain from intercourse for 4 weeks.

Premenstrual syndrome (PMS)

A constellation of symptoms, physical and emotional, which affect many women in days leading up to period; the term 'premenstrual syndrome' is more comprehensive than 'premenstrual tension' and now preferred by women themselves as it has a less sexist, accusatory ring to it. Some 25 per cent of women are not affected by PMS, and the majority of those who are continue to function more or less normally despite feeling slightly 'down' and irritable. For about 1 in 10 women, however, premenstrual mood changes are very marked, ranging from unusual aggressiveness to loss of control over actions and emotions. Suggested causes of PMS include ALLERGY, HORMONE IMBALANCES, nutritional imbalances, and psychological factors; DEPRESSION, for example, seems to be a predisposing factor.

Although emotional symptoms are most talked about because of their knock-on effects in the home and at work, PMS usually includes some enlargement or tenderness of breasts, general fluid retention leading to a slight increase in weight, slight abdominal distension, and early twinges of period pain.

In severe cases, GP may prescribe hormone treatment, tranquillizers, or diuretics. Homeopathic treatment is constitutional, although specific remedies listed below are well worth trying first.

Specific remedies to be take every 12 hours for up to 3 days starting 24 hours before premenstrual symptoms are due
- Symptoms worse first thing in morning, breasts painful *Lachesis 30c*

- Tiredness and lack of energy, clumsiness, cold sweats, breasts swollen and painful, craving for eggs and sweet things *Calcarea 30c*
- Feeling irritable and chilly, constipation, frequent urination, craving sweet or fatty foods *Nux 30c*
- Feeling irritable, chilly, weepy, emotionally flat, turned off by idea of sex, craving sweet or salty foods *Sepia 30c*
- Feeling pessimistic, irritable, and over-sensitive, colicky pains in lower abdomen, frequent urge to urinate or symptoms of cystitis *Causticum 30c*
- Feeling taut, tense, and exhausted, especially if you are overweight, symptoms worse around 3 am *Kali carb. 30c*
- Suddenly bursting into tears, feeling sick, breasts painful, periods irregular *Pulsatilla 30c*
- Feeling bad-tempered and depressed, craving sweet things *Lycopodium 30c*
- Fluid retention, swollen breasts, feeling sad and irritable *Natrum mur. 30c*
- Where craving for sweets is main symptom *Sulphur 30c*

Self-help Among the foods contra-indicated in PMS are heavily salted foods (do not cheat by adding salt at table), junk foods, fatty foods, and tea and coffee. Consumption of dairy products and refined carbohydrates should be limited. Eat plenty of small protein-rich snacks rather than large meals, but make sure most of the protein comes from vegetarian sources (pulses, nuts, wholegrains, etc.). Eat vegetables raw in salads, with sunflower oil dressing.

The following supplements may also be beneficial: Vitamins C, E, and B_6, magnesium, zinc, iron, chromium, evening primrose oil, and pancreatic enzymes. These should be taken continuously for 1 month to start with, then only during fortnight before each period.

If stress is a problem generally, extra premenstrual vulnerability to stress will almost certainly be reduced by taking 30 minutes of outdoor exercise every day, and by learning some simple form of relaxation or meditation (see PART 2). If you smoke, try to give it up.

For more information about PMS contact the Premenstrual Syndrome Advisory Centre (address p. 383).

Pre-menstrual tension (PMT) see
PREMENSTRUAL SYNDROME

Prolapse of uterus or vagina see UTERUS PROBLEMS

Pruritis vulvae see VAGINAL AND VULVAL PROBLEMS

Retroversion of uterus see UTERUS PROBLEMS

For explanation of other symbols, see page 107

Uterus problems see also CANCER OF THE UTERUS

Endometriosis Condition in which fragments of lining of uterus (endometrium) migrate into fallopian tubes, ovaries, vagina, and even into intestine where, still under influence of oestrogen and progesterone, they engorge with blood every month, irritating and scarring surrounding tissue; condition is most common in childless women between age of 30 and 40, but cause is not known, although selenium deficiency and use of tampons have been suggested. Symptoms include heavy periods, dragging period pains which tend to get worse towards end of period (see MENSTRUATION PROBLEMS), difficulty getting pregnant, and perhaps PAINFUL INTERCOURSE, but severe cases are uncommon; in such cases, GP may prescribe combined contraceptive pill or a drug which inhibits ovulation and gives body time to reabsorb dispersed fragments of endometrium; fragments can also be removed surgically; hysterectomy may be advised if ovaries are scarred and no more children are wanted. Constitutional homeopathic treatment is recommended; in the meantime, see MENSTRUAL PROBLEMS (painful periods) and PAINFUL INTERCOURSE for suitable short-term remedies.

Fibroids Non-cancerous growths in or on walls of uterus, sometimes on a stalk and varying in size from a pea to a large plum; tend to occur severally rather than singly and may take a few or many years to develop; small fibroids are often symptomless, but large ones can give rise to heavy, prolonged periods (see MENSTRUATION PROBLEMS), PAINFUL INTERCOURSE, and CYSTITIS (because they press on bladder and prevent it emptying properly); they may also prevent conception, cause MISCARRIAGE or pain during pregnancy, or obstruct delivery; if stalk of fibroid becomes twisted, cutting off blood supply, result is severe PAIN IN LOWER ABDOMEN; appropriate action is ② and *Aconite 30c* every 15 minutes for up to 10 doses.

Fibroids are especially common in women aged 35–40, but cause is not known, although it has been speculated that oestrogens in oral contraceptives may encourage condition. Small fibroids seldom require treatment and tend to disappear after age of 45; troublesome fibroids can be removed surgically following a D and C (scraping of uterus) to confirm diagnosis; sometimes HYSTERECTOMY is advised. Homeopathic treatment is constitutional, although in the short term the remedies below should be tried.

Specific remedies to be taken 4 times daily for up to 3 weeks
- Small fibroids, profuse yellow discharge from vagina *Calcarea iod. 6c*
- Swollen uterus, urge to bear down, watery brown discharge from vagina, painful cramps during periods *Fraxinus 6c*

- Menstrual flow heavier than usual, body feels icy cold, bleeding between periods *Silicea 6c*
- Continuous bleeding *Thlaspi 6c*
- Short scanty periods as menopause approaches, great pain eased by menstrual flow, abdomen very sensitive to tight clothing *Lachesis 6c*
- Where menstrual blood is bright red *Phosphorus 6c*
- Uterus feels as it is being squeezed during periods *Kali iod. 6c*
- Uterus feels swollen and painful, spasmodic contractions of vagina *Aurum mur. 6c*

Prolapse of the uterus or vagina Occurs when ligaments and muscles which hold uterus and vagina in place become weak or slack with age or as result of childbirth, allowing uterus to bulge into vagina and press on bladder or rectum; this causes a heavy, uncomfortable feeling in lower abdomen generally, backache, STRESS INCONTINENCE or difficulty emptying bladder, or straining and discomfort when passing stools. If prolapse is complete, a large part of the vagina or uterus may actually protrude through vaginal opening, causing soreness or ulceration and encouraging infection. Surgery to tighten pelvic floor may be necessary if exercises do not restore muscle tone; a ring pessary, fitted behind pubic bone, may be advised if person is elderly. If symptoms are not too severe, homeopathic remedies below may be of benefit; if there is no improvement within a week or two, see your homeopath.

Specific remedies to be taken 4 times daily for up to 14 days
- Dragging sensation in lower abdomen, made worse by doing jobs which involve bending or lifting, scanty periods, pain on intercourse, depression *Sepia 6c*
- Vagina very hot and dry, pain in lower back, leaden feeling in abdomen and just below ribs, as if abdominal and pelvic contents are about to drop out *Belladonna 6c*
- Sharp spasms of pain, constant urge to pass urine or stool, irritability *Nux 6c*
- Sensation of downward pressure in lower abdomen, pain in small of back, nausea, weepiness, heat and periods make symptoms worse *Pulsatilla 6c*
- Nervousness, irritability, pain and tenderness in lower abdomen, bladder affected, urgent desire to pass stool, itchy vulva which feels as if it needs external support, rest alleviates symptoms *Lilium 6c*

Self-help To strengthen muscles of pelvic floor, try stopping and starting flow of urine several times each time you urinate; this may be difficult at first, but persevere. These exercises are a vital part of orthodox and homeopathic treatment, and particularly important after childbirth. If you are heavier than you should be, try to lose weight.

Retroversion of the uterus In 20 per cent of women uterus lies close to rectum rather than just behind bladder;

---

this is perfectly natural, and has no effect on conception, carrying a baby, or giving birth, but a few women experience backache because of it, especially during periods, or find that deep penetration during intercourse causes pain because penis strikes an ovary (see PAINFUL INTERCOURSE). Uterus can be re-positioned temporarily by inserting a device called a ring pessary into the vagina, or permanently by an operation called a ventrosuspension. See PAINFUL INTERCOURSE for suitable homeopathic remedies.

Self-help Try different love-making positions so that penetration is shallower. Slant-board exercises (see pp. 19–22) may also encourage repositioning of uterus within pelvic cavity.

Trophoblastic tumours Benign or malignant growths which develop in placental tissue, causing MIS-CARRIAGE, or in fragments of placenta remaining in uterus after ABORTION or childbirth; symptoms are irregular bleeding and severe MORNING SICKNESS; diagnosis is by ultrasound scan and by checking urine for excessive levels of HCG (human chorionic gonadotrophic) hormone. Benign tumours, also known as hydatidiform moles, are rare, and malignant tumours extremely rare; the former are removed by D and C (scraping placental tissue out of womb), but the latter may require HYSTERECTOMY and chemo-therapy. For homeopathic approach to malignancy, see CANCER. The remedies given below are for tumours diagnosed as benign; they offer symptom relief until a D and C can be arranged.

Specific remedies to be taken every 4 hours for up to 2 weeks
- Where constitution is strong *Pulsatilla 6c*
- Where constitution is weak *Secale 6c*
- Penetrating pain from base of spine to pubic bone, shooting pains in vagina, bleeding, slightest move-ment makes symptoms worse *Sabina 6c*
- Where urination is painful *Cantharis 6c*

Vaginal and vulval problems
Best insurance against infection is to wash vulva daily with plain water – no soap or bath salts – and avoid vaginal deodorants and medicated douches. Under-wear should be changed daily, and sanitary towels and tampons every 6 hours at least; towels are preferable to tampons if periods are heavy after childbirth or if CYSTITIS is a recurrent problem. Infections occur when acid environment of vagina and its population of healthy bacteria are disturbed – by antibiotics, deodorants, irritants in contraceptive creams, etc.

Bartholinitis Acute infection of Bartholin's gland, which lies at entrance to vagina and secretes fluid which lubricates vagina during intercourse. Symptoms are extreme tenderness, followed by discharge of pus

or formation of ABSCESS; conventionally treated with antibiotics. If homeopathic remedies below do not improve matters, see your GP.

Specific remedies to be taken every 2 hours for up to 10 doses
- Early stage of infection, entrance to vagina hot, red, and swollen *Belladonna 30c*
- Discharge of pus, extreme tenderness *Hepar sulph. 6c*
- Symptoms accompanied by fever and chill, feeling hot and cold by turns *Mercurius 6c*

Bartholin's cyst Condition in which exit from Bartholin's gland (see above) becomes blocked, resulting in swelling and tenderness at entrance to vagina. If the homeopathic remedy below produces no improve-ment, see your GP; if surgical removal of gland is recommended, constitutional homeopathic treatment should be sought after the operation.

Specific remedy to be taken 4 times daily for up to 3 weeks
- *Baryta carb. 6c*

Dryness of vagina May be due to lack of foreplay before intercourse, to MENOPAUSE, or to HORMONAL IM-BALANCES. See MENOPAUSE for suitable homeopathic remedies. KY jelly, obtainable from chemist, is a safe lubricant.

Pruritis vulvae Intense itching or irritation of whole vulval area due to skin problems generally (see ITCHING), HORMONAL IMBALANCES (especially in elderly women), ANXIETY ABOUT INTERCOURSE (especially in very young women), use of tampons, irritants in spermicidal creams, vaginal deodorants, talcum powder, traces of detergent in underwear, etc. Other contributory factors may be a lack of B vitamins, especially B_{12}, poor hygiene, excessive exercise or exertion, and spending too much time sitting down. Condition is not uncommon in DIABETES, and can be an after-effect of rape. If slightly thickened, whitish patches of skin (leucoplakia) develop in itchy areas, see your GP; there is a very small risk of their becoming malignant (see CANCER OF THE VULVA). Where orthodox treatment relies on steroid creams, homeo-pathic medicine treats pruritis vulvae constitutionally; however, the specific remedies and self-help measures given below should be tried first.

Specific remedies to be taken 4 times daily for up to 14 days
- Vulva itches, crotch very sweaty and smelly, matters made worse by heat and washing *Sulphur 6c*
- Increased desire for sex, creeping sensation in vulva which wears off during daytime naps but gets worse at night or when moving around *Caladium 6c*
- Labia visibly swollen, local veins distended *Carbo veg. 6c*

- Localized itching, skin very red, itching relieved by heat *Rhus tox. 6c*
- Itching aggravated by suppressed desire for sex or by frequent sex *Conium 6c*
- Itchiness worse immediately before and after period, general sweatiness and chilliness, especially if woman is overweight *Calcarea 6c*
- Itchiness soothed by hot baths and by moving around out of doors, most uncomfortable first thing in morning *Radium brom. 6c*

Self-help Try not to scratch. Apply Calendula and Urtica ointment to vulva 4 times a day, or bathe vulva with Thuja solution (10 drops of mother tincture to 0.25 1 [½ pint] boiled cooled water). For other local measures, see PRURITIS ANI. To reduce friction during intercourse, lubricate vagina with KY jelly (obtainable from chemist).

Thrush Caused by same fungus, *Candida albicans*, which causes ORAL THRUSH; infection only develops if acid-producing bacteria in vagina are destroyed, as they easily can be by antibiotics, medicated douches, intimate deodorants, etc. Symptoms are itchiness or soreness of vagina and vulva, accompanied by thick, whitish discharge which smells rather like new mown hay or freshly baked bread, more frequent urination than usual and a stinging sensation as urine is passed, and perhaps PAINFUL INTERCOURSE. Orthodox treatment consists of antifungal creams or suppositories. For specific homeopathic remedies and self-help measures, see unusual discharge (below).

Trichomoniasis Vaginal infection caused by single-celled *Trichomonas* organism; symptoms are similar to those of thrush (see above) but vaginal discharge smells unpleasant and is usually copious and greenish. Conventionally treated with drugs such as Metronicazole. For homeopathic remedies and self-help measures, see unusual discharge (below).

Unusual discharge Vagina and cervix are naturally wetter and more slippery around time of ovulation; at other times mucus secreted by walls of cervix is stickier and slightly cloudy. If vaginal discharge is due to thrush (see above), it is thick, curdy, causes itching or intense soreness, but does not smell unpleasant; vaginal deodorants, medicated douches, antibiotics, oral contraceptives, and DIABETES can produce similar symptoms. *Trichomonas* infection (see above) causes quite heavy greenish-yellow discharge which is irritant and smells unpleasant; if LOWER ABDOMINAL PAIN is present as well, this type of discharge suggests PELVIC INFECTION. Heavy, greyish discharge with an offensive smell to it suggests a bacterial infection called *Gardnerella*.

Organisms responsible for genital infections flourish in damp, airless conditions, and are often transmitted by sexual intercourse (see SEXUALLY TRANSMITTED DISEASES), but self-infection is also common, especially if hygiene is poor (leaving tampons in too long, allowing caps to get dirty, inserting barrier devices or checking IUD threads with dirty fingers). Conventional medicine treats such infections with antifungal drugs or antibiotics, as appropriate.

If you suspect you have an infection, select a suitable homeopathic remedy from the list which follows, take it for up to 5 days, and at the same time implement the self-help measures described below; if discharge does not return to normal, see your homeopath or GP.

Specific remedies to be taken 6 times daily for up to 5 days
- Frequent, copious, straw-coloured discharge which causes vulva to itch and smart and stiffens underwear, itchiness relieved by washing in cold water, discharge worse before and after period *Alumina 6c*
- Discharge transparent like egg white and highly irritant, scalded feeling on inside of thighs *Borax 6c*
- Itchy, milky discharge which smells like rye bread, preceded by flushed face and pains in small of back, great weakness *Kreosotum 6c*
- Watery, cloudy discharge which causes smarting and soreness, worse before and after periods and when lying down *Pulsatilla 6c*
- Yellowish, smarting discharge, itchy vulva, sharp stinging sensation in uterus, walking adds to discomfort, abdomen distended, worse during day *Sepia 6c*
- Yellowish, burning discharge *Carbo an. 6c*
- Milky discharge which makes vulva itch, worse after passing urine and before periods *Calcarea 6c*
- Greenish discharge which smarts and stings, suspected *Trichomonas* infection *Bovista 6c*
- Stinging discharge with foul smell, containing some solid matter, feeling chilly and sweaty by turns, *Trichomonas* infection suspected *Mercurius 6c*
- Stringy mucus which is greenish or pinkish and more copious after period, *Trichomonas* infection suspected *Nitric ac. 6c*
- Corrosive, greenish discharge, especially before period, *Trichomonas* infection suspected *Carbo veg. 6c*
- White or yellowish discharge which burns and stings, cramping pains in abdomen or pinching sensation around navel, pain and discharge worse in week before period *Sulphur 6c*

Self-help In general, coffee, alcohol, and sweets are to be avoided; constipation and lack of exercise are not helpful either. Wear cotton underwear and change it every day, and do not use vaginal deodorants, perfumed bath salts, or talcum powder.

If vaginal douching does not put you off, there are several simple ways to soothe vagina and restore its natural acidity (harmful organisms flourish when populations of beneficial acid-producing bacteria are decimated). First, douche vagina with Hypericum and

---

999 Emergency – call GP (or dial 999) immediately. ② Consult your doctor if no improvement within 2 hours

Calendula solution (5 drops of mother tincture of each to 0.25 litre [½ pint] boiled cooled water); do this 3 times a day, and last thing at night apply a cold water compress to lower abdomen. As soon as itchiness and soreness abate, douche vagina 3 times a day with yoghurt solution (1 pot natural live yoghurt to 1.75 litres [3 pints] boiled cooled water) or with a weak solution of fresh lemon juice or vinegar (1 tablespoon to 0.25 litre [½ pint] boiled cooled water); a preparation called Aci-gel is also available from chemist.

Obstinate cases of thrush may respond to extra iron, zinc, Vitamins C and B, and evening primrose oil, and cutting down on carbohydrates and products containing yeast.

Vaginitis Irritation of vagina in absence of infection; sometimes part of a general skin condition (see ITCHING), sometimes a reaction to spermicidal creams, medicated douches, or vaginal deodorants; in younger women it may be a reaction to a difficult sexual relationship; vagina feels sore and itchy. See unusual discharge (above) for self-help measures and homeopathic remedies.

Vulval warts Spot viral infections on labia or around entrance to vagina, often associated with pregnancy or with vaginal infections such as thrush (see above), during which vaginal discharge increases; like penile warts (see PENIS PROBLEMS), vulval warts should not be neglected because they are moderately contagious, easily transmitted to sexual partners, and can become malignant (see CANCER OF THE VULVA), although this is rare; it has also been suggested that they play a part in development of CANCER OF THE CERVIX, so have a yearly smear. GP may prescribe special wart paint or recommend removal of warts by freezing or cauterization. Homeopathic treatment is constitutional; in the meantime select a remedy from the list below, one for yourself and one for your sexual partner.

Specific remedies to be taken 4 times daily for up to 3 weeks
- Fleshy warts, especially if they develop in weeks following orthodox vaccination against smallpox *Thuja 6c*
- Warts are itchy, tendency to suffer from catarrh, shakiness or flutteriness *Medorrhinum 6c*
- Warts associated with sores or ulcers *Nitric ac. 6c*
- Intense itchiness and smarting *Sabina 6c*

Self-help Genital warts can easily spread from warts elsewhere on body; so if you have warts, especially on your hands, always wash your hands before touching your own or your partner's genitals.

SPECIAL PROBLEMS IN MEN

THIS section covers those disorders which affect the male reproductive organs. Infections are the commonest kind of disorder, for although the male urethra is relatively long and less prone to invasion than the female, it has direct communication with the testes, epididymides, and prostate. This means that kidney, bladder, or urethral infections can spread to the organs concerned with reproduction.

The testicles manufacture sperm and also produce the male sex hormone testosterone. They lie outside the body, the left usually lower than the right, because sperm production requires slightly cooler conditions than those which reign inside the body. Normally, both testicles descend into the scrotum, the pouch of skin behind the penis, shortly before birth. At puberty they enlarge and begin to produce sperm.

Each testicle consists of an almond-shaped testis, where sperm are manufactured at the rate of 10,000–30,000 million a month, and a much coiled tube called the epididymis, inside which the sperm mature for about 3 weeks. In all it takes 60–72 days for a sperm to develop fully.

From the epididymides, sperm move into the vasa deferentia and seminal vesicles for storage; in the seminal vesicles a sugar-rich fluid is added to provide the sperm with energy. If mature sperm are not ejaculated, they disintegrate and are reabsorbed into the body, but if psychological conditions are right and orgasm occurs, the seminal vesicles and prostate gland contract powerfully, expelling about 3 ml (half a teaspoonful) of semen into the urethra and out of the end of the penis; this is ejaculation. Once in the female reproductive tract, sperm have a maximum life of 3 days. It is not possible to urinate and ejaculate at the same time because the reflexes which cause the bladder to empty automatically shut off entry of semen into the urethra.

The prostate gland is bulb-shaped and completely encircles the urethra at the point where it leaves the bladder. Its role is to add acids, trace elements, and enzymes to seminal fluid at the moment of ejaculation. These activate the sperm and also give semen its distinct smell. For reasons which are not known, the prostate tends to enlarge and stiffen with age, narrowing the exit from the bladder; this obliges the bladder muscles to work harder to expel urine, and can make urination slow and painful.

The penis relies, for its hydraulic power, on three

For explanation of other symbols, see page 107

cylinders, two hollow and one spongy. These are arranged protectively around the urethra and only fill with blood during sexual arousal. Erection is maintained by strands of muscle at the base of the penis which slow the rate at which blood drains back into general circulation. The head of the penis is most sensitive to touch, the shaft to pressure.

Balanitis see PENIS PROBLEMS

Blood in sperm see PENIS PROBLEMS

Cancer of the penis see also PENIS PROBLEMS
Extremely rare, but most common in elderly men who are uncircumcised or whose standard of hygiene is poor; usually begins as a sore or ulcer on penis, then spreads to lymph glands in groin; to make sure that lumps are not syphilis (see SEXUALLY TRANSMITTED DISEASES) or penile warts (see PENIS PROBLEMS), a biopsy (removal of a tiny tissue sample for analysis) is necessary. Radiotherapy usually achieves a cure if malignancy is detected early enough. For homeopathic approach, see CANCER.

Cancer of the prostate see also PROSTATE PROBLEMS
This is the most common form of cancer affecting male reproductive organs, occurring in about 15 per cent of men aged 40. In men aged 80 or over is very common, but malignancy is slow-growing and usually symptomless; most cases come to light during surgery for an enlarged prostate (see PROSTATE PROBLEMS) or, more rarely, when cancer has spread to bones (see BONE TUMOURS); diagnosis is confirmed by biopsy and a bone scan. If malignancy is confined to prostate and does not cause urination problems, surgery is unlikely to be recommended; current wisdom is to leave well alone, since risk of cancer spreading is relatively low, but regular check-ups are necessary. Radiotherapy is standard treatment for malignancy discovered during prostatectomy. For homeopathic approach, see CANCER.

Cancer of the testicle see also TESTICLE AND SCROTUM PROBLEMS
Relatively rare and slow-growing, but may produce secondaries in lungs and other vital organs if left untreated; most common form of cancer in men aged 20–35; detectable as painless lump or swelling on testis itself rather than on epididymis which lies behind it. Routinely treated by removing affected testis and giving radiotherapy or chemotherapy to make sure all cancer cells are destroyed; fertility and ejaculation are not affected unless adjacent lymph nodes also have to be removed. For homeopathic approach, see CANCER.

For self-examination see TESTICLE AND SCROTUM PROBLEMS.

Hydrocele see TESTICLE AND SCROTUM PROBLEMS

Penis problems

Balanitis Swelling and soreness of foreskin or head of penis, often caused by friction against damp underwear, or by irritants in sheaths and contraceptive creams; can also be caused by *Herpes* virus (see SEXUALLY TRANSMITTED DISEASES). Complaint is most common in men who suffer from diabetes mellitus (see DIABETES), since sugar in urine encourages microbes to flourish. If homeopathic remedy and self-help measures mentioned below do not clear problem up, see your GP; an antibiotic cream will probably be prescribed, but if inflammation keeps recurring, making it difficult or painful to draw back foreskin, GP may recommend CIRCUMCISION.

Specific remedy to be taken every 4 hours for up to 5 days
• *Mercurius 6c*

Self-help In addition to taking the remedy above, bathe foreskin and head of penis with Hypericum and Calendula solution (5 drops of mother tincture of each to 0.25 litre [½ pint] boiled cooled water) every 4 hours. Always keep penis clean and dry, and wash well under foreskin.

Blood in sperm (haemospermia) Pink, red, or brown streaks in semen due to rupture of small veins in urethra during erection; quite common, but harmless, and usually clears up within a day or two; however, if blood appears in urine (see BLOOD IN URINE), see your GP as soon as possible.

Injury Usually the testicles rather than the penis bear the brunt of blows to the groin. Most common injury to penis is getting it caught in trouser zip; if this happens, cut zip free of trousers and go to nearest hospital casualty department; in meantime, bathe wound with Hypericum and Calendula solution (5 drops of mother tincture of each to 0.25 litre [½ pint] boiled cooled water); attempting to undo zip, especially if you are not circumcised, may make matters worse.

Painful penis If pain accompanies erection, cause may be PHIMOSIS (foreskin too tight) or PRIAPISM (erection occurring in absence of sexual excitement); if pain is felt during intercourse, partner's vagina may be too dry; after intercourse, inflammation or soreness may be due to chemicals in sheath, cap, spermicidal creams, etc. Redness or swelling of the head of the penis may be BALANITIS. Painful open sores are likely to be due to herpes (see SEXUALLY TRANSMITTED DISEASES); lumps or bumps caused by penile warts (see below) or syphilis (see SEXUALLY TRANSMITTED DISEASES) are generally painless.

Penile warts (condylomata) Like warts elsewhere on body, virally caused and moderately contagious; not necessarily contracted through sexual intercourse, although susceptible individuals easily become re-infected if partner has genital warts. Since wart-like growths can be first sign of CANCER OF THE PENIS or of syphilis (see SEXUALLY TRANSMITTED DISEASES), ask GP for diagnosis as soon as possible. Conventionally treated by very careful application of specially prescribed wart paint; over-the-counter preparations should be avoided. Homeopathic treatment is constitutional, but while treatment is being sought one of the remedies below should be tried. Your partner should also be examied and treated if necessary.

Specific remedies to be taken 4 times daily for up to 14 days
- Remedy of first resort *Thuja 6c*
- If Thuja produces no improvement, and if foreskin is swollen and warts bleed *Cinnabar 6c*
- Warts accompanied by inability to obtain erection, or by great increase in sexual desire and premature ejaculation *Lycopodium 6c*

Priapism Rare and painful condition in which penis erects and stays erect even though individual is not sexually aroused; cause is sudden, inexplicable obstruction of outflow of blood from penis, or injury to nerves in spinal cord. A priapic erection lasting for longer than 3 or 4 hours can do lasting damage to spongy tissues of penis, making further erection impossible, so appropriate action is ②. Surgery may be needed to assist excess blood in penis to drain back into general circulation. In meantime, give one of the homeopathic remedies below.

Specific remedies to be given every 15 minutes for up to 10 doses
- General feebleness and impotence *Kali brom. 6c*
- Erection usually painful *Cantharis 6c*
- Generally sluggish venous system, individual may have piles or varicose veins *Carbo veg. 6c*

Self-help A 3-week course of Vitamin E is strongly recommended; take 100 units a day to begin with, increasing intake to 600 units a day. If suffering from high blood pressure, see your GP first as Vitamin E can temporarily raise blood pressure.

Thrush Fungal infection mainly found in women but occasionally in men if genital hygiene is poor or sexual partner is infected; yeast grows under foreskin of penis, causing itching and inflammation. Conventional treatment consists of anti-fungal cream.

Specific remedy to be taken 4 times daily for up to 14 days
- *Mercurius 6c*

Self-help Bathe penis in Hypericum and Calendula solution (5 drops of mother tincture of each to 0.25 litre [½ pint] boiled cooled water) 4 times a day for up to 14 days, then apply Calendula ointment.

Trichomoniasis Caused by *Trichomonas* organism which lurks under foreskin of penis, causing soreness and inflammation; condition is far more common in women than in men, and may be result of poor genital hygiene or intercourse with an infected partner. Conventionally treated with drugs such as Metronidazole. See thrush (above) for homeopathic treatment.

Urethritis Inflammation of urethra, often caused by infection transmitted during sexual intercourse; symptoms are a burning sensation when urinating or ejaculating, and a thick yellowish discharge from tip of penis. See CYSTITIS and SEXUALLY TRANSMITTED DISEASES (gonorrhea and non-specific urethritis) for conventional and homeopathic treatment and self-help measures. Intercourse should be refrained from until symptoms disappear; repeated infection can cause urethral stricture (see below).

Urethral stricture Rare condition in which urethra becomes narrowed by scar tissue as the result of injury or infection, making urination and ejaculation painful or impossible (see RETENTION OF URINE); shrinkage of urethra may also force penis into bent position. Occasionally, urethra may narrow as result of nervous spasm. If homeopathic remedies below do not improve matters, see your GP; urethra may have to be stretched under local anaesthetic, or scar tissue may have to be incised or replaced with a graft.

Specific remedies to be taken twice daily for up to 1 month in chronic cases
- Stricture due to scarring *Silicea 6c*
- Sore, burning sensation when passing water *Cantharis 6c*
- Discharge of pus *Mercurius 6c*
- Nervous spasm and discharge of pus *Camphora 6c*

Specific remedy to be taken every hour for up to 10 doses in acute cases
- Painful spasms during urination, tingling or smarting sensation when not urinating *Aconite 30c*

Self-help Bathe penis in cold water twice a day – easiest way to do this is in shower. Avoid spicy foods, and take a 3-week course of Vitamin E, gradually increasing dosage from 100 units to 600 units a day but see note wider priapism in PENIS PROBLEMS.

Priapism see PENIS PROBLEMS

Prostate problems see also CANCER OF PROSTATE
Enlarged prostate Extremely common in men over 45, although cause is not known; symptomless until tissues become sufficiently stiff and enlarged to interfere with expulsion of urine from bladder; at this point sufferer may find it difficult to start stream of urine, especially in mornings, despite urgent signals from bladder, and

may have to get up several times in night; stream of urine is also weak, and there may be blood in it; some sufferers complain of dragging sensation between legs. Symptoms clear up of own accord in 1 in 3 of mild cases; however, if condition persists and is not treated, possible complications include CYSTITIS (bladder infection), acute PYELONEPHRITIS (kidney infection), RETENTION OF URINE (bladder expands to hold more urine, less and less urine passed), and eventually KIDNEY FAILURE. A localised lump rather than general enlargement suggests possibility of CANCER OF PROSTATE; to rule out cancer, a biopsy is necessary.

Excess prostate tissue can be removed surgically by making incision in abdomen or by passing very slender instruments through urethra; most prostatectomy operations completely relieve urinary difficulties, but ability to obtain erection and ejaculate sperm is sometimes lost.

Specific remedies to be taken 4 times daily for up to 21 days
- Difficult or painful urination, with spasms of bladder or urethra *Sabal 6c*
- Where person is senile, urinates frequently at night, complains of pressure on rectum and smarting sensation at neck of bladder *Ferrum pic. 6c*
- Frequent urge to urinate, slow stream of urine, person thin, underweight, prematurely impotent *Baryta 6c*
- Frequent, urgent desire to pass urine *Thuja 6c*
- Loss of potency, shrunken testes, prostate gland feels hard, though hardness may not be due to cancer *Iodum 6c*
- Impotence because erection is lost on penetration, or lack of desire for sex, or pain on intercourse *Argentum nit. 6c*

Self-help Many sufferers find that Lecithin and calcium and magnesium tablets help – both are obtainable from chemists and healthfood shops. Correct dosages are 2 or 3 dessertspoons of Lecithin per day, and one calcium and magnesium tablet 3 times a day for 1 month. Evening primrose oil can also be beneficial.

Prostatitis Inflammation of prostate, usually due to infection spreading from elsewhere in urinary tract; an acute attack causes FEVER, pain and tenderness around base of penis, and difficulty passing urine; if left untreated, prostate may fill with pus and burst, releasing pus into urethra and causing further infection. Condition is most common in elderly men with enlarged prostate (see above), and tends to recur; a mild attack may clear up of its own accord. Conventionally treated by antibiotics; in resistant cases, pus may need to be drained surgically. Homeopathic treatment is constitutional, but in an acute attack the remedies below may help; if there is no improvement within 24 hours, see your GP.

Specific remedies to be taken every 2 hours for up to 10 doses
- Where prostate is enlarged and area around prostate feels cold, or where ejaculation is impossible or intercourse is painful *Sabal 6c*
- Burning sensation at neck of bladder, frequent urge to pass urine *Thuja 6c*
- Thick yellow discharge from penis, urgent need to pass urine, lying on back makes matters worse *Pulsatilla 6c*

Self-help If condition is mild but recurrent, extra zinc and two daily 10–15 ml doses of cold-pressed linseed oil may be beneficial.

Testicle and scrotum problems see also
CANCER OF THE TESTICLE
Problems can be detected early by regular examination of testicles, preferably in a hot bath so that scrotal muscles are relaxed; the testes themselves should feel smooth through skin of scrotum; the epididymides should feel cord-like, with no noticeable bumps or lumps; any nodules, areas of tenderness, or swelling should be reported to your GP.

Enlarged or painful testicle A painless lump in one testicle is most likely to be an epididymal cyst (see below); in rare cases, it may be CANCER OF THE TESTICLE. A painful swelling in one testicle, followed by pain and swelling of scrotum, suggests torsion or epididymitis (see below); both conditions require prompt medical attention, so ②. A blow to the testicles can cause severe pain; if pain does not wear off within an hour or so, or if scrotum is obviously bruised and swollen, ②; surgery may be necessary to prevent internal bleeding causing permanent damage to testes; in meantime, give *Arnica 30c* every 5 minutes for up to 10 doses.

Epididymal cysts These are benign, painless, fluid-filled swellings which develop in one or more of the many tubes leading from testis to epididymis; quite common in men over 40, and can occur in one or both testicles; since epididymis lies behind testis, swelling is usually located in upper rear part of testicle. Surgery is seldom necessary or advised, as it can result in partial sterility. Constitutional homeopathic treatment is recommended, but the remedies below should be tried first.

Specific remedies to be taken 4 times daily for up to 7 days
- Remedy of first resort *Apis 30c*
- If Apis does not reduce swelling *Graphites 6c*

Epididymitis Bacterial infection of epididymis, usually as result of urinary tract infection; results in hot, tender, painful swelling at back of one testicle. Conventionally treated with antibiotics; however, the remedies given below should be tried first. If there is no improvement within 12 hours, see your GP.

Specific remedies to be taken every hour for up to 10 doses
- Testicle extremely hot, red, swollen, tender, and sensitive to slightest jarring *Belladonna 30c*
- Infection onsets very suddenly, dramatic swelling of testicle, pains in scrotum and lower abdomen *Pulsatilla 6c*
- Fever, restlessness, infection comes on after exposure to cold dry winds *Aconite 30c*
- Testicle hot, swollen, and aching as if someone had kicked it, pains shooting up towards bladder *Hamamelis 6c*

Hydrocele Excess fluid in double-layered sheath around testis, causing soft, painless swelling; in most cases, cause is not known, though occasionally condition is precipitated by injury; most common in older men. Condition is usually kept under observation rather than treated, but if swelling is large, GP may recommend drawing off excess fluid under local anaesthetic; if this does not prevent recurrence, surgery may be necessary. If the homeopathic remedies below produce no improvement within a month or so, see your homeopath.

Specific remedies to be taken 3 times daily for up to 3 weeks
- Swelling follows injury *Arnica 30c*
- If Arnica does not help *Bryonia 30c*
- Testicle tends to ache in thundery weather *Rhododendron 6c*

Torsion of the testicle Occurs when one of testicles twists out of its natural position, pinching veins and blocking outflow of blood; result is sharp pain, sometimes sharp enough to cause NAUSEA AND VOMITING, and swelling. Condition is rare, but can happen at any time, even in sleep; in susceptible individuals, double-layered sheath enclosing testis is not as close-fitting as it should be. Twist often undoes itself spontaneously, but if it doesn't, ② as arteries as well as veins may become blocked. While waiting for medical help, take *Aconite 30c* every 5 minutes for up to 10 doses. Standard treatment is surgical exploration as this is the only sure way to prevent torsion recurring.

Varicocele Abnormal distention of veins draining one of testicles, analogous to VARICOSE VEINS in legs; symptoms are swelling, which disappears when lying down, and a dragging pain, especially in hot weather or after exercise; problem is most common in adolescence; in rare cases, increase in local heat can interfere with fertility. Pain and dragging sensation can be relieved by supporting testicles with a jock strap; surgery to remove or bypass distended veins is not always successful.

Specific remedies to be taken 4 times daily for up to 21 days
- Person pale and anaemic, pain made worse by pressure but relieved by cold applications *Ferrum phos. 6c*
- Pain radiates up from testicle into lower abdomen, person also suffers from piles *Hamamelis 6c*
- Heat and lying on painless side make pain in testicle worse, cold applications relieve pain *Pulsatilla 6c*

Undescended testicle see UNDESCENDED TESTICLE p. 334

Urethritis see PENIS PROBLEMS

Urethral stricture see PENIS PROBLEMS

Varicocele see TESTICLE AND SCROTUM PROBLEMS

HORMONES AND METABOLISM

METABOLISM, the sum total of all the chemical processes which occur in the living body, is ultimately controlled by instructions contained in the chromosomes in the nucleus of every cell. But cells must coordinate their activity, and to do this they must communicate. The nervous system provides communication via nerves, delivering messages in microseconds, and the endocrine system provides communication via hormones, which travel around the body in the bloodstream.

Chemically, hormones are either proteins, aminoacid derivatives, or cholesterol derivatives, and they are secreted in response to nervous stimuli – sight, touch, hearing, taste, smell, thoughts, emotions – and in response to various chemicals in the bloodstream, including other hormones. The pituitary gland at the base of the brain, for example, secretes a number of hormones designed to chivvy other hormone-producing glands into action. The hormones produced by these subservient glands circulate in the blood, but if their concentration in the blood falls below or rises above a certain level the pituitary adjusts its output of 'trophic' or stimulating hormones reciprocally. However, the pituitary is not the prime mover of the endocrine world. This role is played by the hypothalamus.

The hypothalamus is a distinct group of cells at the base of the forebrain, with extensive connections to the cortex, brain stem, and hind brain. Stimulating and inhibitory hormones secreted by the hypothalamus in response to nervous impulses from other parts of the brain travel the short distance to the pituitary beneath it, and the pituitary responds by increasing or decreasing its secretory activities.

The anterior lobe of the pituitary secretes growth hormone, prolactin (to stimulate production of breast-milk), and hormones which stimulate the thyroid and adrenal glands, and also the ovaries and testes; its posterior lobe produces antidiuretic hormone (to decrease excretion of water by the kidneys), and oxytocin (to stimulate milk flow and contraction of the womb after childbirth).

The thyroid gland, which lies in the neck at Adam's apple level, produces thyroxin, which controls meta-bolic rate, the pace of chemical activity in every cell in the body; iodine is an essential component of thyroxine. Directly behind the thyroid are the four parathyroid glands; these produce parathormone which, together with calcitonin produced by the thyroid, controls calcium metabolism.

The two adrenal glands, one perched on top of each kidney, secrete the 'fight or flight' hormones adrenalin and noradrenalin in response to stimulation of the sympathetic nervous system. They also secrete steroids, all of which are made from cholesterol. Two of the most important steroids are aldosterone and cortisone. Aldosterone controls the balance of potassium and sodium in the blood, and cortisone plays a crucial part in carbohydrate, protein, and fat metabolism, and many other processes. The adrenal glands also produce small amounts of androgens, masculinizing hormones, in both women and men.

However, the major androgen-producing role in the male body is assumed by the testes, which produce testosterone. In women, femaleness, fertility, and the menstrual cycle are controlled by oestrogens and progestins manufactured in the ovaries. The testes also produce small amounts of oestrogens.

Another very important endocrine gland is the pancreas. Lying under and behind the stomach, it produces two hormones which regulate the level of glucose in the blood, insulin and glucagon; insulin encourages cells to absorb glucose and glucagon encourages stores of glucose to be released into the bloodstream. Both hormones are produced in response to levels of glucose in the blood. If the cells which produce insulin become diseased or un-responsive, the result is diabetes.

Many other parts of the body – the heart, kidneys, stomach, intestines, and placenta – also contain cells which produce hormones.

Acromegaly
Occurs in middle age, producing general thickening and increase in size of bones, structures, and organs; changes include enlargement of hands and feet, head, neck, lower jaw, nose, and ears, thickening of skin and tongue, tingling in hands, sweating, stiffness, deepen-ing of voice, and an increase in body hair, especially in women. Cause is over-production of growth hormone due to a pituitary tumour (see PITUITARY PROBLEMS). Other consequences may be hypopituitarism (see PITUITARY PROBLEMS), visual problems (if tumour in pituitary is large enough to press on adjacent structures in brain), diabetes mellitus (see DIABETES), HIGH BLOOD PRESSURE, and HEART FAILURE. Orthodox treatment consists of drugs to suppress production of growth hormone and/or surgery to remove tumour; unfortunately, physical changes are more or less permanent.

Specific remedies to be taken 3 times daily for up to 21 days once tumour has been removed
• *Conchiolinum 6x* followed by *Hecla 6x* in same dosage

Addison's disease
Occurs when cortex of adrenal glands fails to produce enough steroid hormones (in particular hydrocortisone which, among many other things, suppresses in-flammatory response). Symptoms onset insidiously, beginning with fatigue, INDIGESTION, and loss of appetite (see APPETITE CHANGES); later, person loses weight (see WEIGHT LOSS), develops ANAEMIA, and has increasingly frequent bouts of NAUSEA AND VOMITING, and DIARRHOEA or CONSTIPATION; skin also darkens, as if permanently tanned. Eventually HYPOGLYCAEMIA may set in, or adrenal glands may fail altogether, quickly leading to collapse and symptoms similar to those of GASTROENTERITIS; if this happens, ②.

If Addison's disease is suspected, see your GP; if blood test reveals abnormally low level of steroid hormones, hydrocortisone will be prescribed; how-ever, before taking hydrocortisone, which has to be taken for life, see if one of homeopathic remedies below helps.

Specific remedies to be taken 4 times daily for up to 7 days; if no improvment within 1 week, see your GP
• Constipation, muddy complexion, dry lips and mouth, craving for salt, symptoms made worse by hot sun *Natrum mur. 30c*
• Tremor, apprehension, craving for salt and sweet things *Argentum nit. 30c*
• No stamina, feet sweat profusely and smell un-pleasant, cold weather makes symptoms worse *Silicea 30c*

Aldosteronism
A consequence of over-production of aldosterone by cortex of adrenal glands; symptoms are HIGH BLOOD PRESSURE, muscle spasms in hands and feet, thirst, large volume of urine production, and weakness or

tingling in limbs. Cause of increased aldosterone production may be CIRRHOSIS OF THE LIVER, HEART FAILURE, or some other chronic ailment, or a benign tumour in one or other adrenal gland. Orthodox treatment consists of diuretics, and surgical removal of tumour if necessary, as well as treatment of underlying cause. Constitutional homeopathic treatment is recommended in addition to orthodox treatment.

Cushing's syndrome

Most common in young or middle-aged women and brought on by long-term steroid treatment or by overproduction of steroids by the adrenal glands (perhaps because of an adrenal or pituitary tumour – see PITUITARY PROBLEMS); typical effects include a moon-faced look, WEIGHT GAIN, development of a pad of fat between shoulders, wasting of muscles leading to weakness and fatigue, purplish streaks on skin which resemble stretch marks, easy BRUISING, DEPRESSION, and low sex drive (see LACK OF DESIRE FOR SEX), and in some cases OSTEOPOROSIS, diabetes mellitus (see DIABETES), HIGH BLOOD PRESSURE, or HEART FAILURE. Women who suffer from Cushing's syndrome usually stop menstruating (see MENSTRUAL PROBLEMS), and develop a deep voice and extra body hair; men become impotent and less hairy.

Constitutional homeopathic treatment is recommended in addition to orthodox treatment, which may consist of surgery if a tumour is present, or prescribing drugs other than steroids for conditions such as ASTHMA and RHEUMATOID ARTHRITIS.

Diabetes

May be brought on by damage to the pituitary gland or, more commonly, by malfunction of the pancreas.

Diabetes insipidus is caused by a deficiency of anti-diuretic hormone (ADH); this hormone is produced in the pituitary gland and stimulates the kidneys to reabsorb water from urine, but if pituitary is damaged (by a head injury, surgery, radiotherapy, or a tumour), production of ADH may slow down or stop; kidneys will then allow huge amounts of water – up to 20 litres (35 pints) a day – to be lost in urine and person will be obliged to drink equally large amounts; other symptoms are dry hands and CONSTIPATION. Orthodox treatment consists of synthetic ADH in form of nasal drops, and surgery if there is a pituitary tumour, or diuretics and low salt intake to encourage kidneys to conserve water. If diabetes insipidus is suspected, try the remedies below; if there is no improvement within 1 week, see your GP. If symptoms are severe, 12 .

Specific remedies to be taken 4 times daily for up to 7 days
- Symptoms follow head injury *Arnica 30c*
- Flow of urine day and night *Squilla 30c*
- Flow of urine greater at night *Phosphoric ac. 30c*
- Urination more copious at night, accompanied by an increase in sexual excitement, urine smells like herbs *Murex 30c*
- Person extremely thin and debilitated *Uranium nit. 30c*

Diabetes mellitus occurs when the pancreas secretes insufficient insulin or none at all; without insulin, cells cannot absorb energy-giving glucose from the blood, nor can the liver absorb and store it. Excess glucose is excreted in urine, which has to have a higher water content than normal to carry it, so urination is frequent and passed in large amounts and person is continually thirsty; also, because tissues are starved of glucose, person feels tired and apathetic, and may lose a lot of weight as body breaks down fat and muscle for energy; other likely symptoms are lowered resistance to infection (especially urinary tract infections) because germs flourish in a sugary environment, CRAMP, tingling in hands and feet, blurred vision and possibly erectile difficulties and cessation of periods (see ERECTION PROBLEMS, MENSTRUAL PROBLEMS). Longer-term complications include DIABETIC RETINOPATHY (scarring of retina), damage to peripheral nerves (see NEURALGIA AND NEURITIS), and chronic KIDNEY FAILURE; as a group, diabetics are also more vulnerable to ATHEROSCLEROSIS. In some cases diabetes mellitus is a consequence of another disorder, usually hormonal (see CUSHING'S SYNDROME, THYROID PROBLEMS, ACROMEGALY). Speed at which symptoms onset depends on age at which disease sets in, and degree of malfunction of pancreas.

Insulin-dependent diabetes, also referred to as *juvenile diabetes*, or *Type 1 diabetes* is the form of diabetes mellitus most frequent in young people; it onsets in a matter of weeks or months, and occurs because pancreas produces little or no insulin; incompetence of pancreas may be congenital, or the result of an autoimmune reaction triggered off by a viral infection such as MUMPS or RUBELLA. High incidence of insulin-dependent diabetes in Western countries may have something to do with high consumption of carbohydrates and dairy products. Orthodox treatment consists of daily insulin injections (insulin taken by mouth would be destroyed in stomach), and a strict timetable of meals and snacks so that glucose level in blood remains more or less constant.

Insulin non-dependent diabetes, also known as *maturity-onset diabetes*, or *Type 2 diabetes* is predominantly a disease of middle and old age, most common among people aged 60–70, and onsets very gradually; majority of sufferers are overweight, and about a third have a family history of maturity-onset diabetes; pancreas produces insulin, but not in sufficient quantities to fuel excessive body bulk, and in any case tends to become less efficient with age. This type of diabetes mellitus is usually treated by strict control of diet (substituting small amounts of unrefined carborehydrates for intensely sugary foods such as sweets, chocolates, biscuits, cakes, jams and soft drinks, eating plenty of uncooked vegetables and fruit, and fibre-rich cereals) usually reduces weight to a level that the pancreas can cope with, but if blood still has too much glucose in it, person may be put on hypoglycaemic (glucose-lowering) drugs.

All diabetics are advised to carry some form of identification, giving instructions on what to do in emergencies. If a diabetic develops symptoms of HYPOGLYCAEMIA (sudden loss of energy, hunger, sweating, dizziness, weakness, unsteadiness, headache, irritability, slurred speech, pins and needles), give sugar or glucose by mouth immediately to prevent him or her becoming unconscious, but if this happens despite giving sugar, ⑨⑨⑨. They may be going into a hyperglycaemic coma.

Constitutional homeopathic treatment is recommended in addition to orthodox treatment, and is compatible with it. The remedies below may help while constitutional treatment is being sought.

Specific remedies to be taken 4 times daily for up to 14 days
- Symptoms brought on by nervous exhaustion (grief, working too hard) *Phosphoric ac. 6c*
- Symptoms include digestive upsets, emaciation, weakness, and bedwetting *Uranium nit. 6c*
- Symptoms include swollen ankles *Argentum nit. 6c*
- Skin irritation, restlessness, depression *Codeinum 6c*
- Symptoms accompanied by gout *Natrum sulph. 6c*
- Symptoms include cold, sweaty, smelly feet, and loss of stamina *Silicea 6c*

Self-care Treatment for both insulin-dependent and insulin non-dependent diabetes is largely self-administered, requiring considerable discipline. The British Diabetic Association (address p. 382) can provide valuable support and guidance. You will be expected to test your blood and urine at regular intervals, eat your meals and give yourself insulin injections at set times each day, or strictly follow the calorie intake rules given to you by your GP. Both forms of diabetes benefit from the Blood Sugar Levelling Diet described on p. 352; this consists of three meals a day, with snacks in between, and ensures that your blood is never flooded with unmanageable amounts of glucose. Extra Vitamin C, B_6, B_{12}, chromium, zinc, magnesium and potassium are recommended; also Vitamin E if there are eye complications. Intake of salt and alcohol should be restricted.

If you smoke, try to stop. Always tell anyone who is treating you for non-diabetic ailments – doctors, dentists, nurses, etc. – that you have diabetes. Also, your driving licence and any life or accident insurance policies you have may be invalid if you have not declared your diabetes. If you are dependent on insulin, you should not drive heavy goods or public service vehicles, or work at heights; shift work should also be avoided since it interferes with eating and injection routines. Regular foot care from a qualified chiropodist is recommended in long-standing diabetics.

Dwarfism

Maybe caused by a deficiency of growth hormone from birth or during childhood or adolescence. Fault lies in pituitary gland, but unless a tumour is responsible, reason for malfunction may not be obvious. Some forms of dwarfism are caused by inherited errors of bone formation. Other hormones besides growth hormone may be deficient, causing poor sexual development, although this may also be associated with zinc deficiency. Orthodox treatment consists of injections of growth hormone, or removal of pituitary tumour. Stunted growth is more commonly due to malnutrition and emotional factors, or to conditions such as COELIAC DISEASE and CYSTIC FIBROSIS; see growth charts on pp. 309, 312. Homeopathic treatment is constitutional.

Gigantism

A consequence of pituitary gland producing too much growth hormone while bones, organs, and other structure are still growing; this produces great elongation of limbs and torso, and proportional sideways growth (in adults, who have stopped growing, too much growth hormone produces only sideways enlargement – see ACROMEGALY). If your child is growing too fast (see growth charts pp. 309, 312), see your GP. Orthodox treatment consists of anti-hormone drugs or, if necessary, removal of pituitary tumour. Constitutional homeopathic treatment is advised in addition to orthodox treatment.

Goitre see also THYROID PROBLEMS

Non-toxic enlargement of thyroid gland, usually due to a shortage of iodine in diet; iodine shortage means that thyroid cannot produce enough thyroxine, so pituitary stimulates it to enlarge in a vain attempt to increase thyroxine production; enlargement produces swelling around front of neck. Condition is easily remedied by increasing iodine intake; fish and kelp are good natural sources. The homeopathic remedies below will also help. If, in spite of these measures, swelling does not go down, see your GP.

Specific remedies to be taken every 12 hours for up to 2 weeks
- Obsessive personality, always in a hurry, always feeling hot, dark hair and eyes *Iodum 30c*
- Long-standing swelling of thyroid, lump feels hard *Spongia 30c*
- Person pale, chilly, overweight, with sweaty feet *Calcarea 30c*
- Person who is elderly, but vigorous and full-bodied, with varicose veins *Fluoric ac. 30c*

---

⑨⑨⑨ Emergency – call GP (or dial 999) immediately. ② Consult your doctor if no improvement within 2 hours

Gout

Build-up of uric acid crystals in joints – especially big toe joints, knuckles, knees, and elbows – due to diet, genetic predisposition, lead poisoning, diuretic drugs, or conditions such as PSORIASIS and LEUKAEMIA; uric acid, the unwanted end-product of protein breakdown, is excreted by kidneys, but if kidney function is impaired or if more uric acid is produced than they can cope with, crystals accumulate in spaces between joints, causing gout, or in kidneys themselves, causing HIGH BLOOD PRESSURE and KIDNEY FAILURE.

A first attack of gout usually affects one joint only; joint becomes red, shiny, and excruciatingly painful, often within a matter of hours; moderate FEVER may develop as well. Attack wears off after a few days and may never recur; in most cases, however, attacks do recur, at decreasing intervals and affecting more joints. If untreated, joints may be permanently deformed. Orthodox treatment consists of painkillers and non-steroidal anti-inflammatory drugs, or drugs to increase excretion or reduce production of uric acid. Homeopathic treatment is constitutional, but during an attack one of the remedies below may help.

Specific remedies to be taken every 15 minutes for up to 10 doses
- Person depressed, irritable, weak, and nauseous, affected joint excruciatingly painful, especially at night or when an attempt is made to move it *Colchicum 6c*
- Joints feel bruised and painful *Arnica 30c*
- Affected joints slightly swollen, with a cold feeling in them, discomfort lessened by cold bathing, increased by movement *Ledum 6c*
- Affected joints burn and itch *Urtica 30c*
- Symptoms accompanied by strong-smelling urine *Benzoic ac. 6c*
- One foot hot, other foot cold, symptoms worse 4–8 pm *Lycopodium 6c*
- Pains flit from joint to joint *Pulsatilla 6c*

Self-help To ease pain, apply a hot compress or ice pack to the affected joint, but do not take aspirin as it may interfere with action of anti-gout drugs. To keep bedclothes off joint, improvise a cage or cradle out of a cardboard box. Drink extra fluid (plain water is best, or water with a little sodium bicarbonate in it) to enable your kidneys to excrete as much uric acid as possible, and stick to the Liver Diet (p. 352) for 1 month to reduce protein-processing demands on liver. Extra Vitamin C and magnesium are also beneficial.

Hyperlipidaemia

High levels of fats (including cholesterol) in blood, increasing risk of ATHEROSCLEROSIS, coronary thrombosis (see HEART ATTACK) and STROKE; high levels may be due to an inherited fault in lipid metabolism, over-consumption of saturated fats and cholesterol, too much alcohol, or a generalized ailment such as diabetes mellitus (see DIABETES). In most cases there are no symptoms – condition is diagnosed during investigation of some other ailment; in extreme cases, however, there may be yellowish patches under skin, especially on elbows, between fingers, and around ankles. A low-fat/high fibre diet (minimal amounts of full milk, cream, butter, cheese, eggs, and fatty meat, plenty of fresh vegetables and fruit, and wholegrains) usually achieves some lowering of blood lipid levels; drugs to lower cholesterol level are available. Homeopathic treatment is constitutional.

Hypoglycaemia

Low level of glucose in blood, causing a variety of symptoms in different people; these include sweating, DIZZINESS, trembling, weakness, hunger, slurred speech, blurred vision, tingling in hands or lips, HEADACHE, irritability, aggressiveness, even unconsciousness. All body cells, especially those in the brain, require energy in the form of glucose to function properly, hence the variety of symptoms. Blood glucose level can be lowered by alcohol, paracetamol, progesterone, and oral contraceptives; ADDISON'S DISEASE, hypopituitarism (see PITUITARY PROBLEMS), THYROID PROBLEMS, and CANCER OF THE PANCREAS can also lead to low glucose levels; more commonly, low blood sugar is a symptom of taking too much insulin to correct insulin-dependent diabetes or of overdosing with hypoglycaemic drugs to correct insulin non-dependent diabetes (see DIABETES). In emergencies, orthodox treatment is to give an injection of glucagon (a pancreatic hormone which stimulates liver to release stored glucose) or of glucose; a spoonful of honey or a small glass of milk will boost blood sugar level almost as quickly. However, long-term solution is dietary (see self-help measures below), plus treatment of underlying cause.

Naturopaths, most homeopaths, and a few GPs also recognize a phenomenon called *spontaneous, functional,* or *reactive hypoglycaemia* in which none of the causative factors mentioned above are present, blood sugar level appears to be normal, yet person suffers from typically hypoglycaemic symptoms. In addition to those mentioned above, person may suffer from CONFUSION, forgetfulness, lack of concentration, DEPRESSION, purposelessness, ANXIETY, PHOBIA, or think and behave in a suicidal or anti-social way; on the physical plane, he or she may feel extremely tired, bloated, or cold and sweaty, or have a headache, backache, or joint and muscle pains, or suffer from numb extremities, muscular twitches, abdominal cramps, and even convulsions. Typically such symptoms come on suddenly, often first thing in morning, before breakfast, or 2 hours after exercise or emotional stress. One possible explanation of this form of hypoglycaemia is that although blood glucose level may be normal, level of glucose in brain may be low. Symptoms seem to be helped by eating foods which have a relatively low glycaemic index (low rate of conversion into glucose); these are precisely the foods recommended in the Blood Sugar Levelling Diet on pp. 353–4. Causes of reactive hypoglycaemia appear to be STRESS, excessive consumption of caffeine or refined carbohydrates, food ALLERGY, and smoking. The only sure way of diagnosing condition is to give a glucose tolerance test, over 5 hours if possible.

Homeopathic treatment for both true and functional hypoglycaemia is constitutional.

Self-help If you are prone to hypoglycaemic attacks, make sure your family and work colleagues know what to do if you pass out. Always carry glucose tablets or barley sugar, but keep these strictly for emergencies. Make sure you eat something every 2 hours or so, especially before strenuous exercise, and stick to those foods permitted under the Blood Sugar Levelling Diet on pp. 354–4. Take extra Vitamin C and B complex, and also chromium, magnesium, potassium, zinc and manganese. Get a full 8 hours sleep a night, avoid getting overtired, and exercise regularly, slowly increasing exercise periods.

Obesity

Point at which being overweight restricts movement, places undue strain on heart and joints, or causes embarrassment or social difficulties, to say nothing of feeling heavy and overheating easily; if you are 20 percent or more above your correct weight (see charts opposite), you are on the road to obesity. A rough and ready test is to pinch a fold of flesh just below the navel and see how thick it is; anything above 2.5 cm (1 in) suggests that some weight ought to be lost.

Overeating and lack of exercise are the most frequent causes of obesity and overweight – unexpended calories are simply stored as fat – but behind these there are often unresolved emotional problems; another cause may be a slow metabolic rate – for genetic reasons, the body is very economical in its energy demands – or failure of appetite control mechanism. Putting on weight can also be a response to drugs or any one of the conditions mentioned under WEIGHT GAIN.

Another possible cause of obesity, most often advanced by naturopaths, is delayed transit of faeces and toxins through the bowel. It is not generally appreciated that fat, because it takes a lot of energy to break down, is a convenient dump for all sorts of toxins; more toxins in circulation mean that more fat is laid down to keep them out of circulation. The remedy is a high-fibre diet, and avoidance of as many toxic substances, natural and man-made, as possible (see PART 2).

Disorders to which fat people are more vulnerable than people of normal weight are DIABETES, HIGH BLOOD PRESSURE, CORONARY ARTERY DISEASE, kidney disorders, PNEUMONIA, CHOLECYSTITIS and GALLSTONES, OSTEOARTHRITIS, HERNIAS, HIATUS HERNIA, VARICOSE VEINS, skin disorders, and CANCER; there is also a positive correlation between being fat and being accident-prone, infertile, and dying from operations; still births are commoner among women who are fat.

Only a small minority of obese or overweight people fail to lose weight by taking more exercise (which increases metabolic rate and helps to bring appetite under control) and consuming fewer calories. Most GPs prefer not to prescribe drugs which suppress appetite or increase metabolic rate; procedures such as wiring up the jaw or surgically bypassing intestine where food absorption takes place are of doubtful benefit.

Constitutional homeopathic treatment is recommended in addition to the specific remedies and self-help measures given below.

Specific remedies to be taken every 12 hours for up to 3 weeks, in addition to increasing exercise and cutting down on calories
- Person chilly and flabby, has head sweats, craves eggs and hot food, suffers from indigestion *Calcarea 6c*
- Constipation, chilliness, skin problems such as spotty or greasy skin, eczema, or weeping sebaceous cysts *Graphites 6c*
- Person who is fat, lazy, slovenly, red in face, and complains of burning sensations in stomach or intestines *Capsicum 6c*
- Catarrh, neuralgic headaches, dry, tickling cough at night *Ammonium brom. 6c*
- Person who is pale-faced, oversensitive, and flushes easily, with cold extremities *Ferrum 6c*
- Backache, chilliness, catarrh *Kali carb. 6c*

Self-help Do not crash diet; this only confuses the body's appetite control mechanism, causes water and stored sugar to be lost rather than fat, and robs the body of valuable vitamins and minerals. Instead, eat a balanced diet, applying the twice-a-week rule discussed on p. 24, and be aware of the number of calories you are eating (buy yourself a calorie counter). Stay strictly away from fats and refined carbohydrates, and eat a little often rather than a lot a long intervals. Don't bolt your food. Extra Vitamin C and B complex, and extra chromium, magnesium, manganese, potassium, and zinc are also recommended.

You should aim to lose about 0.5 kg (1 lb) a week, which means either using up 500 more calories per day or eating 500 calories less each day. In practice more exercise *and* fewer calories each day is an easier regime to stick to; exercise has the added advantage of increasing metabolic rate, which makes you feel warmer, which makes it easier for you to control your

Height/weight guide for men

Height ft/in (cm)

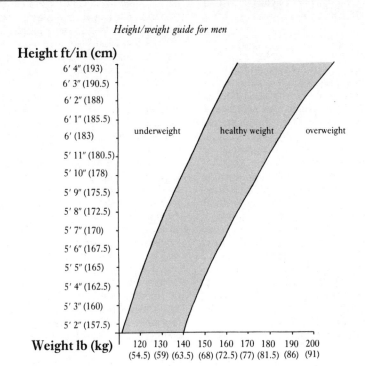

Weight lb (kg)

Height/weight guide for women

Height ft/in (cm)

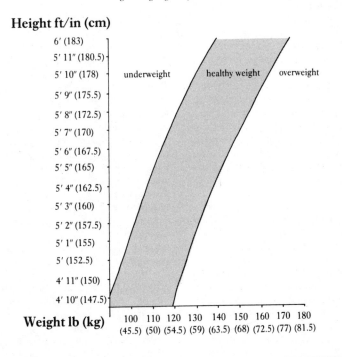

Weight lb (kg)

For explanation of other symbols, see page 107

appetite. Join your local branch of Weight Watchers if you need the support and encouragement of other fighters.

Parathyroid problems

Under- or over-production of parathormone by the four parathyroid glands leads to too low or too high a concentration of calcium in the blood; blood calcium has to be kept within strict limits for nerves and muscles to function normally, and for bones, hair, and nails to form properly.

Hypoparathyroidism (low parathormone production) is a rare disorder but is more common in children than adults, causing HEADACHE, NAUSEA AND VOMITING, FITS, mental retardation, and poor growth of teeth; throat, hands and feet may go into painful spasms (tetany), and face and hands may feel numb or tingly; other symptoms include dry skin, HAIR LOSS, CATARACT, and persistent ORAL THRUSH (and genital thrush – see VAGINAL AND VULVAL PROBLEMS, PENIS PROBLEMS). Cause is not known, but in some cases other hormone-producing glands are affected as well. Condition requires lifelong treatment with Vitamin D, which stimulates absorption of calcium from food in gut; a bad tetany attack may require an injection of calcium. Constitutional homeopathic treatment is also advised.

Hyperparathyroidism (high parathormone production) keeps blood calcium level high, mainly by removing calcium from bones; excess calcium is excreted in urine. Early symptoms may be DEPRESSION and bouts of INDIGESTION (nausea, vomiting, constipation, abdominal pain) but disorder is usually symptomless until well advanced; at this stage, bones fracture easily, and build-up of calcium in kidneys causes KIDNEY STONES, BLOOD IN URINE, and urinary tract infections. Condition does not usually declare itself until middle age; it may be secondary to KIDNEY FAILURE and OSTEOMALACIA, or a consequence of radiotherapy, but more commonly it is caused by a benign tumour in one of glands or general enlargement of all four. Orthodox treatment is removal of tumour, or removal of three out of four enlarged glands. Homeopathic treatment is recommended in addition to surgery.

Pituitary problems

Malfunction of the pituitary gland, which produces eight different hormones, is usually due to a *pituitary tumour*. Most such tumours are benign and all occur – for reasons which are not known – in the anterior (front) lobe of the gland. Disorders such as GIGANTISM, ACROMEGALY, CUSHING'S SYNDROME, and galactorrhea (abnormal milk production – see BREAST PROBLEMS) are caused by excessive production of anterior lobe hormones in response to a type of tumour called an adenoma. Another kind of tumour, a craniopharyngioma, has the opposite effect; it presses on hormone-producing cells in either the anterior or posterior lobe and decreases their output of hormones, causing DWARFISM, diabetes insipidus (see DIABETES), or hypopituitarism (see below); occasionally craniopharyngiomas are malignant. A particularly large tumour may press on nerves to the eyes, causing HEADACHE, visual disturbances, or a SQUINT. Surgical removal or irradiation of pituitary tumours usually gives excellent results, although there is a small risk of damage to healthy part of gland; after surgery, hormone supplements may be necessary. Constitutional homeopathic treatment is also recommended.

Hypopituitarism, also known as Simmond's disease, is the failure of the anterior lobe of the pituitary to produce any of its six hormones; this halts growth (see DWARFISM) and production of breast milk, and inhibits the hormone-producing activities of the thyroid gland, adrenal glands, ovaries, and testes; this in turn causes hypothyroidism (see THYROID PROBLEMS), ADDISON'S DISEASE, general ill health and weakness, arrested sexual development, amenorrhea (see MENSTRUAL PROBLEMS), INFERTILITY, and loss of libido (see LACK OF DESIRE FOR SEX). Most common causes of hypopituitarism are head injuries and pituitary tumours (see above); occasionally, severe blood loss during childbirth is responsible. Treatment consists of hormone tablets or injections (thyroxine, hydrocortisone, testosterone, oestrogen, etc.), and surgery if necessary. Constitutional homeopathic treatment is also advised, although the remedies below may be tried while constitutional treatment is being sought.

Specific remedies to be taken every 12 hours for up to 7 days
- Symptoms onset after head injury *Arnica 30c*
- Symptoms onset after heavy blood loss *China 30c*

Porphyria

An extremely rare inherited disorder in which manufacture of haemoglobin (oxygen-carrying pigment in red blood cells) is faulty, leading to accumulation of chemicals called porphyrins in liver, intestines, skin, and brain. Symptoms are episodic, lasting for a few days, and may include ABDOMINAL PAIN, VOMITING, and CRAMP, or itchy, blistered skin, or depression and mania (see MANIC DEPRESSION). Attacks may be triggered off by certain drugs, alcohol, exposure to sunlight, or pregnancy. Condition is not curable, though it can be managed by avoiding known triggers. Constitutional homeopathic treatment is recommended.

Thyroid problems see also GOITRE

Under- or over-production of thyroid hormone (thyroxine) can slow down or speed up all chemical processes in the body.

Thyrotoxicosis (also referred to as hyperthyroidism, toxic goitre, or Graves' disease) occurs when the whole thyroid gland is overactive, usually because the pituitary gland is producing too much thyroid stimulating hormone, or because there is a 'nodule' (a fluid-filled cyst, a small haemorrhage, or a benign or malignant growth) in part of it; a nodule may be visible as a lump at front of neck, general enlargement as a sizeable swelling. Large amounts of thyroxine are continuously produced and released into the bloodstream, causing a wide variety of symptoms: restlessness, a high level of ANXIETY, inability to relax or sleep properly (see SLEEP PROBLEMS), shakiness and poor control of fine hand movements, sweating, feeling hot even on cold days, rapid heart rate, PALPITATIONS, BREATHLESSNESS, WEIGHT LOSS despite a ravenous appetite, DIARRHOEA, bulging eyes (see EXOPTHALMOS), etc. Accelerated metabolism places extra strain on heart, especially if person already has HIGH BLOOD PRESSURE or ARTERIOSCLEROSIS, and increases risk of ANGINA and HEART FAILURE. Orthodox treatment consists of anti-thyroid drugs, destruction of part of thyroid gland with radioactive iodine, or surgical removal of nodule or large part of gland; blood thyroxine levels must also be checked regularly to ensure that hypothyroidism (see below) does not set in. The homeopathic remedies below may help to bring acute symptoms under control; however, if condition dramatically worsens, 12 .

Specific remedies to be taken every hour for up to 10 doses
- Someone who is obsessive, feels very hot, can't stop hurrying, especially if he or she is dark-haired and dark-eyed *Iodum 30c*
- Constipation, palpitations, earthy complexion *Natrum mur. 30c*
- Flushed face and staring eyes *Belladonna 30c*
- Heart pounding and racing, exopthalmos *Lycopus 30c*

Hypothyroidism is underactivity of the thyroid gland, due in some cases to lack of iodine in the diet or lack of thyroid stimulating hormone from the pituitary; in other cases thyroid defect may be congenital or gland may be missing altogether; in Hashimoto's disease, an autoimmune response develops which destroys thyroid tissue. In adults, the symptoms of low thyroxine production are tiredness, ABNORMAL SLEEPINESS OR DROWSINESS, aches and pains, slow heart rate, CONSTIPATION, feeling cold most of the time, WEIGHT GAIN despite poor appetite, myxoedema (thick, dry, swollen skin), lifeless hair, deep or hoarse voice, loss of hearing, NUMBNESS and tingling in hands, and LACK OF DESIRE FOR SEX; women tend to have heavy periods (see PERIOD PROBLEMS). Babies who are hypothyroid are very torpid, uninterested in food, and may develop JAUNDICE shortly after birth; since thyroxine is essential for growth and mental development, lack of it at this young age can cause cretinism and stunted growth.

Both adults and babies are treated with thyroxine tablets; most babies develop normally if treatment is started before age of three months. However, if hypothyroidism is mild, thyroid gland extract (which contains all the constituents of thyroid tissue, including thyroxine) may be preferable to thyroxine itself; if thyroid gland recovers, thyroid gland extract is more easily discontinued than thyroxine. Constitutional homeopathic treatment is recommended in addition to orthodox treatment.

Specific remedy to be taken every 12 hours for up to 5 days while constitutional treatment is being sought
- *Arsenicum 30c*

Weight Gain
Occurs inexorably when calories consumed are not equalled by calories spent. Too much food and not enough exercise are often features of DEPRESSION – apathy and exercise do not go together, but food and the need for comfort do. Hormonal causes of weight gain (here too emotions and general activity levels play a role) include HYPOTHYROIDISM (always feeling cold, constipation, thinning hair, dry skin), and CUSHING'S SYNDROME (moon-faced look, muscle wasting, easy bruising). Weight gain can also be a symptom of fluid retention (see OEDEMA, KIDNEY FAILURE, HEART FAILURE); most women put on a little weight before their periods due to fluid retention (see PREMENSTRUAL SYNDROME). Some drugs, especially steroids and oral contraceptives, cause weight gain; so, in some people, does giving up smoking.

For orthodox and homeopathic treatment, see conditions mentioned above.

Weight loss
Unexplained weight loss of 0.5 kg (1 lb) or more a week is almost always medically significant. Steady weight loss can be a symptom of thyrotoxicosis (sweating, feeling hot and restless, diarrhoea, increased appetite – see THYROID PROBLEMS), diabetes mellitus (great thirst, frequent urination, tiredness, normal appetite – see DIABETES), TUBERCULOSIS (mild fever, tiredness, dry cough with blood or pus in sputum), BRUCELLOSIS ('flu-like symptoms, which drag on, depression, joint pains), PEPTIC ULCER or CANCER OF THE STOMACH (pain in upper abdomen), CROHN'S DISEASE or CANCER OF THE COLON (abdominal pain, diarrhoea, perhaps blood in stools), MALABSORPTION (diarrhoea, pale, bulky stools which float), or AIDS (see SEXUALLY TRANSMITTED DISEASES). See entries above for homeopathic treatment.

SEXUAL PROBLEMS

PROBLEMS of sexual identity and problems arising from chromosomal anomalies lie outside the scope of this book and are, more properly, the province of the psychotherapist and psychosexual counsellor. However, constitutional homeopathic prescribing can help to relieve tension and anxiety where these are part of the picture.

Erection, orgasm, and ejaculation are reflexes, but there is nothing automatic about them. They can be helped or hindered by thoughts and emotions. They can be helped by trust, relaxation, and fantasy. They can be hindered by guilt, sexual taboos, and fear of inadequacy even when all the right sensual stimuli are there, even when all the nerves, blood vessels, glands, and hormones involved in sexual response are perfectly normal. Male orgasm is a more reliable response than female orgasm, during intercourse that is; during masturbation both sexes' capacity for orgasm is about equal.

Sexual anatomy and the techniques of sexual intercourse are described at length in many books, but as anyone who has been in a long-term sexual relationship knows, sexual intercourse is a great deal more than the art of applying the right techniques to the right erogenous zones. Indeed, sexual intercourse is only one aspect of sexuality. To concentrate on it to the exclusion of dress, humour, flirting, seduction, affection, and so on is like insisting that music begins and ends with Beethoven and Haydn.

There is no reason why sexual drive and sexual function should not continue into our 80s or even 90s, with, as one wag put it, this important proviso: those who enjoy the party tend to leave last! Intercourse does make demands on the heart, but if you can climb two flights of stairs without suffering from palpitations or getting painfully out of breath, you should be quite safe. Penis size has very little to do with female satisfaction, primarily because it is the outer third of the vagina which is the most sensitive.

Much has been written about the mismatch of the male and female 'sexual response cycle' as a source of sexual dissatisfaction; both are described in terms of an excitation phase, a plateau phase, orgasm, a resolution phase, and a refractory phase. The most common complaint is that he climaxes too fast, she too slowly – however, anthropologists have pointed out that this may be a cultural rather than a physiological phenomenon. What does seem to be a physiological phenomenon, however, is that very few men over the age of 25 reach orgasm more than once in a love-making session. Quite a few women do. Foreplay is a way of prolonging the man's excitement and plateau phase and bringing the women to plateau phase or even orgasm before penetration. Men are not responsible for women's orgasms; both sexes are responsible for their own.

What a person expects during sexual intercourse and what actually happens may be rather different. This is often a cause of problems. For example, orgasm is not always dramatic or obvious – some people moan or cry out, others are silent; nor is it experienced the same way on every occasion. Synchronized climaxes happen a lot in novels but not in the real world – psychologists would say that 'coming' together is an intermittent reward that serves to strengthen rather than diminish sex drive. Techniques that please one person may not excite someone else – we are all different in our capacity for pleasure.

What a person wants from intercourse may be unreasonable – this too can be a source of conflict. Love-making seldom solves problems in other areas of life, nor does it always shut them out. Quite the reverse, in fact. Job worries, money problems, identity problems, depression, boredom, fatigue, and so on have a habit of getting into bed with us.

Sexual education begins with the way in which we treat our children. Hitting or beating a child, or denying physical affection, may make it very difficult for that child to have loving sexual relationships; his or her sexuality may be tinged with sadism or masochism. Many films and advertisements on television subtly suggest that sex equals power and possession, that sex is not real sex unless it is violent and exploitative. In the author's view, parents should do everything possible to combat this distortion.

Like every other part of the body the genitals are susceptible to infection, especially to sexually transmitted infection. There are specific homeopathic remedies for such ailments, but in these days of global travel and high mobility the giving of antibiotics for some of these conditions is, the author feels, justifiable on medical and social grounds. However, a susceptibility to sexually transmitted infections indicates an underlying miasm which constitutional treatment may help to dispel.

Anxiety about intercourse
Can be due to lack of knowledge, fear of AIDS, herpes, and other SEXUALLY TRANSMITTED DISEASES, lack of physical affection in childhood, or parental strictures against exploring genitals or masturbating. Escaping into drugs or alcohol generally makes problem worse. Where anxiety is bound up with general insecurity or difficulty forming intimate relationships, constitutional homeopathic treatment is recommended; in the meantime, the remedies below may be helpful.

Specific remedies to be taken every 12 hours for up to 5 days

- Man who is torn between intense desire for sex and fear of sexual failure, general insecurity *Lycopodium 30c*
- Woman who is very emotional, cries and blushes easily, hates being in hot stuffy rooms *Pulsatilla 30c*
- Phobias and irrational thoughts, obsessive fear of 'catching something' *Argentum nit. 30c*
- Difficulties caused by grief or disappointment in a previous relationship *Ignatia 30c*

Ejaculation problems

Rarely due to any physical disorder, although SPINAL CORD INJURY, urethral stricture (see PENIS PROBLEMS), or surgical removal of prostate gland or testis may interfere with ejaculatory mechanism. Ejaculation can occur without orgasm, and if refractory period (time between one climax and the next) is short orgasm can occur without ejaculation; capacity for repeated ejaculation decreases rapidly after puberty – only 5 per cent of 40-year-olds are capable of ejaculating more than once during a love-making session. Ejaculation during dreams, 'wet dreams', is quite normal.

There is nothing abnormal about 'premature' ejaculation – climaxing before or as soon as penis enters vagina – but it does suggest anxiety, however caused, lack of concern for partner's satisfaction, and perhaps ignorance of female sexual response and of techniques for delaying orgasm. If it happens regularly, it can lead to profound sexual dissatisfaction for both partners; woman begins to feel used, cheated, angry – all of which may depress her desire for sex (see LACK OF DESIRE FOR SEX); man begins to feel self-conscious, dreads climaxing too soon, and may become so anxious about his sexual performance that even erection becomes difficult (see ERECTION PROBLEMS). Rapid orgasm and ejaculation is common at beginning of many relationships; as trust and affection increase and anxiety wears off, timing of orgasm is easier to control. In isolated cases urethritis (see PENIS PROBLEMS), prostatitis (see PROSTATE PROBLEMS), or a nervous disorder may make it difficult to delay orgasm and ejaculation, but if early ejaculation is causing problems and has no physical basis, try the self-help measures below; if you still feel you need expert help, ask your GP about sex therapy; it may be necessary for you *and* your partner to attend sessions since problem is seldom one-sided. Constitutional homeopathic treatment is strongly recommended; in the meantime, the remedies below are useful dissolvers of anxiety and tension.

Specific remedies to be taken every 12 hours for up to 5 days
- Feeling short-tempered and impatient, craving excitement, use of drugs such as cocaine *Nux 30c*
- Increased desire for sex accompanied by lack of self-confidence and expectation of failure *Lycopodium 30c*

Self-help Relax before you make love, and don't make love when you are tired or in a hurry. When orgasm is near, you or your partner should firmly squeeze penis just below glans; this will not affect erection, but will delay orgasm and ejaculation.

Erection problems

Physical causes include injury or surgery to spinal cord or genitals, chronic illnesses such as DIABETES, various nervous disorders, many groups of drugs (tranquillizers, diuretics, anti-depressants, barbiturates, drugs for high blood pressure and stomach ulcers, recreational drugs such as alcohol, marijuana, cocaine), fatigue, and sometimes lack of appropriate stimulation. But in 90 per cent of cases inability to have or sustain an erection is due to psychological factors; STRESS, a state of general mental and emotional turmoil induced by pressures of modern living, or ANXIETY ABOUT INTERCOURSE easily inhibit erectile response. Most men have erectile difficulties at some time in their lives, often with women they feel strongly about, but a single failure or even occasional failure does not spell 'impotence'. However, if fear of failure becomes a self-fulfilling prophecy, try the self-help measures and homeopathic remedies below; constitutional homeopathic treatment is strongly recommended where stress and anxiety are the culprits. If you go to see your GP, you may be offered testosterone or anti-anxiety drugs. Sex therapy is also an option.

Specific remedies to be taken every 12 hours for up to 5 days
- Surge of desire, anticipation of failure, penis cold and small *Lycopodium 30c*
- Erection not firm enough for penetration, general weakness, penis cold and small, especially if intercourse has been very frequent or if erectile difficulties have come on recently *Agnus 30c*
- Following bruising injury to penis *Arnica 30c*
- Following injury which has bruised spinal cord *Hypericum 30c*
- Erection does not last, great surge of sexual feelings after long abstinence, legs feel cold and cramped *Conium 30c*
- Erectile difficulties associated with dribbles of semen during sleep, increased desire for sex, erotic fantasies *Selenium 30c*
- Erection occurs when half asleep but disappears on waking up, even when sexually excited penis remains flaccid *Caladium 30c*

Self-help Try making love in different places and at different times, and try out different forms of foreplay; forget intercourse for a while and concentrate on giving and receiving pleasure with all your senses and with every part of your body except your genitals.

For explanation of other symbols, see page 107

Excessive desire for sex

Rarely has a physical cause but may be aggravated by certain drugs; not a problem unless compulsion to have intercourse (see OBSESSIONS AND COMPULSIONS) becomes a burden to person concerned or makes unreasonable demands on a partner. Constitutional homeopathic treatment may be necessary, but the remedies below should be tried first; if urge to have sex does not become more controllable within 3 weeks, see your GP.

Specific remedies for men, to be taken every 12 hours for up to 5 days
- Intense desire to have intercourse, ejaculation during erotic dreams *Phosphorus 30c*
- Local irritation of penis *Camphora 30c*
- Profuse ejaculation of semen, great exhaustion, absence of erotic dreams *Picric ac. 30c*
- Man very easily aroused, especially after alcohol or cocaine *Nux 30c*

Specific remedies for women, to be taken every 12 hours for up to 5 days
- Woman who has enormous sexual appetite, despises men, suffers from depression *Platinum 30c*
- Woman who behaves in a highly emotional way, makes obscene remarks, strips off and exposes genitals, suffers from paranoia *Hyoscyamus 30c*
- Woman who is always seeking excitement and has inflated sense of her own importance *Gratiola 30c*

Specific remedies for partners exhausted by sexual demands, to be taken every 4 hours for up to 3 days
- Apathy, lethargy, indifference *Phosphoric ac. 30c*
- Physical exhaustion, chilliness, over-sensitivity *China 30c*

Lack of desire for sex

Root cause is usually psychological – STRESS, DEPRESSION, fear of getting pregnant, performance anxiety (see ERECTION PROBLEMS, PREMATURE EJACULATION, LACK OF ORGASM), and frequently boredom – rather than hormonal or physical (see Special Problems in Women pp. 239–51 and Special Problems in Men pp. 251–5). Labels such as 'frigidity' and 'impotence' are old-fashioned and extremely unhelpful. There is no 'normal' level of desire for sex (libido) in men or women, although in both sexes it is the 'male' hormone testosterone which sustains it; testosterone levels can be depressed by poor liver or kidney function, PITUITARY PROBLEMS, fatigue, pain, illness, depression, and stress, and also by tranquillizers, opiates, drugs used to treat high blood pressure, appetite suppressants, and alcohol.

In men testosterone production, and therefore libido, slowly declines with age; this leads to less urgency for coitus, slower erection, and delayed orgasm, all of which can add to sexual enjoyment rather than detract from it. In both sexes the ability to be mentally aroused lasts longest. For some women libido goes right down before a period (see PREMENSTRUAL SYNDROME); temporary loss of interest in sex is perfectly natural after childbirth or gynaecological surgery; in some women oral contraceptives and hormone replacement therapy have a lowering effect on sex drive. In general, if sex is pleasurable before the MENOPAUSE it will continue to be pleasurable after it; indeed, for some women, cessation of fertility and relief from some of the pressures of home-making are a boost to libido. If sex drive falters after the menopause or after HYSTERECTOMY and this causes relationship problems, GP may prescribe testosterone.

Treatment of underlying conditions mentioned above is obvious first step to restoring libido. Where cause is mainly psychological, sex therapy can be very helpful. Homeopathic approach is constitutional, provided there are no physical problems, but the remedies below should be tried first.

Specific remedies for men, to be taken every 12 hours for up to 5 days
- Loss of sex drive or positive aversion to sex, premature ejaculation or no ejaculation, especially if herpes is diagnosed *Graphites 30c*
- Premature ejaculation or inability to have an erection *Lycopodium 30c*
- Irritability, self-criticism and extreme sensitivity to real or fancied criticism from others, despair, thoughts of death *Nitric ac. 30c*
- Formation of allergies *Apis 30c*
- Apathy and indifference *Phosphoric ac. 30c*

Specific remedies for women, to be taken every 12 hours for up to 5 days
- General weakness, especially after prolonged or frequent intercourse *Agnus 30c*
- Irritability, feeling chilly, exhausted and indifferent to sex, energy revives after brisk exercise *Sepia 30c*
- Loss of libido associated with grief or repressed emotions *Natrum mur. 30c*
- Loss of libido following periods, vagina feels raw and sore *Causticum 30c*
- Formation of allergies *Apis 30c*
- Lumps in breasts *Conium 30c*
- Weepiness and depression *Pulsatilla 30c*
- Apathy and indifference *Phosphoric ac. 30c*

Lack of orgasm

Orgasm during intercourse is a much more reliable response in men than in women; as anthropologists have pointed out, this may be related to the fact that until a few decades ago women were not supposed to enjoy sex to the extent of having orgasms; now that they are, not having orgasms can create the kind of performance anxiety which causes ERECTION PROBLEMS and EJACULATION PROBLEMS in men. Even if the right sensory information goes to the brain, orgasm can be blocked by ANXIETY, ANGER, guilt, mistrust, or determination not to lose control. In isolated cases, lack of orgasm is caused not by psychological blocks but by drugs or damage to vital nerve pathways.

For majority of women, clitoris is primary focus of sensations which lead to orgasm, with vagina and labia important but secondary; on most occasions clitoris is not sufficiently stimulated by thrusting movements of penis in vagina to trigger off orgasm; only 30 per cent of women are regularly orgasmic through vaginal stimulation alone.

If lack or infrequency of orgasm, your own or your partner's, worries you or is beginning to cause problems, try the self-help methods below; constitutional homeopathic treatment might also help, although the remedies listed below or under ERECTION PROBLEMS should be tried first. If situation does not improve, and GP has ruled out physical causes, you might consider sex therapy.

Specific remedies for women, to be taken every 12 hours for up to 5 days
- Inability to let go of emotions *Natrum mur. 30c*
- Fatigue and lack of energy *Agnus 30c*
- Difficulty follows grief or painful end to a love affair *Ignatia 30c*

Self-help Try to de-emphasize orgasm by making other phases of response cycle more pleasurable. Tell or show your partner where your most sensitive areas are and what you find most exciting, and allow yourself to fantasize – fantasies can take the brakes off!

Masturbation worries
May be justified if masturbation is causing problems within a marriage or within a valued relationship, or if self-stimulation is compulsive (see OBSESSIONS AND COMPULSIONS), associated with extremely sadistic fantasies, or a symptom of inability to socialize. Worries about masturbation sapping health, leading to homosexuality, retarding development of adult sexual relationships, or undermining ability to have orgasm during intercourse are unfounded. Studies have shown that people who continue to masturbate once they are in a sexual relationship are less likely to seek help for sexual problems than people who don't; for some couples, mutual or self-masturbation is part of intercourse or sex play. However, if urge to masturbate is causing anxiety, see your GP and ask about sex counselling or psychotherapy. Constitutional homeopathic treatment can help to defuse anxiety and tension; in the meantime the remedies below may be helpful.

Specific remedies to be taken every 12 hours for up to 5 days

- Sinking feeling in stomach, untidiness, being oblivious to what other people think of appearance or behaviour *Sulphur 30c*
- Irritability, resentment, bottled up emotions, masturbating to get your own back on the world *Staphisagria 30c*
- Obesity, feeling sweaty and chilly by turns, masturbating to release tension or relieve boredom *Calcarea 30c*
- Increasing isolation and withdrawal, feeling worn out after masturbation or intercourse, constipation *Natrum mur. 30c*
- Erections have nothing to do with desire for sex *Picric ac. 30c*
- Masturbation followed by great weakness *Phosphoric ac. 30c*
- Masturbation associated with increase in sexual appetite *Calcarea phos. 30c*

Painful intercourse (dyspareunia)
In women intercourse may be painful due to vaginal or vulval infections, which cause unusual discharge or itchiness (see VAGINAL AND VULVAL PROBLEMS), CYSTITIS (frequent urge to urinate), or VAGINISMUS (spasm of muscles at entrance to vagina); pain on deep penetration or in certain positions may be a symptom of endometriosis or retroversion of the uterus (see UTERUS PROBLEMS), or of cervical erosion (see CERVICAL PROBLEMS). Dryness of vagina can cause discomfort and soreness for both partners; vaginal secretions tend to become scantier after MENOPAUSE, but sometimes lack of lubrication is due to ANXIETY ABOUT INTERCOURSE, or too perfunctory foreplay; KY jelly usually helps. Resuming intercourse too soon after having a baby can be painful, as can intercourse for the first time ever.

In men a burning sensation when ejaculating or urinating, and perhaps unusual discharge from penis, suggests urethritis (see PENIS PROBLEMS) or prostatitis (see PROSTATE PROBLEMS); pain during intercourse may be balanitis (see PENIS PROBLEMS) or herpes (see SEXUALLY TRANSMITTED DISEASES), especially if head of penis is red, itchy, sore, or blistered. Soreness or itchiness around head of penis after intercourse suggests sensitivity to spermicidal creams or vaginal secretions; problem is easily solved by using a sheath; if rubber of sheath causes an allergic reaction, switch to a non-allergenic brand. Occasionally tip of penis may be irritated by friction against trailing threads of partner's IUD; this can be solved by asking GP to shorten threads. Erection and intercourse can also be painful if foreskin is too tight (see PHIMOSIS); if foreskin has recently been removed (see CIRCUMCISION), intercourse may be painful for several months until glans becomes less sensitive.

For orthodox and homeopathic treatment, see causative conditions mentioned above. If none of the homeopathic remedies given seems to meet the case,

For explanation of other symbols, see page 107

try one of the remedies below; if there is no improvement within 3 weeks, see your GP or homeopath.

Specific remedies to be taken every 4 hours for up to 2 weeks

- Vulva and vagina feel very sensitive, pain in ovary during intercourse, 'honeymoon' cystitis *Staphisagria 6c*
- Vagina very sensitive, severe pain in left ovary after intercourse, vulval warts *Thuja 6c*
- Vulva and vagina feel itchy and twitchy, burning sensation in uterus and ovaries after intercourse, increased desire for sex *Platinum 6c*
- Dry vagina, constipation, emotional upset *Natrum mur. 6c*
- Heavy, dragging sensation in lower abdomen, intercourse causes pains which shoot up through vagina and uterus to navel *Sepia 6c*

Sexually transmitted diseases (STDs)

Diseases whose main means of transfer is through sexual intercourse. Fear of AIDS and herpes (see below) is changing attitudes to casual sex. It pays to be choosy about who you have sex with, especially if you or your partner have other partners. Be fastidious about genital hygiene, don't ignore unusual discharges, itches, bumps, or sores in the genital area, and if you think you have an infection, DON'T PASS IT ON; tell your sexual contacts so that they can tell theirs, go and see your GP or your local STD clinic, and refrain from intercourse until you are symptom-free.

If you trust a person enough to want to go to bed with them, have the courage to ask, perhaps with a half smile, 'Do you have anything I could catch?' If you cannot bring yourself to do this, at least check that your intended partner has no obvious signs of infection; the best place to do this, and the most fun, is in the bath or shower. Risk of infection can also be reduced by using a condom, whether this is necessary from the contraceptive point of view or not.

AIDS (acquired immune deficiency syndrome)
Human immunodeficiency virus, HIV for short, is responsible for a spectrum of conditions of which AIDS is only a part. These are: HIV positive (virus present in blood but no noticeable symptoms); PGL or persistent generalized lymphadenopathy (lymph glands remains swollen and sometimes painful for at least 3 months following HIV infection); ARC or AIDS-related complex (a range of relatively mild signs and symptoms including seborrhoeic dermatitis, malaise, fever, night sweats, profound fatigue, recrudescent acne, cold sores around mouth, shingles, weight loss, diarrhoea); and full-blown AIDS (symptoms include FEVER, malaise, HEADACHE, BREATHLESSNESS, dry COUGH, ORAL THRUSH, abdominal tenderness, DIARRHOEA, swollen lymph glands, a subcutaneous form of CANCER called Kaposi's sarcoma, rapid WEIGHT LOSS, cerebral abscess, FITS, ENCEPHALITIS, MENINGITIS, PNEUMONIA (including *Pneumocystis carinii*) DEPRESSION, PSYCHOTIC ILLNESS, dementia, personality changes).

It is thought that HIV causes changes in the gastro-intestinal tract, leading to malabsortion of one or several nutrients essential for immune function and absorption of microbes and microbe products not normally admitted into the bloodstream. Recently it has emerged that AIDS may be related to syphilis (see below); AIDS symptoms are similar to those of advanced syphilis and blood tests in AIDS patients are often positive for syphilis.

HIV is transmitted from person to person through blood and blood products, and through any bodily secretion. Groups most at risk are homosexual men and drug users who share needles; it is through drug use and bisexual behaviour, and through heterosexual relationships with people from countries where AIDS is endemic, that AIDS is slowly spreading into the heterosexual population. Where blood has not been properly screened and heat-treated, people receiving transfusions, organ transplants, or Factor VIII injections for haemophilia are at risk; babies can be infected during pregnancy, at birth, or through breast milk if mother is HIV positive.

About 30 per cent of people diagnosed as HIV positive develop AIDS within 7 years; the percentage of HIV positives who develop ARC within the same timescale is about the same; other people with the virus develop PGL or remain symptom-free. *Everyone* who has the virus can transmit it to others through activities which involve exchanging blood or body fluids; for most people, this means sexual activity, with some forms of sex being safer than others (see self-help measures below).

If you think you have been exposed to HIV or if you develop any of the symptoms mentioned above, see your GP and ask for a blood test. If test is positive, most constructive approach is holistic; accept treatment (usually antibiotics) offered by GP, adopt immunity-boosting habits outlined in PART 2, implement the self-help measures described below, and seek constitutional treatment from an EXPERIENCED HOMEOPATH.

Self-help Always use a condom during vaginal or anal sex. If possible, avoid surgery, blood products, and injections in developing countries or countries where AIDS is endemic. Never share razors, toothbrushes, or other articles which may have blood on them, burn sanitary towels or if this is not possible put them in a double bag, flush tampons down the lavatory, always cover wounds, and after accidents carefully wipe all blood off skin and furniture, then clean furniture with diluted bleach (1 part bleach to 10 parts water) using a disposable cloth, and carefully dispose of all swabs and dressings.

---

999 Emergency – call GP (or dial 999) immediately. ② Consult your doctor if no improvement within 2 hours

If a child is HIV positive, warn him or her against blood-mixing rituals, ear-piercing, tattooing, and giving blood in science classes. He or she should also be trained to take the precautions outlined above. The sharing of toys, and of pens and pencils which have been chewed or sucked, should be kept to a minimum.

Various organizations offer information and support to AIDS sufferers and to those diagnosed as HIV positive (addresses p. 385).

Gonorrhea ('clap') Bacterial infection spread by oral, vaginal, or anal intercourse with person who is incubating infection or already has symptoms; condition is related to promiscuity and affects twice as many men as women; incubation period is 3–5 days, followed by discomfort when urinating and increasingly thick and copious discharge of pus from tip of penis; occasionally, however, the man may have no symptoms; in women, there may be no obvious symptoms, or unusual discharge from vagina. If rectum is infected, there may be a feeling of wetness inside rectum or pus in faeces; after oral intercourse, throat may feel sore. Unchecked, infection can spread, causing rashes and joint problems, PELVIC INFECTION, or stricture of the urethra (see PENIS PROBLEMS).

If gonorrhea is suspected, see your GP or visit your local STD clinic immediately; if diagnosis is positive, take penicillin or other antibiotics offered, refrain from intercourse until you are symptom-free, then seek constitutional homeopathic treatment in order to boost resistance to further infection. There are specific remedies for treating gonorrhea, but these should only be taken under guidance of an EXPERIENCED HOMEOPATH.

Herpes (herpes genitalis) Caused by same type of virus which causes COLD SORES around mouth; transmitted by oral-genital or genital-genital contact with someone who is incubating virus or who already has symptoms; virus incubates for about 10 days, then causes itchiness and crop of small blisters on penis or vulva; these quickly become moist and ulcerated, glands in groin become swollen and tender, and slight FEVER develops; symptoms usually clear up within 2 weeks, but for 50 per cent of sufferers virus goes to ground in bundle of nerve cells at base of spine and causes further attacks, milder and less and less frequent, whenever health is below par. Herpes can be fatal to babies, so if infection is active at time of birth, baby will have to be delivered by caesarian section.

If herpes is suspected, see your GP or visit your local STD clinic – an anti-viral ointment will probably be prescribed – and refrain from intercourse until ulcers heal. Alternatively, you can treat yourself, using the self-help measures and homeopathic remedies below. Constitutional homeopathic treatment may help to prevent recurrence.

Specific remedies to be taken 4 times daily for up to 14 days
- Bad ulcers which bleed, especially at night, whole genital area very tender and painful *Sempervivum 6c*
- Skin of genitals very dry, lesions hot and puffy, with pearl-like blisters *Natrum mur. 6c*
- Genitals burn and itch, discomfort aggravated by cold or damp, general restlessness *Rhus tox. 6c*
- Genitals burn and sting, skin cracked, with red, itchy rash *Capsicum 6c*

Self-help Avoid intercourse during an attack or if you feel tingling or tenderness which heralds an attack. Always wash your hands with soap and water after touching ulcers, and expose ulcers to air as much as possible. Ulcers can be bathed in Hypericum and Calendula solution (5 drops of mother tincture of each to 0.25 litre [½ pint] boiled cooled water) 4 times a day, or Calendula ointment can be applied. Frequent warm baths with salt added to the water are soothing and speed healing.

Non-specific urethritis (NSU) Infection and inflammation of urethra due, in 45 per cent of cases, to organisms called *Chlamydia*, which are half way between a virus and a bacteria; in other cases cause of infection cannot be pinpointed. Three-quarters of sufferers are men. Infection is usually, though not invariably, spread through sexual contact and may take 1–5 weeks to incubate. In men, first sign is tingling sensation at tip of penis, especially after urinating first thing in morning; this is followed by clear discharge from penis, scanty at first, then thicker and heavier. In women, there may be no symptoms at all, or slightly increased discharge from vagina.

If infection is suspected, see your GP or visit your local STD clinic at once; take antibiotics prescribed, and do not have intercourse until course of antibiotics is finished and you are symptom free; your partner should take antibiotics too, even if he or she has no symptoms. Constitutional homeopathic treatment is recommended after antibiotics.

Pubic lice ('crabs') Crab-shaped species of louse about 2 mm (1/10 inch) long which lives in pubic hair and in hairs around anus, sucking blood and causing itching, especially at night. Adults move from one body to another during sexual contact, but symptoms of infestation may take several weeks to appear because eggs (nits) laid by adults take a week or two to hatch. If pubic lice are suspected, see your GP or visit your local STD clinic; a special cream or ointment will be prescribed to kill the lice, and you may be advised to shave pubic hair to get rid of nits, which cannot be removed by normal washing.

Reiter's syndrome A combination of CONJUNCTIVITIS, joint pains (see OSTEOARTHRITIS, RHEUMATOID ARTHRITIS), and acute urethritis (see CYSTITIS) or DIARRHOEA; probably due to an infection-triggered change in immune system; may be acute or chronic, and in majority of cases is sexually transmitted. Orthodox treatment consists of antibiotics in acute stage, and non-specific anti-inflammatory drugs. If the homeopathic remedy given below does not produce some improvement within 2 weeks, constitutional treatment should be sought. For self-help measures, see conditions mentioned above.

Specific remedy to be taken every 4 hours for up to 2 weeks
- *Sulphur 6c*

Syphilis Bacterial infection transmitted during oral, anal, or vaginal intercourse. Though once a killer, disease is now very rare and is almost always cured before it reaches serious stage; two-thirds of sufferers are men, usually homosexual; blood tests in AIDS patients are also positive for syphilis. Incubation period is 9–90 days; first stage, highly infectious, is a painless sore or chancre on penis, anus, or vulva which disappears in a few weeks; second stage, also highly infectious and lasting for only a few weeks, is a non-itchy rash all over body, including palms of hands and soles of feet, accompanied by swollen lymph glands and moist warts around anus or under arms. Disease then becomes latent, but may re-emerge years later to attack heart valves and walls of arteries supplying brain and vital organs.

Any sores on penis, vulva, or around anus should be promptly investigated by GP or local STD clinic; it is essential that antibiotics are taken, and that all sexual contacts are traced and treated; intercourse should be refrained from until course of antibiotics is finished and symptoms have disappeared. Afterwards, constitutional homeopathic treatment is recommended.

Thrush see SPECIAL PROBLEMS IN WOMEN, SPECIAL PROBLEMS IN MEN

Trichomoniasis see SPECIAL PROBLEMS IN WOMEN, SPECIAL PROBLEMS IN MEN

Vaginismus
Unusual condition in which muscles around entrance to vagina go into spasm, making intercourse, vaginal examination, or use of tampons painful or impossible; spasm may be accompanied by arching of back and drawing together of thighs. If problem has a physical basis, your GP will probably refer you to a gynaecologist; if psychological, sex therapy may be the answer. Constitutional homeopathic treatment may also be beneficial, but the remedies below should be tried first.

Specific remedies to be taken every 12 hours for up to 5 days
- Extreme sensitivity of vulva and vagina, constipation *Plumbum 30c*
- Extreme sensitivity of vulva and vagina, made worse by sitting, irritable bladder *Staphisagria 30c*
- Where spasms are a hysterical reaction to grief or a broken love affair *Ignatia 30c*
- Vagina feels burning hot and as heavy as lead, sensation made more unpleasant by slightest jarring *Belladonna 30c*
- Extreme sensitivity of vulva accompanied by pleasurable itching, general restlessness and insomnia, attention-seeking behaviour *Coffea 30c*
- Painful periods, copious early flow of dark blood which ceases on lying down, heart condition *Cactus 30c*

INFECTIONS, INFESTATIONS, AND IMMUNE SYSTEM

INFECTIONS are an almost daily occurrence, but if we are healthy our immune system deals with them before we notice any symptoms. Most microorganisms enter the body through the nose and mouth – in the air, in our food, sometimes on dirty fingers. Some enter through cuts and abrasions. Others invade the urinary or reproductive tract through the urethra or vagina.

Many of the microorganisms with which we share this planet are harmless. Some permanently inhabit the inside and outside of the human body; a few even produce substances useful to it and prevent harmful bacteria from finding a foot-hold. This is true of certain bacteria in the large intestine and vagina. Some

bacteria are harmless in one part of the body but damaging in others; this is true of *E. coli*, benign while it is in the colon or rectum but harmful if it is transferred to the urethra, vagina, or mouth.

Each kind of microorganism, whether it is a bacterium, virus, fungus, or blood parasite, carries special chemical markers known as antigens. Some strains of lymphocyte (the kind of white blood cell produced in the lymph nodes, spleen, bone marrow, adenoids, tonsils, and the wall of the gut) recognize antigens and stimulate other lymphocytes to produce proteins called antibodies, which then disable the carrier organism; other lymphocytes directly attack and destroy the invading organism. For about six months after birth babies are protected by their mothers' antibodies; after that, the immune system is sufficiently mature to start manufacturing its own.

Artificial immunity can be given by injecting large numbers of antibodies or small quantities of antigen to provoke the production of antibodies; this is orthodox immunization. Homeopathic immunization does not involve introducing live or dead viruses or antibodies into the body; instead remedies are prepared from disease tissue or secretions using the traditional dilution and succussion method. Like other homeopathic remedies, they contain, in highly potent form, the essence of the source material used, in this case the essence of the disease organism and its toxins. The body reacts to such remedies, known as nosodes, by sharpening up its immune response. If you are worried about the side effects of orthodox immunization or are likely to come into contact with potentially serious infections, consult your homeopath.

The production of antibodies in response to antigens, the so-called immune response, is not the body's only line of defence. The body's first-line trouble-shooters are neutrophils and macrophages, two kinds of white blood cell which constantly patrol the bloodstream and tissue fluids and respond immediately to the chemical and thermal signals sent out by tissues when they become inflamed. If inflammation is suppressed, white cell activity is impaired. Neutrophils and macrophages gobble up and digest offending microbes, foreign particles, and other noxious elements. The resulting pus is a mixture of necrotic tissue, dead bacteria, and dying white blood cells.

Infections can be treated by killing the germs which cause them or by helping the immune system to deal with them, or both, depending on general health and the virulence of the infection. Antibiotics can deal with bacteria, but not viruses; after a course of antibiotics live yoghurt, eaten daily for at least 5 days, helps to repopulate the gut with beneficial bacteria. Homeopathic remedies, improved nutrition, fresh air, exercise, and rest can restore the coping ability of the immune system. In some cases homeopathic remedies and antibiotics may be necessary. Constitutional homeopathic treatment is always advisable after serious infections.

Occasionally, as the result of ageing or exposure to certain viruses, bacteria, chemicals, and environmental factors, the body loses some of its ability to discriminate between self and non-self or fails to recognize and destroy its own abnormal cells. The first kind of impairment leads to autoimmune diseases such as rheumatoid arthritis and systemic lupus erythematosus; the second leads to cancer.

Allergies – distressing reactions to certain drugs, chemicals, foods, and other substances which seem to be tolerated by the majority of people – are the down side of having an immune system.

Allergy

An allergy is conventionally thought of as an excessive reaction between an antigen (allergen) and an antibody. Some people, through their genetic inheritance, produce large numbers of the kind of antibodies which cause the release of large quantities of histamine when they bind to certain antigens (allergens); histamine causes large quantities of fluid to leak out of blood vessels and tissues, resulting in the distressing symptoms of allergy – local swelling, redness, and itching. Into this category of allergic reaction come HAY FEVER AND ALLERGIC RHINITIS, COELIAC DISEASE, certain forms of ASTHMA and CONJUNCTIVITIS, ECZEMA, and URTICARIA. In a few people the histamine reaction occurs throughout the body (anaphylaxis) and can cause death from SHOCK or suffocation.

At the other extreme allergies are known to cause headaches and feelings of fullness in the head (see HEADACHE), excessive drowsiness after eating (see ABNORMAL SLEEPINESS OR DROWSINESS), insomnia (see SLEEP PROBLEMS), ringing in the ears (see TINNITUS), recurrent SINUSITIS and ear infections (see LABYRINTHITIS, MIDDLE EAR INFECTION), SORE THROAT, NAUSEA AND VOMITING, DIARRHOEA, CONSTIPATION, flatulence, ABDOMINAL PAIN, chronic fatigue, aching joints and muscles, binge eating (see BULIMIA), ANXIETY attacks, DEPRESSION, tearfulness, unusually aggressive behaviour, apathy, CONFUSION, HYPERACTIVITY, inability to concentrate. . . In such cases mechanisms other than the classic antigen-antibody response are almost certainly involved.

Among the many substances known to cause allergic reactions are dust, house dust mites, fur and feathers, tree and grass pollens, various plants, wool and other fabrics, nickel and other metals, gases and vapours given off by gas appliances, household cleaners, paints, solvents, and plastics, pesticide residues, non-stick coatings, various drugs, including penicillin, and of course many foods and food additives.

Desensitization treatment – carefully controlled exposure to progressively stronger doses of the allergen concerned – only works if one or two substances are involved, and should only be tried if other measures fail. In the author's experience, all forms of desensitization carry a risk. In some people desensitization 'works' for a while, then the allergy returns more violently than before and is more difficult to treat. Suppressing allergy symptoms with antihistamines, steroids, and decongestants is not recommended, unless symptoms are making life unbearable; the specific homeopathic remedies given under the conditions mentioned above should be tried first.

Broadly speaking, there are two kinds of allergy,

fixed allergies and cyclic allergies. A *fixed allergy* is one which declares itself before the age of 2. One school of thought attributes this kind of allergy to a 'leaky bowel': the walls of the bowel are such that certain proteins easily pass into the bloodstream, where they are identified as 'foreign' and trigger off antibody production. The bowel may be leaky from birth, or leakiness may develop as a result of inflammation or *Candida* infestation (see CANDIDIASIS). The permanent presence in the blood of large numbers of antibodies which would not normally be there seems to encourage allergic reactions. Most fixed allergies involve single substances.

If you suspect a food, a sensible first step would be to restrict consumption and take one of the remedies listed in the General Remedy Finder (pp. 68–71) under Food and Drink – ten remedies are listed under 'milk makes symptoms worse', for example. If this produces good results, you could then confirm your suspicions by trying the elimination and challenge test (see below). If the results are equivocal and allergic symptoms persist, you should seek constitutional treatment; if appropriate, your homeopath may recommend bowel cleansing and *Acidophilus* capsules to reduce the permeability of the bowel. If these measures do not work, desensitization may be necessary.

Cyclic allergies tend to occur in older people, and only declare themselves after repeated exposure to certain substances – usually several substances are involved. Exposure may not always cause a reaction because, up to a point, the body develops tolerance; this is known as 'allergy masking'. In the author's experience, cyclic allergies are often a symptom of much deeper imbalances. In some people, identifying and eliminating one substance or group of substances uncovers a sensitivity to others; it is as if removing one allergy obliges the body to find another way, and sometimes a more unpleasant way, of expressing its imbalances. That is why initial treatment should be constitutional. If this fails, avoidance of specific substances is the logical next step, provided nutrition is not compromised by cutting out too many foods; if this is likely, vitamin and mineral supplements may have to be taken under supervision, and safe foods eaten in strict rotation to prevent new allergies developing. Desensitization, orthodox and homeopathic, is a last resort.

Food allergies may be fixed or cyclic, and can declare themselves in many ways – as rashes, stomach upsets, mood swings, hyperactivity, aggression, general tiredness, apathy, and malaise, and as cravings. If you suspect you have a food allergy the first items to be suspicious of are: foods which upset you; foods which you crave or find difficult to resist; foods you would miss if you were asked to give them up; foods which make you feel better after having eaten them. In this context 'foods' include beverages.

Testing for allergies Orthodox and complementary medicine offer a number of tests, and there are simple tests which you can do yourself (see self-help measures below). Skin tests, also known as patch tests, are a good way of assessing sensitivity to inhaled or contact allergens but not to food substances; a single drop of allergen extract is placed on the skin and the skin is then gently scratched with a needle; if an angry wheel develops, there is an allergy. Radio absorption testing (RAST) detects antigen-antibody reactions in a blood sample by means of radioactive isotopes. Cytotoxic testing, which is expensive but accurate in 70–80 per cent of cases, involves taking a small sample of blood and examining the activity of white blood cells when exposed to suspect substances. Sublingual testing involves placing a small amount of the suspected allergen under the tongue to see if it causes a reaction; the allergen is then diluted to see at what dilution the allergic response disappears. Applied Kinesiology and Touch for Health practitioners detect allergies by placing suspect substances on the tongue and then testing the strength of various muscles, sometimes with very clear-cut results, sometimes not; weakness is taken as an indication of allergy. Dowsing with a pendulum can sometimes produce good results, and sometimes yield nothing; much depends on the dowser's ability to keep his or her mind clear.

Self-help There are a number of simple tests you can do yourself. If you suspect you have a food allergy, test the foods mentioned above, eliminating them one at a time. NEVER ELIMINATE MORE THAN ONE FOOD AT A TIME. This is called 'elimination and challenge' testing. Eliminate each food for at least 4 days, then reintroduce it within 12 days. If you feel better after not eating it and worse when you reintroduce it, you are probably allergic to it. Once you have established which foods are safe, take care to eat them on a rotational basis; if you eat them too frequently, you may develop intolerance to them again.

You might also try the pulse test. This involves taking your pulse before you eat a particular food and again afterwards to see if your pulse rate rises rapidly or not. If it does, you are probably allergic to that food. To take your pulse, place your fingers lightly on the thumb side of the inside of your wrist for 30 seconds, and count the number of beats. This test only works if you are calm and breathing quietly to start with, and if your pulse rate is not too variable. If your pulse rate is more or less the same on five successive occasions when you have been sitting calmly for 15 minutes or so, the test may well work for you.

If you suspect that paints, plastics, or household chemicals may be the culprit, try the 'sniff test'. Go for an hour's walk in the fresh air, and when you get home quickly go round the house sniffing anything which gives out a strong smell. The smell which affects you most may well be the one you are allergic to.

---

⑨⑨⑨ Emergency – call GP (or dial 999) immediately. ② Consult your doctor if no improvement within 2 hours

Amoebic dysentery see DYSENTERY

Anthrax

A bacterial infection spread by contaminated animal products, extremely rare today, but at one time a hazard among dock workers; anthrax of lungs or intestines used to be fatal, anthrax of the skin less so. Antibiotics are essential.

Specific remedies
- Once infection is diagnosed *Echinacea* mother tincture, 1 to 10 drops every 2 hours
- To prevent infection if exposure is likely *Anthracinum 30c* every 12 hours for up to 3 doses

Autoimmune disease

This occurs when, for a variety of reasons, body identifies certain of its own cells as non-self and attacks them as if they were hostile invaders. Most common of all autoimmune diseases is RHEUMATOID ARTHRITIS; other examples are SYSTEMIC LUPUS ERYTHEMATOSUS, MYASTHAEMIA GRAVIS, ANKYLOSING SPONDYLITIS, POLYARTERITIS NODOSA, TEMPORAL ARTERITIS, and haemolytic and pernicious ANAEMIA. Change in immune response can be triggered off by almost any virus, by certain bacteria (*Streptococcus*, for example), by certain drugs (methyldopa, for example, used to treat raised blood pressure), or by the presence in the bloodstream of cells which are not normally in circulation. Although what goes wrong with 'self' and 'non-self' recognition mechanism is not entirely understood, it seems that the body actually produces a small number of self-hostile lymphocytes which, under normal circumstances, are continually policed and destroyed by other lymphocytes; the 'triggers' mentioned above may subvert this process, allowing self-hostile lymphocyte numbers to increase. Some autoimmune diseases correct themselves after a number of years. Orthodox treatment is usually palliative; homeopathy also treats the symptoms, but most homeopaths try to promote health at a more fundamental level, giving advice on diet and nutrition, prescribing vitamin and mineral supplements, recommending various measures to eliminate body toxins, and identifying and eliminating allergens (see ALLERGY).

Blood poisoning (septicaemia)

Occurs in people whose resistance to infection is already low or being overtaxed; harmful bacteria enter bloodstream – from an ABSCESS or other infection site, or through a wound – and begin to multiply unopposed, producing powerful toxins; FEVER sets in, accompanied by NAUSEA, faintness, and an accelerated pulse rate, and skin becomes pale, cold, and clammy. If toxins continue to build up, person may go into septic SHOCK (earlier symptoms give way to drowsiness, confusion, unconsciousness).

If early symptoms of blood poisoning are present, ②

and select a remedy from the list below. If person goes into shock, ⑨⑨⑨, give First Aid (see p. 103) and *Aconite 30c* every 5 minutes.

Specific remedies to be given every 15 minutes for up to 10 doses
- Blood poisoning after wounds or surgery *Arnica 30c*
- Where a wound has turned septic *Lachesis 6c*
- High fever, slow pulse rate *Pyrogenium 6c*
- Sensation of being separated from body *Baptisia 6c*
- Dull headache, backache, chills, weakness, depression *Ignatia 6c*
- Blood poisoning from a boil or abscess *Gunpowder 6c*

Bornholm's disease

A viral infection which causes bouts of violent, stabbing CHEST PAIN, with FEVER, HEADACHE, COUGH, and loss of appetite; lasts 3–4 days, but full recovery may take 2 weeks. Orthodox treatment is to give painkillers. Plenty of fluids should be drunk. If remedies below seem inappropriate, select one from COUGH.

Specific remedies to be taken every 2 hours for up to 10 doses
- Chest pain made worse by coughing or slightest movement *Bryonia 30*
- Symptoms worse in sultry, thundery weather *Rhododendron 6c*

Brucellosis

A viral infection caught from infected milk, and also from infected animals; symptoms are similar to those of INFLUENZA and last about 2 weeks, though more severe illness may develop and last for several months. If condition is suspected, ⑫. In Britain pasteurized cow's milk is brucellosis-free; if you are unsure whether goat's milk, sheep's milk, etc. has been pasteurized, boil it for 2 minutes before using. Constitutional homeopathic treatment is recommended in addition to antibiotics or steroids.

Cancer

Every day, as part of the continuous growth and repair process which takes place in the human body, some 500 billion new cells are formed. Occasionally defective cells are produced, some of which may escape the policing activities of the immune system and begin to multiply extremely fast. Rapid, uncontrolled growth is a characteristic of cancer cells. A rapidly dividing colony of cancer cells becomes a tumour, invading normal tissue; if cancer cells spread to other parts of the body via the blood or lymph, secondary tumours may develop; this spreading process is known as metastasis.

What causes the formation of defective cells in the first place? Chromosome damage is one possible explanation; inherited or acquired defects in the immune system are another; ageing may also be a factor, because as we age our immune system becomes less efficient and chromosome copying mistakes occur. Cell function can be altered by radiation (including strong sunlight), by viruses, by tobacco smoke, asbestos fibres, and other airborne irritants, by waterlogging due to retention of sodium in cells, by toxic wastes which accumulate as the result of constipation. . .

Overall, cancer affects more men than women, and older people rather than youngsters, but there are exceptions; brain tumours and certain forms of leukaemia, for example, are no respecters of youth. Incidence can also be influenced by nutritional habits, climate, and cultural practices.

Although cancer is not a modern disease, its incidence is increasing. This is partly due to external factors such as smoking and pollution, but also to increased life expectancy. We are not dying young from infectious diseases, as we used to, but living to a ripe old age and succumbing to degenerative diseases instead.

The role of the psyche in all this is difficult to assess. For years psychologists have been pointing out that there is a 'cancer personality', rooted in unresolved conflict between mother and child; typically the child deals with his or her frustration by becoming too adult too soon, by repudiating affection and denying his or her own needs. Sooner or later these unsatisfied needs reassert themselves, usually as the result of the loss of a loved object or person. Though cancer is not the only expression of buried needs, diagnoses of cancer in people who have lost a close relative or friend within the previous 18 months are well above chance. It should also be said that the age-cancer link may have something to do with the generally low esteem in which old people are held in our society.

That said, most experts agree that there is no single cause for cancer. At least two factors – heredity and diet, for example, or pollution and personality – need to come together in the same individual for cancer to develop.

Early warnings The symptoms listed below are not infallible signs of cancer; nine times out of ten they have a quite different cause. But whereas most infections run a natural course and then clear up, cancer does not; it causes persistent change for the worse. If you have any of the following symptoms, ask your GP to investigate.

1. A persistent lump or thickening anywhere on the skin
2. Unexplained swelling in a limb
3. A mole or wart which starts to bleed, get bigger, or change colour
4. Sores or 'bites' which do not heal
5. Unusual bleeding from mouth, anus, genitals, or nipples, bleeding between periods, or altered bleeding during periods

6. Persistent indigestion or a change in bowel habits unrelated to alterations in diet
7. Unexplained weight loss of more than 0.5 kg (1 lb) per week
8. Hoarseness lasting for more than one month
9. Increasing difficulty swallowing or passing urine

Treatment No single branch of medicine offers a certain cure for every type of cancer. All forms of therapy should be considered – listen to everyone, take what appeals to you, and avoid fanatics. Depending on the kind of cancer you have and the stage it has reached, you may need several forms of treatment. For example, it might be sensible to buy time with orthodox treatment while you rebuild your immune system with homeopathy.

The homeopathic view of cancer is that it represents a profound breakdown in health at all levels. Home prescribing is not really appropriate in such circumstances. Instead you should seek the help of an EXPERIENCED HOMEOPATH, who will probably prescribe specific remedies as well as constitutional treatment. In some cases, injections of potentized mistletoe (Iscador) may be given. Some homeopaths also use Bach Flower Remedies as part of cancer treatment. Vitamins and minerals may also have a role to play.

A deficiency of Vitamin C has been found in conjunction with certain tumours; high levels of Vitamin A have some protective effect against cancer in smokers – high doses of Vitamin A are used in therapy but can give rise to toxic side effects; Vitamin E and selenium, both anti-oxidants, are also believed to have protective effects, although in high doses they can weaken the immune system; Vitamin B complex, potassium, iron, zinc, magnesium, copper, manganese, and calcium may also be relevant in some cases; digestive enzymes may be given to try to halt the activities of 'trophoblastic' cancer cells; treatment with Vitamin B_{17}, also known as laterile, is the subject of great controversy, its detractors claiming that it is worthless and dangerous because B_{17} contains cyanide, its supporters that it is safe provided no more than 1 gm is given orally per day and that it helps to relieve pain – in theory only cancer cells are susceptible to the cyanide because normal cells contain protective enzymes.

There are various dietary therapies for cancer, most based on strict vegan or lacto-vegetarian regimes. However, drastic changes in diet are not appropriate except in the early stages of cancer; in the later stages you may be too run down. The Gerson diet – strictly vegan initially, with juices and coffee enemas to detoxify the liver – has shown good result with cancers such as malignant melanoma, which are difficult to treat; it is not suitable if you have already had chemotherapy (see below).

Orthodox medicine offers surgery, radiotherapy, chemotherapy, and hormone treatment as appropriate.

Unfortunately orthodox sucesses with childhood leukaemia have not been repeated with the more common forms of cancer. Surgery removes malignant tissue and also an area of healthy tissue around it; radiotherapy uses radioactive radium or cobalt to destroy cancer cells *in situ* – cancer cells are more easily destroyed by radiation than normal cells; chemotherapy involves treatment with strong drugs, often called cytotoxic drugs because they interfere with cell reproduction and metabolism – again, normal cells are less interfered with than cancer cells.

Psychological treatment is now regarded as a valuable adjunct to orthodox and alternative treatment. Cancer sufferers are taught to relax and create a vivid mental picture of their cancer being dissolved by the combined energies of their own immune system and whatever treatment they are receiving; this technique is called 'positive visualization'.

To find out more about treatment options, contact Cancer Contact, Cancer Help Centre, (addresses p. 382).

Candidiasis see also ORAL THRUSH, VAGINAL AND VULVAL PROBLEMS, PENIS PROBLEMS

Low-grade infection caused by *Candida albicans*, a weakly infective fungus which lives in warm, moist conditions; broad-spectrum antibiotics, steroids, immuno-suppressive drugs, oral contraceptives, pregnancy, and eating over-refined carbohydrates or foods containing yeasts or moulds all adversely affect competing populations of healthy bacteria in the body, allowing *Candida* to thrive. Illness and nutritional deficiencies (iron and zinc in particular) can have a similar effect.

Many ailments besides ORAL THRUSH and genital thrush (see VAGINAL AND VULVAL PROBLEMS, PENIS PROBLEMS) are thought to be related to high concentrations of *Candida*; these include general fatigue and lethargy, HEADACHE, MIGRAINE, joint pains, urethral syndrome (see CYSTITIS), vaginitis (see VAGINAL AND VULVAL PROBLEMS), PELVIC INFECTION, PRURITIS ANI, skin problems such as URTICARIA and ATHLETE'S FOOT, MOUTH ULCERS, INDIGESTION, DIARRHOEA, CONSTIPATION, DISTENDED ABDOMEN, ALLERGY to various foods and chemicals, a craving for alcohol and sweets, LACK OF DESIRE FOR SEX, DEPRESSION, irritability, and lapses of memory and concentration. Anti-fungal drugs are unlikely to form part of orthodox treatment of the conditions mentioned above, partly because there are more obvious drugs of first resort and because there is as yet no widely available test specifically for *Candida*. However, many practitioners of complementary medicine, including homeopaths, recognise a '*Candida* syndrome' and recommend the self-care measures given below; these help many people, but not everyone. Constitutional homeopathic treatment is recommended.

Self-help First of all, stop taking any drugs (see above) which might be encouraging *Candida* to flourish; if necessary, discuss alternatives with your GP. Cut down consumption of refined carbohydrates, provided you are not underweight. Also reduce consumption of foods containing yeasts and moulds (see pp. 351–2). To keep gut bacteria healthy, drink Acidophilus milk occasionally, or take Acidophilus tablets. Eat more foods rich in biotin and be liberal with the garlic and fresh leafy vegetables. Take extra Vitamin A, B, C, zinc, iron, and magnesium.

Cholera

Bacterial infection of the gut, spread by polluted water or raw fruit and vegetables, causing ABDOMINAL PAIN, almost continuous DIARRHOEA, vomiting, and great thirst; there is no fever. Orthodox treatment consists of antibiotics and, if necessary, an intravenous drip to replace lost fluids; recovery takes about 2 weeks. See GASTROENTERITIS for appropriate homeopathic remedies.

Immunization Vaccination against cholera is only compulsory for visitors to a few countries in Africa and tropical Asia; injection must be given at least 6 days before travelling, and is only 50 per cent effective for 6 months. Homeopathic immunization (see p. 17) is also available.

Self-help Drink plenty of boiled water with salt and sugar in it (1 teaspoon salt and 1 teaspoon sugar to 1 litre [2 pints] water).

Dysentery

Spread by faecal-oral route, and rare in developed countries, but whether caused by *Shigella* bacillus or by amoebae, symptoms are the same: DIARRHOEA, with BLOOD IN FAECES, and ABDOMINAL PAIN. *Bacillary dysentery* may require antibiotics, *amoebic dysentery* a combination of drugs, which commonly cause vomiting. See GASTROENTERITIS for specific homeopathic remedies.

Fever see also FEVER pp. 305–6, 321

Running a temperature above normal range of 36–37°C (96.8-98.6°F) is usually a sign that the body is fighting some kind of infection. Particularly serious are PNEUMONIA (temperature above 40°C [104°F], breathlessness, coughing, rust-coloured sputum), MENINGITIS (fever, headache, nausea, vomiting, stiff neck, light hurts eyes), and PUERPERAL FEVER (marked fever shortly after childbirth); all three require prompt medical attention, so ②.

Fever can also accompany such ailments as acute PYELONEPHRITIS (rapid onset of high fever, pain in small of back), TUBERCULOSIS (slight fever, weight loss, fatigue, dry cough, shortness of breath, chest pain), BRUCELLOSIS (flu-like symptoms after drinking unpasteurized milk), and of course various tropical diseases; to be on safe side, 12 .

For explanation of other symbols, see page 107

Other conditions which cause temperature to rise are acute BRONCHITIS (wheezing, coughing, yellow-green phlegm), INFLUENZA (headache, general aches and chills, runny nose), GASTROENTERITIS (headache, diarrhoea, vomiting), PHARYNGITIS and TONSILLITIS (sore throat, difficulty swallowing), CYSTITIS (painful urination, frequent urge to urinate), MEASLES (rash, runny nose, cough, red eyes), RUBELLA (red rash, pea-like bumps on back of head), CHICKENPOX (rash followed by itchy blisters), and PELVIC INFECTION (lower abdominal pain, foul-smelling vaginal discharge).

Prolonged exposure to sun, especially if humidity is high, can cause HEATSTROKE, sending body temperature rocketing to 40°C (104°F) or more; person looks flushed, has hot, dry skin and a fast, thudding pulse, and may lose consciousness; give First Aid (see p. 101).

Homeopathic remedies for fever appear under FEVER p. 321; however, if underlying condition is known – influenza, cystitis, etc. – select a remedy from those listed under appropriate condition.

Fleas

Prefer pets to humans, usually hatching in animal's bedding or carpets and sofas; bites are red and circular, and itch intensely for about 48 hours. Pets should wear a flea collar or be regularly sprayed; areas which harbour eggs should also be sprayed. If infestation is really bad, call in a professional fumigator. Apply Urtica ointment (obtainable from homeopathic pharmacies – see addresses p. 388) to bites.

Food poisoning see also SALMONELLOSIS

Usually a reaction to toxins produced by *Salmonella* or *Staphylococcus* bacteria – these thrive in food which has not been properly cooked or food which is kept warm; violent reactions to specific foods (to shellfish, for example), to poisonous foods (certain fungi, for example), or to foods contaminated by toxic metals (mercury, for example) are also referred to as food poisoning. In most cases, symptoms resemble those of GASTROENTERITIS; suitable homeopathic remedies appear under this heading.

Gastroenteritis (gastric flu) see also

DYSENTERY, SALMONELLOSIS, FOOD POISONING
Inflammation of digestive tract, usually caused by a virus transmitted by personal contact; can also be caused by contaminated food or water, by specific foods which produce an extreme allergic reaction (see ALLERGY), by a sudden change in diet (abroad, for example), or by any illness or drug which alters natural balance of bacteria in gut. Symptoms vary in severity, but usually pass off within 48 hours; a bad case will cause repeated NAUSEA AND VOMITING, DIARRHOEA, cramping ABDOMINAL PAIN, FEVER, and exhaustion; a mild case may be limited to vague nausea and a loose stool or two. In infants and elderly people, 'stomach upsets' can be serious as they easily lead to dehydration and even SHOCK. Best treatment is rest and plenty of fluids, though GP may prescribe drugs to control vomiting and diarrhoea.

If above symptoms persist for more than 48 hours, or are accompanied by severe abdominal pain for more than 1 hour, ⑨⑨⑨ and give *Lachesis 6c* every 5 minutes for up to 10 doses; condition may not be gastroenteritis but APPENDICITIS.

Specific remedies to be taken every hour for up to 10 doses
- Burning pain in abdomen, person feels chilly, restless, anxious, thirsty for sips of water, symptoms worse between midnight and 2 am *Arsenicum 6c*
- Symptoms worse at night, with no two stools alike, fatty foods make diarrhoea worse, person tearful *Pulsatilla 6c*
- Frothy yellow stools, flatulence, person feels chilly and exhausted, draughts or light pressure on abdomen make symptoms worse *China 6c*
- Diarrhoea made worse by moving, pale-coloured stools, no pain or vomiting *Phosphoric ac. 6c*
- Diarrhoea, burning sensation as stools are passed, vomiting, craving for ice-cold water which is vomited up as soon as it becomes warm in stomach *Phosphorus 6c*
- Severe diarrhoea, stools greenish and full of mucus, especially in early morning, cramping pains in abdomen, weakness *Podophyllum 6c*
- Person cold, clammy, and prostrate, fanning brings relief *Carbo veg. 6c*
- Burning diarrhoea which drives person out of bed at around 5 am, anus red and itchy *Sulphur 6c*
- Stools dark, bloody, putrid-smelling, and nearly liquid, abdomen distended, person feels limp and wrung out, lying on right side makes symptoms worse, *Salmonella* infection suspected *Baptisia 6c*
- Colicky pain relieved by pressing on abdomen or bending double, stomach upset associated with extreme anger *Colocynth 6c*
- Diarrhoea, blood and mucus in stools *Mercurius corr. 6c*
- Constant abdominal pain relieved by passing stools, diarrhoea brings on attack of piles, chilliness, irritability *Nux 6c*
- Unremitting nausea, foul-smelling, greenish-yellow stools full of fermenting food *Ipecac 6c*

Self-help Rest, and drink plenty of fluids – add 1 teaspoon salt (no sugar) to 1 litre (2 pints) boiled water. Milk is not recommended, as it sometimes causes secondary lactose intolerance. Take no food until stomach settles down, and then stick to a light diet for a few days. Be meticulous about personal hygiene so as not to pass bug on to rest of family.

Glandular fever (infectious mononucleosis)

Viral infection, spread by personal contact, which begins rather like INFLUENZA (fever, sore throat, headache, general achiness); within a day or two glands become swollen and painful, tonsils enlarge and become dirty-looking, and JAUNDICE or a rash similar to that of RUBELLA may develop. Though these symptoms wear off in 2–3 weeks, full recovery may take some time (see POST-VIRAL SYNDROME). Since antibiotics are ineffectual against viruses, only treatment is rest and plenty of fluids. Your GP will do a blood test to confirm diagnosis, but this is not always reliable as glandular fever can involve many viruses, not just one. Constitutional homeopathic treatment is recommended if condition drags on.

Specific remedies to be taken every 4 hours for up to 10 doses during acute phase
- Sudden onset of high fever, person excited, incoherent, and red in the face *Belladonna 30c*
- Feeling chilly and shivery, sticking tongue out makes glands in neck feel painful, cold air and mental exertion make symptoms worse *Cistus 6c*
- Headache, weakness, muscular pains, ulcers in throat make swallowing difficult *Ailanthus 6c*
- Dark red tonsils, swallowing causes pains which shoot up towards ears, food and hot drinks make swallowing more painful *Phytolacca 6c*
- Glands distinctly swollen, especially if sufferer is a child and a late developer *Baryta carb. 6c*
- Chilliness, sweating, sour taste in mouth, feeling mentally and physically worn out *Calcarea 6c*
- Offensive perspiration, glands feel tender *Mercurius 6c*

Prevention Glandular fever nosode 30c, taken once a day for up to 10 days, would be a sensible precaution if family, friends, or colleagues are affected.

Self-help Rest is the best medicine – avoid strenuous exercise and do only 75 per cent of what you are actually capable of. Take extra Vitamin C, B complex, and zinc, and evening primrose oil.

Hepatitis see HEPATITIS p. 227

Hydatid disease

Caused by swallowing eggs from tapeworms which infest dogs and sheep; eggs settle in liver, lungs, and brain, and develop into sacs full of larvae (cysts); as cysts slowly enlarge they press on tissues of host organ; in the brain, this can cause FITS, and in the lungs shortness of breath; surgical removal is only cure. Since eggs are transmitted by faecal-oral route, prevention depends on washing hands thoroughly after handling animals, especially before eating.

Hydrophobia see RABIES

Influenza

Caused by many different strains of virus, and spread by droplet infection; affects respiratory tract, causing a SORE THROAT, COUGH, and sometimes CHEST PAIN, but also produces muscular aches and pains generally, chills, HEADACHE, and FEVER. Incubation period is 1–2 days, fever lasts 2–3 days, and full recovery may take 1–2 weeks. Young children, elderly people, smokers, diabetics, and people who suffer from chronic lung disease are likely to be hit hardest; possible complications are acute BRONCHITIS and PNEUMONIA. One attack confers only limited immunity. Provided there are no complications, best treatment is bed rest and plenty of fluids; antibiotics are not appropriate unless there is secondary infection. If temperature is not back to normal within 4 days, see your GP.

Specific remedies to be taken every 2 hours for up to 10 doses
- Chills up and down spine, feeling tired, weak, and shaky, but not thirsty, bursting headache, passing urine seems to relieve symptoms *Gelsemium 6c*
- Feeling dried out, hot, and irritable, especially when moving about, tremendous thirst at infrequent intervals, headache made worse by coughing, wanting to be in quiet of own home *Bryonia 30c*
- Eyes and nose hot and streaming, chills, exhaustion, feeling thirsty for sips of water *Arsenicum 6c*
- Suddenly feeling knocked out and gone to pieces, high fever, drugged, stupid look on face *Baptisia 6c*
- Severe pains in limbs, as if bones were broken, bursting headache, shivering, eyeballs feel sore *Eupatorium 6c*
- Symptoms come on suddenly, especially in dry, cold weather, person very apprehensive *Aconite 30c*
- Severe pain in back of thighs, chills, rapid pulse, slightly raised temperature, restlessness, bed feels too hard *Pyrogenium 6c*
- Restlessness, muscles feel stiff and painful *Rhus tox. 6c*
- Feeling very chilly, slightest movement increases cold feeling, nose stuffed up during day and runny at night, fluids seems to make symptoms worse, stomach upset *Nux 6c*
- Pain in throat extends to ears, glands swollen and tender *Phytolacca 6c*
- Symptoms come on suddenly, very high temperature, excited or incoherent behaviour, flushed face and staring eyes *Belladonna 30c*
- Bursting, throbbing headache *Glonoinum 6c*

Immunization/prevention Since each flu outbreak or epidemic is caused by a slightly different virus, immunization – whether orthodox or homeopathic – can only be partially effective. Some GP's advise annual vaccination for diabetics, bronchitics, etc. Homeopathy offers *Flu nosode 30c*, or a combination of this and *Bacillinum nosode 30c*, to be taken once every 3 weeks during winter months.

For explanation of other symbols, see page 107

Legionnaire's disease

Caused by bacteria which lurk in air-conditioning systems, and possibly water; initially symptoms resemble those of INFLUENZA or PNEUMONIA, with the added discomfort of DIARRHOEA, VOMITING, and ABNORMAL SLEEPINESS OR DROWSINESS; possible complications include KIDNEY FAILURE, RESPIRATORY FAILURE, and SHOCK, so hospital treatment is essential; antibiotics are part of treatment. Recovery takes 3–4 weeks. For appropriate homeopathic remedies, see INFLUENZA, PNEUMONIA.

Leprosy

A bacterial disease caught through prolonged contact with an infected person, now limited to tropical countries; disease damages skin and nerves, especially those of hands and feet, causing numbness and paralysis; fingers and toes with no sensation in them are easily injured. Leprosy can now be cured with modern drugs, but treatment is slow and may have to be continued for many years. There are specific homeopathic remedies for leprosy, but these should only be taken under the guidance of an EXPERIENCED HOMEOPATH.

Lice see HEAD LICE, PUBIC LICE

Lockjaw see TETANUS

Malaria

Caused by single-celled parasites of the genus *Plasmodium*, spread from person to person by *Anopheles* mosquitoes; mosquito bites and draws blood from an infected person, then bites a non-infected person, at same time injecting parasites into bloodstream; parasites settle in liver, where they begin to multiply; 9–30 days after bite, thousands of them enter bloodstream, and first symptoms of malaria appear, typically HEADACHE, fatigue, and NAUSEA; 24 hours later, person begins to feel cold and shivery, then FEVER sets in, accompanied by rapid breathing, then there is profuse sweating and a fall in temperature; this sequence of events takes 12–24 hours, after which person is left feeling extremely weak, with great tenderness in liver area. Appropriate action, as soon as malaria is suspected, is ②. Unless drugs are taken immediately another attack is likely within 2–3 days (parasite population takes 2–3 days to build up again). If parasite is *P. falciparum*, acute phase is likely to last 2–3 days, and be very severe, but recurrence is unlikely. Untreated malaria can lead to ANAEMIA and blocked blood vessels in vital organs (parasites damage red blood cells and cause them to stick together).

The homeopathic remedies which follow should be given in addition to orthodox drugs.

Specific remedies to be given 4 times daily for up to 6 days

- Thirst before or after acute phase but not during it, chilliness not helped by warmth, sweating and weakness, attack preceded by restlessness and pains in joints *China 6c*
- Chills, fever and sweating, thirst, pains in spine *China sulph. 6c*
- Burning fever, great weakness and prostration, fluid retention, person thirsty for sips of water *Arsenicum 6c*
- If none of the remedies above seems suitable *Sulphur 6c*

Prevention If you are visiting a country where malaria is endemic, ask your GP for a supply of anti-malarial drugs; these have to be taken for several weeks before travelling, while you are in the country, and for several weeks afterwards. If for some reason you cannot take these drugs, arm yourself with *China sulph. 6c* or *Arsenicum 6c*, and take two doses daily while you are in malarial areas.

Polio see POLIO p. 134

Post-viral syndrome (PVS)

Extremely low energy levels following viral illnesses such as GLANDULAR FEVER; theory is that some viruses alter immune system, causing body to react to stress, chemicals, bacteria, toxins. etc. in ways it did not react before. This may be mechanism behind condition known as *myalgic encephalomyelits* (also known as Royal Free disease, after the London hospital where it was first identified), which begins like a normal viral illness and then becomes so debilitating that a normal pattern of life is impossible – symptoms include extreme physical and mental tiredness, muscle and joint pains, HEADACHE, ABDOMINAL PAIN, cold extremities, pallor, pins and needles or NUMBNESS, inability to concentrate, forgetfulness, difficulty understanding written words, panic attacks, unstable emotions, uncontrollable bouts of weeping, and DEPRESSION.

There is no single, simple treatment for PVS. The most important requisite is rest – do 50-75 per cent of what you normally do, and stop as soon as you feel tired. Some GPs offer gammaglobulin injections. Best course would be to put yourself under the care of an EXPERIENCED HOMEOPATH; the route to recovery is likely to consist of constitutionally prescribed remedies, attention to diet and nutrition, vitamin and mineral supplements, and perhaps bowel cleansing or anti-*Candida* treatment, or identification and elimination of allergies.

Specific remedy to be taken every 12 hours for up to 3 days while waiting for constitutional treatment
- *China 30c*

Psittacosis

Flu-like infection caught from handling large numbers

of parrots and budgerigars; culprit is *Rickettsia*, a micro-organism half way between a bacteria and a virus, which invades lymph system and lungs; 'flu symptoms may be accompanied by BREATHLESSNESS and NOSEBLEEDS; incubation period is 1–2 weeks, and severe cases may last for 2–3 weeks, with risk of RESPIRATORY FAILURE. Antibiotics may be necessary, and artificial respiration if breathing becomes extremely difficult. See PNEUMONIA for suitable homeopathic remedies.

Rabies (hydrophobia)

Contracted through being bitten or scratched by an animal infected with rabies virus; once in human body, virus may be neutralized or may attack central nervous system, causing FEVER, irrational behaviour, and violent spasms of the throat made worse by sight of water; without intensive care in hospital (which may involve tracheotomy, artificial ventilation, and sedation), dehydration can cause death within a few days. Only 1 in 10 people bitten by a rabid animal actually develops rabies, but complacency on this score is dangerous since incubation can take anything from 2 weeks to 2 years.

If you think you have been bitten by a rabid animal (one that behaves oddly or aggressively, growls all the time, has froth around mouth), ② and inform the local police; it is customary to start course of anti-rabies vaccinations immediately, although these will be discontinued if animal is found not to be rabid. Suspect animals are usually captured rather than destroyed and kept under observation for 10 days; if they survive, they are not rabid.

Specific remedies to be taken every 2 hours for up to 10 doses if symptoms of rabies develop
- Remedies of first resort *Belladonna 30c* followed by *Stramonium 6c* in same dosage
- Person tears at clothes around throat *Lachesis 6c*
- Symptoms aggravated by water, intense fear of water *Hydrophobinum 6c*

Prevention While visiting countries where rabies is endemic, take *Hydrophobinum 30c* once a day for 7 days, then *Belladonna 6c* twice daily for 6 months.

For special risk groups e.g. vets, orthodox immunization may be necessary.

Rheumatic fever see RHEUMATIC FEVER p. ●●●

Salmonellosis (salmonella poisoning) see also FOOD POISONING

Usually contracted by eating tainted meat (meat that has not been butchered, frozen, thawed, cooked, or reheated properly) or eggs, but can also be caught through contact with an infected person or someone who has been handling tainted meat. Symptoms are similar to those of GASTROENTERITIS – DIARRHOEA, FEVER, ABDOMINAL PAIN, and vomiting – but in severe cases *Salmonella* bacteria invade bloodstream as well as

gut causing inflammation and ABSCESS development in kidneys, gallbladder, heart, or joints. Such cases are fortunately rare, most *Salmonella* infections being fairly mild; main risk is dehydration from vomiting and diarrhoea.

If diarrhoea lasts for more than 3 days, and is accompanied by fever, pain, and vomiting, ⌐12⌐. Your GP may prescribe drugs to control vomiting and diarrhoea, and possibly antibiotics to destroy residual bacteria. Otherwise treatment is bed rest and plenty of fluids. For specific homeopathic remedies, see GASTROENTERITIS.

Septicaemia see BLOOD POISONING

Scabies

Intensely itchy rash on trunk, with itchy red lumps on hands, wrists, genitals, or buttocks; scratching causes sores and scabs; culprit is scabies mite or 'itch mite', a parasite which burrows under skin to lay eggs, which hatch into more mites; transmitted by personal and sexual contact, or caught from infested clothes or bedding; mites thrive where there is overcrowding and poor hygiene. If the self-help measures and the homeopathic remedy given below do not improve matters within 1 week, see your GP; he or she will probably prescribe an insecticide lotion.

Specific remedy to be given every 12 hours for up to 3 days to *all members of family/household* whether infected or not, provided they do not suffer from eczema
- *Sulphur 30c*

Self-help Apply oil of Lavender (obtainable from chemist) to lesions. Launder all clothes and bedding in household; if certain items cannot be laundered, stop using them and thoroughly air them for at least 4 days. Mites cannot survive for more than a day or two away from human skin.

Shingles (herpes zoster)

Caused by same virus which causes CHICKENPOX; virus may lie dormant in a nerve root in spine for many years until reactivated by STRESS; when this happens, virus multiplies and attacks the nerve, causing searing, knife-like pains along its course; a few days later, skin above nerve erupts in itchy blisters; these generally heal within 1 week, but nerve pains may last for many weeks. If facial nerve is affected, face may be temporarily paralysed; if optic nerve is affected, cornea may be seriously damaged (see CORNEAL ULCER).

If nerve pain and rash occur on trunk, ⌐24⌐; if face or eyes are involved, ②. Orthodox treatment includes analgesics and antiviral ointments with antiviral tablets and infusions for eye involvement.

Specific remedies to be taken every 2 hours for up to 10 doses while waiting to see GP

For explanation of other symbols, see page 107

- Red, blistered, itchy skin, especially if scalp is affected or person is young, warmth and moving about make symptoms more bearable *Rhus tox. 6c*
- Burning pains worse between midnight and 2 am, isolated skin eruptions becoming more numerous and merging together, person restless, anxious, exhausted, and chilly, symptoms alleviated by warmth *Arsenicum 6c*
- Severe pain, skin burns and itches and forms brown scabs, person middle-aged or elderly *Mezereum 6c*
- Nerve pains and itching, slightest touch or movement makes symptoms worse, and so does eating *Ranunculus 6c*
- Left side of body affected, with some swelling, aggravated by warmth but relieved by cold *Lachesis 6c*

Prevention Anyone who is elderly or infirm and has been in contact with a chickenpox or shingles sufferer should take 3 doses of *Variolinum 30c* at 12-hour intervals as a preventive.

Self-help Take as much bed rest as possible to begin with. Sponge blisters with Hypericum and Calendula solution (5 drops of mother tincture of each to 0.25 litre [½ pint] boiled cooled water). Hot and cold compresses also relieve nerve pains.

Smallpox
A virulent, highly infectious disease which has now been eradicated worldwide; today smallpox virus only exists in a small number of research laboratories, and vaccination programmes have ceased, although a few countries still insist that visitors carry a vaccination certificate. In sensitive people, skin eruptions, NEURALGIA AND NEURITIS, and INDIGESTION may be the long-delayed consequences of smallpox vaccination many years ago.

Tapeworms
Transmitted in infected beef, pork, or fish which has not been thoroughly cooked, and possibly by birds and flies; once in human intestine, mature embryo develops a head which fastens itself to wall of jejunum (upper part of small intestine), then grows into a long, segmented worm, feeding on pre-digested contents of intestine; mature segments containing thousands of embryos occasionally break off and appear in faeces. If infected person is reasonably healthy, only symptoms will be occasional ABDOMINAL PAIN, itching around anus (see PRURITIS ANI), and slight WEIGHT LOSS; undue hunger is unlikely unless person is already suffering from malnutrition or MALABSORPTION.

If analysis of faeces confirms presence of tapeworm, GP will prescribe a drug to kill it.

Tetanus (lockjaw)
Occurs when body is invaded by *Clostridium* bacteria, whose toxins attack nerves in spinal cord; symptoms are painful CRAMP and rigidity in muscles of spine, limbs, abdomen, chest, and throat; cases are rare, thanks to immunization and injection procedures, but can be fatal if chest and throat spasms interfere with breathing. *Clostridium* bacteria live in soil and enter body through wounds, even through small cuts and grazes; incubation period can be anything from 2 days to several months. Orthodox treatment consists of antibiotics, and drugs to combat bacterial toxins and relax rigid muscles; person may also need assistance with breathing. Homeopathic remedies below should be taken in addition to orthodox remedies.

Specific remedies to be taken every hour for up to 10 doses during tetanus attack
- At first signs of muscle spasm *Aconite 30c*
- Head thrown back, muscles of jaw and throat in spasm and jerking *Cicuta 6c*
- Tetanus following a puncture wound or injury to a nerve, site of injury still very tender *Hypericum 30c*
- Where jaw is locked *Oenanthe 6c*

Immunization/prevention Always clean wounds thoroughly using Hypericum and Calendula solution (5 drops of mother tincture of each in 0.25 litre [½ pint] boiled cooled water). If wound has been contaminated with soil and you have not been immunized or received a tetanus booster injection in the last 5 years, take *Hypericum 6c* three times daily for 3 weeks as a preventive. In infancy, immunization against tetanus is part of DTP (diptheria, tetanus, whooping cough) vaccine; in author's opinion, side effects of tetanus immunization at this age are far outweighed by dangers of not being immunized. Thereafter booster injections should be given every 5–10 years.

Threadworms see THREADWORMS p. 333

Toxocariasis
Caught by swallowing eggs of thread-like *Toxocara* worms which live in intestines of dogs and cats; symptoms, if any, may be mild FEVER or slight BREATHLESSNESS, but if worm attacks eye, sight may be lost; most victims are children. Orthodox medicine offers anti-parasitic drugs and homeopathy can boost general immunity through constitutional treatment, but real solution is prevention.

Prevention Discourage pets from licking you, wash your hands thoroughly after grooming them, wash their eating utensils separately from your own, and always wash your hands before eating or preparing food. Do not allow children to play in parks or gardens fouled with faeces.

Toxoplasmosis
Another infection caught from contact with faeces of dogs and cats; micro-organism responsible is *Toxo-*

plasma, which invades digestive and nervous system, and can affect developing foetus; in rare instances, infection can cause MENINGITIS and HYDROCEPHALUS; more commonly, it causes vague ABDOMINAL PAIN and slightly swollen glands, or no symptoms at all. Your GP will prescribe a course of drugs to kill *Toxoplasma*, but to boost general immunity constitutional homeopathic treatment is also recommended. For prevention, see TOXOCARIASIS.

Tuberculosis (TB)

Now rare in Western countries but still common in Asia, Africa, and Caribbean, and becoming so among AIDS sufferers; tuberculosis bacillus (a type of bacteria) is spread by droplet infection or through milk which has not been TB-tested, and mainly affects lungs, but also brain (see MENINGITIS), kidneys, or bones. A single attack may confer immunity, but residual bacteria can lie dormant for many years until reactivated by general ill health or undernourishment; the initial attack may produce no symptoms at all, or be mistaken for a mild case of INFLUENZA; symptoms of the secondary stage (once known as consumption) include slight FEVER, night sweats, fatigue, WEIGHT LOSS, a dry COUGH which eventually produces pus or bloody sputum, BREATHLESSNESS, and sometimes CHEST PAIN, but these tend to onset extremely slowly.

If TB is suspected, see your GP; a prolonged course of antibiotics may be necessary, together with rest and time off work, and a better diet. If brain is affected, symptoms will be those of MENINGITIS (severe headache, stiff neck, intolerance of light); appropriate action is ②.

Although the homeopathic remedies below can be self-prescribed, sufferers are advised to put themselves under the care of an EXPERIENCED HOMEOPATH.

Specific remedies to be taken every 2 hours for up to 10 doses when symptoms are acute
- Fever and weight loss *Bacillinum 6c*
- Fever, head sweats, hands and feet feel cold and clammy, person weak and apprehensive *Calcarea 6c*
- Person wrung out and exhausted, chilly and worried, thirsty for sips of water *Arsenicum 6c*

Immunization BCG vaccination is offered shortly after birth to babies considered most at risk, and again in early teens. If BCG is contra-indicated because of eczema, asthma, or immune system deficiencies, *Tuberculinum 30c* nosode can be given. See your homeopath.

Self-help Increase level of potassium-rich foods in diet (raw vegetables and fruit) and ensure good levels of protein (from wholegrains and pulses as well as fish and meat). Get plenty of rest and fresh air.

Typhoid fever

A highly contagious bacterial illness spread through contaminated food and water supplies, or passed from person to person (some people carry typhoid fever but do not succumb to it); bacteria rapidly inflame walls of intestine and enter bloodstream, causing what seems to be a bad attack of INFLUENZA at first, although this is followed by persistent high FEVER, DIARRHOEA, intestinal bleeding, general weakness, DELIRIUM, and sometimes a pink rash on abdomen. If typhoid fever is suspected, and particularly if there is BLOOD IN FAECES, ②. Person will need to be isolated and given antibiotics.

Specific remedies to be taken every 2 hours for up to 10 doses
- Yellow-coated tongue, bitter taste in mouth, loose stools, restlessness *Baptisia 6c*
- Shooting pains in head, throat, chest, abdomen and limbs, made worse by slightest movement *Bryonia 30c*
- Exhaustion, feeling chilly, worried, restless, and thirsty for small sips of hot drinks *Arsenicum 6c*

Immunization/prevention If visiting tropical or sub-tropical parts of the world, ask your GP for orthodox vaccination; this consists of two injections which give protection for 3 years. If you have been in contact with a typhoid sufferer, take *Typhoidinum 30c* daily for 10 days as a preventive.

Self-help If medical help is not immediately available, person should stay in bed and take only water with a little salt and sugar in it (½ teapoon salt and 1 teaspoon sugar to 1 large cup of water); this allows walls of intestine to heal. Best way of reducing temperature is to give 10-minute tepid sponge-downs every 2 hours. Do not give aspirin or paracetamol as these may aggravate intestinal inflammation/bleeding.

Yellow fever

Viral infection endemic in South and Central America and parts of Africa, and spread by mosquitoes; virus attacks liver, causing symptoms which resemble those of INFLUENZA, and in severe cases JAUNDICE, NAUSEA AND VOMITING, and ABDOMINAL PAIN; person may also become very depressed, confused, or comatose. As with many viral ailments, treatment can only be palliative; one attack confers lifelong immunity.

Specific remedies to be taken every hour for up to 10 doses during acute attack
- Person feverish, vomiting, jaundiced, restless *Aconite 30c*
- Pain in abdomen, retching and vomiting, symptoms made worse by slightest movement *Bryonia 30c*
- Person exhausted, restless, and chilly, thirsty for sips of water *Arsenicum 6c*

Immunization Orthodox immunization lasts for about 10 years, and is compulsory if you are visiting certain countries; injection should be given 10 days before travelling.

For explanation of other symbols, see page 107

FERTILITY AND PREGNANCY

ANYONE searching for evidence of miracles need look no further than the process of conception. Every month, as each ripe egg is released from its ovary and enters the Fallopian tube, the mucus at the entrance to the womb becomes less sticky. If intercourse takes place, millions of vigorously swimming sperm make their way through the mucus, into the womb, and into the Fallopian tubes. Here they congregate around the egg, causing it to spin round with the movement of their beating tails. Eventually one sperm penetrates the egg, the nuclei of sperm and egg fuse, and the process of cell division begins. The fused nuclei split into two cells, then four, then eight, then sixteen, all containing the 46 individual packages of information or chromosomes which will create a new and totally unique human being.

Seven days after fertilization the ball of cells embeds itself in the wall of the uterus. At 20 days the placenta begins to form, at 30 days the spinal cord, at 6 weeks the heart, and by 13 weeks all the body organs are formed. At 5 months the baby can be felt to move. At 6 months the lungs become functional and the nostrils open. At 7 months the baby should be in the head down position ready for birth.

A full-time pregnancy usually lasts 38 weeks, counting from the moment of conception to the time the baby is born. Conception usually takes place halfway between periods if your cycle is 28 days and regular. However, since many women's periods are not exactly 28 days, pregnancy is usually measured as being 40 weeks from the first day of the last period. Common pointers to pregnancy are missing a period, more than usually tender or swollen breasts and darker nipples, nausea, tiredness, a frequent urge to pass urine, and sometimes loss of appetite or cravings for unusual foods. To confirm your pregnancy you should have a pregnancy test. This can be done by your GP, a family planning clinic, or a pregnancy testing service. If you use a home pregnancy testing kit from the chemist, read the instructions very carefully, and if you are still in doubt see your GP.

Your chances of having twins are about 1 : 80! Identical twins develop from the same egg and share the same placenta; non-identical twins develop from different eggs and have a placenta each. Only three pairs of twins in every ten are identical. Triplets are much rarer, only occurring in 1 : 6,400 pregnancies. According to recent evidence, efforts to determine the sex of a baby by having intercourse at a particular time during ovulation or by altering the acid-alkaline balance of the vagina do not work.

Once you have established that you are pregnant, do go for regular antenatal check-ups, even it it means frustrating waits in hospital antenatal clinics or in your GP's waiting room. Normally your GP will share your antenatal care with a midwife and a hospital consultant. If you want to have your baby at home, write to the Supervisor of Midwives at your local Maternity Unit, stating you intend having a home birth and asking her to provide you with a midwife.

Antenatal care is important since it allows you to find out at an early stage if there are any problems. Ultrasound (a sound picture of the baby in the womb) is thought to be harmless to mother and baby and can be used to monitor the size, shape and position of the baby at any stage of pregnancy. Amniocentesis (taking a sample of the amniotic fluid around your baby) is usually carried out between 16 and 18 weeks, but only if a previous baby has been abnormal or there is a family history of congenital problems, or it the mother is over 35. An earlier test, chorion villous biopsy, can be done at 10 weeks in some centres. Conditions such as spina bifida or Down's syndrome can be detected in this way. However, the procedure does involve a slight risk of miscarriage. You should also consider carefully what your attitude would be if your baby was found to be abnormal. Would you want to terminate the pregnancy or not?

Here, in brief, are some of the dos and don'ts of pregnancy. Treat your baby as a person from the word go – moderate exercise – swimming and walking in the fresh air are very good, but anything which involves repeated compression of the spine, such as horseriding or trampolining, should be avoided; always keep 25 per cent of your energy in reserve. Do go to antenatal classes – they will teach you what to expect and how to breathe in order to cope with pain during labour. Don't wear tight clothes. Get as much sleep as you can and avoid late nights. Don't sit in hot baths for too long; 10 minutes is about the maximum, especially if you faint easily or have a tendency to bleed. Avoid serious travelling if you can, especially if you have had a threatened miscarriage or there are complications, or you suffer from travel sickness; most airlines do not like you to fly after 32 weeks or so, so if you must fly, check with the airline first. Stop working before 28 weeks (when maternity benefit can be claimed) if your work is very strenuous.

The old idea that an expectant mother needs to 'eat for two' has been comprehensively demolished in recent years. Everything depends on the efficiency of the mother's metabolism. The 'twice a week rule' is a good one to follow (see p. 24), with an increase in iron and calcium foods and also a modest increase in protein intake, preferably in the form of oily fish, nuts, seeds, pulses and wholegrains. The latter, with generous helpings of raw vegetables and fruit, will help to guard against constipation. Tea, coffee, and alcohol should be avoided. Chamomile tea should also be avoided, especially in the later stages.

As for sex during pregnancy, there are no rules really, except to say that if you do not feel like it your partner should respect your wishes. Intercourse during the first 16 weeks should be avoided if you have had a threatened miscarriage or previous miscarriages; it is also unwise if there is still occasional vaginal bleeding, or if you are excessively nervous and worried about the effects of intercourse on your pregnancy. In the later months of pregnancy, deep penetration should be avoided. There are women who claim that orgasms in the later stages of pregnancy make labour less painful.

Homeopathic remedies during pregnancy During the first three months of pregnancy, the most vulnerable time, you should AVOID ALL MEDICATION if you possibly can – that means prescription drugs, recreational drugs, over-the-counter preparations from chemists and healthfood shops, vitamin and mineral supplements, and homeopathic remedies. There is no evidence that homeopathic remedies cause any problems during pregnancy, but to be on the safe side they should not be taken in potencies less than 6c except for Tissue Salts. It is probably best to avoid low potency Apis altogether and take 30c if you need to.

There are many schools of thought among homeopaths as to the most appropriate treatment of pregnancy. There are homeopaths who only treat if there are symptoms to treat; others recommend a 'miasmatic clear-out', giving nosodes for all the diseases or weaknesses which appear in the family history; others favour a systemic clear out using Sulphur, Calcium carb., Lycopodium, and Tissue Salts; others favour constitutional treatment for both the mother and the father; others give Caulophyllum in the last stages of pregnancy to stimulate the womb.

In fact pregnancy is a very good time to treat someone because constitutional features tend to declare themselves very strongly due to the general mobilization of the Vital Force. Also by treating the mother's symptoms the baby can be treated as well. Indeed some of the mother's symptoms are the baby's. My treatment approach depends on the length of time I have known the parents and the family, the family's medical history, the health of the mother during pregnancy, and sometimes the health of the father too. Where possible I advise preconceptual constitutional treatment for both parents.

For minor complaints during pregnancy, homeopathic remedies should be tried first. If you feel very unwell, see your GP before taking anything.

Abdominal pain in pregnancy

Griping, pinching sensations in the lower abdomen, most common during the first trimester of pregnancy, and sometimes described as 'colic'. If pain persists for more than 3 hours, especially if it is associated with vaginal bleeding, an ECTOPIC PREGNANCY should be suspected; appropriate action is ②.

Specific remedies to be taken ½-hourly for up to 6 doses
- Griping sensation behind navel, bowels full of trapped wind, symptoms brought on by anger *Chamomilla 6c*
- Constipation, ineffectual straining to pass stools *Nux 6c*
- Bowels feel as if they are being clutched by a hand, hot, bloated feeling, discomfort made worse by jarring *Belladonna 30c*
- Bowels feel as if they are being pinched between two stones, pain relieved by bending double or pressing hand hard against abdomen *Colocynth 6c*

Abortion see TERMINATION OF PREGNANCY

Anaemia during pregnancy see also ANAEMIA pp. 184–6

Ideally, of course, anaemia should be corrected before conception. However, iron deficiency anaemia and folic acid deficiency anaemia can develop quite quickly during pregnancy; symptoms are pallor, fingernails which look unhealthily white, tiredness, weakness, fainting, breathlessness, even palpitations. Vitamin B_{12} deficiency anaemia, which mainly affects vegetarians, is of more insidious onset; in addition to the symptoms above there may be abdominal pain, weight loss, yellowing of the skin, and tingling in hands or feet. The main dangers of anaemia are to the mother rather than the foetus; low iron and haemoglobin levels can predispose her to post-natal infections and POST-NATAL DEPRESSION.

The forms of anaemia mentioned above usually respond to dietary change or nutritional supplements (see PART 6). Green leafy vegetables contain plenty of folic acid. Vitamin B_{12} is a constituent of animal products and of brewer's yeast. Iron can be taken in the form of iron tablets, with extra Vitamin C or tissue salts Ferr. Phos. and Calc. Phos. to aid absorption and assimilation. It is not necessary, or advisable, to take iron supplements during pregnancy if you are not anaemic.

Antepartum haemorrhage

Bleeding from the vagina any time after the 28th week of pregnancy; before then, bleeding is classified as a threatened MISCARRIAGE. Sometimes due to a burst varicose vein in the vagina or damage to the cervix; more seriously, blood loss may be due to PLACENTA PRAEVIA, in which part of the placenta becomes detached from the wall of the womb, preventing an adequate flow of nutrients to the foetus and slowing foetal growth; in severe cases, this can be fatal to mother and foetus.

Any bleeding after the 28th week requires prompt investigation; the best course is ②, or ⑨⑨⑨ if bleeding is very heavy. You will probably be admitted to hospital; situation may be stabilized by a blood transfusion, or it may be necessary to induce labour or deliver the baby by Caesarean.

For explanation of other symbols, see page 107

Specific remedies to be taken every 5–10 minutes for up to 10 doses until help arrives.
- Sudden onset of bleeding, fear for baby's life *Aconite 30c*
- Bleeding brought on by injury *Arnica 30c*
- If *Arnica* does not stop bleeding *Bryonia 30c*
- Blood bright red and hot *Belladonna 30c*
- Bleeding profuse and continuous, feeling sick *Ipecac. 30c*
- Blood partially clotted, slightest movement seems to increase blood loss, shooting pains in vagina *Sabina 30c*
- Blood loss temporarily stopped, feeling exhausted and very much on edge *China 30c*

Backache during pregnancy
Lower back pain is common in pregnancy as extra weight accumulates forward of the spine and as the ligaments of the pelvis begin to stretch in preparation for birth. Extra care should be taken when bending, lifting, or twisting; when standing and walking, the baby's weight should not be allowed to pull the pelvis too far forward; when side-lying, a pillow buttress for the abdomen takes some of the strain off the lower back.

Specific remedies to be taken 4 times daily for up to 7 days
- Back feels weak and tired, dragging pains in middle and lower back *Kali carb. 6c*
- Hard, tense feeling in lower abdomen, head feels hot *Belladonna 6c*
- Hard, tense feeling in lower abdomen, feeling hot all over, symptoms worse in stuffy rooms *Pulsatilla 6c*
- Hard, tense feeling in lower abdomen, feeling chilly *Nux 6c*

Specific remedy to be taken 2-hourly for up to 10 doses
- Backache due to injury or strain *Arnica 30c*, followed by *Rhus tox. 6c* every 6–8 hours for up to 7 days if backache persists.

Self-help If you are prone to backache even when you are not pregnant, take tissue salts Calc. Fluor. and Calc. Phos. 3 times daily for 5 days out of 7 during pregnancy.

Bleeding see MISCARRIAGE, ANTE-PARTUM HAEMORRHAGE

Breast discomfort during pregnancy
Distention of the breasts during the first few months of pregnancy is quite normal, and due to hormone changes; in the last two or three months, feelings of fullness and discomfort are due to incoming milk. However, if discomfort is accompanied by FEVER and tender glands under the armpits, MASTITIS should be suspected, in which case 12.

Specific remedies to be taken 4-hourly for up to 5 days
- Mild discomfort caused by enlargement *Conium 6c*
- Breasts feel hard and tense *Bryonia 6c*
- Breasts feel hard and tense, with red streaking of skin *Belladonna 6c*

Breech and other malpresentations
Before 36 weeks it is sometimes possible to turn a baby in the womb – that is, turn the head down and the buttocks up, or turn the body so that the baby is facing the mother's buttocks – by giving three doses of *Pulsatilla 30c* at 12-hour intervals. If this fails, it may be possible to manipulate the baby into the normal position. If the malpresentation persists, the baby may have to be delivered by forceps or Caesarean.

Cardiovascular problems during pregnancy
Pregnancy puts extra strain on the heart and circulatory system. It is not uncommon, for example, for heart murmurs to develop during pregnancy; these represent slight alterations in blood flow through the heart and are usually not serious, but your GP will probably want to investigate. If you have an existing heart problem, rest as much as possible during pregnancy, don't smoke, learn some form of relaxation or meditation (see PART 2), and follow the dietary suggestions given under ATHEROSCLEROSIS. If you have a congenital heart defect, see your GP; he or she will probably send you to see a specialist. If one of your heart valves is damaged (see VALVULAR DISEASE), antibiotics may be prescribed to prevent infection, which could prove fatal, but if you are unable or unwilling to take antibiotics, take 3 doses of *Silica 6c* for 5 days out of 7 throughout pregnancy. To relieve the strain which delivery puts on the heart, you may need an episiotomy (an incision in the vulva so that the baby's head slips out more easily).

High blood pressure during pregnancy can be due to general anxiety; constitutional homeopathic treatment, rest, relaxation, and the diet suggestions given under HIGH BLOOD PRESSURE will almost certainly help. If high blood pressure is accompanied by headaches, blurred vision, nausea, vomiting, intolerance of light, and swollen ankles, the chances are that you are developing PRE-ECLAMPTIC TOXAEMIA so ②.

Palpitations are not uncommon during pregnancy; they are a sign that the heart is having to work harder to pump an increased voume of blood. For some information see PALPITATIONS.

Specific remedies to be taken every 2 hours for up to 10 doses
- Palpitations onset suddenly after a shock of some sort, fear of dying *Aconite 30c*
- Palpitations brought on by heat or rich, fatty food, general weakness *Pulsatilla 6c*

- Palpitations worse at night, especially when lying on left side *Lycopodium 6c*
- Heartbeats seem to shake whole body, constricted feeling in chest, heat and sympathy make discomfort worse *Natrum mur. 6c*

Swollen ankles, most common in the sixth and seventh month of pregnancy, tend to occur in women who take too little exercise and whose lymphatic drainage is poor; rest and walking usually improve matters. More seriously, puffy ankles can be a sign of HIGH BLOOD PRESSURE or developing PRE-ECLAMPTIC TOXAEMIA. Provided your GP rules out the latter, constitutional homeopathic treatment would be beneficial.

Swollen or inflamed vulva has similar causes to swollen ankles.

Specific remedies to be taken 4 times daily for up to 7 days
- Bearing down sensation as if contents of womb are about to escape through vagina, sensation makes you cross your legs *Sepia 6c*
- Itchy, raw, scalding sensation after passing water, soothed by washing *Mercurius 6c*
- Vulval swelling associated with constipation, in-effectual straining to pass stools and always feeling there is more to come, urge to urinate *Nux 6c*
- Vulva and vagina excessively tender and itchy, but too sensitive to scratch *Coffea 6c*
- Swelling due to venereal disease *Thuja 6c*

Varicose veins are usually aggravated rather than caused by pregnancy, as the weight of the uterus begins to bear down on the veins of the pelvis. Usually one leg is more affected than the other; exercise tends to make distended veins more painful, and in severe cases they may burst. Get as much rest as possible, with legs raised above hip level, and avoid constricting clothing.

Specific remedies to be taken every 4 hours for up to 2 weeks
- Remedy of first resort *Pulsatilla 6c*
- If Pulsatilla does not work, and skin is marbled, with knotted, painful veins *Carbo veg. 6c*
- One foot hot, the other cold *Lycopodium 6c*

Cervical incompetence
Weakness of the cervix which causes it to open up at some time after the 12th week of pregnancy and cause MISCARRIAGE; weakness may be due to damage caused by previous deliveries or by D and Cs (stretching of the cervix in order to remove a foetus, fibroids, or cysts from the uterus). Standard treatment is a minor operation in which a suture is put around the cervix, like a purse string, and tightened; it is removed at 38 weeks, unless labour begins earlier.

Constipation during pregnancy see also
CONSTIPATION p. 223
The hormone which maintains pregnancy, pro-gesterone, decreases the tone of the bowel muscles, and the growing foetus also presses on the large intestine; the net result is delayed transit of faeces. If constipation does not respond to the homeopathic remedies or self-help measures below see your GP. On no account take laxatives – they may cause MISCARRIAGE or premature labour.

Specific remedies to be taken 4 times daily for up to 14 days
- Dull headache, feeling of fullness in rectum, fre-quent but unsuccessful straining to pass stools *Nux 6c*
- Hard, knobbly stools, never emptying bowels properly, piles or inflammation around anus *Sulphur 6c*
- Hard, dry, burnt-looking stools, especially during morning, discomfort made worse by movement and cold drinks, thirst for large quantities of fluid at infrequent intervals *Bryonia 6c*
- Large, hard stools, rectum feels as if there is a hard ball inside it, pains which shoot up rectum *Sepia 6c*
- No desire to pass stools unless rectum is full, even soft stools are difficult to pass *Alumina 6c*
- Hard, small stools, passed with difficulty, never emptying bowels properly, ineffectual straining, passing a lot of wind *Lycopodium 6c*

Self-help Drink more, increase the amount of fibre in your diet, take more exercise, and never suppress the urge to pass stools. If these measures fail, try taking psyllium husks or linseeds, once a day to begin with, then three times a day; the correct dose is 1 teaspoon husks (1 desertspoon linseeds) stirred into a cup of water and drunk immediately, followed by 2 more cups of water. Most healthfood shops stock both psyllium husks and linseeds.

Cramp during pregnancy see also CRAMP
p. 203
Cramp in the calves is common during pregnancy, and very exhausting if it occurs at night as well as during the day.

Specific remedies to be taken every 4 hours for up to 7 days
- Cramp worst in calves, but relieved by warmth and walking *Veratrum 6c*
- Cramp in calves and soles of feet, numbness or pins and needles in arms and hands, rest relieves discomfort, cold makes it worse *Nux 6c*
- Cramp mainly affects left leg but wears off when pressure is applied *Colocynth 6c*
- Legs feel cold and numb, but better for cold applications *Ledum 6c*

Self-help If cramp is persistent, take Mag. Phos. tissue salt as well as one of the remedies above.

For explanation of other symbols, see page 107

Cravings and aversions during pregnancy

Strong food likes and dislikes during the first 3–4 months of pregnancy are very common, but not compulsory! If health is good, there is nothing to worry about. However, if cravings or aversions persist, try one of the remedies listed in the General Remedy Finder (pp. 68–71) under 'Drinks' and 'Food'. The remedy you choose should be taken in 6c potency 3 times daily for up to 6 days.

Diabetes during pregnancy see also DIABETES pp. 257–8

Can declare itself during pregnancy, especially if previous babies have weighed 4 kg (9 lbs) or more at birth. If urine tests during regular antenatal check-ups reveal high levels of glucose, you will be given a glucose-tolerance test; if this is positive, your GP will prescribe dietary and/or insulin treatment as necessary (see DIABETES pp. 257–8). Constitutional homeopathic treatment is also recommended.

Pre-existing or not, diabetes during pregnancy requires careful management since risks to mother and baby are twice as high as normal; risk of neonatal death is also much higher. If diabetes is severe, you may need to spend the last 10 weeks of pregnancy in hospital; induction or a Caesarean may be recommended at 36 weeks.

Self-help Control of diabetes takes considerable self-discipline, especially where diet is concerned. Your GP may give you a detailed diet sheet, but if not, follow the Blood Sugar Levelling Diet on p. 353

Diarrhoea during pregnancy see also DIARRHOEA p. 225

The danger of diarrhoea during pregnancy is that it may trigger off a MISCARRIAGE. If three or more successive bowel movements are very loose and watery, ②. In the meantime, select a remedy from the list below.

Specific remedies to be taken every hour for up to 10 doses
- Cramping pains in abdomen, yellow-green stools which look like chopped egg *Chamomilla 6c*
- Cramping pains in abdomen, stools yellow-green and watery, slimy tongue and bitter taste in mouth, no thirst, symptoms worse at night *Pulsatilla 6c*
- Diarrhoea follows over-chilling after exertion *Dulcamara 6c*
- Diarrhoea makes you rush to the lavatory first thing in morning, no abdominal pain *Sulphur 6c*

Ectopic pregnancy

Development of foetus in one of Fallopian tubes or in abdominal cavity rather than in uterus; symptoms are persistent abdominal pain and bleeding, as placenta burrows into surrounding tissues to establish foetal blood supply; cause may be some abnormality of the Fallopian tubes due to previous operations or infections, or the presence of an IUD. If there is bleeding and abdominal pain lasting for more than 3 hours, ②; you will be sent to hospital, and may need an operation to remove the developing pregnancy, and possibly the tube as well. If the other tube is in good shape, you stand a good chance of becoming pregnant again, and in the normal way.

Specific remedies to be taken ½-hourly for up to 10 doses if ectopic pregnancy is suspected
- Feeling very worried and afraid *Aconite 30c*
- Abdominal pain accompanied by bleeding *Arnica 30c*

Emotional disturbance during pregnancy

Pregnancy is an emotional time for many women; moods fluctuate very rapidly; joy, fear, anger, and so on seem to be more intense than usual. Hormone changes are partly responsible, but cognitive processes are also involved. In the author's experience, very strong emotions in the mother affect the baby, so if you find your emotions distressing, take one of the remedies below.

Specific remedies to be taken every 12 hours for up to 3 days
- Fear/apprehension – fear of dying, pale face, palpitations, fainting fits *Aconite 30c*
- Fear/apprehension – feeling of anguish, trembling, breathlessness, face dark and flushed *Opium 30c*
- Fear/apprehension – diarrhoea, feeling chilly all the time *Veratrum 30c*
- Fear/apprehension – face red and hot *Belladonna 30c*
- Grief – feeling sad, constricted feeling in chest, lump in throat, headache *Ignatia 30c*
- Grief – indifference to people and surroundings, lack of energy *Phosphoric ac. 30c*
- Anger – breathlessness, fidgeting, diarrhoea, bilious attacks *Chamomilla 30c*
- Anger – irritability, being over-critical *Nux 30c*
- Anger – wanting to be left alone, worrying about money *Bryonia 30c*
- Joy – inability to sleep, going 'over the top' *Coffea 30c*

Excessive salivation during pregnancy

Profuse salivation during first trimester of pregnancy, distressing because one wants to spit all the time; most sufferers cope by carrying a large box of tissues around with them; the remedies below are also recommended.

Specific remedies to be taken 4 times daily for up to 7 days
- Profuse salivation, dribbling on to pillow at night, sweet, metallic taste in mouth *Mercurius 6c*
- Excessive salivation accompanied by nausea, aversion to food, tongue looks white or yellow *Pulsatilla 6c*

- Symptoms as for Pulsatilla, but tongue clean *Ipecac. 6c*
- Too much saliva, feeling weak, chilly, restless, and worried *Arsenicum 6c*
- Too much saliva, forehead cold and sweaty, feeling weak and apathetic *Veratrum 6c*

Fainting during pregnancy see also FAINTING p. 128

Can occur for no obvious reason, or may be due to extra circulatory load, blood loss, poor diet, previous illness, or wearing clothes which are too tight around the waist.

Specific remedies to be taken every 12 hours for up to 3 days
- Fainting associated with sadness or grief *Ignatia 30c*
- Fainting associated with irritability *Chamomilla 30c* or *Nux 30c*
- Fainting due to general overloading of cardio-vascular system, fear and apprehension *Aconite 30c*
- Fainting due to heat *Belladonna 30c*
- Faints brought on by movement *Bryonia 30c*
- Fainting due to illness or blood loss *China 30c*

False pains

In the last few months of pregnancy the muscles of the uterus start to tone up and contract at infrequent intervals in preparation for labour (see pp. 292–3); there is no cause for alarm unless contractions are prolonged or increasing in frequency, or unless there is a discharge of blood or fluid from the vagina.

Specific remedies to be taken every hour for up to 10 doses in the following order:
- *Pulsatilla 6c, Coffea 6c, Nux 6c, Secale 6c, Caulophyllum 6c*

Fluid retention during pregnancy see CARDIOVASCULAR PROBLEMS DURING PREGNANCY

Foetal growth problems

If you fail to gain weight, or start losing weight, or if the baby stops moving, ② – all of these symptoms suggest that the placenta is not functioning properly. Possible causes include PRE-ECLAMPTIC TOXAEMIA, ANTE-PARTUM HAEMORRHAGE, high blood pressure (see CARDIOVASCULAR PROBLEMS), DIABETES, smoking, and drugs.

Haemorrhoids during pregnancy see PILES DURING PREGNANCY

Heartburn during pregnancy

Affects nearly 50 percent of all women. The preg-nancy-maintaining hormone progesterone causes the muscles which close the entrance to the stomach to slacken; this allows stomach acid to splash up into the oesophagus, causing a burning sensation. Upward pressure of the womb on the stomach in later pregnancy aggravates reflux problems.

Specific remedies to be taken 4 times daily for up to 7 days
- Burning sensation behind breastbone, great thirst, drinking causes shuddering and marked flatulence *Capsicum 6c*
- Sight or smell of food causes nausea, cold feeling in pit of stomach, craving for fizzy drinks *Colchicum 6c*
- Craving for ice-cold drinks which are vomited up as soon as they become warm in stomach, craving for salt *Phosphorus 6c*
- Heartburn worse around 11 am, gnawing sensation in stomach, craving for sweets, marked thirst but little appetite, drinking milk makes heartburn worse *Sulphur 6c*

Self-help Eat small meals at frequent intervals; this will go a long way towards easing discomfort. If you suffer from heartburn at night raise the head of your bed by a few inches; this is not recommended, however, if you have swollen ankles.

High blood pressure during pregnancy see CARDIOVASCULAR PROBLEMS DURING PREGNANCY

Hydramnios

An excessive amount of fluid (amniotic fluid) around the baby during later months of pregnancy; more common in mothers who are carrying twins or who have DIABETES or PRE-ECLAMPTIC TOXAEMIA; may be symptomless or accompanied by increasing breathless-ness, indigestion, a dull ache in the abdomen, and swelling of the legs, thighs, and face; sometimes symptoms onset suddenly, with nausea, in which case there is a risk of premature labour. Appropriate action is ②; in the meantime, rest and take one of the remedies below.

Specific remedies to be taken every 15 minutes for up to 6 doses if symptoms onset suddenly
- Fear and apprehension *Aconite 30c*
- Face hot and flushed *Belladonna 30c*

Specific remedies to be taken 4 times daily for up to 7 days if symptoms are of more gradual onset
- Increased breathlessness, puffy legs and face *Arsenicum 6c*
- If symptoms include constipation or frequent urination or vomiting *Nux 6c*
- Symptoms come on after loss of fluid or blood *China 6c*
- If none of the above remedies seems appropriate *Sulphur 6c*

Indigestion during pregnancy see also
HEARTBURN DURING PREGNANCY

Often a feature of late pregnancy, when the digestive tract and its veins and arteries become compressed by the expanding uterus; breathing may also be affected (see RESPIRATORY CHANGES DURING PREGNANCY).

Specific remedies to be taken 15 minutes before meals for up to 3 days
- Remedy of first resort *Nux 6c*
- If Nux does not prevent indigestion, and main problem is bloating and flatulence *China 6c*
- If fatty foods are the problem, with vomiting and lack of thirst, and stuffy rooms make indigestion worse *Pulsatilla 6c*

Infertility

If you have been having regular, unprotected intercourse for 12 months and have not become pregnant, you or your partner may be infertile. Infertility is quite common – one in eight couples researchers say, although a recent GP survey put the figure rather lower, at 3.3 per cent of 35-year-olds – and in most cases can be traced to a specific problem in the woman or the man.

Female infertility may be due to damage to the uterus (from infection or fibroids), to retroversion of the uterus (see UTERUS PROBLEMS), or to the presence of a wall or septum in the uterus, a congenital defect; mucus produced by the cervix may be too viscous for the sperm to penetrate or it may contain antibodies which kill the sperm; one or both Fallopian tubes may be blocked, as the result of gonorrhea (see SEXUALLY TRANSMITTED DISEASES), endometriosis (see UTERUS PROBLEMS), or TUBERCULOSIS; one or both ovaries may be affected by OVARIAN CYSTS or endometriosis, and fail to produce the necessary hormones; or chronic ill health, STRESS or emotional trauma may depress production of follicle stimulating hormone by the hypothalamus and so prevent eggs maturing in the ovaries (see HORMONE IMBALANCES). Investigation will be by physical examination initially, at which time a full medical history will be taken; you may also be asked to keep a temperature chart – a slight rise in temperature in mid-cycle indicates that ovulation is occurring. If ovulation is not the problem, the next step is to take a sample of semen from your cervix shortly after intercourse to see what effect your cervical mucus has on the sperm. If this is not the problem you will be given blood tests to check hormone levels, followed by X-rays and a small operation to see if your Fallopian tubes and ovaries are normal.

Specific remedies to be taken every 12 hours for up to 7 days while waiting for constitutional treatment
- Breasts tender, with areas of hard swelling, desire for sex suppressed for some reason *Conium 30c*
- Tenderness in lower abdomen over right ovary, dry vagina *Lycopodium 30c*
- Previous miscarriages before 12 weeks *Sabina 30c*
- Irregular periods, womb feels as if it is about to drop out of vagina, feeling chilly, weepy, and irritable, aversion to sex *Sepia 30c*

If a pituitary problem has been diagnosed, take *Agnus 6c* up to 3 times daily for 3 weeks out of 4 (if your periods are regular, stop during the week of your period).

Male infertility may be due to a low sperm count (causes include mumps, too much heat around testicles, varicocele, steroids, drugs, alcohol, excessive smoking, lead or carbon-monoxide poisoning, and X-rays), or sperms may be deformed or unable to swim vigorously; testicles or vasa deferentia may be damaged by gonorrhea or syphilis; stress, overwork, tiredness, and psychological factors can case ERECTION PROBLEMS and EJACULATION PROBLEMS.

Diagnosis is by physical examination and history taking; a sample of semen will be needed to check sperm numbers and quality; if no sperm are found, a testicular biopsy (analysis of a small sample of tissue from the testes) may be necessary.

Specific remedies to be taken every 12 hours for up to 7 days while waiting for constitutional treatment
- Ineffectual erection, lack of energy, absent-mindedness *Agnus 30c*
- Inability to sustain erection, cramp and coldness in legs *Conium 30c*
- Increased desire for sex but intercourse spoiled by anticipation of failure, general insecurity *Lycopodium 30c*
- Dragging sensation in genitals, no desire for sex *Sepia 30c*

Self-help If infertility is due to a low sperm count, try to abstain from intercourse in the week leading up to ovulation; this will allow sperm numbers to build up, increasing the chances of conception.

Orthodox treatment of infertility is by drugs – to ensure ovulation, increase sperm production, boost certain hormones and suppress others. There are also various implantation techniques. Occasionally, such drugs result in multiple pregnancy. Some abnormalities can be corrected by surgery. Otherwise, the options are artificial insemination or test-tube fertilization, both of which require careful thought, and considerable effort and commitment.

Before embarking on orthodox treatment, the author advises nutritional therapy (see Preconceptual Care p. 23) and constitutional homeopathic treatment.

---

999 Emergency – call GP (or dial 999) immediately. 2 Consult your doctor if no improvement within 2 hours

Miscarriage

The main causes of miscarriage – defined as losing a baby before 28 weeks – are foetal abnormality, structural problems in the uterus, CERVICAL IN-COMPETENCE, HORMONE IMBALANCES, and falls; however, miscarriage as the result of a fall is rare – the baby is well protected inside the womb. Losing a baby after 28 weeks is, technically speaking, a stillbirth if the baby is dead; a premature baby is a live baby born after 28 weeks but before term.

A miscarriage is inevitable if the foetus dies in the womb; this is technically a *missed miscarriage* if there are no symptoms – and MORNING SICKNESS and fullness in the breasts disappear and at your next check-up your GP will find that your uterus has not increased in size. Usually, however, there are obvious signs – discharge of blood and solid matter from the vagina – and crampy pains in the lower abdomen and back; if part of the foetus is retained in the uterus – this is an *incomplete miscarriage* – pain and bleeding may persist for several days. Scanty brown or bloody discharge at around the time when periods are due is not uncommon; this is a *threatened miscarriage*, but in most cases the baby is not lost and the pregnancy proceeds normally.

Any vaginal bleeding during pregnancy is potentially serious, so best course is ⑫. If bleeding is associated with abdominal pain, ② and give one of the remedies listed under ECTOPIC PREGNANCY. If you pass any solid matter, keep it for the doctor to see. In the meantime, rest. Since it is usually necessary to remove the remains of the foetus and placenta from the uterus under general anaesthetic in order to prevent infection and anaemia, don't eat or drink while waiting to see your GP. Have constitutional homeopathic treatment afterwards.

Specific remedies to be taken every hour for up to 10 doses while waiting to see your GP
- Bleeding and pain after a blow, a fall, or a particularly violent movement *Arnica 30c*
- Feeling feverish, restless, thirsty, and very worried, dry skin *Aconite 30c*
- Steady loss of bright red blood, cramping pains in abdomen, weakness, nausea *Ipecac. 30c*
- Appearance of dark, coagulated blood towards end of third month or at times when periods would normally occur, tearing pain between lower back and vagina, nausea and vomiting, diarrhoea *Sabina 30c*
- Face hot and dry, distended abdomen, bearing down sensation in vagina *Belladonna 30c*
- Feeling very nervous and agitated, unable to sleep, vulva and vagina extremely sensitive *Coffea 30c*
- Intermittent bleeding which is more profuse each time it occurs, blood dark and coagulated, cramping pains *Pulsatilla 30c*
- Profuse discharge of thick, blackish blood, feeling weak, exhausted, and afraid of dying *Secale 30c*
- Missed miscarriage, no symptoms *Sepia 30c* followed by *Coffea 30c*

Morning sickness

Many women, especially first-time mothers, experience nausea and vomiting in the second and third month of pregnancy, and not just in the mornings; symptoms usually wear off by 14–16 weeks, although a few women go on to develop 'hyperemesis', severe vomiting which causes fluid and chemical imbalances and may require hospital treatment.

As a first resort, try the self-help measures below; if these do not help, try one of the homeopathic remedies given below or see your homeopath. If you are vomiting most of your meals, see your GP; anti-vomiting drugs are available, but there is increasing reluctance to prescribe them.

Specific remedies to be taken 2-hourly for up to 3 days
- Nausea worse in morning, vomiting small amounts of food with mucus in them *Nux 6c*
- Non-stop nausea, everything vomited up, liquids and solids *Ipecac. 6c*
- Nausea in evening, wearing off at night *Pulsatilla 6c*
- Nausea a few hours after eating, suddenly vomiting everything *Ferrum 6c*
- Vomit full of milky mucus, especially if temperament is melancholy, irritable, and weepy *Sepia 6c*
- Breasts hard and swollen *Conium 6c*
- Heartburn, keeping nausea at bay by constant eating, getting up at night to eat, aversion to meat and fat, cabbage aggravates symptoms *Petroleum 6c*
- Diarrhoea, burning sensation in abdomen, feeling restless and exhausted *Arsenicum 6c*
- Aversion to bread, fat, and slippery foods, craving for salt, feeling very thirsty *Natrum mur. 6c*
- If none of the above remedies seem appropriate *Sulphur 6c*

Self-help Eat small, frequent meals, avoiding greasy foods, and get plenty of rest. If you feel sick in the mornings, a dry biscuit before you get up might help. Using fresh ginger in cooking can also help. An acupressure device called a Seaband, worn around the wrist, may also be effective (obtainable from Seaband UK, Church Walk, Hinkley, Leics.).

Oedema during pregnancy see
CARDIOVASCULAR PROBLEMS DURING PREGNANCY

Piles during pregnancy see also PILES p. 230
Varicose veins in the rectum and around the anus are related to constipation and pressure of the uterus on the veins of the pelvis (see CONSTIPATION DURING PREGNANCY, CARDIOVASCULAR PROBLEMS DURING PREGNANCY).

Specific remedies to be taken 4 times daily for up to 7 days
- Remedy of first resort *Pulsatilla 6c*

- If Pulsatilla does not work, and if piles are aggravated by drinking wine or coffee and you are constipation-prone, even when not pregnant *Nux 6c*
- Burning, fiery pains in rectum, soothed by heat *Arsenicum 6c*
- Distended veins look bluish, burning pains after passing stools *Carbo veg. 6c*
- Anal fissures with cutting pains *Chamomilla 6c*

Placenta praevia

Condition in which placenta is attached to the wall of the uterus close to the cervical canal rather than higher up; in this position, it can more easily become detached or damaged, causing bleeding (see ANTE-PARTUM HAEMORRHAGE), but no pain; if bleeding is severe, a blood transfusion and an emergency caesarian section may be necessary. However, as uterus grows, placenta is usually pulled upwards, decreasing risk of complications.

Pre-eclamptic toxaemia (PET)

A complication of late pregnancy, associated with raised blood pressure (see CARDIOVASCULAR PROBLEMS). In mild cases, there may be no obvious symptoms apart from raised sphygmomanometer readings. In severe cases, symptoms are headaches, blurred vision, intolerance of light, nausea and vomiting, and swollen ankles due to fluid retention; protein may appear in urine. If blood pressure is not brought under control, the symptoms of eclampsia – convulsions, drowsiness, unconsciousness – develop, threatening the life of mother and baby.

Eclampsia is now rare, thanks to better antenatal care, but PET is quite common, especially in first pregnancies. PET is routinely treated by drugs to lower blood pressure; in some cases it may be necessary to induce the baby early.

If convulsions develop or if other symptoms are severe, (999) and give one of the emergency remedies below. The other remedies given below are interim palliatives only – THEY ARE NO SUBSTITUTE FOR EXPERT MEDICAL CARE.

Specific remedies to be taken every 5 minutes for up to 10 doses while waiting for help
- Face hot, dry, and flushed, staring eyes, congestive headache *Belladonna 30c*
- Severe symptoms accompanied by great fear *Aconite 30c*
- Severe symptoms aggravated by grief *Ignatia 30c*
- Severe symptoms aggravated by fright *Opium 30c*

Specific remedies to be taken 3 times daily for up to 3 days
- Stinging pain in legs, aggravated by heat *Apis 30c*
- Feeling chilly, exhausted, and anxious *Arsenicum 30c*

Self-help The most sensible thing you can do is cut down on salt and rest as much as possible.

Respiratory changes during pregnancy

Respiratory symptoms such as shortness of breath and coughing are not uncommon in the last months of pregnancy, especially if the baby is large and the mother small. Diaphragm and rib movements which pull and push air into and out of the lungs are, to some extent, hampered by upward pressure of the uterus; the lungs also become congested because of pressure on veins and arteries, making gaseous exchange less efficient. Digestion is often affected too, for similar reasons (see INDIGESTION DURING PREGNANCY).

If coughing is severe, (2); in the meantime take *Aconite 30c* every 5 minutes for up to 10 doses, especially if fear is the overwhelming emotion. If you are short of breath even when at rest, [12].

Coughing
Specific remedies to be taken 4 times daily for up to 7 days
- Coughing after meals, shortness of breath *Nux 6c*
- Frequent, dry, exhausting cough which gets worse at night, salty taste in mouth *Sepia 6c*
- Cough accompanied by nausea and vomiting *Ipecac. 6c*
- Cough accompanied by involuntary passing of urine, alleviated by drinking cold water *Causticum 6c*

Shortness of breath
Specific remedies to be taken every 5 minutes for up to 10 doses as soon as symptoms come on
- With palpitations, fainting, fear *Aconite 30c*
- With weakness, swollen ankles, face pale and anguished looking, feeling chilly and restless *Arsenicum 6c*
- With nausea, fainting *Ipecac. 6c*

Rhesus incompatibility

Rhesus factor is one of several factors used to type blood; a mother who is Rh− (Rhesus negative) will make antibodies against her own baby if the baby's blood (and the father's) is Rh+ (Rhesus positive) and mixes with hers during pregnancy; if this happens, the mother's antibodies will start to destroy the baby's red blood cells, and the baby will be born jaundiced (see NEONATAL JAUNDICE). Risks to second or third Rh+ babies are higher, the mother's immune system having been primed by the first.

However, stillbirths and neonatal problems due to Rhesus incompatibility are now rare, thanks to maternal blood tests during pregnancy and to the practice of giving Anti-D serum injections to Rh− mothers of Rh+ babies immediately after delivery (or after MISCARRIAGE, ANTE-PARTUM HAEMORRHAGE, or TERMINATION OF PREGNANCY, which can also result in a mixing of foetal and maternal blood); because Anti-D serum kills Rh+ red blood cells, full-scale antibody production is forestalled.

---

(999) Emergency – call GP (or dial 999) immediately. (2) Consult your doctor if no improvement within 2 hours

Rubella (German measles) during pregnancy see also RUBELLA p. 330

Can cause congenital defects (see BIRTH DEFECTS) if contracted during the first trimester of pregnancy; can be prevented by immunization at age of 13, though immunization is not necessary if you have already had the disease and therefore have immunity to it; immunity can be confirmed by a blood test, a wise precaution since many viruses produce symptoms similar to those of German measles. Conception should be avoided for 3 months after immunization.

If you become pregnant and have not had German measles/been immunized, take *Rubella nosode 30c* immediately, 3 doses at 12-hour intervals to begin with, then 1 dose every 3 weeks until you are past the 12th week of pregnancy.

If you contract German measles during pregnancy, you may wish to consider a TERMINATION OF PREGNANCY; you should discuss this with your GP.

Skin changes during pregnancy

These are caused by raised hormone levels; if neither of the remedies below seems suitable, see remedies given under ACNE and CHLOASMA.

Specific remedies to be taken 4 times daily for up to 7 days
- Brown/dirty yellow freckling over bridge of nose *Sepia 6c*
- Skin dry, itchy, hot, and scurfy, made worse by washing *Sulphur 6c*

Sleep problems during pregnancy see also SLEEP PROBLEMS pp. 121–3

ANXIETY about pregnancy and birth, HEARTBURN, the urge to urinate, general discomfort, the baby kicking . . . all of these can break sleep during pregnancy; then worrying about not sleeping makes sleeping more difficult, and so a vicious circle is set up.

Specific remedies to be taken before going to bed for up to 5 nights and hourly if still awake
- Over-excitement, mental over-stimulation, excessive joy *Coffea 30c*
- Feeling you will never get to sleep again, especially after some form of grief *Ignatia 30c*
- Feeling very afraid *Aconite 30c*

Self-help If you cannot get comfortable in bed, tuck a pillow under your abdomen, into the small of your back, between your knees, or wherever you feel you need support. For other self-help measures see pp. 122–3. If you still cannot sleep, don't be tempted to take sleeping pills, especially in the first 16 weeks of pregnancy; get up and read a book or do housework, and make up for lost sleep later, enlisting your partner's help if necessary.

Termination of pregnancy

As the law now stands, termination is illegal unless two doctors agree that it is necessary for one of the following reasons: the baby is abnormal; there is a risk to the physical or mental health of the baby; the health of the mother or of other children may be jeopardized if the pregnancy continues. Termination is also illegal after 28 weeks.

If pregnancy is unwanted and bringing up a child yourself is totally unfeasible, you have two choices: termination or adoption. Adoption preserves life; on the other hand, pregnancy and labour are not without risks, the baby has to be given up shortly after birth, and you may come to regret that you took no part in his or her growing up. Termination also has its pros and cons; it is less risky than carrying a baby to term, although there is a slight risk of CERVICAL INCOMPETENCE in subsequent pregnancies; guilt, sometimes severe, is a common reaction.

If your GP is not sympathetic to termination, the British Pregnancy Advisory Service, Family Planning Association, Brook Advisory Centre, or National Council for One-Parent Families (addresses pp. 385, 384) will give you all the advice and information you need.

Termination involves a D and C (dilation and curettage, or suction removal of the contents of the womb); this is a 15-minute procedure done under general anaesthetic and seldom involves a hospital stay of more than 12 hours.

Specific remedies to be taken every 4 hours for up to 3 days after operation
- Feeling very upset, with lump in throat and tight feeling around chest *Ignatia 30c*
- Where symptoms are more physical – i.e. abdominal pain, cystitis *Staphisagria 30c*

Toothache during pregnancy see also TOOTHACHE p. 169

The best preventive is good dental care and adequate calcium before conception and during pregnancy.

Specific remedy to be taken as required for up to 10 doses
- *Sepia 6c*

Urinary problems during pregnancy

These are usually caused by pressure on the bladder, urethra, and pelvic floor muscles, and can be aggravated by tight jeans, non-cotton underwear, bubble baths, etc.

Cystitis causes a burning sensation on passing water and a frequent urge to urinate. If none of the remedies given below seems appropriate, more remedies – and self-help measures – are given under CYSTITIS pp. 233–4.

Specific remedies to be taken up to 2-hourly for up to 3 days

---

- At first sign of discomfort, especially if weather is cold and windy and you are feverish, restless, and apprehensive *Aconite 30c*
- Slightest tension causes leakage of urine, scalding sensation during and after urination, lack of thirst, heat and lying down make discomfort worse *Pulsatilla 6c*
- Bladder and urethra feel itchy and irritable, dribbles of urine passed frequently and with some difficulty *Nux 6c*
- Urge to pass urine most frequent at night, burning and soreness after passing urine, urgency, urine copious and almost colourless *Sulphur 6c*
- Passing copious amount of cloudy urine at frequent intervals, burning sensation, urge to pass urine most frequent at night *Phosphoric ac. 6c*
- A bad attack of cystitis, with constant burning and urgency *Catharis 30c*

Incontinence of urine during pregnancy is due to extra strain on the muscles which close the sphincter from the bladder. See INCONTINENCE OF URINE and STRESS INCONTINENCE for more information.

Specific remedies to be taken 4 times daily for up to 14 days
- Remedy of first resort *Pulsatilla 6c*
- Bearing down sensation as if contents of womb are about to fall out of vagina *Sepia 6c*
- Incontinence made worse by coughing *Causticum 6c*

Retention of urine (see also RETENTION OF URINE p. 238) is not uncommon in later pregnancy, and tends to come on gradually; urine flow becomes scantier, with intermittent pain in the bladder area; scanty flow can also contribute to cystitis (above). If pain becomes severe and urination impossible, ②; your GP will pass a small tube called a catheter into the bladder to drain off the urine. The remedies given below are only suitable in the early stages of retention, when urination starts to become difficult.

Specific remedies to be taken ½-hourly for up to 10 doses
- Remedy of first resort *Nux 30c*
- If Nux does not bring relief *Pulsatilla 30c*

Varicose veins during pregnancy see CARDIOVASCULAR PROBLEMS DURING PREGNANCY

CHILDBIRTH AND POST-NATAL PROBLEMS

MORE and more women today feel that birth should not be a high-tech affair unless there are definite indications for it. Hospitals are notoriously unrelaxed, noisy, insensitive places in which to give birth, but they have their merits. The author saw a young mother in her second pregnancy nearly die because the womb inverted as the placenta was delivered; this is very rare and could not possibly have been foreseen, but the mother would certainly have died if she had been at home.

The ideal solution would be to make hospitals homelier and more responsive to real need. In special birthing units mothers could be attended by their own midwife, give birth in the way which suits them rather than the hospital, and have members of their family present at the birth if they wish. Emergency medical help would be available within minutes.

If complications are expected, it is best to have the baby in hospital. If you have strong views on specific procedures or specific drugs, approach your consultant at some point during the antenatal period – do this privately if you cannot get to see him or her on the NHS – and make your wishes clear. This is also the time to ask if there would be any objection to your using homeopathic remedies; these will not interfere with any drugs you may be given.

First stage of labour In the last week or so of pregnancy the baby's head slides down into the pelvis – this relieves pressure on the diaphragm and stomach but increases pressure on the bladder and rectum – and the whole vulval area becomes moister. You will probably have felt twinges of pain (see FALSE PAINS) in the last few weeks of pregnancy, but as labour approaches these will become more insistent, more frequent, and more regular; you may also feel trembly and chilly. Now is the time to telephone your GP or the hospital. A sure sign that labour has started is the 'show', a discharge of blood and fluid as the protective plug of tissue in the cervix is shed. At the same time or shortly afterwards the membranes around the baby may rupture, resulting in a trickle or sudden flood of fluid, the 'waters'. As labour proceeds, your pulse will become harder and faster, and your mouth may feel dry; restlessness, nausea, and sometimes vomiting are quite common, especially at transition, where things may come to a halt before second stage begins.

During this first stage of labour the cervix or neck of the uterus opens and is pulled upwards so that uterus, cervix, and vagina form a single tube or 'birth canal'.

Once in hospital you will be given a vaginal examination to assess how close you are to giving birth, and possibly an enema to empty your bowels; the old-fashioned habit of shaving the pubic hair is not necessary to prevent infection.

This first stage of labour usually lasts about 12 hours in a first pregnancy and 6 hours in a second, but there are no hard and fast rules; sometimes the first stage takes up to 24 hours, sometimes a few minutes.

Second stage of labour This usually lasts an hour or so in first pregnancies, and about half an hour the second or third time around. Contractions become stronger and you feel the urge to push; push with the contractions and rest between them. If your bowels feel as if they are going to open, this is because the baby's head is pushing against your rectum; don't let this stop you from pushing. As the head comes down the birth canal and is ready to escape from the pelvis, go into panting respiration. The midwife or other helper will control the head so that it slips through the vagina without stretching it too much or causing splitting. If there is a fear that the vagina will be badly torn, you may need an episiotomy (an incision in the skin of the vagina under local anaesthetic). However with good control and gentle massage of the vaginal skin an episiotomy is often not necessary, though in some cases it is to the advantage of mother and baby; this is something you should discuss with the midwife or consultant beforehand.

Once the head emerges, the shoulders and body soon follow. The baby can then be delivered on to your tummy. Breathing is started by clearing the baby's airways of mucus and tipping his or her head down. The cord need not be clamped and cut until it has stopped pulsating, unless it is round the baby's neck.

Third stage of labour This takes another 30 minutes or so, and is marked by an increase in bleeding, as the placenta or 'afterbirth' is delivered. The midwife usually pulls gently on the cord while pushing gently on the womb. You may be given an injection of Syntometrine (derived from the same source as the homeopathic remedy Secale) to make the womb contract and prevent excessive bleeding. This is a good time to bond with the baby, have a quiet cuddle and offer the breast.

Baby check Immediately after birth the midwife or doctor will check to see that your baby is all right, although a more thorough check will be done later. The baby's facial features will be checked for Down's syndrome, genitals inspected for doubtful sex, and fingers and toes counted; the back will be checked for signs of spina bifida (hairy patches or missing skin at the base of the spine), and the navel for signs of diaphragmatic hernia; the anus will be examined to make sure that it is open; a finger will be put in the baby's mouth to check for cleft palate; hips and feet will be checked for congenital dislocation or club foot.

After the birth Once the baby has been settled, you will be washed or asked to take a shower. Bathing your vaginal area with Arnica solution (10 drops of mother tincture to 0.25 litre [½ pint] warm water) will take away some of the soreness and promote healing. After that you should be allowed to sleep, or at least be very quiet and tranquil. At this time well-meaning visitors and telephone calls can be very exhausting.

You will probably not feel very hungry for a day or two. Thin vegetable soup is good on the first day, with salads and fruit on the second, and a return to your normal diet on the third. Tea, coffee, chamomile tea, and wine are best avoided. The most important nutrients in the weeks after birth are iron (to make up for lost blood), protein (to aid healing), and calcium (if you are breastfeeding). To get back into shape, cut down on starchy foods.

A mixture of blood, fluid, and mucus are discharged from the womb in the days immediately following delivery. After pains are common at this time, and tend to be worse if labour has been relatively easy. It is quite normal to feel very weary and stiff. Some women also find themselves perspiring at lot. Within 12–15 days the womb returns to its normal size. After an episiotomy or a tear, the vulva and vagina will take several weeks to heal.

Periods usually restart 6–8 weeks after delivery, but may not reappear for several months, especially if you are breastfeeding. If you are worried, see your GP.

Breastfeeding Breast milk contains, in ideal proportions, everything your baby needs – not only carbohydrates, proteins, fats, vitamins, and minerals, but also antibodies against many infections, including those which cause diarrhoea. In Western countries breastfeeding tends to prevent obesity; in many Third World countries it prevents the opposite marasmus or wasting diseases. There is mounting evidence too that breastfeeding for the first 4–6 months helps to prevent allergy-formation, especially if there is a family history of allergy. Cot deaths, constipation, intestinal obstruction, hypocalcaemic convulsions and tooth decay also occur less frequently in breast-fed babies than in bottle-fed. Child abuse is also less common, probably because of the strong emotional bond which grows out of the physical contact between mother and baby. From the mother's point of view the breast is much cheaper than the bottle and always handy. Lactation also helps to balance her hormone secretions.

Bottled milk contains additives such as pH adjusters, anti-oxidants, carageen, hydroxypropyl starch, emulsifiers, and thickening agents. Though some constituents – zinc for example – are in the same proportion as those found in breast milk, they are less well absorbed.

Try to breastfeed in the first 24 hours if you can, because this is the most sensitive time for your baby. Your milk will be very watery to begin with, but rich in protective antibodies. As your baby sucks on the pigmented area around the nipple messages go to your pituitary gland telling it to produce oxytocin, a hormone which stimulates the glands in your breasts to produce milk. Proper milk comes in on the second or third day, at which time you may experience sudden chills or notice that blood and fluid loss becomes scantier.

For explanation of other symbols, see page 107

Feed on demand if you can, otherwise your milk production may drop or cease altogether. Breastfeeding is not a reliable means of contraception though, even if you are feeding on demand, so if you need contraception, see your GP. Combined oral contraceptives should be avoided as they interfere with the volume and composition of breast milk.

If you cannot breastfeed, don't feel guilty or despairing about it, but have a really good try first. Not everyone takes to breastfeeding like a duck to water. There is a knack to it, so don't be afraid to ask your nurse or midwife what to do or contact the La Leche League (addresss p. 384). If the bottle turns out to be best, you can always kick your partner out of bed in the middle of the night to feed junior!

Breastfeeding problems

Failure to breast feed Very full breasts are difficult for the baby to suck; if this is the case, expressing some milk before feeding will solve the problem. Sometimes the milk is too watery or it may have a salty or bitter taste which the baby does not like; this can be due to emotional problems in the mother, or maternal malnutrition, or the mother may be taking salty or strongly spiced foods, strong tea, chamomile tea, or drugs, which give an odd taste to her milk. Sometimes the mother needs to be nurtured by another female figure (her own mother, for example) before she can produce enough milk. Difficulties may also increase with successive babies. Constitutional homeopathic treatment can sometimes help, but in the meantime one of the remedies below should be tried.

Baby refusing milk or vomiting

Specific remedies to be taken 4 times daily for up to 3 days
- Poor quality milk, mother large and prone to chills and sweats *Calcarea 30c*
- If downward movements while nursing cause baby to scream *Borax 30c*
- If baby is thin, with a large, sweaty head, and vomits after feeds *Silicea 30c*
- Sudden excessive milk production in a young, healthy mother *Aconite 30c*
- Breasts hard and swollen *Bryonia 30c*
- Overproduction of milk, mother young, timid, and weepy *Pulsatilla 30c*

Engorgement If the baby refuses to feed or if you decide to stop breastfeeding the breasts can become painfully distended with milk. Expressing milk provides immediate relief, but one of the remedies below should also be taken.

Specific remedies to be taken every 4 hours until engorgement passes
- Feeling weepy and sensitive to cold, hating to be in stuffy rooms *Pulsatilla 30c*

- Extreme sensitivity to cold, cold sweats, tendency to be overweight *Calcarea 30c*

Exhaustion from breastfeeding is an unusual reaction, but can occur because of the fluid loss which breast feeding entails. In addition to the remedy below you could try expressing some milk so that your partner can give one of the night feeds.

Specific remedy to be taken every 4 hours for up to 10 doses
- *China 30c*

Hardness of the breasts

Specific remedies to be taken every hour for up to 10 doses
- Suspected breast abscess or mastitis *Bryonia 30c*
- Suspected breast abscess or mastitis, with red streaks on skin *Belladonna 30c*
- If neither Bryonia nor Belladonna help *Calcarea 30c*

Loss of milk

Specific remedies to be taken 4 times daily for up to 3 days
- Remedy of first resort if milk production stops *Agnus 6c*
- If Agnus fails and milk stops after exposure to cold, breasts swollen, sore, and sensitive *Dulcamara 6c*
- If Dulcamara fails *Pulsatilla 6c*
- If due to grief *Ignatia 6c*
- If due to anger *Chamomilla 6c*
- If due to shock or fright *Aconite 30c*
- If due to jealousy *Hyoscyamus 6c*
- If due to extreme joy *Coffea 6c*

Sore or cracked nipples After each feed bathe the nipples with Arnica solution (10 drops mother tincture to 0.25 litre [½ pint] boiled cooled water), then dry them thoroughly and apply Calendula cream (from chemist or health food shop). One of the remedies below should also be taken.

Specific remedies to be taken every 4 hours for up to 6 doses
- Nipples inflamed and very tender to the touch *Chamomilla 6c*
- Sore nipples, especially if associated with grief *Ignatia 6c*
- Sore nipples, especially if mother is timid and weepy *Pulsatilla 6c*
- Pain and soreness made worse by exposure to cold *Aconite 6c*
- Cracked nipples which cause smarting, burning pain *Sulphur 6c*
- Nipples cracked and sore, with blisters on them *Graphites 6c*
- Cracked nipples associated with plentiful milk production and distended breasts, although milk is poor and baby dislikes it *Calcarea 6c*
- Ulcerated nipples *Silicea 6c*

Delayed periods after childbirth

Periods usually restart within 6–8 weeks of birth, but may be delayed for several months if you are breast feeding on demand. Orthodox treatment is to give drugs to stimulate ovulation or recommend a D and C to make sure that none of the products of conception remain in the womb. Before such measures are taken, try one or other of the remedies below.

Specific remedies to be taken every 12 hours for up to 7 days
- Lack of thirst, weepiness, feeling worse in hot, stuffy surroundings *Pulsatilla 30c*
- Feeling chilly, tired, depressed, irritable, and turned off by sex, constipated *Sepia 30c*

Emergency childbirth

If labour comes on suddenly and proceeds very fast (see description of labour pp. 292–3), and there is no time to get the mother to hospital, you must be prepared to deliver the baby yourself. Don't panic – birth is a natural event and in most cases proceeds perfectly normally with only minimum assistance from those in attendance.

Make sure the room is warm, and put fresh sheets on the bed, with a large plastic sheet underneath to keep the mattress clean. Up to 0.5 litre (1 pint) of blood and fluids will be lost during the birth; this is quite normal. Boil a pair of scissors and a length of string to sterilize them. Wash your hands thoroughly, taking care to scrub under your finger nails.

The baby's head will appear first, followed by the shoulders. As soon as the shoulders are out, support the head, but do not pull on it or the umbilical cord. Once the body and legs have emerged, gently wipe the mucus away from the nose and mouth and tip the baby's head downwards. This should start the baby breathing, but if it doesn't do so within 1 minute, begin artificial respiration (see First Aid pp. 87–7).

Once the cord stops pulsating, tie it with the sterilized string in two places, one about 10 cm (4 in) away from the baby's tummy and the other about 20 cm (8 in) away;) then cut the cord between the pieces of string with the sterilized scissors. Swaddle the baby in a clean sheet and give him or her to the mother to hold.

Within about 30 minutes of the birth, the placenta should appear; gently massage the mother's stomach to assist delivery of the placenta, but do not pull on the cord. If bleeding continues after delivery of the placenta, (999), give reassurance, and massage the mother's stomach every few minutes until help arrives.

Once the placenta has been delivered and the baby has settled, encourage the mother to take a shower, and bathe the whole vulval area with Arnica solution (10 drops of mother tincture to 0.25 litre [½ pint] warm water). If there are large tears in vulva or near back passage, suturing will be necessary.

Homeopathic remedies during emergency childbirth The remedies listed below represent only a small proportion of those traditionally used by homeopaths to assist childbirth, but they should be used only if no other help is available. Prolonged or difficult labour requires medical attention.

Contractions

Specific remedies to be given every 17 minutes for up to 7 doses
- Moderate or severe back pain, bearing down sensation on cervix, no dilation *Coffea 6c*
- Sensation of constant pressure in womb, constant bearing down sensation, forcing pains, mother very distressed *Secale 6c*
- Mother very restless, chilly, and tearful, labour very slow *Pulsatilla 6c*
- Severe pains which suddenly cease, with cervix undilated, urge to pass urine or stool *Nux 6c*

Prolonged labour

Specific remedies to be given every 15 minutes for up to 7 doses
- Mother exhausted, muscles of uterus no longer able to push, death of baby suspected *Secale 6c*
- Severe backache, muscles of uterus exhausted, mother of strong constitution, or if death of baby is suspected *Pulsatilla 6c*
- Pain stops suddenly due to emotional upset, face red, hot, and puffy *Opium 6c*
- Mother delirious *Hyscyamus 6c*

Labour pains see also EMERGENCY CHILDBIRTH
Psychoprophylactic techniques, especially breathing techniques, learnt at antenatal classes help many women to control pain during labour. In hospital, pain control options include nitrous oxide gas and air, a local anaesthetic if forceps delivery is necessary, or an epidural (injection of anaesthetic into the space around the lower part of the spinal cord). The danger with an epidural is that the mother may not be able to push properly, so the baby may have to be delivered by forceps; the mother may also have a violent headache afterwards and low blood pressure. The drug Pethidine is sometimes given, but not immediately before birth as it can cause respiratory distress in the baby and make the mother very spaced out.

Hypnotherapy and acupuncture deserve wider use in labour – for information, contact addresses on p. 386 – but they are not widely available yet. Homeopathic remedies are more widely accepted. Those most commonly used are listed below, but there are many others; if possible, consult your homeopath beforehand.

Specific remedies to be given every 5 minutes for up to 10 doses
- Labour proceeding normally but contractions so violent they are almost unbearable, woman cries out with pain, and is nervous and restless between contractions *Coffea 30c*
- Pains accompanied by frequent urge to pass water or stool, woman very irritable and impatient *Nux 30c*
- Woman in great anguish, talking incoherently, limbs twitching, eyes staring *Belladonna 30c*

Specific remedies to be taken after an epidural
- *Arnica 30c* ½-hourly for up to 7 doses, followed by *Hypericum 6c* every 4 hours for up to 5 days

Malpresentation
Normally babies emerge from the birth canal with their face pointing towards the mother's back; malpresentation occurs when the baby faces forwards or fails to turn into the head-down position in the last few weeks of pregnancy. The face-forward or occipito-posterior position usually causes prolonged labour and severe backache, 'backache labour'; the buttocks-down or 'breech' position can make delivery extremely difficult since the buttocks do not enlarge the birth canal sufficiently for the head to follow easily. In these and other forms of malpresentation the baby may have to be delivered by Caesarean.

Specific remedy to be given hourly for up 3 doses
- *Pulsatilla 30c*

Post-delivery problems
After pains These are a sign that the womb is contracting back to its normal size; discomfort tends to be worse if labour has been relatively easy. If the remedies below produce no improvement within 24 hours, contact your GP or midwife; if you begin to run a temperature, [12].

Specific remedies to be taken every 2 hours for up to 10 doses
- Sharp pains, especially if woman is over-sensitive and has lost a lot of sleep *Coffea 6c*
- Pains associated with frequent urge to pass water or stool *Nux 6c*
- Pains made worse by drinking coffee *Chamomilla 6c*
- If part of placenta has been retained *Pulsatilla 6c*

Appetite changes Strange cravings or difficulty controlling appetite in the weeks immediately after delivery are due to hormone changes, as pregnancy ends and lactation begins.

Specific remedies to be taken every 12 hours for up to 3 days
- Craving for salt and salty foods *Natrum mur. 30c*
- Craving for sweets and sugary foods *Lycopodium 30c*
- Indigestion after fatty foods *Pulsatilla 30c*

If you are having difficulty losing weight, increase the amount of exercise you take, and reduce your salt, fat, and carbohydrate intake. Constitutional homeopathic treatment is recommended, but in the meantime one of the remedies below may help.

Specific remedies to be taken 4 times a day for up to 7 days
- Insatiable appetite, feeling hotter than usual, diarrhoea first thing in morning *Sulphur 6c*
- Not losing weight, constipation, feeling chilly, irritable, and apathetic *Sepia 6c*
- Fluid retention and a craving for salt *Natrum mur. 6c*
- Not losing weight, especially if woman tends to be pale, chilly, sweaty, and clumsy *Calcarea 6c*

Constipation

Specific remedies to be taken every 4 hours for up to 10 doses
- Ineffectual straining to pass stool *Nux 6c*
- Stools hard, brown/black, and burnt-looking *Bryonia 6c*
- Feeling chilly, exhausted, and irritable as well as constipated *Sepia 6c*

Discharge from uterus (lochia) Following delivery of the placenta, a quantity of blood, fluids and mucus is discharged from the womb, pure blood at first, and then a milky mixture of mucus and fluid. If discharge is very scanty or very copious, see your midwife; in the meantime try one of the remedies below.

Specific remedies to be taken every hour for up to 10 doses
- Scanty discharge, red in colour, made even scantier by strong emotions or exposure to cold *Aconite 30c*
- Scanty discharge, diarrhoea, abdominal pain, headache or toothache *Chamomilla 30c*
- Scanty discharge, distended abdomen *Colocynth 30c*
- Scanty discharge, delirious behaviour *Belladonna 30c*
- Scanty discharge, desire for sex *Platinum 30c*
- Copious bloody discharge *Secale 30c*
- If no response to Secale and whole vulval area is extremely sensitive *Platinum 30c*
- Discharge very slow *Calcarea 30c*
- Discharge very slow, woman feels worn out *China 30c*
- Excessive discharge after over-exertion *Arnica 30c*
- Profuse discharge made worse by chamomile tea *Coffea 30c*
- Profuse discharge made worse by coffee and alcohol *Nux 30c*
- Profuse milky discharge *Pulsatilla 30c*
- Profuse milky discharge which then becomes bloody *Calcarea 30c*

- Bearing down sensation in womb, milky discharge which becomes streaked with pus, or feeling generally chilly, with cold, clammy extremities *Sepia 30c*
- Sweating, increased saliva, offensive-smelling discharge, sensitivity to heat and cold *Mercurius 30c*
- Excessive milky discharge with putrid smell *Carbo an. 30c*

Exhaustion The effort of giving birth leaves most women extremely tired and stiff and very drained emotionally; this is perfectly normal. Rest and quiet are the best healers. However, one of the remedies below may be helpful; if there is no improvement within 3 days, and there are no complications, consult your homeopath.

Specific remedies to be taken 4 times daily for up to 3 days
- Exhaustion follows profuse sweating or loss of blood *China 30c*
- Exhaustion accompanied by profuse sweating *Carbo veg. 30c*
- Exhaustion accompanied by hair loss *Calcarea 30c*
- Distended abdomen, bearing down pains *Sepia 30c*
- Distended abdomen, spasmodic abdominal pain *Colocynth 30c*

Incontinence Bladder control may temporarily be lost as the result of trauma to the muscles of the pelvic floor. Stopping and starting the flow of urine several times as you pass water will help to tighten these muscles. If, despite these exercises and taking the remedy below, there is no improvement within 3 days, see your homeopath.

Specific remedy to be taken 4 times daily for up to 3 days
- *Belladonna 30c*

Injury to vulva or vagina Overstretching, tears, or incisions and stitches in this area should be bathed three or four times a day with Arnica solution (10 drops of mother tincture to 0.25 litre [½ pint] warm water) to aid healing.

Piles These are the result of extreme pressure on the pelvic veins. If the remedy below produces no improvement within 3 days, see your homeopath.

Specific remedy to be taken every 4 hours for up to 3 days
- *Pulsatilla 6c*

Post-maturity
The risks of stillbirth and brain damage rise significantly after 40 weeks in utero; if the placenta starts to fail, the baby may die from lack of oxygen; lack of oxygen can also cause brain damage. Since the baby's head is also larger and harder than normal, labour is often more difficult, making forceps delivery or Caesarean section more likely. Constitutional homeopathic treatment is recommended, but if there are lots of 'false' pains after 41 weeks, take *Caulophyllum 30c* every 12 hours for 3 doses.

Post-natal depression see also DEPRESSION
Many women feel 'down' after giving birth, and for many reasons – hormonal changes, tiredness (possibly due to a drop in blood sugar levels), previous episodes of post-natal depression, strains within the marriage or relationship, anxiety about coping with a new baby, financial problems, the sudden realisation that life has changed for good. . . In a few women such feelings, initially a natural response to a new situation, last for much longer than a few weeks and seriously undermine their ability to cope. Symptoms include tiredness, an increase or decrease in appetite, feeling that one is a failure, feeling very aggressive towards the baby when he or she cries and guilty afterwards, withdrawing from family, friends, and all forms of social contact, and not least feeling that everything is unreal, that the whole world is made of cardboard. A few women completely lose touch with reality, in which case their behaviour can be said to be psychotic (see PSYCHOTIC ILLNESS) rather than depressed; if this happens ② and give *Aconite 30c* ½-hourly until help arrives. Otherwise, select a remedy from the list below; if there is no improvement within a week or so, seek constitutional treatment from an experienced homeopath or see your GP.

Specific remedies to be taken 4 times daily for up to 3 days
- Not interested in anything, sex least of all, feeling tired, irritable, and chilly, constipated, yellow-brown discoloration across bridge of nose, morale very good during pregnancy but very low afterwards *Sepia 30c*
- Talking excitedly and incoherently, face red and flushed, eyes staring *Belladonna 30c*
- Persistent obscene thoughts, unusual talkativeness and suspicion, inappropriate laughter, breaking off encounters abruptly and running away *Hyoscyamus 30c*
- Depression brought on by grief *Ignatia 30c*
- Feeling very weepy, not at all thirsty, and worse for heat *Pulsatilla 30c*
- Woman withdrawn, irritable, full of guilt and resentment, refuses to be consoled or comforted, says she just wants to be left alone *Natrum mur. 30c*

Self-help Mild post-natal depression can be helped by getting more sleep, and by getting out of the house away from the baby. Don't bottle up your feelings; talk things over with a confidante. Taking extra zinc and trying the Blood Sugar Levelling Diet for a month or so might also help.

Post-partum haemorrhage
In hospital the drug Syntometrine (derived from the same source as Secale) is given to staunch bleeding

after delivery. If you are not in hospital, (999) and take one of the remedies below.

Specific remedies to be taken every 5 minutes for up to 10 doses

- Remedy of first resort *Secale 30c*
- Blood dark and clotted, labour pains continue *Pulsatilla 30c*
- Profuse bleeding, backache which feels like period pain, tingling sensation in vagina, body feels as if it is getting larger *Crocus 30c*
- Exhaustion from blood loss during labour *China 30c*
- Continuous, profuse bleeding, bright red blood, nausea and vomiting, feeling cold and clammy, gasping for breath *Ipecac. 30c*
- Dark clots of blood lost intermittently, haemorrhage associated with outburst of anger *Chamomilla 30c*
- Bright red blood which clots easily, pulse hard and full, face burning hot *Ferrum 30c*
- Slightest movement causes bleeding, blood mixed with fluid, blood dark and clotted as well as bright red *Sabina 30c*
- Profuse bleeding with intermittent after pains, blood hot and bright red, feeling of pressure in abdomen *Belladonna 30c*

Premature birth
Birth before 37 weeks can be caused by conditions such as PRE-ECLAMPTIC TOAXAEMIA, PLACENTA PRAEVIA, ANTE-PARTUM HAEMORRHAGE, and HIGH BLOOD PRESSURE DURING PREGNANCY but in many cases the cause is not known. Premature babies are at risk of RESPIRATORY DISTRESS SYNDROME and NEO-NATAL JAUNDICE due to the immaturity of their lungs and liver; nevertheless even babies of 26 weeks can be viable, given intensive care. If labour begins several weeks before you expect it, (999); in some cases, drugs are given to relax the uterus and prevent labour. If the delivery goes ahead, take *Aconite 30c* four times daily for up to 7 days afterwards

Puerperal fever
This is caused by infection of the genital tract shortly after birth, although any fever within 2 weeks of childbirth is dangerous since it can cause INFERTILITY or SEPTICAEMIA. Puerperal fever is now rare thanks to improved hygiene during delivery and of course antibiotics. However, if you begin to run a tempera-ture, [12], and take one of the remedies below.

Specific remedies to be taken every hour for up to 10 doses

- Sudden rise in temperature, skin hot and dry, pain in uterus, vivid thoughts about dying *Aconite 30c*
- Sudden onset of fever, face hot and red, eyes staring, delirium, distended abdomen, great thirst, bowels feel as if they are being clutched by a giant hand *Belladonna 30c*

- Profuse sweating, great sensitivity to heat and cold, offensive-smelling discharge from vagina, increase in saliva, mucus or blood in stools, symptoms worse at night *Mercurius 30c*
- Vaginal discharge suddenly stops, constipation, nausea and vomiting, irritability *Nux 30c*
- Womb feels very sore, slightest movement aggra-vates soreness, irritability, feeling very apprehensive and pessimistic about the future *Bryonia 30c*

Retained placenta
Normally the placenta is shed within about half an hour of birth, or sooner if the drug Syntometrine is given; if retained for more than an hour, it may have to be removed by hand under general anaesthetic. The homeopathic remedies below aid contraction of the womb and expulsion of the placenta.

Specific remedies to be given every 5 minutes for up to 10 doses

- Intermittent bleeding, retention of urine, lower abdomen hot, red, sore, and painful to the touch, especially if woman is of a mild, tearful disposition *Pulsatilla 30c*
- Bearing down sensation continues, pains strong and continuous but ineffectual, muscles of uterus no longer able to contract, woman throws bedclothes off and craves fresh air *Secale 30c*
- Vagina feels dry and hot, profuse bleeding, woman red in face, moaning, very distressed, and sensitive to slightest jarring *Belladonna 30c*
- Vulva and vagina extremely sensitive, severe cramp-ing pains in abdomen, constant ooze of dark blood *Platinum 30c*

Sex after childbirth
Intercourse should not be resumed until the vagina has healed; this takes at least 10 days, and several weeks after a tear or an episiotomy. However, many couples prefer to wait for at least 6 weeks, when a full post-natal check-up is routinely done. The vagina will be very sensitive at first, and possibly dry, in which case a lubricant such as KY jelly should be used. Pelvic floor exercises will help to tone up the muscles around the vagina; when you pass water, try to stop and restart the flow of urine several times. Many factors can cause loss of libido at this time – pain, lack of sleep, emotional exhaustion, anxiety, fear of another pregnancy. . . It is possible to become pregnant again even before your periods restart, so some form of contraception will be necessary for a few months even if you are planning to have another baby; breastfeeding cannot be relied on to prevent ovulation.

The remedies listed below are helpful in that they boost energy levels generally. However, if loss of libido persists for more than a few months, constitutional homeopathic treatment should be sought; if the problem lies in the relationship between you and your partner, sexual counselling might be more helpful (addresses p. 385).

Specific remedies to be taken every 12 hours for up to 2 weeks

- Feeling very battered, bruised, and low in energy *Arnica 30c*
- Feeling exhausted after loss of blood, sweat, or other body fluids *China 30c*

- Feeling emotionally fragile and weepy, especially in stuffy rooms *Pulsatilla 30c*
- Aversion to sex, chilliness, irritability, depression *Sepia 30c*

Stretch marks (striae)

The best treatment for these is Vitamin E (100 units a day for 5 days a week) for up to 3 months; you could also try Calc. Fluor tissue salts, 3 tablets 3 times a day for 5 days a week for up to 3 months.

SPECIAL PROBLEMS IN INFANTS

THERE can be little doubt that breast feeding gives a baby the best possible start in life. However, milk is not 'let down' immediately a baby is born. For three days or so after birth the breasts secrete a clear, yellowish fluid called colostrum, which gives the baby valuable antibodies and hormones. The baby's sucking causes extra large amounts of a hormone called oxytocin to be released from the pituitary; this stimulates milk production and also helps the walls of the uterus to contract.

The balance of minerals, vitamins, and proteins in cow's milk is not ideal for babies. It contains many times more sodium, potassium, magnesium, calcium, and phosphorus than the baby needs, three times as much protein, which overtaxes acid secretion in the baby's stomach, resulting in indigestion and a proliferation of harmful bacteria, and only a third of the Vitamin C and a tenth of the Vitamin D.

At birth the the head is very large compared with the body – about a quarter of body length is head. This is because the brain develops well in advance of the body. At birth the brain weighs about a quarter of its adult weight, at six months about 50 per cent, and at twelve months about 60 per cent. By contrast, birth weight is only 5 per cent of young adult weight, although this doubles within six months and triples within twelve. Head circumference is measured 3–4 days after birth and serves as a baseline for growth and for detecting any abnormalities.

The pace of brain development is most easy to observe in the way a baby looks at things. In the first few weeks, a baby sees and reacts to objects about 20 cm (8 in) away from the face. By the age of three months the eyes are sufficiently coordinated to be able to track slowly moving objects, provided they are no more than 30 cm (12 in) away. At four months full accommodation or focusing occurs. At six months objects are watched with great attention until they disappear from sight and are then 'forgotten'; the realization that people and things continue to exist when the eye can no longer see them comes much later. At twelve months a baby recognizes familiar people as soon as they come within a range of 6 m (20 ft).

Even newborn babies 'corner' their eyes towards certain sounds. In tests babies have shown themselves to be far more sensitive to the human voice than to pure tones and household noises; in other words they possess an innate ability to distinguish speech sounds from other sounds, an ability fundamental to language acquisition. The first recognizable syllables, usually produced towards the end of the first year, are preceded by burbling and babbling as the pitches and rhythms of speech are tried out. Other tests have shown that even very young babies have a good memory for smells – they recognize mum by her smell.

Physical development is most obvious between 16 and 28 weeks, when the neck and trunk muscles develop, allowing the baby to sit up and look around and take experimental swipes at nearby objects. By 40 weeks most babies are experienced crawlers, eager for horizons beyond the cot and the pram. Shortly afterwards there are wobbly attempts to stand, though unsupported standing is not usually achieved until about a year old.

The things to watch out for particularly in infants are fever and dehydration. Temperature quickly rises in response to infection, hot weather, too many blankets, and so on, and measures to reduce it should be taken very swiftly (see FEVER pp. 305–6). To take a baby's temperature, put the bulb of the thermometer under the armpit for 3 minutes. Persistent diarrhoea or vomiting can easily cause dehydration; usually the cause of diarrhoea is premature introduction of solids or too much sugar in feeds.

Daily immersion in soap and water is not essential for a baby. The essential areas to clean thoroughly are eyes, face, hands, and bottom, the tradition 'topping and tailing' method.

Granules are the most convenient way of giving homeopathic remedies to babies; they quickly dissolve on the tongue and cannot be spat out as easily as pilules. Alternatively, crush a pilule between two clean spoons, dissolve it in a little warm water, and drop it on to the tongue with a dropper.

For explanation of other symbols, see page 107

Asphyxia of the newborn

Failure of a newborn baby to breathe, more common in small-for-dates babies, overdue babies, and babies whose mothers have received pethidine in labour. Baby doesn't move or cry, and turns blue; after 5 minutes of not breathing brain damage is likely, and after 10 minutes baby will die.

If baby is being delivered at home, ⑨⑨⑨ and start mouth-to-mouth resuscitation (see First Aid pp. 86–7), removing any fluid or mucus from baby's mouth first; once the baby is breathing, give one of the emergency homeopathic remedies below.

If mouth-to-mouth resuscitation does not work, artificial respiration may be necessary (a tube is inserted through the baby's mouth and into the lungs, and attached to a respirator); in meantime, give *Carbo veg. 30c* in the dosage specified below.

Specific remedies to be given every 2 minutes until baby loses blue tinge and is breathing and crying normally
- Baby collapsed, limp, cold, nearly dead *Carbo veg. 30c*
- Baby cold, blue, gasping for breath, failing pulse *Laurocerasus 6c*

Birth defects see CONGENITAL DISORDERS

Birthmarks

Caused by local pigmentation of skin or by an accumulation of tiny blood vessels (naevi) close to surface of skin.

Pigmented spots, also known as 'cafe au lait' spots because they are coffee-coloured, are usually permanent; they are much larger than ordinary moles, irregular in shape, and may have hairs growing out of them.

There are three types of naevi (marks caused by collections of tiny blood vessels): *capillary naevi*, which are flat pink or pink-brown spots – these usually fade within 18 months; *strawberry naevi*, which are strawberry-red, raised, about 2.5 cm (1 in) across, and grow rapidly at first, then slow down and grow with the child – most fade after 3 years; and *port wine stains*, mulberry-coloured, slightly raised, and often extensive patches on face or limbs – these generally persist into adult life. Disfiguring or unsightly birthmarks can be treated by cosmetic surgery or disguised with skin-coloured creams.

If a strawberry naevus bleeds, apply pressure and give *Phosphorus 6c* every 5 minutes until bleeding stops, then give 3 doses of *Phosphorus 30c* at 12-hour intervals. For a strawberry naevus which does not bleed, give 3 doses of *Thuja 30c* at 12-hour intervals and apply Thuja mother tincture every day for 3 weeks. If these measures do not help, see your homeopath.

Bronchiolitis

Viral infection which causes swelling of the membranes lining the smaller airways (bronchioles) in the lungs. Usually occurs in children under 18 months old, often after COLDS, and is most dangerous in children under six months old. If, within 2–3 days of starting a cold, child begins to wheeze, has difficulty breathing, looks blue around lips, and refuses food, ② as there may be a danger of HEART FAILURE or PNEUMONIA.

Specific remedies to be taken every 10 minutes for up to 10 doses until help arrives
- Child hoarse, wheezy, blue in face, exhaled breath feels cold, attack comes on in evening *Carbo veg. 30c*
- Child exhausted with trying to breathe, too weak to cough up loose phlegm, nostrils sucked in with effort of breathing, vomiting *Antimonium tart. 30c*

Circumcision

Surgical removal of foreskin of penis; usually an elective procedure but occasionally necessary in cases of balanitis (see PENIS PROBLEMS), PHIMOSIS, or repeated swelling of foreskin when urine is passed. Do not attempt to pull back the foreskin until the child is at least 3 years old, as it may tear and lead to PHIMOSIS. As soon as child can comfortably move it back, he should be taught to wash underneath it in the bath. If there is any irritation, apply Hypericum and Calendula solution (5 drops of mother tincture of each in 0.25 litre [½ pint] warm water).

Colds

Quite common in young babies, but not harmful unless they interfere with feeding, or spread to throat, lungs, ears, or brain. See COLDS pp. 163, 317 for suitable homeopathic remedies and self-help measures. Decongestant nose drops (1% saline solution or 0.5% Ephidrine, both obtainable from chemist) can be given just before feeding or sleeping if a stuffy nose is causing problems, but always in strict accordance with instructions on bottle and never for more than a day at a time as they can damage sensitive lining of nose. Homeopathic remedies should always be tried first.

Colic

Sharp tummy pain which causes baby to pull legs up, scream, and go red in face; may be a reaction to dairy products, wheat, cabbage, or citrus fruit in mother's diet, or mother's tension and ANXIETY; in a bottle-fed baby it may be due to air-swallowing because hole in teat is too small. Most common form of colic is *3-month colic*, typically coming on in evening and lasting anything from a few minutes to several hours; burping or laying baby over knee or shoulder usually has little effect. If baby turns very pale and limp, or vomits, or has DIARRHOEA, a more serious condition should be suspected; to be on safe side, ⑫.

Specific remedies to be given every 5 minutes for up to 10 doses
- Symptoms relieved by firm pressure on stomach *Colocynth 6c*

---

⑨⑨⑨ Emergency – call GP (or dial 999) immediately. ② Consult your doctor if no improvement within 2 hours

- Symptoms relieved by warmth and gentle pressure *Magnesia phos. 6c*
- Baby very irritable, screams at slightest movement *Bryonia 30c*
- Baby impossible to please, but seems to improve when carried around *Chamomilla 6c*
- Where mother is breast-feeding and grieving or emotionally upset *Ignatia 6c*

Self-help If mother's exhaustion is affecting baby, try to arrange for someone else to do the household chores for a day or two and encourage her to remain in bed. Resting will encourage milk production, and drinking more fluids will encourage a better milk supply in evenings and at night. If mother is irritable from lack of sleep, give *Nux 30c* every 8 hours for up to 5 days.

Congenital disorders

Disorders which are present at birth, usually requiring surgery within first year of life; while there is a slight tendency for congenital disorders of the heart and central nervous system to run in families, most other congenital disorders are the result of genetic or developmental accidents. However, there is evidence that some can be prevented by good preconceptual care (see p. 23) and by good nutrition and avoidance of alcohol, drugs, and nicotine during pregnancy. Where there is a hereditary component, genetic counselling can help to put the risks in perspective.

Biliary atresia Condition in which bile ducts are partially missing, preventing bilirubin and bile acids processed by liver from emptying into duodenum; as a result, bilirubin builds up in blood, causing JAUNDICE, and eventually CIRRHOSIS OF THE LIVER. If faulty duct lies outside liver, chances of surgically repairing or bypassing it are good; if small ducts inside liver are affected, death within a year or so is inevitable unless child receives a liver transplant.

Cleft palate Cleft extending along midline of palate from behind teeth to nasal cavity; often there is a gap in the upper gum and lip as well (see hare lip below). At first, baby may regurgitate milk through nose when feeding, but after a month or so he or she learns to suck and swallow with reasonable efficiency; in severe cases a palate plate may have to be used for feeding. Cleft is usually repaired when child is about a year old, before he or she starts learning to speak; any speech problems which develop can usually be corrected by speech therapy. Condition sometimes affects more than one child in same family; nutritional deficiencies before and during pregnancy may play a part.

Club foot (talipes) Condition in which one or both feet are bent inwards and downwards, or upwards and outwards; can be corrected by manipulating foot each day – GP can teach mother how to do this – or by repeatedly splinting foot until it is in proper alignment with ankle; surgery is only necessary in very severe cases. Condition tends to run in families, although deficiencies of Vitamin B_2, B_3, B_5, folate, manganese, iron, and zinc before and during pregnancy have also been implicated.

Congenital dislocation of the hip Condition in which head of femur lies outside socket in pelvis because socket is too shallow; can occur in one or both hips and is often a family trait; hip gives a clicking sound when manipulated as part of routine tests immediately after birth. Hip may require splinting for up to 9 months, or mother may be advised to use double nappies folded into a rectangle rather than a triangle to keep baby's thighs well apart and thigh bones firmly in their sockets. If condition is not detected until child begins to walk, surgery and several months of wearing a plaster cast may be necessary; late correction is not always successful, and child may be left with a permanent walking problem.

Congenital heart defects Symptoms which indicate that baby's heart is not functioning as it should are cyanosis (skin develops bluish tinge) or very rapid, distressed breathing when baby is active or feeding, weak crying or only short bouts of crying, FEEDING PROBLEMS (baby is too breathless to suck properly), and fails to thrive (see SLOW WEIGHT GAIN). In most cases, cause is not known; chances of a parent passing a congenital heart defect on to his or her children are less than 5 per cent, and then defect is unlikely to be serious; occasionally cause may be a chromosome abnormality such as DOWN'S SYNDROME, or heart may be damaged in early months of pregnancy by drugs or infections such as RUBELLA; deficiencies of Vitamins A, B_5, E, folate, iron, zinc, and chromium before and during pregnancy have also been implicated; alternatively, circulatory changes that ought to take place shortly after birth, when baby's oxygen comes from lungs rather than placenta, fail to take place.

  Hole in the heart is the most common heart disorder at birth – the hole in question may be between the two atria (upper chambers) or between the two ventricles (lower chambers); surgery to close a large hole is usually done between age of five and ten. Some conditions, such as *tetralogy of Fallot* (four separate abnormalities), *patent ductus arteriosus* (non-closure of duct between aorta and pulmonary artery), and *transposition of the great vessels* (where blood from lungs passes back into lungs instead of into aorta) require surgery before age of five. Valve defects such as *congenital aortic stenosis* and *congenital pulmonary stenosis*, which reduce blood flow to body and lungs, are usually operated on when child is older, as is *constriction of the aorta*. If condition is extremely severe, surgery may be necessary in infancy, but success rate is lower. If at all possible, condition is treated with drugs until child is strong enough to undergo open-heart surgery.

For explanation of other symbols, see page 107

Diaphragmatic hernia Condition in which part of intestine or even stomach protrudes upwards into chest cavity through hole in diaphragm, pressing on baby's lungs and causing breathlessness. Surgery may be necessary shortly after birth to close hole in diaphragm and reposition intestine in abdomen; however, if condition is not severe, it tends to repair itself within a year or so; meanwhile baby should be fed in an upright position and thickening agents added to feeds. Deficiency of Vitamin A, folate, and zinc before and during pregnancy may play a part in this disorder.

Hare lip Can occur on its own or in conjunction with cleft palate (see above); one or both sides of upper lip may be split, sometimes with split extending to base of nose or into nostril; upper gum may also have a cleft in it. In mild cases, lip is merely notched. Defect tends to run in families, though cause is not known; recently it has been suggested that a deficiency of Vitamin B_2, B_3, B_5 and folate acid before and during pregnancy may be a contributing factor. Corrective surgery at around three months is usually very successful.

Hirschsprung's disease Absence of nerve cells in colon and rectum; this means that muscles in bowel walls cannot contract in order to push faeces out; result is severe CONSTIPATION, a distended stomach which becomes as tight as a drum, and VOMITING; vomit is green and may have blood in it. Nutritional deficiency during pregnancy is one possible cause. Condition is diagnosed by barium enema and X-ray, and rectal biopsy (removing a small sample of tissue for analysis). Surgery, which involves removing affected section of large intestine and rejoining cut ends, is usually very successful.

Hydrocephalus (water on the brain) Build up of fluid (cerebrospinal fluid) inside brain, causing brain to swell and forcing soft bones of skull apart; condition can be detected in womb by X-rays and ultrasound; in such cases, baby may have to be delivered by CAESARIAN SECTION. Shortly after birth a fine tube is inserted into brain through a small hole drilled in skull and connected to a main blood vessel returning to heart; this continuously drains fluid from brain, and over a period of months size of baby's head returns to normal. If tube becomes blocked for any reason, baby will become irritable and start to vomit; if this happens, (999). If degree of hydrocephalus is severe at birth, baby will almost certainly be brain damaged; growth will be stunted and baby will succumb to infection sooner rather than later. Many hydrocephalic babies also suffer from some degree of spina bifida (see below). Hydrocephalus can also onset in late infancy due to infections which damage brain or to a BRAIN TUMOUR.

Imperforate anus Absence of connection between rectum and anus or presence of a membrane in anal canal which prevents bowels being opened; discovered immediately after birth by inserting finger or thermometer into back passage, or within 12 hours of birth, when baby fails to pass meconium (greenish-black, tarry substance passed shortly after birth). Baby will need surgery to remove membrane or join rectum to anus; if muscles of anus are poorly developed, making it unlikely that child will ever develop proper bowel control, colostomy (making a permanent opening in abdomen so that faeces can be voided into a bag) may be recommended.

Intestinal atresia and *intestinal stenosis* Absence or severe narrowing of part of small intestine; within hours of birth baby begins to vomit, bringing up green bile with or without blood in it, and abdomen swells with retained wind. Diagnosis is confirmed by X-ray. Immediate surgery is necessary to cut and join blind ends of intestine or widen constricted section; results are generally excellent.

Oesophageal atresia Absence of part of oesophagus; instead of being swallowed, secretions from mouth and nose pool in gullet and overflow into baby's windpipe and lungs; breathing may be blocked and baby may start to turn blue; attempts to breathe cause a bubbling sound in throat, and any attempt to feed baby results in coughing and spluttering. Diagnosis is confirmed by trying to pass tube down gullet. Immediate surgery is necessary to cut and join blind ends of oesophagus; in meantime, airway is kept clear by suction.

Pyloric stenosis Abnormal thickening of walls of pylorus, (short tube which joins stomach to duodenum), blocking flow of nourishment into intestine where absorption takes place; stomach contracts violently in effort to force feed through narrowed pylorus, which results instead in explosive VOMITING, also known as 'projectile vomiting'; vomit is a mixture of milk curds and mucus, and smells unpleasant; baby fails to put on weight (see SLOW WEIGHT GAIN), becomes fretful and restless, and passes small, infrequent stools; greatest danger is dehydration. Until diagnosis can be confirmed, give small, frequent feeds. Since condition may be due to spasm of digestive tract rather than to stenosis, it would be worth giving *Belladonna 30c* every 15 minutes for up to 6 doses, followed by *Nux 6c* in same dosage, after a first attack of projectile vomiting. If vomiting continues, see your GP. Results of surgery to relieve stenosis are usually excellent; 4 doses of *China 6c* at 2-hour intervals are recommended before the operation.

Spina bifida Mild or severe malformation of bones of spine, leaving part of spinal cord unprotected; nerves in spinal cord may also be defective; condition can be detected in womb by amniocentesis (taking a sample of amniotic fluid for analysis). In mild cases, site of

---

999 Emergency – dial 999 immediately. (2) Consult your doctor if no improvement within 2 hours

abnormality is marked by nothing more than a dimple in skin, and baby may hardly be handicapped at all. At the other extreme, unprotected part of spinal cord is merely covered with a fragile reddish-purple membrane containing cerebrospinal fluid, and nerves to legs, bowel, and bladder are not properly formed; paralysis of the legs and incontinence of urine and faeces are almost inevitable; MENINGITIS may develop if membrane around spinal cord is damaged and infections enter cerebrospinal fluid. Very few spina bifida children escape some degree of paralysis of the legs, although many eventually achieve bladder control. Damage to membrane around spinal cord can be repaired surgically, but damage to cord itself is irreversible. Support offered by Association for Spina Bifida and Hydrocephalus (address p. 384) is invaluable to many parents; as the association's name implies, spina bifida often occurs in conjunction with hydrocephalus (see above).

Cot death (Sudden Infant Death Syndrome – SIDS)

Happens to 13–15 in every 10,000 babies, usually between age of six weeks and four months; girl babies, first babies, breast-fed babies, and babies born into fairly affluent families do not succumb as often as boy babies, second, third, and fourth babies, bottle-fed babies, and babies born into poorer families. Suffocation by pillows, blankets, etc. is very rarely the cause. However, there does seem to be a link between SIDS and various respiratory problems – FEEDING PROBLEMS which are respiratory in origin, ASPHYXIA OF THE NEWBORN (when baby fails to breathe at birth), cyanotic attacks (breathing difficulties which cause skin to turn blue), and minor respiratory tract infections, especially those occurring in winter. One cot death in four is attributed to a combination of factors, including brain malfunction, respiratory tract abnormalities, and sudden severe infection. In other cases, death may occur because nervous control of breathing is jeopardized by larynx descending into throat – this happens when infant is about three months old; atmospheric pollution (carbon monoxide, lead, organo-phosphate pesticides) at this critical age is known to affect nervous control of breathing. Other speculative causes include ALLERGY to cow's milk, botulism (a particularly nasty form of FOOD POISONING), hyperthermia from being in over-heated rooms, hyperthyroidism (see THYROID PROBLEMS), and a deficiency of biotin, Vitamin E, selenium, or potassium. World Health Organization, in its attempt to reduce incidence of SIDS worldwide, recommends that women should not get pregnant too young, that number of pregnancies should be limited, with 2–3 years between pregnancies, that mothers should not smoke or take drugs, and that babies should be breast-fed for 4–6 months.

Cradle cap see SEBORRHOEIC ECZEMA

Crying and screaming

A baby's way of communicating hunger, thirst, discomfort, pain, loneliness, boredom, anxiety. . . If cause of crying is not understood, parents become angry and worried and their feelings communicate themselves to the baby, who reacts by crying more – the classic vicious circle. If you cannot work out why your baby is crying, talk to your GP or health visitor.

Generally speaking, the more lustily a baby bawls, the more healthy he or she is; a healthy newborn baby may spend waking hours crying, but by age of six months a lot of waking time is spent gurgling and playing. So if crying is feeble or infrequent, especially in a newborn baby, or if a six-month old baby does nothing but cry when he or she is awake, something may be wrong. Other danger signs are FEVER, runny nose, COUGH, DIARRHOEA, VOMITING, and SLOW WEIGHT GAIN. An unusually high-pitched cry, coupled with vomiting, a bulging fontanelle (soft spot on top of head where bones of skull meet), and intolerance of light, may be a sign of brain infection, possibly MENINGITIS; appropriate action is ⑨⑨⑨.

Most frequent cause of crying is hunger; if baby stops crying when fed, increase frequency of feeds; if baby starts crying less than 2 hours after being fed, increase size of feeds. FEEDING PROBLEMS can also cause crying. If a few sips of water between feeds relieve crying, cause may be thirst.

Babies also cry because of COLIC (screaming attacks in evening, especially around age of three months), TEETHING (usually from six months onwards), or NAPPY RASH, or because nappy pins are sticking in, or bath water is too hot, or fingers get caught in shawls, or because they get worried by too much noise, very bright lights, too much laughter, too much hugging, too much tickling. . . Crying when passing water is quite normal; if observed closely, a baby usually cries just before passing water, which helps to raise pressure in bladder and so expel urine. Excessive crying may also be an early sign of HYPERACTIVITY.

If baby stops crying when picked up, he or she may simply be feeling bored or excluded; even if you cannot give your undivided attention, place the cot where he or she can watch what you are doing. Babies are very accurate sensors of tension in the family, especially of tension and tiredness in the mother; crying then becomes a way of expressing emotional discomfort and asking for reassurance.

Self-help Only a parent who has had to care for a constantly crying baby knows how exhausting it is. For the sake of her health and sanity, the mother should try to rest while the baby is sleeping, even if that means letting the housework slide. She also deserves an evening out and a good night's sleep at least once a week; if she is breast-feeding, milk can be expressed beforehand and left in a bottle. For suggestions about how to get a good night's sleep for both self and baby, see SLEEP PROBLEMS pp. 121–3 and 308–9. Parents who feel ragged from loss of sleep might also benefit from constitutional homeopathic treatment.

A crying baby often responds to rhythmic sounds (a tape recording of mother's heartbeat, for example), or to being rocked. Sucking a dummy or a thumb also has a soothing effect; dummies should be changed every week or so as they quickly become germ-ridden.

Only a very thin line separates parents who manage to cope with a continually crying baby and those who don't. If you have ever battered your baby, or feel that you might, seek help immediately, and don't be afraid to do so; talk to your GP, health visitor, or the Social Work Department of the NSPCC (address p. 384). CRY-SIS (address on p. 384) also offers support. If you have good reason to believe that someone is battering his or her baby, tell one of the agencies mentioned above; you will be helping both baby and parent in the long run. A word of caution, however; some cases of 'baby battering' have been found to be due to copper deficiency, which produces X-ray images very similar to those seen in genuine cases.

Dehydration see GASTROENTERITIS, DIARRHOEA, VOMITING

Diaphragmatic hernia see CONGENITAL DISORDERS

Diarrhoea

Potentially serious in very young babies as it quickly leads to dehydration. Diarrhoea is one of symptoms of GASTROENTERITIS (fever of 38°C [100°F] or more, with or without VOMITING, lack of enthusiasm for feeds, torpor); if gastroenteritis is suspected, or if stools are mixed with blood, or if diarrhoea persists for longer than 12 hours, call your GP. In meantime, give frequent sips of water to prevent dehydration and select a remedy from the list below.

Occasionally diarrhoea in infants is caused by too much sugar (too little water added to fruit juices or too much sugar added to fruit purees, for example); some drugs are also given in a very sugary base. Gripe water can also cause diarrhoea. Liquid stools in a baby who has just been weaned usually indicate that he or she is still unable to cope with solids; wait 2–3 weeks, then reintroduce them.Occasionally diarrhoea is due to too early reintroduction of milk after an attack of GASTROENTERITIS.

Specific remedies to be given every hour for up to 10 doses
- Diarrhoea comes on after exposure to cold wind *Aconite 30c*
- Diarrhoea brought on by food which has gone off slightly, or diarrhoea which gets worse when baby is given cold food or drinks, with baby exhausted, breathless, and emaciated *Arsenicum 6c*
- Diarrhoea associated with teething, greenish stools, baby irritable and difficult to please *Chamomilla 6c*

- Diarrhoea associated with colic *Colocynth 6c*
- Diarrhoea caused by over-feeding *Nux 6c*
- Baby passes watery stools after eating or drinking, and even during washing *Podophyllum 6c*
- Diarrhoea caused by sour fruit or by drinking cold drinks when overheated, slightest movement makes diarrhoea worse *Bryonia 30c*

Doubtful sex

A baby's sex is usually evident at birth from appearance of genitals; in a few cases, however, appearance is ambiguous, and true sex has to be confirmed by examining chromosomes in cells scraped from inside of baby's mouth. Surgery is usually recommended, so that outward appearance conforms to chromosomal sex; a succession of operations may be necessary over a period of years. Sex of baby is determined when sperm fertilizes egg, but sex organs develop between weeks 7 and 12 in response to hormones secreted by the foetus; if these are not secreted or secreted in insufficient amounts, sex organs may not form properly. Parents who have had a child whose sex is doubtful and who want more children are advised to seek genetic counselling; good preconceptual care (see p. 23) is also important.

Down's syndrome

Caused by presence of extra chromosome (47 instead of 46) contributed by mother or father. Most Down's children have small facial features, with upward-slanting eyes (at one time such children were called 'mongols'), a large tongue, a flattish back to the head, and short hands with a near-horizontal crease in the palm; degree of mental handicap varies, but most Down's children are lively, responsive, and affectionate; some, given special schooling and family support, go on to do simple but useful jobs in a sheltered environment. Congenital heart defects and intestinal atresia (see CONGENITAL DISORDERS) are more frequent among Down's babies than among the population at large, and so is LEUKAEMIA. Ear, nose, and throat infections are also a particular problem; here constitutional homeopathic treatment can be invaluable.

Down's syndrome can be detected by amniocentesis during weeks 16–18 of pregnancy or at 10 weeks by chorion villous biopsy at some centres; procedure is advised for women aged 35 or over, incidence of syndrome being significantly higher in older mothers. Suggestion that syndrome may be partially caused by nutritional factors makes good preconceptual care (see p. 23) especially relevant; excessive levels of lead, cadmium, aluminium, and copper, and a deficiency of selenium, have been implicated. Chances of there being more than one Down's child in same family are remote. Parents of Down's babies are advised to contact the Down's Syndrome Association (address p. 357).

---

(999) Emergency – call GP (or dial 999) immediately. (2) Consult your doctor if no improvement within 2 hours

Eczema see SEBORRHOEIC ECZEMA, ECZEMA p. 140

Eye inflammation

Usually a combination of a mild infection and blocked tear ducts (see WATERING EYES); if tear ducts cannot be unblocked by gently massaging skin on either side of nose, paediatrician will use a probe to open them. Wipe eyes every 4 hours with Hypericum and Calendula solution (5 drops of mother tincture of each in 0.25 l [½ pint] boiled cooled water) and give *Argentum nit. 6c* every 2 hours for up to 10 doses. If inflammation persists, see your GP; an eye swab may have to be taken. In rare cases, eyes may be inflamed because of gonorrhoea (see SEXUALLY TRANSMITTED DISEASES) during pregnancy.

Failure to thrive see SLOW WEIGHT GAIN,
FEEDING PROBLEMS

Feeding problems

Modern wisdom is that babies should be fed on demand and allowed to feed until satisfied. Breast-feeding may need to be every 2 hours at first (see pp. 293–4 for pros and cons of breast-feeding and bottle feeding). Time to introduce solids is when baby's hunger increases, causing more frequent waking at night; this usually happens from four months onwards, although breast-feeding should continue until about six months.

Consult your GP or health visitor if baby loses interest in food or stops gaining weight (see SLOW WEIGHT GAIN). Regurgitation of small amounts of food is quite normal, but this should happen less and less once solids are introduced. However, if baby actually vomits (brings up large amounts of half-digested food), and this happens several times within 24 hours, or if VOMITING is accompanied by FEVER or DIARRHOEA, 12. Possible causes include a digestive tract abnormality (see CONGENITAL DISORDERS), GASTROENTERITIS, LACTOSE INTOLERANCE, and INTUSSUSCEPTION; see VOMITING for further information.

Breast-fed babies Baby should be put to the breast as soon as possible, and certainly within 24 hours of birth, and then fed on demand, if possible, until age of four to six months. If breasts are too full for baby to suck comfortably, some milk should be expressed before feeding. If milk is too watery, salty, or bitter, baby will probably cry and draw away from the breast. Self-help measures and homeopathic remedies for distended breasts, sore nipples, loss of milk, unpleasant-tasting milk, etc. appear under BREAST-FEEDING PROBLEMS on p. 294.

Bottle-fed babies Carefully follow mixing instructions on container. Feed which is too dilute will result in small, firm, dark green stools; feed which is not sufficiently diluted will make baby thirsty because salt content is high for its volume; in both cases baby is likely to express discomfort by crying. If baby nods off while feeding, wake him or her up.

Weaning Best policy is to introduce solids one by one at first, just in case there are any intolerances. Best foods to wean on are rice, potatoes, vegetables (especially carrots and greens), fruit, avocados, and fish or lean meat, all well pureed of course. Avoid wheat, nuts, corn, and mushrooms, which are not digested well, and keep dairy products to a minimum. If any food produces wind or other upsets, note it down and wait for a month or two before reintroducing it. If there is a family history of food intolerance, delay introduction of wheat and dairy products until age of twelve months.

Fever

Generally a sign that body is marshalling its resources to fight and destroy infection; however, in very young babies, whose temperature regulation mechanism may not be mature, temperature quickly rises in response to hot weather, hot rooms, or too many clothes or blankets.

Automatically reaching for aspirin, paracetamol, etc. when a baby has a temperature is to be condemned; aspirin should not be given to young children because of risk of Reye's syndrome, a rare but fatal disease which seems to be linked to taking of aspirin. In most cases the homeopathic remedies listed below effectively bring temperature down; sometimes simply undressing the baby or giving tepid sponge-downs brings temperature back to normal. Junior paracetamol should only be given if fever rises above 39°C (102°F) and homeopathic remedies are not working, if baby is prone to FEBRILE CONVULSIONS (fits which come on when temperature rises above normal), or if fever is preventing baby from sleeping.

If, despite all efforts, baby's temperature remains above 39°C (102°F) for more than 2 hours, call your GP. Also, if your baby has a history of febrile convulsions, call your GP as soon as fever develops. If baby goes into convulsions, or if skin develops bluish tinge, (999).

Conditions such as CROUP AND STRIDOR (crowing intakes of breath), acute BRONCHITIS and BRONCHIOLITIS (rapid breathing, gasping for breath), PNEUMONIA (dry cough, wheezing, rapid breathing), and MENINGITIS (unusual drowsiness or irritability, unusual high-pitched cry) are accompanied by fever, and require prompt medical attention; appropriate action is (2). Fever can also be an indication of GASTROENTERITIS (diarrhoea, perhaps vomiting as well) or of one of the childhood fevers (see MEASLES, CHICKENPOX, etc); appropriate action is 12. MIDDLE EAR INFECTION (sudden waking, crying, pulling at affected ear) and throat infections (refusing solids) can also be accompanied by fever; keep infant under close observation, and if there is no improvement within 24 hours, call your GP.

Specific remedies to be given every hour for up to 10 doses as soon as fever comes on
- Sudden rise in temperature after exposure to cold dry wind, baby restless, shivery, and thirsty *Aconite 30c*
- Sudden onset, baby very thirsty, with burning hot skin and staring eyes, unusual noises and movements *Belladonna 30c*
- Baby very restless and thirsty for small drinks at frequent intervals, symptoms worse between midnight and 2 am *Arsenicum 6c*
- Slightest movement causes baby to cry out, large quantities of fluid gulped down *Bryonia 30c*

Self-help Tepid sponging is a very effective method of bringing temperature down. Spread a clean towel on the floor in a warm room, undress the child, and lay him or her on the the towel; sponge face, arms and legs, and front of body with tepid water, then pat dry with a second towel; turn baby over, wet-sponge arms, legs, and back, and pat dry. Repeat this procedure, front and back, six times. If temperature has not come down within 2 hours, repeat the process. Give baby as much to drink (dilute, unsweetened apple juice, for example) as he or she seems to want.

Sometimes, simply undressing baby and and giving frequent small drinks does the trick.

If fever is not due to overheating nor accompanied by any other obvious symptoms, a low-level infection may be the cause. If this is the case, give Ferrum Phos. (see Tissue Salts p. 35) every 30 minutes for up to 4 doses, then every 2 hours for up to 4 doses. If there is no improvement within 48 hours, see your GP.

Gastroenteritis
Potentially serious in very young babies since inflammation of stomach and small intestine causes DIARRHOEA and VOMITING, and therefore dehydration; stools are green and watery, baby develops slight FEVER, tends to feed poorly, and becomes miserable and tetchy. Signs of dehydration are a dry mouth, sunken eyes and fontanelle (spot on top of head where cranial bones meet), and irritability. Condition is less common among breast-fed babies who are, to some extent, protected against bacteria and viruses by antibodies in mother's milk; bottle-fed babies not only miss out on this protection but are also exposed to germs harboured by bottles, teats, and other feeding utensils.

If remedies below do not produce some improvement within 12 hours, or if signs of dehydration develop, call your GP.

Specific remedies to be given every 1–2 hours (depending on severity) for up to 10 doses

- Milk makes symptoms worse, stools green and watery, baby limp and passive, upper lip looks very pale *Aethusa 6c*
- Baby cold, weak, restless, and obviously miserable *Arsenicum 6c*
- Symptoms come on in cold wet weather, or after catching a chill, stools greenish-yellow and slimy *Dulcamara 6c*
- Colicky stomach pain, with legs drawn up, gentle pressure seems to relieve pain *Colocynth 6c*
- Copious vomiting and diarrhoea *Nux 6c*
- Baby chilly, apathetic, and makes a fuss if touched, stools yellow and frothy, a lot of wind *China 6c*
- Baby very thirsty for cold water, which is vomited up as soon as it becomes warm in stomach *Phosphorus 6c*
- Diarrhoea, with undigested food in stools, baby seems better after passing stools but shows no obvious pain on doing so *Phosphoric ac. 6c*

Self-help If you are bottle-feeding, make sure all utensils are sterilized each time you use them; avoid touching teats once they have been sterilized, and never put them in your mouth. Stop feeding for 24 hours, and give water with a little glucose and salt in it (1 teaspoon glucose and ½ teaspoon salt to 0.5 litre [1 pint] boiled cooled water) instead; on the second day give quarter-strength feed, the next day half-strength, and the next day three-quarters-strength; on the fifth day, go back to normal strength, but feed a little and often rather than a lot all at once.

If you are breast-feeding, give extra spoonfuls of boiled cooled water (made up as above) between feeds.

These measures should produce some improvement within 24 hours, but if they don't, call your GP.

Head banging
Usually means that baby needs more love and attention; banging head on side of cot is an expression of anger and hurt feelings; if parents open up more, baby will probably redirect anger against them, at least for a while. Just occasionally, head banging may be due to EARACHE. Sides of cot should be padded to prevent injury.

Specific remedies to be given last thing at night for up to 5 nights
- First choice *Millefolium 30c*
- Where head banging is part of general withdrawal from people and becomes an obsession *Silicea 30c*
- Baby very angry, impossible to please, soothed by being carried around but enraged by being put back in cot *Chamomilla 30c*

Intussusception
Condition in which small intestine telescopes into large intestine, causing violent ABDOMINAL PAIN and screaming. Usually occurs around six months of age

---

and is more common in boys than girls. In intervals between pain, child is limp and pale, and may vomit. Stools may be red and jelly-like. If intussusception is suspected ② and give nothing by mouth, except homeopathic remedies; if intestine cannot be manipulated back into place, an operation may be necessary.

Specific remedies to be given every 15 minutes while waiting for help to arrive
- First choice: colon seen as a pad during colic *Belladonna 30c*
- Pain relieved by bending child double *Colocynth 6c*
- Pain not relieved by bending child double *Nux 6c*
- Child restless and passing red, jelly-like stools *Rhus tox. 6c*

Jaundice see NEONATAL JAUNDICE

Lactose intolerance
Failure of small intestine to produce enzyme which breaks down lactose (milk sugar); lactose ferments in gut, causing VOMITING and frothy DIARRHOEA; condition is more common among Asian and African people, who have a low tolerance for dairy products. Symptoms disappear if milk is removed from diet, and reappear if milk is reintroduced. May occur temporarily after GASTROENTERITIS. Condition can be managed by keeping infant on lactose-free diet (avoiding dairy foods) or by giving enzyme supplements (see your GP), but it is not curable. If intolerance is severe, homeopathic remedies should be given as drops rather than lactose granules or pilules.

Meningitis see also MENINGITIS pp. 131 and 326
Potentially more serious in infants and toddlers than in older children and adults as there is a slight risk of BRAIN DAMAGE if condition is not detected and treated in early stages. First symptom is FEVER of 39°C (102°F) or more; early signs of head pain are unusual irritability or quietness, and turning eyes away from light; infant will also hold neck rigid or arched back despite attempts to push head foward; other symptoms may be VOMITING and convulsions (see FEBRILE CONVULSIONS, FITS), an unusual high-pitched cry, and a purplish rash on trunk; in very young babies, fontanelle (meeting point of skull bones on top of head) may bulge due to pressure of cerebrospinal fluid around brain.

If meningitis is suspected, ⑨⑨⑨; baby may need antibiotics and intravenous drip. Chances of complete recovery, with no residual mental handicap, are good.

Specific remedies to be given every 5 minutes until help arrives
- Symptoms onset after head injury *Arnica 30c*
- Baby restless, panicky, thirsty, skin feels very dry *Aconite 30c*
- Baby very hot, making unusual noises and movements, pupils wide and staring *Belladonna 30c*
- Baby obviously in great pain, unusually quiet, unable to look into light *Bryonia 30c*

Nappy rash
Usually caused by ammoniacal reaction between urine and faeces, or by irritating chemicals in faeces; not thoroughly rinsing soap or detergent out of nappies is another possible cause. Baby's buttocks, thighs, and genitals become sore, red, spotty, and weepy in areas touched by soiled nappies; in boys, foreskin may become inflamed, making urination painful; rash may become secondarily infected with *Candida* fungus if baby has been given antibiotics or if breast milk has antibiotics in it, or if mother has ORAL THRUSH or genital thrush (see VAGINAL AND VULVAL PROBLEMS).

If homeopathic remedies listed below produce no improvement, see your homeopath.

Specific remedies to be given 4 times daily for up to 5 days
- Rash dry, red, and scaly *Sulphur 6c*
- Skin itchy, with little blisters *Rhus tox. 6c*
- Nappy area very moist and sweaty, baby produces more saliva than usual *Mercurius 6c*
- Rash area raw and bleeding *Medorrhinum 6c*
- Nappy rash in a fat baby who suffers from copious head sweats at night *Calcarea 6c*

Self-help Simplest and most effective treatment is to allow baby to spend as much time out of nappies as possible, provided room is warm and dry; rash almost always clears up when exposed to air. After washing rash area with warm water only (no soap), pat dry with sterile cotton wool, and apply Calendula ointment. If you are using washable nappies, be extra careful about rinsing out all soap or detergent; if rash persists, try disposable nappies, and if one brand doesn't seem to help, try another. At all events, change nappies more frequently.

Neonatal jaundice
Many babies, especially babies born before term, develop a yellowish tinge within 2–3 days of birth due to immaturity of liver, which cannot process the yellow pigment bilirubin (a by-product of continuous breakdown of red blood cells) fast enough. Both skin and white of eyes turn yellow, and baby may become lethargic and half-hearted about feeding; in an otherwise healthy baby, jaundice fades after a few days. Standard treatment is to give baby plenty to drink to flush out excess bilirubin; if bilirubin level remains high, baby may be exposed to ultraviolet light to make bilirubin water soluble so kidneys can eliminate it (there is a risk of very high bilirubin levels causing brain damage); in very severe cases, baby may need a blood transfusion.

In a few cases, jaundice may be due to haemolytic ANAEMIA caused by RHESUS INCOMPATIBILITY (baby's red blood cells come under attack from mother's antibodies) or bile duct atresia (see CONGENITAL DISORDERS); former is referred to as haemolytic jaundice, and appears within 24 hours of birth; latter is known as obstructive jaundice, and usually onsets a week or so after birth, accompanied by DIARRHOEA and loss of weight. Haemolytic jaundice may require a blood transfusion, or no treatment at all, but outlook for obstructive jaundice is poor unless bile ducts can be surgically repaired.

Special remedies to be given every 2 hours for up to 10 doses when first signs of jaundice appear
- First choice *Chamomilla 6c*
- If Chamomilla is not effective *Mercurius 6c*
- If jaundice is due to rhesus incompatibility *Crotalus 6c*

Respiratory distress syndrome (RDS)
Most common in premature or very small babies, and in large babies whose mothers suffer from DIABETES; condition is caused by a deficiency of surfactant, a chemical which increases surface tension inside tiny air sacs in lungs and keeps them expanded; if air sacs start to collapse – this tends to happen within a few hours of birth – blood becomes starved of oxygen and overloaded with carbon dioxide; baby becomes short of breath, exhales with a grunting sound, sucks chest in when inhaling, and develops a bluish tinge. If baby has been delivered at home, (999) and give *Carbo veg. 30c* every 5 minutes for up to 10 doses. In hospital, baby will need artifical respiration in intensive care unit until lungs are capable of producing adequate amounts of surfactant.

In later stages of pregnancy surfactant levels of babies thought to be most at risk can be checked by sampling amniotic fluid; if level is low, mother is given an injection of ACTH (adrenocorticotrophic hormone) to stimulate the production of surfactant. At one time, when intensive neonatal care was not as widely available as it is today, babies often died of RDS or, if they survived, suffered permanent brain or lung damage.

Screaming see CRYING AND SCREAMING

Seborrhoeic eczema
Common during first 3 months of life, affecting scalp, face, neck, armpits, or nappy area; scurfy patches on scalp are known as 'cradle cap'; these may become yellow and soggy-looking, and extend to eyebrows and ears; on face and elsewhere condition causes red blotches and pimples which become angry-looking when baby cries or gets hot; cause is not known, but condition is occasionally triggered off by NAPPY RASH (whereas nappy rash is confined to nappy area, eczema may involve abdomen and thighs as well). Severe seborrhoeic eczema can lead to infantile eczema (see ECZEMA pp. 140, 320), but most cases heal of their own accord. If homeopathic remedies and self-help measures given below produce no improvement within 3 weeks, see your homeopath. Antibiotics and steroids should be avoided unless general health is suffering, and then only used for as short a time as possible.

Specific remedies to be given every 4 hours for up to 14 days
- Affected areas of skin weepy, encrusted, and easily become infected *Graphites 6c*
- Eczema mainly affects scalp and face, lesions thickly encrusted, swollen glands *Viola 6c*
- Skin dry and scaly, but not infected, Calendula ointment seems to have no effect *Lycopodium 6c*
- Scabby patches on scalp which ooze and mat hair together *Vinca 6c*

Self-help Keep affected areas clean with regular washing and thorough drying. After washing, apply Calendula ointment. Gently rub skin with olive oil to loosen scales before washing.

Skin problems
A rash in nappy area clearly suggests NAPPY RASH; if elsewhere, and affected areas are scaly and itchy, infantile eczema (see ECZEMA pp. 140, 320) may be the culprit; SEBORRHOEIC ECZEMA produces scurfy patches on scalp or red blotching on face, or in armpits or groin, but is not usually itchy. If spots are accompanied by FEVER, |12|, especially if baby is under three months of age; ailments which cause both rash and fever are listed on p. 321.

Sleep problems
Generally speaking, newborn babies spend most of their time sleeping or dozing, waking only for feeds, nappy changes, and cuddles. By end of first year, most babies are awake for 8 hours out of 24, although they may spend 2–3 hours sleeping during the day; by the time they are seven to ten months old most babies, and their parents, sleep through the night without waking. Ideally, a baby should be allowed to sleep whenever he or she is tired, wherever that happens to be; a certain amount of background noise is no bad thing.

Most night-time sleep problems in babies under six months old are caused by hunger, so first resort should be the breast or the bottle. If this does not have a sedative effect, problem may be wind or a dirty nappy; winding baby or changing nappy usually does the trick. Discomfort of COLIC or NAPPY RASH, or running a temperature, can also cause night-time grizzling. In the long run, taking baby back to bed with you, or giving too many cuddles in middle of night, may create more problems than it solves.

Occasionally babies wake in middle of night because they have kicked all their bedclothes off and feel cold; a sleeping bag or sleeping suit usually solves the problem.

Once need for night-feeding stops, around age of seven to ten months, baby should sleep through the night; if he or she starts crying, don't immediately rush in to give reassurance; he or she will probably go back to sleep within a few minutes. If attention is always given on demand, baby may start to exploit the

---

(999) Emergency – call GP (or dial 999) immediately. (2) Consult your doctor if no improvement within 2 hours

situation! That said, changes in routine can be very upsetting to babies, and at such times they genuinely need extra cuddling and reassurance.

Specific remedies to be given every 30 minutes starting 1 hour before baby's bedtime and every 30 minutes if baby wakes; 10 doses is maximum
- If baby has had a shock or a fright *Aconite 30c*
- Baby irritable and impossible to please, only stops crying when picked up and carried around *Chamomilla 30c*
- Baby too excited or overwrought to sleep *Coffea 6c*
- Baby who wakes crying around 4 am and refuses to be pacified *Nux 6c*

Self-help Make sure baby's room is warm, but not too warm (around 20°C [68°F] is about right), and relatively quiet.

Baby should be woken up and given a late-night feed when parents go to bed. If baby wakes up hungry in middle of night, feed him or her immediately – if you are bottle-feeding, have everything ready you are likely to need. Give a proper feed, not water, as water will only temporarily allay hunger. If you find it difficult to get back to sleep, drink some chamomile tea – keep a thermos of it next to the bed. If you and your partner can take turns night-feeding, so much the better.

If sleepless nights are really getting you down, and baby is over 12 weeks old and going about 5 hours between feeds during the day, it may be worth leaving baby to cry for about 20 minutes before you take action; hunger crying is likely to continue, but habit crying will probably stop.

If baby sleeps through the night but wakes very early, best thing to do is change nappy and give him or her some toys to play with, while you go back to sleep for an hour or two. You could also try adjusting baby's internal 'clock' by making bedtime 15 minutes later each night until he or she wakes at a civilized hour.

Babies are very conservative and like to have a routine, so try to keep things in the same sequence and at roughly the same times each day. Avoid overexcitement in hour or so before baby's bedtime. Have toys and mobiles nearby.

Slow weight gain

Most babies lose weight, often as much as 140 g (5 oz), in first few days, but by ten days old they should have regained their birth weight; they should weigh twice as much by five months and three times as much at one year old (see chart opposite). Steady weight gain, without troughs or plateaus, is the desideratum; even a low birth weight baby should make steady progress, albeit on a lower level.

Breast-fed babies who are losing weight should be fed on demand, if possible, and be allowed to suck for as long as they want; if bottle-feeding, check that you are giving correct amount and concentration of feed

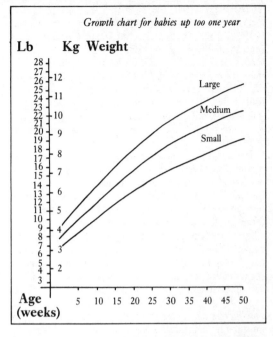

Growth chart for babies up too one year

(see FEEDING PROBLEMS). If baby is over three months old, he or she may need solids; this should be discussed with your health visitor or GP.

If slow weight gain is associated with periodic VOMITING, or with undue sleepiness, irritability, or reluctance to feed, see your GP; if it is associated with loose, pale, smelly stools, baby may have a digestive problem such as LACTOSE INTOLERANCE or COELIAC DISEASE; these problems also require attention of GP. Constitutional homeopathic treatment may also help.

Umbilical hernia

Soft bulge of tissue around navel due to weakness in abdominal wall; bulge can be pushed back into tummy but tends to reappear when baby cries. There is little danger of underlying section of intestine becoming strangulated (see HERNIAS). Most such hernias are painless and heal of own accord during first year; if surgery is necessary, it is usually done between age of three and five. If homeopathic remedies below do not produce some improvement within 2 months, see your GP.

Specific remedies to be given 3 times a day for up to 3 weeks
- Infant or toddler who is overweight, very quiet, prone to head sweats at night, especially if he or she likes to eat earth or worms *Calcarea 6c*
- Infant or toddler who is thin and weedy, with a large head and sweaty feet *Silicea 6c*
- In all other cases *Nux 6c*

For explanation of other symbols, see page 107

Vomiting

Regurgitation of small amounts of feed is quite normal (see FEEDING PROBLEMS), but if nearly all food is regurgitated and vomiting has been going on for more than 24 hours, call your GP. Repeated vomiting is very dehydrating for a young baby; if signs of dehydration are present (dry mouth, sunken eyes, depressed fontanelle), (2) and try to give sips of water with a little glucose and salt dissolved in it (1 teaspoon glucose and ½ teaspoon salt to 0.5 l [1 pint] boiled cooled water.)

If vomiting is accompanied by bouts of screaming, or if vomit is greenish-yellow, cause may be OBSTRUCTION or INTUSSUSCEPTION; appropriate action is (2), and *Aconite 30c* every 5 minutes for up to 10 doses. Vomiting can also be a symptom of GASTROENTERITIS (with fever and frequent, watery stools), WHOOPING COUGH (slight fever, runny nose, paroxysms of coughing), and pyloric stenosis (see CONGENITAL DISORDERS); in latter case, baby may vomit with such force that stomach contents are propelled some distance across room. If any of these conditions is suspected, 12 .

Specific remedies to be given every hour, or every 15 minutes if vomiting is severe, for up to 10 doses
- For vomiting generally *Ipecac 6c*

- Waxy pallor, no crying, bluish rings around eyes *Phosphoric ac. 6c*
- Vomit full of green or yellow curds, perhaps because baby has developed intolerance of milk, baby exhausted and very distressed *Aethusa 6c*
- Vomiting in a fat, flabby baby who is prone to sour-smelling head sweats during sleep, fontanelle slow to close, teeth late in coming through *Calcarea 6c*
- Marked distention of abdomen *Lac can. 6c*
- Vomiting accompanied by constipation, stools pale, dry, and crumbly *Magnesia carb. 6c*
- Baby's stomach full of wind and rumbling which obviously cause pain *Natrum carb. 6c*
- Baby refuses breast, has sweaty head and cold smelly feet *Silicea 6c*
- Vomiting caused by fruit or food which has gone off slightly *Arsenicum 6c*
- Vomiting caused by fright *Aconite 30c*
- Vomiting brought on by rich or fatty foods, baby irritable and wants to be left alone *Bryonia 30c*
- Vomiting accompanied by craving for cold water, which is vomited up as soon as it becomes warm in stomach *Phosphorus 6c*

Water on the brain see CONGENITAL DISORDERS

AILMENTS AND DISEASES IN CHILDHOOD

MANY of the conditions which affect children between the age of one and twelve today are rites of passage rather than serious illnesses, a tuning up of the body's immune system, and of its mental and emotional defences, in readiness for adult life. Homeopathic remedies can play an important part in the 'tuning up' process. To echo the trampoline analogy in PART I, they help to train the body to bounce back from illness. They also recommend themselves to parents who are concerned about the side effects of some prescription drugs.

An infant becomes a child at around the age of twelve months when he or she begins to talk, and also tries to stand up for the first time. At this age most children weigh about three times their birth weight. A year later they weigh about four times birth weight. After that weight gain and height gain slow down to around 2.3-3.0kg (5-6lb) and 5cm (2in) per year; at puberty physical development speeds up again. Smaller than average children may have smaller than average parents – growth is partly governed by genetics – but nutritional or hormonal deficiencies can also lead to smallness. Congenital illnesses which affect the heart, lungs, and digestive system can also hinder

growth. Emotional deprivation can hinder it too. Abnormal tallness is more unusual, and in most instances is due to over-secretion of growth hormone, a tendency which may be inherited. Childhood ends at puberty, which occurs a little later in boys than in girls; for most girls puberty begins between the age of 11 and 13, but for most boys it arrives six months to a year later.

Until about the age of seven the fastest growing system in a child's body is the lymphatic system, a sophisticated chain of defences against infection. Swollen lymph glands, especially in the neck, are a sign that the system is being tested and that invading bacteria and viruses are being identified and destroyed. Most adults are not vulnerable to the germs which cause the diseases we think of as 'childhood diseases' precisely because they fight and conquer them in childhood, when their lymphatic system is at its most active. Many childhood diseases – mumps, measles, rubella, whooping cough – are more serious in adults than in children.

Development of the nervous system depends partly on a process called myelinization. Myelin is a fatty substance which forms a sheath around certain nerve fibres, and speeds up the rate at which electrical impulses travel along them. Those parts of the brain responsible for planning and thinking ahead myelinize between the age of six and ten. Some nerve tracts, those concerned with fine control of movement, for example, do not fully myelinize until the age of four.

A three-year old throwing a ball clearly has more control of his shoulder and arm than of his wrist and fingers. Catching a ball is a different matter; it requires split-second timing and coordination. Throw a ball to a two-year old, and he will look at you, not at the ball; he will make no movement to catch it. His brain and nervous system cannot process information about distance, speed, and body movements in space quickly enough to enable him to make an attempt at catching. But by the age of five most of his catching attempts will be successful, if a little jerky; if he drops or misses the ball sometimes it is probably because he is trying to keep his eye on three things at once, on the ball, on his hands, and on the thrower!

Children's paintings and drawings are also pointers to mental development. Most one- and two-year olds enjoy making their mark on the world with pencils and coloured crayons. Slowly the scribbles take on a more deliberate, intentional character; though still unrecognizable, they are clearly symbolic of something. By the age of three the squiggles turn into faces; by the age of six or seven the faces acquire bodies and limbs, even if the proportions are a little odd; by the age of eight or ten there are attempts at pattern and perspective.

There are many ways of assessing whether a child is developing normally. Comparing your child's height and weight with those of children of a similar age is one way; comparing the ages at which he or she acquires certain skills is another. But it must be stressed that there is a great deal of variation in the ages at which children reach a certain height or weight or level of performance. What is more important is the overall pattern or sequence of events. A child may be consistently under average height and weight for his or her age, but nevertheless gain a consistent number of inches and pounds in the years between infancy and puberty. What is important is sustained growth throughout childhood, with no plateaux or troughs. The growth charts on page 312 plot weight and height against age in the juvenile population at large. As you can see, the range of acceptable weights and heights becomes wider as age increases. If your child's weight or height lies outside this range, or if the rate of his or her growth stops climbing in a more or less straight line, you should consult your GP.

With mental and physical skills too it is a normal sequence one is looking for as much as precocity or delay. Certainly the majority of children have begun to say Mama and Dada by the age of twelve months, but some children say their first words as early as nine months or as late as fifteen. Most children can do up buttons by the age of four, but some can't; they may still be mastering the knack of putting arms through sleeves. With this caveat in mind, here are some of the milestones which most children can be expected to reach between the age of one and five. A delay of a few months is not significant; longer delays may be significant if growth and general health are poor.

Age	Milestones
12 months	child says Mama and Dada, and can also stand unsupported for a minute or two
15 months	child begins to walk, and also to use a spoon for eating
18 months	child understands simple commands, and begins to imitate parents' actions around the house
20 months	child able to control bowels
2 years	child able to put simple sentences together and control bladder during the day
2½ years	child able to jump up and down; also learns to dress and undress, but needs a lot of supervision
3 years	child begins to coordinate mind and body to do puzzles
3½ years	child stops bedwetting, begins to draw recognizable pictures, and loses fear of being separated from parents
4 years	child able to hop on one foot, and dress and undress without help, including buttons and shoes; also begins learning to read and write
5 years	child able to catch a ball and use a skipping rope

Abdominal migraine (cyclical vomiting)

Periodic attacks of abdominal pain in which the child is very pale and wants to lie down, feels nauseous, vomits, or has a high temperature. May be a precursor of adult MIGRAINE. Often caused by STRESS and therefore responds in the long term to constitutional treatment.

Specific remedies to be taken every hour for up to 10 doses

- Sharp cutting pains relieved by bending double, especially if brought on by anger outburst *Colocynth 6c*
- Pain worse for heat or slightest movement, provided appendicitis, peritonitis, and intestinal obstruction have been ruled out *Bryonia 30c*
- Cramps and diarrhoea, alleviated by heat and pressure *Magnesia phos. 6c*
- Constant nausea and diarrhoea *Ipecac. 6c*
- Attack brought on by rich, fatty food, worse for being in hot room, child tearful and clinging *Pulsatilla 6c*

For explanation of other symbols, see page 107

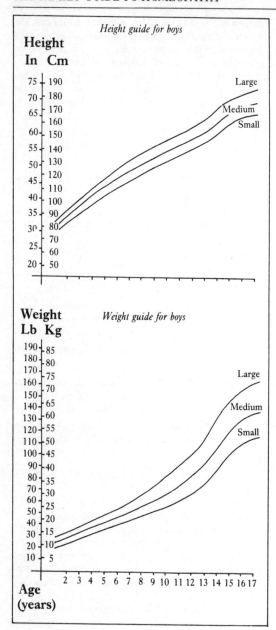

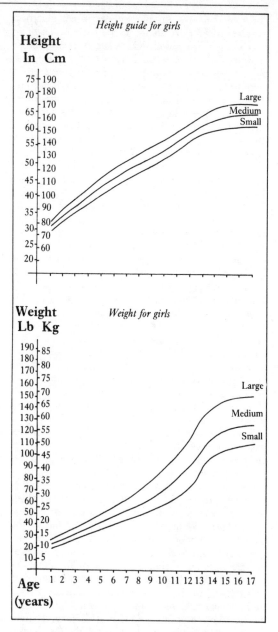

Self-help Let the child rest in bed, with a hot water bottle to soothe the pain, and give plenty to drink.

Abdominal pain (stomach ache)

May be due to APPENDICITIS (severe, continual pain, especially over appendix area, not relieved by vomiting), OBSTRUCTION (severe, continual pain, not relieved by vomiting bile, stomach distended, constipation or diarrhoea depending on severity of obstruction, sometimes fever), FOOD POISONING (diarrhoea and vomiting), GASTROENTERITIS (fever), swollen glands in the stomach, CONSTIPATION, wind, COLDS and other infections of the upper respiratory tract, urinary tract infections (frequent or painful urination), PEPTIC ULCER, food ALLERGY, and psychological discomfort (see STRESS, ANXIETY, INSECURITY).

If slightest movement causes agony and screaming, child may be suffering from a burst appendix; appropriate action is (999), and *Lachesis 6c* every 5 minutes for up to 10 doses until help arrives. If child is in severe pain and vomiting green-yellow bile, cause may

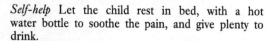
(999) Emergency – call GP (or dial 999) immediately. (2) Consult your doctor if no improvement within 2 hours

be obstruction; again, (999), but in this case give *China 6c* every 5 minutes for up to 10 doses.

If pain is associated with a lump in the groin or testicle, child may be suffering from a strangulated inguinal HERNIA or torsion of the testicle (see TESTICLE PROBLEMS); in either case, (2).

Specific remedies to be given every 5 minutes while waiting for help to arrive
● Child frightened and panicky *Aconite 30c* or *Bryonia 30c*

Abnormal sleepiness see ABNORMAL SLEEPINESS OR DROWSINESS p. 125

Adenoids
Glands behind the nose which develop between fourth and sixth year of life and form part of lymphatic chain of defence against infection. Enlargement can cause obstruction of nose, throat, and eustachian tubes, which in turn can cause nasal-sounding speech and difficulty breathing. Infection causes COUGH, as CATARRH drips on to vocal cords, and may spread up eustachian tubes to ears, causing chronic MIDDLE EAR INFECTION, GLUE EAR, or DEAFNESS. In cases of severe obstruction or chronic infection, surgical removal of adenoids may be necessary. If condition is less severe, it would be well worth seeking constitutional homeopathic treatment; however, if child has been deaf more or less continuously for at least 4 months, see your GP.

Specific remedies to be taken 4 times daily for up to 3 weeks
● Enlarged adenoids, recurrent tonsillitis, coupled with poor mental and physical development *Baryta 6c*
● Enlarged adenoids, child overweight, with cold and clammy skin, prone to head sweats, also a late walker and talker *Calcarea 6c*
● Symptoms as above, but child of normal weight and irritable *Calcarea phos. 6c*
● Adenoids causing obstruction, child always hungry, feels faint mid-morning, dislikes baths *Sulphur 6c*
● Thick, yellow, bland discharge from nose and throat, child tearful and timid *Pulsatilla 6c*
● Swollen adenoids following orthodox immunization, especially if child is thin, has a large head, and tends to have sweaty feet *Silicea 6c*
● Clear discharge from nose and throat *Agraphis 6c*
● Blockage of eustachian tubes, copious saliva, dislike of heat and cold *Mercurius dulc. 6c*

Anaemia see also ANAEMIA pp. 184–6
Shortage of oxygen-carrying components in blood. Often accompanies COELIAC DISEASE or STILL'S DISEASE. Symptoms include tiredness, BREATHLESSNESS, PALPITATIONS, loss of appetite (see APPETITE CHANGES), pale fingertips, pale skin inside eyelids, very blue whites of eyes (sclera). A common cause, especially in children born pre-term, is iron deficiency. If iron deficiency is suspected, [48]. GP will do blood test and prescribe iron if necessary. See p. 347 for foods containing iron.

Anaphylactoid purpura
Blotchy purple rash on the legs and buttocks due to leakage of blood from small blood vessels, brought on by an abnormal reaction to an infection (usually a streptococcal throat infection), a food, or a drug. Rash comes and goes, but does not fade when pressed. Often associated with ABDOMINAL PAIN and arthritis; can also lead to acute NEPHRITIS (kidney damage, blood in the urine). If condition is suspected, (2). Early constitutional treatment is also recommended.

Specific remedies to be taken 4 times daily for up to 5 days
● *Lachesis 6c* followed by *Crotalus 6c* if there is no improvement

Asthma see also ASTHMA p. 176–7, BREATHING DIFFICULTIES, BREATHLESSNESS, WHEEZING
Narrowing of the small airways in the lungs, causing child to wheeze, cough, choke, and fight to breathe; extremely distressing and occasionally fatal. Seldom occurs without some family history of ALLERGY or respiratory disease. Often associated with ECZEMA, HAY FEVER AND ALLERGIC RHINITIS, and allergies to house dust, house dust mites, grass pollens, animals, cigarette smoke. Sometimes triggered off by BRONCHITIS or BRONCHIOLITIS. Attacks can be brought on by exercise, emotion, rapid changes in the weather, some prescription drugs (beta blockers for heart disease, for example), and various allergens present in food and the environment (see environmental hazards pp. 32–3). Wheezy bronchitis during the first year of life (COLDS that settle on the chest, causing thick phlegm and coughing), plus a family history of asthma or allergies, should alert you to the possibility that your child might develop asthma. Immediate constitutional treatment from an experienced homeopath could minimize that risk. That said, most young children who develop asthma grow out of it by the age of seven.

In acute attacks, conventional treatment is Ventolin, given by inhaler or nebulizer. Ventolin opens the airways, allowing mucus to be expelled, and must be used in strict accordance with your GP's directions. In severe acute attacks, aminophylline or steroids may be prescribed. In fact there is an increasing tendency to use steroids early in acute attacks. Intal may be prescribed over a long period to desensitize membranes.

The homeopathic approach to chronic asthma is constitutional (both Ventolin and Intal are compatible with constitutional treatment). Remedies for acute attacks are listed below.

If neither conventional nor homeopathic remedies control an acute attack and the child's condition gets worse, or if there is any sign that the child's extremities are turning blue (cyanosis), or if the respiratory rate is beginning to climb above 50 or 60 breaths per minute if child is very young or above 40 breaths per minute if child is aged four or over, or if the ribs are being sucked inwards, or if the child becomes unusually drowsy or has difficulty speaking, ②.

Specific remedies to be taken every 10 minutes for up to 10 doses
- Attack comes on suddenly, especially after shock or exposure to cold, dry wind *Aconite 30c*
- Attack comes on suddenly in middle of night, child unable to lie down, blue extremities *Sambucus 6c* and ⑨⑨⑨
- Attack comes on between midnight and 2 am, child feels restless, chilly, wants sips of hot drinks *Arsenicum 6c*
- Coughing, gagging, fighting for air, made worse by talking or eating *Carbo veg. 30c*
- Lots of phlegm coughed up, child complains of great weight on chest and feeling sick all the time *Ipecac. 6c*
- Attack comes on during or after stomach upset, child very irritable *Nux 6c*
- Child coughing a lot, very thirsty, wants to be held and comforted *Phosphorus 6c*
- Attack comes on around 4 am, especially if child is worried or anxious about something *Kali carb. 6c*
- Attack comes on between 4 and 5 am, especially in damp weather, child clutches chest while coughing *Natrum sulph. 6c*
- Child irritable, finds fault with everything, wants to be picked up and carried *Chamomilla 6c*
- Greenish phlegm coughed up, child tearful *Pulsatilla 6c*

Self-help Avoid feathers, animals, and dust around house and in child's room. Child's bedding should be a plastic-covered mattress, foam pillow, and cotton blankets. Child's room should also be as bare as possible, with linoleum on the floor rather than carpet. An air ionizer (see p. 30) may also be beneficial. Keep child out of rooms you are cleaning, and if you smoke, confine your smoking to a room the child rarely enters and use a proprietary cleaner to remove all traces of cigarette ash. As for diet, avoid all food additives, cut right down on sugar and fat, and make sure child has plenty of Vitamin B$_6$ and B complex, Vitamins C and E, zinc, selenium, and linseed oil. In an acute attack, sit the child up and give as much comfort and reassurance as you can. A humidifier (see p. 30) will help the child to cough up phlegm. In especially difficult cases, a form of psychotherapy called family therapy may also be beneficial.

Autism
Withdrawal from all forms of social contact. Child retreats into own world, refuses to be cuddled, avoids eye contact, shows poor language development, becomes obsessed with things or routines, goes in for repetitive movements such as body rocking and head banging. Condition can last into adult life, with behaviour becoming increasingly violent. See SCHIZOPHRENIA. Cause or causes not really known. One theory is that the child-parent bond goes wrong, locking the child into a permanent state of fear and conflict – he or she wants affection but is always too afraid to ask for or respond to it. An imbalance in body chemistry caused by nutritional deficiency may also have something to do with it. There is also a theory that head banging, and the groaning and grimacing that sometimes go with it, may be an attempt to relieve head pain caused by over-compression of the skull during birth. Accordingly, treatment options include behaviour therapy for both child and parents, nutritional therapy, and cranial osteopathy. Homeopathy can offer constitutional treatment, and the short-term remedies given below.

Specific remedies to be taken up to 4 times daily for up to 3 weeks
- Child irritable, restless, lashes out when approached, repeatedly bangs head on wall, clearly finds noise very upsetting *Chamomilla 6c*
- Child retreats into shell, sits on floor and counts things over and over again, has head sweats at night, and sweaty, smelly feet *Silicea 6c*
- Child mutters, is suspicious of unfamiliar objects, goes into fits of laughter, plays with genitals *Hyoscyamus 6c*

Self-help Add Vitamins B$_3$, B$_5$, B$_6$, and C to the diet, also zinc and manganese. Avoid copper. Contact the National Autistic Society (address p. 384).

Bedwetting see also TOILET TRAINING PROBLEMS
Towards the end of their second year most children begin to know what a full bladder or bowel feels like and either ask to go to the toilet immediately or delay going until a convenient moment. Daytime control of the bladder is usually achieved between the age of eighteen months and three years, and night-time control a year or so later, between the age of two and a half and three and a half. Dry nights should come naturally after this. However, some children take longer to develop bladder control than others. About 10 per cent of four- and five-year-olds regularly bedwet, and a further 10 per cent do so on occasions.

Doctors distinguish between primary bedwetting and secondary bedwetting. Primary bedwetting means that a child has never been completely dry for very long. This may be purely physiological, the nervous system not being mature enough to signal urgency or close the sphincter from the bladder, or it may be psychological, the child never having learned to like being dry because nappy changes were infrequent. Secondary bedwetting means that the child has been dry for a significant period, but has started to wet again. Causes include ANXIETY, problems in the family or at school, food ALLERGY, food additives, a slight degree of spinal maladjustment, urinary infections, and WORMS. If infection or infestation is suspected 48; a urine test may be necessary. Constitutional treatment can help to boost the child's general resistance to infection.

Specific remedies to be taken at bedtime for up to 14 nights
- Wetting during dreams *Equisetum 6c*
- Wetting early in night, especially if child goes to bed cold after a hair wash *Belladonna 6c*
- Child sleeps deeply but wets during dreams in early part of night and cannot wake fast enough to get to toilet *Kreosotum 6c*
- Wetting in first sleep, worse when child has a cough, and worse in dry, clear weather *Causticum 6c*
- If above remedies fail, and there are no indications for any other remedy *Plantago 6c*

Self-help With older children, it is important to make them feel that they can handle the problem; one way of doing this is to encourage them to change soiled sheets themselves, leaving fresh sheets out for them each night. If the cause is spinal maladjustment, osteopathy or chiropractic may produce improvement.

Behavioural problems

Any persistent form of behaviour which disrupts family life, progress at school, or relationships with age mates, can be called a 'behavioural problem'. See HYPER-ACTIVITY, TANTRUMS, AUTISM, SLEEP PROBLEMS, FEED-ING PROBLEMS, LEARNING DIFFICULTIES, PHOBIA, DEPRESSION, INSECURITY.

Some problems can be avoided by consistent but caring discipline. A balance has to be struck between over-strictness and over-permissiveness. Children need some rules of conduct, if only to make them feel secure, but they should be told why such rules exist – for their own safety or the safety of others, for example. Inevitably, rules get broken. When this happens, a child should be given a chance to mend his or her behaviour; try to encourage an acceptable alternative form of behaviour and carefully explain, again, what the rule is for, and that punishment will follow if the rule is broken again. Never threaten punishment and then not carry it out. If you decide to punish, do it immediately; the 'wait until your father gets home' approach is not really fair on the child because it creates a sense of fear and dissociates the crime from the punishment. If you smack a child, which should only rarely be necessary, never smack him or her around the head. Afterwards, make it clear that you still love the child and give a cuddle.

Bow legs and knock knees

Both of these conditions right themselves by the fifth year of life, provided diet is not deficient in Vitamin D or calcium. Bow legs are quite common when children begin to walk and support their own weight; later the knees turn inwards to compensate. By the age of four, however, the legs straighten and assume their adult shape.

Breath-holding see FITS

Breathing difficulties

Sudden difficulties may be due to acute ASTHMA (wheezing and phlegm), PNEUMONIA (dry cough and high fever), CROUP AND STRIDOR (deep, crowing intakes of breath), ACUTE EPIGLOTTIS (choking and high fever), inhaling a foreign body or noxious chemicals (see First Aid pp. 94–5), or to viral infections such as BRONCHITIS and BRONCHIOLITIS. May also be a sign of a congenital heart defect (see CONGENITAL DISORDERS), CYSTIC FIBROSIS, swollen or infected ADENOIDS, or congenital 'floppy' larynx. For last condition, consult an ear, nose and throat specialist.

If child's lips or tongue turn blue, or if breathing rate climbs above 50-60 breaths per minute in a very young child or over 40 breaths per minute in a child aged four or over, or if he or she is drowsy or has difficulty speaking, (999).

Bronchitis see BRONCHITIS pp. 178–9

Cerebral palsy (spastic paralysis)

Stiff, uncontrollable, or paralysed muscles due to brain abnormality or BRAIN DAMAGE during birth, or in rare cases to brain damage caused by MENINGITIS or FITS. Condition not hereditary. Muscles may be floppy to begin with and not stiffen up until child is at least six months old. First signs may be delayed milestones (see p. 311). Extent of spasticity can vary from one limb to whole left or right side of body. Associated conditions include DEAFNESS, SQUINTING, FITS, CONSTIPATION, and MENTAL HANDICAP. However, despite their physical difficulties, most spastic children are just as bright as their peers and should not be classified or treated as mentally subnormal. Physiotherapy and speech therapy should begin as early as possible. Later, surgery may be necessary to correct deformities. Occupational therapy and special schooling may be appropriate if there is some degree of mental handicap. Home homeopathic treatment should be supervised by an EXPERIENCED HOMEOPATH. Suitable remedies include those listed under BRAIN INJURY and those listed below.

Specific remedies to be taken 4 times daily for up to 14 days
- Affected limbs cold, stiffer when covered up *Secale 6c*
- Stiffness and paralysis accompanied by stubborn constipation *Plumbum 6c*

Specific remedy to be taken every 4 hours for up to 2 weeks
- Muscular spasms markedly worse *Arnica 6c*

Self-help Stiff, jumpy muscles are often relaxed by hot baths and massage.

Chafing
Sore, red skin caused by friction against clothing.

Specific remedies to be taken 4 times daily for up to 5 days
- Chafing worst in groin *Chamomilla 6c*
- Affected areas very sore and painful *Mercurius 6c*
- Soreness made worse by walking *Aethusa 6c*
- Recurrent bouts of chafing *Lycopodium 6c*

Self-help Apply Hypericum and Calendula ointment (see Building a Home Medicine Chest p. 35) to affected areas, and make sure all clothes worn next to the skin are loose-fitting, made of cotton, washed with soap powder rather than detergent, and thoroughly rinsed and dried.

Chest infections see PNEUMONIA, BRONCHITIS, BRONCHIOLITIS, CYSTIC FIBROSIS

Chicken pox
A very infectious viral disease spread by droplets from the nose, mouth, or rash of an infected child or from an adult with SHINGLES. If your child has been in contact with someone suffering from chicken pox or shingles, give *Varicella 30c* or *Rhus tox. 30c* once a day for 10 days as a preventive.

Incubation period is 13-17 days from contact with infected person. First stage is low FEVER and feeling generally unwell; this usually lasts for 24 hours. Second stage is eruption of rash and a temporary increase in fever. Third stage is decrease of fever and gradual healing of spots, which takes 6-10 days. Child remains infectious until all spots have healed. If scratched, spots can become infected and leave lasting pockmarks. Most children recover completely, but there is a small risk of the chicken pox virus (*Herpes zoster*) staying in the system and manifesting later as shingles. If spots are confined to hands, feet, and inside of mouth, child may be suffering from hand, foot and mouth disease (not the same as foot and mouth in cattle) rather than chicken pox.

If you suspect your child has chicken pox, 24 or contact your homeopath. If fever is still high 2 days after rash appears, or if child is clearly very poorly and chesty, ② as there may be a risk of PNEUMONIA or shingles.

Specific remedies to be taken every 2 hours for up to 10 doses
- Low fever and general discomfort during first stage *Aconite 30c* or *Belladonna 30c*, or a daily dose of Ferrum Phos. (see Tissue Salts p. 35)

- Large blisters develop, child whines and doesn't want to be left alone *Antimonium tart. 6c*
- Rash, fever, child very restless *Rhus tox. 6c*
- Rash, fever, child very clingy, tearful, not thirsty in spite of high temperature *Pulsatilla 6c*
- Rash, fever, child very thirsty and hungry but refuses to eat *Sulphur 6c*
- Temperature down, spots beginning to heal but some infected *Mercurius 6c*

Self-help Rub honey or Vitamin E cream on spots, provided skin is not broken. Oatmeal baths or sponge-downs with a solution of baking soda (4 teaspoonfuls bicarbonate of soda to 2.25 litres [4 pints] warm water) will help spots to dry and heal.

Clumsiness
Poor coordination and accident-proneness may be due to ANXIETY, LACK OF CONFIDENCE, lack of concentration, immaturity of the nervous system, effects of orthodox drugs or ADDICTION to recreational drugs or alcohol, neurological or muscular disorders (usually associated with headaches and general unwellness), and in rare cases to CEREBRAL PALSY or bismuth poisoning (see toxic metals pp. 30, 349).

Specific remedies to be taken 4 times daily for up to 14 days
- Poor coordination, child oversensitive and inclined to burst into tears if someone else is hurt *Causticum 6c*
- Poor coordination, child lacks self-confidence and tries to attract attention by doing outrageous things *Lycopodium 6c*
- Poor coordination, child overweight, with a chilly skin and sweaty head *Calcarea 6c*

Self-help Clumsy children often benefit from some form of disciplined exercise – judo, dancing, etc. If clumsiness is the result of showing off, show that you are not impressed; quietly point out the risk of injury to the child and to others.

Coeliac disease
Inability of cells lining upper part of small intestine to break down gluten, a protein found in wheat, oats, barley, and rye. At present the disease cannot be positively diagnosed except by biopsy, removing a tiny sample of tissue for analysis; this is not a pleasant procedure, but will shortly be replaced by blood or urine tests.

Intolerance to gluten seems to run in families, but is less often seen in children who are breast-fed or introduced relatively late to foods containing gluten. In susceptible children, the disease develops by the age of two, usually 3–6 months after gluten is introduced into the diet. Signs are failure to gain weight (see growth charts p. 312), CONSTIPATION, or on the contrary bulky, offensive-smelling stools passed with great frequency, lack of muscle tone, a blown-out stomach, and general pallor and apathy. The only effective treatment is to remove gluten from the diet on a temporary or permanent basis. Early constitutional treatment from an EXPERIENCED HOMEOPATH may make permanent avoidance of gluten unnecessary.

The above symptoms are not solely those of coeliac disease, however. ALLERGY (especially to cow's milk, soya products, and fish), LACTOSE INTOLERANCE in the wake of GASTROENTERITIS, CYSTIC FIBROSIS, immune deficiencies, and even emotional deprivation can produce similar symptoms. Do not put your child on a gluten-free diet until you are sure of the diagnosis. For further information contact the Coeliac Society of the United Kingdom (address p. 382).

Colds see also COLDS p. 163

Extremely common in childhood, especially once child goes to school or playschool and is exposed to new germs. Positive side is that colds gradually build up immunity. Most colds begin with a tight feeling in the throat, followed by sneezing and a runny nose; mucus is clear at first, becoming thicker, and yellow or greenish; mucus dripping on to vocal cords irritates them, causing a COUGH, and if swallowed can cause stomach ache (see ABDOMINAL PAIN). Most colds run their course within 7–10 days. Some 'colds' may be a symptom of ALLERGY (mucus stays clear) or common childhood illnesses and fevers (see FEVER p 321), or part of a pattern of symptoms associated with ASTHMA or CYSTIC FIBROSIS. Recurrent colds, especially if they descend to the chest and develop into BRONCHITIS or TONSILLITIS, or lead to acute MIDDLE EAR INFECTION, warrant constitutional treatment as the child's immune system may not be as robust as it should be.

If child has a temperature of 39°C (102°F) or over, or is taking more than 40 breaths per minute, or has difficulty breathing or speaking, or is very drowsy, or starts to turn blue around the lips, ②.

Specific remedies to be taken every 2 hours for up to 10 doses
- First stage of cold, especially if child recently exposed to draught or cold wind *Aconite 30c*
- Child has high temperature, red face, staring eyes, feels very thirsty, symptoms come on after a hair wash or haircut *Belladonna 30c*
- Thick, greenish catarrh, child tearful, clinging, not at all thirsty *Pulsatilla 6c*
- Cold begins as sore throat, child complains of earache and is very sensitive to draughts, lymph glands in neck swollen and tender, saliva glands working overtime *Mercurius 6c*
- Cold comes on after child has got wet or damp after being hot *Dulcamara 6c*
- Cold resembles 'flu, child heavy-eyed, weak and shivery, complains of aches and chills *Gelsemium 6c*
- Thick, yellow catarrh, rattly breathing, child irrit-able, clammy, wants to stay indoors away from wind and draughts with legs and arms covered *Hepar sulph. 6c*
- Child irritable, wants to be left alone, very thirsty and gulps down large quantities of fluid, constipated, stuffed up nose and dry lips *Bryonia 30c*
- Streaming nose, lots of sneezing, constipation, irritability, child most ill around 4 am *Nux 6c*

Self-help If child suffers from lots of colds, turn down central heating, give the house a daily airing, and invest in a humidifier (see p. 30). If you smoke, try to confine your smoking to one room and clean all curtains and furniture in the house with a proprietary cleaner to remove all traces of cigarette ash, which is an irritant. Reducing the quantity of dairy foods (milk, cheese, yoghurt, butter) in the diet, and increasing intake of Vitamin C and zinc, may also help.

Constipation see also CONSTIPATION pp. 223–4

Definitions vary, some doctors defining constipation as the failure to pass a stool every day, others regarding a bowel movement every four or five days as acceptable, provided stools are not too hard or painful to pass. Nevertheless the longer faeces remain in the bowel the more opportunity there is for toxic substances to be reabsorbed into the bloodstream and passed to the liver, causing poor liver function and other problems. Constipation may be a sign of Hirschsprung's Disease (see CONGENITAL DISORDER) in babies or very young children, ANAL FISSURE, hypothyroidism (see THYROID PROBLEMS), or parental over-emphasis on regular bowel habits (see TOILET TRAINING PROBLEMS). Persistent constipation requires constitutional treatment. If the remedies listed below fail to work within 48 hours, [12]. Laxatives and suppositories should only be used on your doctor's instructions.

Specific remedies to be taken 4 times daily for up to 14 days
- Stools difficult to pass even when soft, child has no desire to pass stool unless rectum is completely full, itchy eyes, dry skin *Alumina 6c*
- Stools large, dry, and hard, mouth and tongue dry, child very thirsty *Bryonia 6c*
- Child irritable and chilly, feels urge to pass stool but is unable to, or if able to feels there is more to come *Nux 6c*
- Sudden stomach cramps, urge to pass stool but stool slips back up inside *Silicea 6c*
- Child feels better when constipated *Calcarea 6c*
- Small, hard stools with ineffectual straining and a lot of wind *Lycopodium 6c*
- Lazy bowel, no desire to pass stool for days on end, when passed stool takes form of little hard balls, child loses appetite, is drowsy during day and wakeful at night, and very sensitive to noise *Opium 6c*

For explanation of other symbols, see page 107

Self-help Increase amount of fibre in child's diet, avoid cooking in aluminium utensils or foil, and increase fluid intake, especially if constipation is acute and child's temperature is higher than normal.

Convulsions see FITS in First Aid, also FITS pp. 128–9, 321–2

Cough see also COUGH pp. 179–80

Coughing expels foreign bodies and irritating mucus from the trachea and airways of the lungs. The membranes lining the whole respiratory tract are extremely sensitive and react to all kinds of inhaled particles by producing mucus, which is then coughed up, the colour of the sputum or phlegm being an indication of the nature or degree of irritation or infection. Catarrh from the nose or sinuses can also drip on to the vocal cords, causing coughing. Coughing is one of the signs of WHOOPING COUGH (violent bouts of coughing with whooping noise, sometimes vomiting), MEASLES (in the early stage), ASTHMA (difficult breathing, flaring of nostrils or sucking in of lower ribs in effort to breathe, blueness around lips), CROUP AND STRIDOR (crowing intakes of breath), inhaling a foreign body, BRONCHIOLITIS, acute PNEUMONIA and BRONCHITIS (difficulty breathing, temperature above 39°C [102°F]), INFLUENZA and other viral infections, TRACHEITIS, and SINUSITIS. Cigarette smoke may also be the culprit.

If cough lasts for more than 10 days or is accompanied by FEVER, or if you suspect the early stages of measles, [12]. If coughing is associated with difficulty breathing, blue tongue or lips, unusual drowsiness, fast breathing (over 40 breaths per minute), or difficulty speaking, (2). Do not use cough suppressants, especially if you do not know the cause of the cough. Recurrent coughs require constitutional treatment.

Specific remedies to be taken every 4 hours up to 10 doses in acute attack
- Dry, irritating cough, sudden onset *Aconite 30c*
- Bouts of dry, tickly coughing which may end in a whoop or sneeze, bursting, congested feeling in head, Adam's apple tender *Belladonna 30c*
- Hard, dry cough which causes child to hold chest or head, child thirsty for cold drinks but more soothed by hot ones *Bryonia 30c*
- Breathlessness, wheezing, chest feels weighed down, child blue and rigid during coughing bouts, persistent nausea, clean tongue *Ipecac. 6c*
- Violent, tickly cough from chest, with retching and gagging, and pain below ribs, worse at night and out of doors *Drosera 6c*
- Barking, croaky cough, with hoarseness, alleviated by eating and drinking and lying with head low, child chokes and panics on waking *Spongia 6c*
- Croaky cough, temperature higher than normal,

worse in cold, dry weather and aggravated by draughts, child chilly, irritable, craves hot drinks *Hepar sulph. 6c*
- Racking, tickly cough from larynx, aggravated by talking, by changes in temperature, and by lying down, child craves cold drinks but vomits as soon as fluid becomes warm in stomach *Phosphorus 6c*
- Dry, irritating cough with wheezing, worse at night, perhaps brought on by anger, child very irritable *Chamomilla 6c*
- Cough with stringy phlegm *Kali bichrom. 6c*
- Dry cough with retching, child feverish, chilly, worse for exposure to cold, oversensitive and very irritable *Nux 6c*
- Cough dry at night, moist in morning, with yellow or greenish phlegm, child tearful, miserable, not thirsty, more poorly in warm, stuffy rooms *Pulsatilla 6c*
- Dry, tickly cough at back of throat, made worse by talking and by cold air, and worse at night, preventing sleep, child feels better with head under blankets *Rumex 6c*
- Cough worse around midnight, with wheezing, child cold, restless, anxious, worn out, thirsty, finds sipping hot drinks soothing *Arsenicum 6c*
- Rattling cough from chest, which sounds full of phlegm, child too weak to clear phlegm, very pale, blue around lips, feels he or she must sit up or suffocate (999) as child may require hospitalization, and in meantime *Antimonium tart. 6c*
- Dry cough, raw throat, hoarseness, no phlegm, child finds cold drinks soothing, may pass urine involuntarily *Causticum 6c*
- Sweetish-tasting phlegm and sore throat during day, dry, violent cough during evening, child breathless, hardly able to talk, symptoms made worse by talking or laughing *Stannum 6c*
- Dry, hacking cough at night, made worse by bringing up phlegm *Sticta 6c*
- Dry, hard cough, with lumpy sputum and wheezing, worse between 3 and 5 am, child feels weak and chilly *Kali carb. 6c*

Self-help Avoid dry atmosphere in home, turn down central heating, and humidify child's room (see p. 30). If there is a smoker in the house, meticulously remove all traces of cigarette ash. Hot lemon and honey drinks will soothe a raw throat.

Croup and stridor

Stridor is medical shorthand for 'crowing', grunting, and wheezing brought on by sudden narrowing of the larynx due to infection or obstruction. The most appropriate action in such circumstances is (999) and First Aid (see p. 86), and *Belladonna 30c* every 5 minutes until help arrives.

Occasionally stridor is a symptom of ACUTE EPIGLOTTITIS (bacterial infection accompanied by high fever), which may require hospitalization and assist-

---

(999) Emergency – call GP (or dial 999 immediately. (2) Consult your doctor if no improvement within 2 hours

ance with breathing. If a foreign body has been inhaled, it should be located and removed or it may settle in the lungs and cause PNEUMONIA.

Croup is stridor following a cold. A child with croup becomes hoarse, breathless, and develops a hollow, crowing COUGH, usually worse in the middle of the night. If croup is accompanied by high FEVER, treat as for ACUTE EPIGLOTITIS.

Specific remedies
- Child wakes in night, coughing, breathless and frightened *Aconite 30c* immediately, and again ½ hour later if child still awake
- If above symptoms persist after Aconite, give *Spongia 6c* and *Hepar sulph. 6c* alternately every hour for up to 3 doses each

Self-help If child has croup, give the main meal of the day at lunch time, and a light supper in the evening. Humidify child's room (see p. 30) or, during coughing attack, take child into the bathroom, close the windows and switch off the extractor fan, and turn on all the hot taps. Never leave a small child unaccompanied.

Cyclical vomiting see ABDOMINAL MIGRAINE

Cystic fibrosis
Hereditary condition affecting pancreas and lungs. Under-production of digestive enzymes by the pancreas leads to poor absorption of nutrients from the gut, and sticky mucus secreted in the lungs stagnates and leads to chest infections. First sign may be retention of meconium (first faeces) in newborn baby, sometimes requiring surgical removal, followed by SLOW WEIGHT GAIN and passage of large, greasy, offensive stools. Cystic fibrosis can be managed – by giving pancreatic extracts and keeping the child on a low fat diet, combined with physiotherapy to keep the lungs as free from mucus as possible – but not cured. Constitutional homeopathic treatment can help. If there is cystic fibrosis in your family, it would be wise to seek genetic counselling before conceiving. For more information contact the Cystic Fibrosis Trust (address p. 357).

Self-help Vitamins A, D, E, and K, and also zinc and selenium may be beneficial.

Dental problems see TOOTH DECAY, TEETHING

Diabetes see DIABETES pp. 257–8

Diarrhoea see DIARRHOEA p. 225
May be due to GASTROENTERITIS (vomiting and fever), ABDOMINAL PAIN, FOOD POISONING, certain drugs, ENCOPRESIS (soiling pants with faeces), ANXIETY, or food ALLERGY. Details of homeopathic treatment are given on p. 225.

If child refuses to drink, has sunken eyes, is abnormally sleepy, does not pass urine as often as usual, complains of constant stomach ache, or has been vomiting for more than 6 hours, ②.

Diptheria
Acute bacterial infection of the throat (larynx, pharynx, tonsils), once common but now rare due to immunization and improved hygiene. Toxins produced by diptheria bacteria destroy mucous membranes lining throat, giving them a grey, veil-like appearance, and causing swelling of underlying tissues. As membranes slough off and tissues swell, breathing may be obstructed. Toxins can also damage nervous system (see NEURITIS) and affect heart. First signs are FEVER, HEADACHE, SORE THROAT, and swollen glands in neck; later signs may be obstructed breathing, irregular pulse, vomiting, and difficulty swallowing or focusing. Incubation is 2–6 days, but child remains infectious for at least 10 days after onset of fever.

If diptheria is suspected, [12]. Conventional treatment is penicillin and injections of anti-toxin serum.

Specific remedy to be taken ½-hourly until help arrives
- *Mercurius cyan. 6c*

Immunization Both homeopathic and orthodox medicine offer immunization based on the diptheria bacteria (*Corynebacterium diptheriae*) or its toxins. Orthodox immunization is usually part of 'triple' immunization, which boosts resistance to TETANUS and WHOOPING COUGH as well as diptheria.

Dyslexia
Child has normal IQ but finds reading and spelling difficult and unrewarding, confusing similar letters such as d and b, and p and q. Performance can be improved by special remedial exercises and constitutional homeopathic treatment.

Specific remedy to be taken 3 times daily for up to 3 weeks while remedial or constitutional treatment is being sought
- *Lycopodium 6c*

Self-help Extra zinc may be helpful. For further information contact the British Dyslexia Association (address p. 383).

Earache see EARACHE pp. 158–9

Ear wax see also EAR WAX p. 159
General opinion today is that wax protects outer ear from infection and is unlikely to conceal infection. On the contrary, inflammation caused by infection is likely to melt earwax. Syringing is not advised unless wax is completely blocking ear and causing DEAFNESS.

Eczema see also ECZEMA pp. 140, 308,
SEBORRHOEIC ECZEMA
An allergic reaction to incompletely digested protein or to toxins in the blood due to the liver's inability to break down certain foods properly. First signs are patches of dry skin, which then become red, scaly, and very itchy. In severe cases, little blisters form, which weep and can become infected if scratched. Condition usually starts between age of two months and two years, but often disappears around age of seven, although child may manifest other allergic reactions such as HAY FEVER AND ALLERGIC RHINITIS or ASTHMA. The homeopathic view is that eczema is not a skin disease but a disease of the whole metabolic system manifesting itself via the skin. The skin erupts in an effort to rid the body of toxins in the bloodstream. A family history of TUBERCULOSIS often indicates a predisposition to eczema and related conditions.

Conventional treatment is by antihistamines, which give some respite from itchiness and scratching, or by antibiotics, if skin becomes infected. As a rule steroid ointments should only be used if itching is so severe that it prevents the child sleeping and begins to affect his or her general health, or if the skin is severely infected. Steroid ointments certainly suppress the condition, but they do not cure it. EXPERT CONSTITUTIONAL HOMEOPATHIC TREATMENT is advised, although the remedies given below are also effective in the short-term, but watch out for aggravations; if redness and itchiness flare up, stop the remedy at once.

Specific remedies to be taken 4 times daily for up to 5 days
- Skin dry, itchy and red, especially so in bed or after bathing, child untidy and boisterous, suffers from diarrhoea in morning *Sulphur 6c*
- Skin blistered, especially on wrists, markedly worse in damp conditions *Rhus tox. 6c*
- Skin looks dirty and unwashed, eczema worse on legs *Psorinum 6c*
- Skin weepy, pus honey-coloured, condition worst behind ears and on palms of hands *Graphites 6c*
- Infected, oozing crusts, especially on scalp *Mezereum 6c*
- Skin bubbling, with yellow crusts, worse at night *Petroleum 6c*

Self-help Make sure child wears only cotton – not wool or man-made fibres – next to skin, and use emulsifying ointment rather than soap in bath. Oatmeal baths, which can be bought in sachet form, may also be beneficial. A blue light in the child's room gives the illusion of coldness, reducing scratching at night, and cold packs give temporary relief from itching. Dietary treatment – either a general diet to improve liver function (see Liver Diet p. 352) or a specific elimination and challenge diet – can be very effective and is part of constitutional treatment. Only minor dietary changes should be made on your own initiative,

however, as too restricted a diet can make metabolic problems worse. Consult your homeopath or a dietary therapist if in doubt. In the meantime, a children's strength multivitamin and mineral supplement, plus zinc and evening primrose oil, may be beneficial.

Encopresis
Child soils pants with faeces even when he or she has been toilet-trained for some time. Usual cause is CONSTIPATION, with fluid matter trickling past constipated mass in rectum. Treat as for constipation. If soiling matter is solid, problem may be emotional, and constitutional treatment would be appropriate.

Epilepsy see EPILEPSY pp. 127–8

Fears see INSECURITY

Febrile convulsions see also FITS pp. 128–9 and 321–2
Fits brought on by FEVER. There is no evidence that febrile convulsions cause permanent brain damage, but if they recur without fever, constitutional treatment should be sought. In acute attack ⑨⑨⑨ if homeopathic remedies fail to take effect within two minutes. It may be necessary for GP to give a tranquillizer by rectum to stop convulsions. If child loses consciousness, put him or her in recovery position (see First Aid pp. 90–1).

Specific remedies to be given every minute for up to 3 doses or until fit subsides
- First signs of fit *Aconite 30c*
- Fit accompanies gastroenteritis *Aethusa 6c*
- Fit preceded by staring eyes and excited, incoherent behaviour *Belladonna 30c*
- Child very pale, has sunken fontanelle *Zinc sulph. 6c*

Self-help See FEVER for care of feverish child.

Feeding problems
Despite the guilt and rejection felt by many parents whose children refuse to eat, or won't eat properly, or play up at mealtimes, there is evidence that children have a more efficient metabolic and digestive system than adults, and use even small quantities of food more efficiently. It has been demonstrated that over a period of time, left to their own devices, children tend to eat foods which balance each other and make up a perfectly nutritious diet, provided they are not offered junk foods. As long as your child is growing and healthy (see milestones p. 311), faddy eating should not be a cause for concern.

Self-help The following tactics help to establish good eating habits: provide as nutritious and as varied a diet as possible (see children's diets pp. 24–5); if child picks at food during mealtimes, don't force him or her to eat and don't make a big issue out of not eating, but make it

⑨⑨⑨ Emergency – call GP (or dial 999) immediately. ② Consult your doctor if no improvement within 2 hours

clear there will be no snacks between meals; if child is too tired or too hungry to eat, consider adjusting mealtimes; if child is very young and seems to be hungry outside mealtimes, offer nutritious snacks, but not junk food; never offer or withhold food, especiaally sweet things, as a bribe or a punishment; allow very young children to feed themselves in their own way – allow them to use their fingers if they want to, don't make them wait once the meal is on the table, let them leave the table as soon as they have finished, and never make them stay at table as a punishment.

Fever

Fever, signalled by body temperature rising above the normal range of 36–37°C (96.8–98.6°F), is the body's way of making invading germs easier to attack and destroy. Dosing with paracetamol may bring temperature down for a while, but will not assist the germ-fighting process, and may even lead to complications. Paracetamol may be given to ensure a good night's sleep or if temperature goes above 39°C (102°F) and child is prone to FEBRILE CONVULSIONS.

A temperature above 39°C (102°F) is always a cause for concern in a child, so don't hesitate to call your GP if you are worried. If a cause cannot be found, and you are unsure about which homeopathic remedy to give, consult your homeopath. If fever is associated with BREATHING DIFFICULTIES, or with HEADACHE, NAUSEA AND VOMITING, intolerance to light, and a stiff neck, or with a purple rash on the elbows, ankles, and buttocks, ② as child may have PNEUMONIA, MENINGITIS, or ANAPHYLACTOID PURPURA.

Fever without rash Causes include APPENDICITIS (abdominal pain), MIDDLE EAR INFECTION (earache, child keeps pulling at affected ear), COLDS (running nose, sneezing), MEASLES (early stages), TONSILLITIS, LARYNGITIS and PHARYNGITIS (sore throat, hoarse voice, coughing), INFLUENZA (sudden chills and aches), BRONCHITIS (a cold that turns into a chesty cough), PNEUMONIA (breathing problems), GASTRO-ENTERITIS (diarrhoea), MUMPS (painful swelling between ears and angle of jaw), MENINGITIS (headache, nausea with or without vomiting, stiff neck, intolerance of light), urinary tract infections (pain on passing urine, or wanting to urinate more frequently than usual), HEATSTROKE, and some tropical diseases.

If symptoms are those of meningitis, or if respiratory rate climbs above 40 breaths per minute, ②. If child is coughing, wheezing, struggling to breathe or speak, breathing very fast, or turning blue around the lips, ⑨⑨⑨.

Fever with rash Causes include ANAPHYLACTOID PURPURA (purple blotches on elbows, ankles, and buttocks, sore throat two weeks before onset of rash), MEASLES (red spots, runny nose, red eyes, dry cough), RUBELLA (red spots and pea-like bumps at back of head), CHICKEN POX (red, itchy spots which develop

into blisters and then crust over), ROSEOLA INFANTUM (pink rash, swollen neck glands), and occasionally drugs.

If temperature stays above 39°C (102°F) for longer than 6 hours, or if child goes into convulsions, ⑨⑨⑨.

Specific remedies to be given every hour for up to 10 doses in acute situations
- Fever comes on suddenly and is worse around midnight, child pale-faced, restless, and thirsty *Aconite 30c*
- Child feels chilly and won't drink despite fever, feels worse in hot rooms, complains of sharp, stinging pains, may also be delirious *Apis 30c*
- Fever worse between midnight and 2 am, child restless, anxious, exhausted, chilly, thirsty for small sips of water, complains of burning pains in limbs, head feels better for cold but limbs feel better for heat *Arsenicum 6c*
- Fever comes on suddenly and violently, child has hot, flushed skin, pounding pulse, staring eyes, and becomes delirious *Belladonna 30c*
- Child very thirsty at long intervals, irritable, wants to be left alone, feels worse for moving, especially if he or she has a headache, asks to be taken home although already at home *Bryonia 30c*
- Fever comes on gradually, child has red cheeks, a weak and rapid pulse, feels shivery despite frequent sweats, and has a throbbing headache, soothed by cool applications *Ferrum phos. 30c*
- Child feels shivery and 'fluey, with aching muscles and heavy eyelids, not thirsty despite fever, headache made worse by movement *Gelsemium 6c*
- Child feels worse for changes in temperature, is very thirsty, salivates and sweats profusely, breath smells foul and sweat offensive, tongue lolls out *Mercurius 6c*
- Child looks well despite fever, behaves apathetically, seeks sympathy, craves cold drinks which are vomited up as soon as they become warm in stomach, may also have chest infection *Phosphorus 6c*

Self-help Take child's temperature every four hours, check for any pain which might suggest a chest, ear, or throat infection, and give plenty to drink and nothing to eat until fever subsides. If temperature is 39°C (102°F) or above and child is susceptible to FEBRILE CONVULSIONS, undress child and give a 10-minute tepid sponge-down every two hours, or train a fan on the child's body – both measures help the body to cool down. Aspirin and Disprin should be avoided.

Fits see also EPILEPSY, FEBRILE CONVULSIONS
Not all involuntary, convulsive movements are epileptic fits or traceable to injury or infection of the brain.

For explanation of other symbols, see page 107

However, if your child goes into convulsions and loses consciousness put him or her in the recovery position (see First Aid pp. 90–1) and ⑨⑨⑨. During the fit, be gentle and make sure the child comes to no physical harm. Orthodox treatment is to give tranquillizers by rectum.

Specific remedies to be given every minute for up to 3 doses while waiting for help
- At first sign of attack *Aconite 30c*
- If attack continues *Cicuta 6c*

Breath-holding attacks An angry or injured toddler can cry to the point where he or she stops breathing and becomes unconscious. This is not a true fit.

Specific remedies to be taken every 5 minutes for up to 6 doses as soon as child recovers consciousness
- Breath-holding due to injury *Arnica 30c*
- Breath-holding due to bad temper *Chamomilla 6c*

Self-help Extra calcium is recommended if child is prone to breath-holding attacks.

Epileptic fits (including petit mal, grand mal, and temporal lobe epilepsy) See EPILEPSY for description and treatment. In acute attacks give *Cicuta 6c* every 2 minutes.

Febrile convulsions Convulsions associated with FEVER. See p. 320 for description and treatment.

Infantile spasm Also known as 'salaam attacks' because child doubles up at waist in an attitude of prayer. Attacks last for up to 2 seconds and may come on twice or three times a day. Causes include BRAIN DAMAGE at birth, lack of oxygen or sugar in blood going to brain, brain infection, and metabolic diseases such as PHENYLKETONURIA; can also be an after effect of whooping cough vaccine. Unfortunately, attacks can cause or aggravate brain damage.

Self-help Extra magnesium is recommended.

Flat feet see also FOOT PROBLEMS
All babies have flat feet, with arches developing by the age of five or six, so diagnosis of flat feet cannot be certain until that age. Make sure child's diet contains adequate calcium and Vitamin D.

Foot problems see also FLAT FEET, ATHLETE'S FOOT
Causes include FRACTURES (child unable to walk), SPRAINS or bruising (child can walk, but finds it painful), ATHLETE'S FOOT (itching between toes, skin broken or peeling), SPLINTERS (foot very painful, inflamed, and swollen), WARTS or hard skin on the soles of the feet (pain only on standing or walking),

congenital malformations (bent toes, for example), and shoes and socks that are too tight.

See First Aid for fractures, sprains, and splinters. If a fracture is suspected, ⑨⑨⑨ and give *Arnica 30c* every 5 minutes for up to 6 doses.

Foot care is important because problems which affect a child's gait or posture for any length of time tend to affect the rest of the body, especially the back, and because deformities caused by footwear can cause a lot of suffering in later life.

Self-help Allow toddlers to go barefoot until they really need outdoor shoes; or if they need something warm to wear indoors, let them wear loose-fitting socks with grip soles. Buy lightweight shoes to begin with and make sure socks are not too tight – tight socks can deform growing bones as surely as tight shoes. Have your child's feet measured regularly, every 3 months or so, if possible by a trained shop assistant. Don't pass shoes down to younger children as they may not be the right fitting. Avoid shoes that are too tight – there should be an empty finger's width or so at the tips to give the feet room to grow. Shoes that are too loose are no good either, because the toes have to be screwed up to keep them on.

German measles see RUBELLA

Glue ear see also GLUE EAR p. 159
Muffled hearing due to build-up of sticky fluid in middle ear and poor transmission of sound by middle ear bones. Caused by repeated episodes of MIDDLE EAR INFECTION. Persistent glue ear may need to be treated by making an incision in the eardrum, draining off some of the fluid, and inserting a grommet to drain the rest. The grommet, a small plastic tube, falls out of its own accord within a year or so and the eardrum heals. Repeated grommets may lead to weakening of the drum. While grommet is in place there is added risk of infection, so child should not swim or bathe without wearing moulded earplugs; on no account should child be allowed to dive.

Persistent middle ear problems require constitutional treatment. See MIDDLE EAR INFECTION and GLUE EAR p. 159 for specific remedies.

Specific remedies to be taken 3 times daily for up to 14 days before or after insertion of grommet
- Discharge from ear, neck glands swollen, child overweight, flabby, prone to head sweats at night *Calcarea 6c*
- Thick, sticky strings of mucus down back of throat, pain behind nose or in sinuses *Kali bichrom. 6c*
- Crackling noises in affected ear, honey-like discharge from ear *Graphites 6c*
- Thick, yellow, stringy mucus down back of throat, blockage of eustachian tube on affected side *Hydrastis 6c*

---

⑨⑨⑨ Emergency – call GP (or dial 999) immediately. ② Consult your doctor if no improvement within 2 hours

Growing pains

Aching, heavy pains in the calves and thighs, usually experienced between age of six and thirteen, and usually worse at night. Cause not known, but growth is certainly not the cause. May respond to constitutional treatment.

Specific remedies to be taken nightly for up to 14 nights to relieve bouts of pain
- Dragging pains in ankles and knees, worse for walking, especially if child is overweight, pale, clammy, has head sweats at night, and was a late walker *Calcarea 30c*
- Pains worse in cold, wet weather, aggravated by heat and exertion but better when pressure is applied *Guaiacum 30c*
- Child feels weak, pains come on after prolonged stress and feel as if bones are being scraped, worse after exertion *Phosphoric ac. 6c*

Self-help Two tablets of *Calc. Fluor.* and *Calc. Phos.* 3 times a day are often beneficial. Make sure diet is not lacking in calcium and Vitamin D.

Growth disorders

Compare your child's growth with the growth charts on pp. 309 and 312. If your child's height or weight lies outside the acceptable range for his or her age, consult your GP. See also remarks on child development on pp. 310–11. Transient fluctuations in height and weight are common, since growth tends to take place in little spurts. Some weight loss after illness is also quite usual. Weighing your child once a month or once every 2 months should enable you to keep tabs on his or her development.

The causes of abnormal growth range from the hormonal to the congenital. Excessive growth may be diagnosed as OBESITY or GIGANTISM, stunted growth as DWARFISM, hypothyroidism, (see THYROID PROBLEMS), CYSTIC FIBROSIS, COELIAC DISEASE, STILL'S DISEASE, THALASSAEMIA, sickle cell ANAEMIA, or a congenital heart defect (see CONGENITAL DISORDERS). Conventional treatment is by surgery, hormones, or anti-hormone drugs. Homeopathic treatment is constitutional, although the remedies listed below may produce some improvement.

Specific remedies to be given every 12 hours for up to 10 days, then keep child under observation for 1 month; if no improvement, consult your GP
- Child stunted, suffers from chronic catarrh, improves markedly at seaside *Medorrhinum 30c*
- Immaturity associated with constant tonsillitis, swollen neck glands, and emotional insecurity *Baryta 30c*
- Child flabby and overweight, prone to sour-smelling head sweats, late in walking, fontanelle late in closing *Calcarea 30c*

- Child thin, with a large head, sweaty head and feet, sweat very pungent *Silica 30c*

Self-help Extra zinc may produce some improvement.

Headache see HEADACHE pp. 129–30

Head lice

Insects which parasitize human scalp and lay eggs (nits) the size of a pinhead on hair shafts behind ears and around nape of neck. Easily passed from person to person. A mature louse lays 100 eggs a month; these hatch and grow into sexually reproductive individuals within 2 weeks. Lice prefer clean hair to greasy hair and dandruff, and cause intense irritation and scratching, and swollen glands at the back of skull and around neck. Men are seldom affected, for hormonal reasons. If child is infested, the whole family must be treated as well. Constitutional homeopathic treatment may render child less attractive to lice.

Self-help Alert school doctor. Burn all headgear, and wash all bedding, clothing, chair covers, brushes, and combs which might harbour lice or nits. Nits can be picked out of the hair by hand or combed out with a metal comb wetted in vinegar, but treatment with malathion shampoo is more thorough. Follow instructions carefully, drying hair naturally, as beneficial effect is destroyed by hair dryers, and also by chlorine (avoid swimming pools).

Hepatitis see also HEPATITIS p. 227

Children are usually affected by type A viral hepatitis, spread from faeces to mouth by poor hygiene. Because the liver is infected, the whole metabolism of the body is upset. Incubation is 2–6 weeks. Symptoms are those of INFLUENZA and JAUNDICE, plus ITCHING, loss of appetite (see APPETITE CHANGES), pale stools, dark urine, and sometimes NAUSEA AND VOMITING, lasting for about a month. Recovery can take weeks or months. Conventional treatment is immunization of contacts; antibiotics are not effective. Homeopathic treatment is highly recommended during the acute stage (if you are unsure which remedy to take, seek the guidance of an EXPERIENCED HOMEOPATH), with constitutional treatment afterwards to speed recovery.

Specific remedies to be given 4 times daily for up to 7 days
- Pain in liver area, aggravated by lying on right side, unpleasant taste in mouth, increased flow of saliva *Mercurius 6c*
- Sharp pain in liver area, alleviated by lying on right side but made worse by movement, child very thirsty *Bryonia 30c*
- Stools yellow, pain extending from right shoulder blade to base of right rib cage *Chelidonium 6c*
- Pale stools, with a lot of flatulence and wind *China 6c*

Self-help Bed rest and plenty of fluids, especially honey-sweetened drinks (i.e. drinks containing carbohydrates) and thin vegetable soups, are recommended. See that hands are thoroughly washed before eating or preparing food. Do not allow child's towel, flannel, crockery, or cutlery to be used by other members of the family, and thoroughly disinfect lavatory, bath, and handbasin each time child uses them.

High temperature see FEVER

Hyperactivity
A constellation of symptoms which add up to a recognizable pattern of overactive behaviour, more readily diagnosed in the United States than in Britain. Dozens of adjectives are used to describe hyperactive children – restless, excitable, unpredictable, demanding, boisterous, aggressive, destructive, and so on – but the links between physiology and behaviour are not fully understood. Three times as many boys as girls are hyperactive, for reasons which are not clear. Difficulties with speech, hearing, balance, and eye-hand coordination are not uncommon. Intelligence range is similar to that in the non-hyperactive population. Many hyperactive children are fair-haired, attractive, ticklish, have very blue eye whites and hair down the spine, and love the limelight.

Overactivity may begin in the womb. In babies, signs of hyperactivity are head banging, cot rocking, colic, prolonged bouts of crying and screaming, general restlessness, great thirst, copious saliva, and fitful sleep. Hyperactive infants are often slow to crawl. Hyperactive toddlers are excitable, cry easily and often, burst into TANTRUMS if their demands are not instantly met, can't sit still or concentrate on anything for more than a few seconds, must be always on the move, run everywhere and even walk on their toes, touch everything and anything in reach and often break or destroy it, sometimes turn their destructivness on themselves, and have a high pain threshold. Hyperactivity is above average among juvenile delinquents.

Possible causes include lead poisoning (see toxic metals p. 349), food ALLERGY, HYPOGLYCAEMIA, minimal BRAIN DAMAGE at birth, intestinal *Candida* infection (see CANDIDIASIS) passed from mother to child at birth, drug reactions, overtiredness, too much TV, and unhappiness at home or at school. There also seems to be a link with baby battering. There is also a higher incidence of hyperactivity among children whose mothers smoke or suffer from PREMENSTRUAL SYNDROME, or whose families have a history of allergy. EXPERT CONSTITUTIONAL HOMEOPATHIC TREATMENT is recommended.

Self-help One support group advises the following measures, in order of priority. Contact the Hyperactive Children's Support Group (adress p. 384).
1 Avoid food additives

2 Make sure child is not suffering from HYPOGLYCAEMIA
3 Check for food allergies (see p. 272)
4 Check for chemical allergies (see p. 272)
5 Check for toxic metals in environment (see pp. 30–1, 349).

If child becomes violent after a particular food or beverage, give ½ teaspoon bicarbonate of soda in a small glass of water or milk immediately, and repeat every 2 hours, though not more than three times. Dietary supplements, especially essential fatty acids, Vitamin B complex, Vitamin C, and zinc may also be necessary. Also check child's sensitivity to local tap water – it may contain unacceptable levels of fluoride, chlorine, or lead – and change to bottled water if necessary, or use a water filter (see pp. 217–8).

Indigestion see also INDIGESTION pp. 218–8
Heartburn, BELCHING, flatulence, nausea, or just vague discomfort after eating. In children, if symptoms persist for more than 2 or 3 hours, cause may be GASTROENTERITIS. See also ABDOMINAL PAIN and ABDOMINAL MIGRAINE. Conventional treatment is by antacids or bland diets. Chronic indigestion requires constitutional treatment, although the remedies listed below may also be useful.

Specific remedies to be given every 15 minutes for up to 6 doses when indigestion comes on badly
- Pain comes on half an hour after eating, worse after over-eating, child irritable *Nux 6c*
- Burning pains and vomiting after eating over-ripe fruit or ice cream, worse between midnight and 2 am, child chilly, breathless, thirsty for hot drinks *Arsenicum 6c*
- Indigestion after an outburst of anger, gas and cramps in stomach, child complains of bitter taste in mouth and feels worse after hot drinks *Chamomilla 6c*
- Sour belching, especially after an emotional upset *Ignatia 6c*
- Discomfort considerably relieved by belching *Carbo veg. 6c*
- Indigestion brought on by rich food, especially if child is tearful, not thirsty, and feels worse in stuffy rooms *Pulsatilla 6c*

Self-help Indigestion may be caused by a particular food, in which case try to identify what it is and avoid it. Encourage child to eat slowly and chew properly, and set a good example yourself. Try to prevent child running about too soon after meals. Slippery Elm Food, obtainable from chemists, may also help to settle stomach.

Insecurity see also SCHOOL PHOBIA, PHOBIA
Most young children have fears and apprehensions of some kind. They may be afraid of the dark, of baths, of

---

shadows under the bed . . . they may dread their parents' anger, being told off by teachers, being left with strangers, going to the dentist. . . Irrational as such fears may seem to adults, they are very real to the child concerned and should not be dismissed lightly or ridiculed. Give as much reassurance as you can. A very timid child may benefit from constitutional treatment.

Specific remedies to be given every 12 hours for up to 2 weeks
- Child afraid of parent's or teacher's anger *Nux 30c*
- Insecurity after an incident which caused great emotional distress *Ignatia 30c*
- Child nervous, scared of the dark, gives in easily, mentally and physically sluggish *Calcarea 30c*
- Child insecure but covers up by acting over-confidently, craves sweet things *Lycopodium 30c*
- Child weak, trembly, heavy-eyed, especially before performing in public or sitting exams *Gelsemium 30c*
- Child afraid of dark, thunderstorms, lavatories, etc., but easily reassured *Phosphorus 30c*

Knock knees see BOW LEGS AND KNOCK KNEES

Lack of confidence
Some degree of nervousness and uncertainty in unfamiliar situations is quite natural in toddlers but less so in older children. By the age of four or five a child should be standing up for himself or herself, and not giving in too easily. Passivity, timidity, and withdrawal are usually signs of INSECURITY.

Specific remedies to be taken every 12 hours for up to 2 weeks
- Child timid, tearful, clinging, often feels too hot, especially in stuffy rooms, easily gives in to others *Pulsatilla 30c*
- Symptoms as above but child more stubborn, has a big head and thin body, often feels chilly, sweats on head and feet *Silicea 30c*
- Child apprehensive, feels tension in stomach, hates to be left alone, very sensitive to noise *Kali carb. 30c*
- Child oversensitive, cries easily when others hurt themselves, hates sweet things, bedwets, has warts *Causticum 30c*

Learning problems
Poor concentration and slow progress at school can be due to hearing problems (see Ears pp. 157–61), poor eyesight (see Eyes pp. 149–57), DYSLEXIA, ALLERGY, HYPERACTIVITY, AUTISM, MENTAL HANDICAP, and sometimes to ANXIETY about problems at home (rows between parents, financial worries, etc.). A child can also be disruptive at school (and at home) because he or she is actually very bright and is bored. Constitutional treatment can be effective, but there are no specific short-term remedies.

Self-help Check out the possible causes mentioned above. Encourage child to develop non-academic skills (riding, swimming, dancing, gymnastics, drama, etc.) to improve self-confidence. If lack of concentration is the problem, give extra Vitamin B_1.

Left-handedness
Although the world is set up for the convenience of right-handed people, a child who begins to develop fine control with his or her left hand should not be discouraged but given extra help with writing, tying shoelaces, using scissors, and so on. Handedness is probably determined in the womb, during the very early stages of development of the central nervous sytem, but it is known that more breech-born babies (babies born buttocks first) become left-handed than their normally born peers.

Leukaemia see also LEUKAEMIA p. 194, CANCER
Literally 'white blood', cancer of the blood. Most common form of leukaemia in children is *acute lymphatic leukaemia*, in which production of infection-fighting white blood cells (lymphocytes) in lymph glands suddenly and massively increases. Most of these cells are immature or defective, but once in blood stream they infiltrate bone marrow, interfering with production of both red and white blood cells, and also with liver, spleen, brain, and spinal cord. Symptoms are those of ANAEMIA (pallor, tiredess), purplish rash, limb pains, MOUTH ULCERS, bad HEADACHE, swollen neck glands, an enlarged spleen, and vulnerability to infections such as PNEUMONIA, and onset is very rapid, taking just 1 or 2 weeks. Diagnosis is by bone marrow biopsy (removing a small sample of tissue from the centre of a bone for analysis). Can be brought under control by chemotherapy, radiotherapy, and steroids, but there is a risk of relapse. Complementary treatments include dietary therapy, vitamin and mineral supplements, and visualization (using the imaging powers of the mind to fight the disease). See CANCER for homeopathic treatment.

Lice see HEAD LICE

Limping
If limp disappears when child is barefoot, suspect shoes or socks that are too tight, or a nail sticking through shoe. Veruccae (see WARTS) can also cause limping. See First Aid pp. 104–5 for treatment of SPRAINS (pain and limping, leg and ankle look normal) and splinters. For FRACTURES and DISLOCATIONS (limping and severe pain following injury to leg or hip, leg looks odd) (999), give First Aid (see pp. 96 and 99) and give *Arnica 306c* every 15 minutes until help arrives.

Limping can also be a sign of RHEUMATIC FEVER or STILL'S DISEASE (painful, red, swollen joints), OSTEO-MYELITIS (pain and tenderness over a bone), INFECTIVE ARTHRITIS (joint swelling and pain caused by an infection), congenital dislocation of the hip, especially if child has just learnt to walk (see CONGENITAL DISORDERS), CEREBRAL PALSY (stiffness in and poor control of affected limb), ANAPHYLACTOID PURPURA, and even of INFLUENZA. If child limps for more than two days without apparent reason, 48 .

Masturbation
Not usually a 'problem' in children under twelve, simply part of a child's general exploration of his or her body. Excessive playing with the genitals may indicate that all is not well emotionally, in which case constitutional treatment should be sought.

Measles
Highly infectious viral disease spread by droplets in coughs and sneezes. More serious in adults than children, although one infection usually confers immunity for life. Until age of six months babies are protected by their mothers' antibodies. Incubation is 10–11 days, followed by pre-rash stage and rash stage. Child is infectious from first day of pre-rash stage until five days after rash appears. Contact your GP to confirm diagnosis. Complications include acute MIDDLE EAR INFECTION, BRONCHITIS and other chest infections, ENCEPHALITIS, and in rare cases FEBRILE CONVULSIONS. If FEVER persists or child still feels ill after rash begins to fade, or if child complains of EARACHE, 12 . If remedies listed below produce no improvement, or if you are uncertain which remedy to give, contact your homeopath.

Pre-rash stage Lasts 3–4 days. First signs are inflamed throat, runny nose, dry COUGH, red, watering eyes, and a high temperature, followed within 24 hours by Koplik's spots (raised, white, salt-like spots) inside mouth. Koplik's spots confirm that infection is measles.

Specific remedies to be given every 2 hours for up to 10 doses
- Cold symptoms and high fever *Aconite 30c* or *Belladonna 30c*
- Symptoms as for Aconite or Belladonna, but eyes red and watering, and eyelids swollen *Euphrasia 6c*
- Child feverish but not thirsty, very tearful and miserable, thick green catarrh, light hurts eyes, dry cough at night, lots of phlegm coughed up in morning, upset stomach or diarrhoea *Pulsatilla 6c*

Rash stage Lasts 2–3 days. Spots are dark red, flat or raised, and appear first on forehead, around hair line, and behind ears, then spread downwards to rest of body. As rash fades, temperature returns to normal and spots turn brownish and flaky.

Specific remedies to be given every 4 hours for up to 10 doses
- Rash slow to appear, child irritable, has high temperature and is very thirsty, dry hacking cough, headache made worse by coughing *Bryonia 30c*
- Rash slow to clear, spots turn purplish *Sulphur 6c*

Immunization Orthodox medicine offers injection of live modified virus in second year of life, homeopathic medicine *Morbillinum 30c* nosode (see p. 12 for definition of nosode). If your child has not been immunized and comes into contact with a measles sufferer, contact your homeopath. If child is already incubating measles, orthodox immunization may suppress rash and lead to more serious illness in adolescence. If child's immune system is already suppressed for some reason (by an existing illness or by antibiotics, for example) 12 an injection of gammaglobulin, which protects for 2 weeks, may be the best course.

Self-help Keep child away from others if possible, and in a well-ventilated room. Draw curtains if light hurts eyes. Give plenty of bottled or filtered water to drink until fever subsides, and keep child on light diet, with plenty of Vitamin C, until runny nose and cough clear up. Bathe eyes with saline solution (1 teaspoon salt dissolved in a glass of warm water). See FEVER p. 321 for other self-help measures.

Meningitis see also MENINGITIS pp. 131 and 307
Inflammation of membranes or meninges surrounding brain and spinal cord, caused by bacterial or viral infections. Infection may be primary, or a complication of infections such as TUBERCULOSIS, PNEUMONIA, ear infections, SINUSITIS, and MUMPS. Meninges can also be damaged by FRACTURES of the skull. Symptoms include HEADACHE, FEVER above 39°C (102°F), NAUSEA AND VOMITING, FEBRILE CONVULSIONS, a stiff neck, and intolerance of light, followed by ABNORMAL SLEEPINESS OR DROWSINESS and coma. If child is very young, see symptoms given under MENINGITIS in infants, p. 307. Recovery from viral infection is usually total. Bacterial infection is more serious, especially if general resistance is low; consequences may be a brain abscess, BRAIN DAMAGE, DEAFNESS, and even death. If meningitis is suspected, ②.

Specific remedies to be given every 15 minutes until help arrives
- Symptoms come on after head injury *Arnica 30c*
- Child restless, frightened, thirsty, skin very dry *Aconite 30c*
- Child very hot, delirious, pupils wide and staring *Belladonna 30c*
- Child in great pain, finds slightest eye movement excruciating, emotionally very low, lapses into unconsciousness *Bryonia 30c*

---

999 Emergency – call GP (or dial 999) immediately. ② Consult your doctor if no improvement within 2 hours

Mental handicap

One child in fifty is assessed as educationally subnormal and likely to benefit from going to a special school. Most normal schools lack the time and expertise to be of real help to such children, whereas special schools generally achieve an increase in confidence and emotional stability. Constitutional homeopathic treatment can help to improve concentration and persistence.

Specific remedies to be given every 12 hours for up to 3 weeks
- Very childish behaviour (scampering, hiding, kicking), recurrent tonsillitis and swollen neck glands *Baryta 6c*
- Child has poor memory and concentration, always seems to be in a hurry or afraid of someone behind, often feels too hot, has chronic catarrh, seems to improve in sea air *Medorrhinum 6c*
- Child irritable, tearful, bored by favourite people or things, happier doing some form of strenuous exercise *Sepia 6c*

Self-help Multivitamin and mineral supplements can sometimes alleviate behavioural problems. Also, the possibility of food ALLERGY contributing to learning problems would be worth investigating.

Mumps

Viral infection of saliva glands (parotid and submaxillary), spread by droplets in coughs and sneezes. Not as infectious as measles or chicken pox, and more common in spring and summer. More than one attack is rare. Complications include ENCEPHALITIS, PANCREATITIS, and inflammation of the testes or ovaries. Despite folklore to the contrary, mumps seldom causes sterility or permanent damage to testes or ovaries. Incubation is 14–28 days. Infection onsets with moderate FEVER, HEADACHE, and pain in front of the ears as first one parotid gland then the other becomes swollen. The submaxillary glands beneath the jaw may also be affected. Glands subside within 10 days, during which time child remains infectious.

If child develops severe headache, shrinks away from bright light, or is stupid and drowsy, ② as there may be a risk of ENCEPHALITIS. If testicles or ovaries are painful, ⒓ and give *Pulsatilla 6c* every 4 hours for up to 10 doses.

Specific remedies to be given every 4 hours for up to 10 doses
- Onset of fever, child very restless *Aconite 30c*
- High fever, right parotid gland more painful than left, child red in face, eyes wide and staring *Belladonna 30c*
- Saliva thick and sticky *Pilocarpin mur. 6c*

- Submaxillary glands swollen and hard as stones, child complains of ear pains on swallowing *Phytolacca 6c*
- Glands on right side of jaw most affected, saliva smells unpleasant, child sweaty, tongue lolling *Mercurius 6c*

Immunization Mumps is now routinely immunized against in Britain as part of MMR (Measles, Mumps and Rubella) vaccine. Homeopathy can offer *Parotidinum 30c* nosode (see p. 12 for definition of nosode) or *Rhus tox. 30c* during incubation period. Dose is 1 daily for up to 10 days.

Self-help Avoid acid beverages (lemon, orange, grapefruit juice, for example) as these painfully stimulate the salivary glands.

Muscular dystrophy (MD)

An inherited condition in which the muscles degenerate and weaken, resulting in CLUMSINESS, frequent falls, difficulty climbing stairs, etc. It is not known whether the muscles themselves are the problem, or the nerves supplying the muscles. Fat gradually replaces muscle fibres, making affected muscles look plumper than normal. Child may take longer than usual to walk normally but not be diagnosed as having MD until age of three or four. Prognosis is confinement to a wheelchair before teens, and death a few years later due to failure of heart or chest muscles (see HEART FAILURE, RESPIRATORY FAILURE). Most common form of MD is Duchenne's, affecting mainly boys and causing curvature of the spine; to stand up from a lying position, a Duchenne's child literally climbs up his legs with the help of his arms, his back being too weak to straighten on its own. The author has not treated MD nor, to his knowledge, are there any reports of treatment in the homeopathic literature. Parents are advised to seek help from the Muscular Dystrophy Group of Great Britain and Northern Ireland (address p. 383)

Nailbiting

May be a sign of INSECURITY, boredom, or repressed ANGER, but too much fuss about unsightly nails can make the habit worse. Encourage the child to use a nailfile so that he or she has no bits to pick or gnaw at. If habit is part of a larger behaviour picture, constitutional homeopathic treatment should be sought.

Nephritis see also GLOMERULONEPHRITIS p. 235

Inflammation of the kidneys, often brought on by abnormal immune reaction to infection, especially to streptococcal infections of the throat (see SORE THROAT) and SCARLET FEVER. Kidneys cease to function, blood pressure rises, child develops HEADACHE, feels extremely ill, and may vomit or go into FITS.

Urine has bloody or smokey appearance, and is passed in less volume than usual. Retained fluids cause OEDEMA (tissue swelling), especially around eyes, giving child telltale 'bags' under the eyes. Recurrent attacks can lead to chronic KIDNEY FAILURE. Conventional treatment is by antibiotics, and diuretic and hypotensive drugs. Constitutional homeopathic treatment is recommended to prevent recurrence.

Specific remedies to be given every hour for up to 10 doses in acute situation
- Oedema *Apis 30c*
- Attack comes on after scarlet fever or acute sore throat, burning pains on passing water *Cantharis 30c*
- Child anxious, restless, chilly, wants frequent drinks of water, has marked oedema *Arsenicum 30c*

Self-help The simplest and most effective measures are bed rest, reducing salt and protein in the child's diet, and cutting down on fluids. Less salt, protein, and fluids give ailing, inflamed kidneys less to cope with. Also, eliminate as many sources of aluminium as possible (see p. 349).

Nephrotic syndrome see also
GLOMERULONEPHRITIS
Damage to kidneys, resulting in decreased flow of urine, excretion of protein in urine, and loss of protein from the blood, causing fluid to seep out of blood vessels and accumulate in surrounding tissues, especially under eyes and around abdomen (see OEDEMA). Usually occurs in children aged two to four. Unchecked, condition can lead to chronic PYELONEPHRITIS. Symptoms take a few weeks to develop. Most appropriate action is [12]. Child will almost certainly be admitted to hospital, given steroids to halt damage to kidneys, and put on a high protein/low salt diet, with a low fluid intake. Constitutional homeopathic treatment may prevent recurrence.

Specific remedies to be taken every 2 hours for up to 8 doses during acute attack
- Fluid retention all over body, child chilly, exhausted, restless, anxious, wants frequent drinks of water *Arsenicum 6c*
- Child pale, bloated, vomiting, has nosebleeds, passes stools with undigested food in them *Ferrum 6c*
- Frequent urge to pass water, fever, headache *Ferrum phos. 6c*

Nits see HEAD LICE

Nose, blocked or runny
Usually accompanies COLDS and INFLUENZA, but may also be a symptom of HAY FEVER AND ALLERGIC RHINITIS. Can also be caused by inhaling chemicals or foreign bodies, in which case see First Aid pp. 94–5.

Obesity see also OBESITY pp. 260–2
Many children, especially toddlers, are chubby rather than obese. Obesity is unlikely to be diagnosed unless child's weight is near the top of the acceptable range for his or her age on relevant age/weight chart (see p. 312), or unless child is both unusually short and unusually overweight for his or her age. An obese child usually has rolls of fat on upper arms and thighs. Unless a hormonal cause can be established, treatment involves changing diet (less salt and fat, fewer snacks and refined carbohydrates, no more than 0.4 litre [¾ pint] milk per day) and increasing exercise. For more information on children's diets, see p. 24–5. Some children overeat because they have emotional problems, because they feel insecure or unloved; eating can be a form of self-punishment as well as self-comfort. Try to find out what lies behind the overeating.

Osteomyelitis
Inflammation of a bone due to infection or injury. Acute cases often follow injury. If resistance is high, body seals off affected area as an ABSCESS. If resistance is low, condition may become chronic and flare up again and again, putting child at risk of SEPTICAEMIA or permanent deformity of adjacent joints as infection spreads and pus enters bloodstream. Symptoms are painful, red, swollen skin over affected bone. If you suspect osteomyelitis, [24]. Child will almost certainly be put on antibiotics (essential in such cases) and referred for surgery to remove diseased tissue from affected bone. While waiting for treatment, give *Gunpowder 6c* every 2 hours for up to 12 doses. After surgery, constitutional homeopathic treatment may help to prevent recurrence.

Phenylketonuria (PKU)
Accumulation of the amino acid phenylalanine in brain due to defect in metabolism of proteins (proteins in diet are broken down into amino acids, which are then built up into proteins the body needs). Unchecked, condition can cause mental deficiency. All babies in Britain are routinely given the Guthrie test for PKU shortly after birth. If test is positive, child is put on special diet until age of 12. Risk of PKU can be minimized by mother going on low phenylalanine diet before conception. For further information, contact the National Society for Phenylketonuria and Allied Disorders (address p. 383).

Phimosis see PHIMOSIS p. 338, PENIS PROBLEMS p. 252

Pneumonia see also PNEUMONIA p. 182
Infection of the lungs caused by various bacteria and viruses.

Bronchopneumonia In this form of pneumonia large areas of lung tissue become flooded with inflammatory secretions, drastically reducing oxygen uptake. Common in CYSTIC FIBROSIS, a complication of COLDS, BRONCHITIS, MEASLES, and WHOOPING COUGH, and in some cases a reaction to foreign bodies lodged in lungs. If preceded by a cold, usually onsets 3 days after development of cold symptoms. Signs are high FEVER (temperature above 39°C [102°F]), dry COUGH, fast breathing, and in severe cases WHEEZING and blueness around lips (cyanosis). Scarring of lung tissue can cause permanent damage.

Lobar pneumonia Infection confined to one lobe of lungs. Onsets suddenly with burning FEVER (temperature up to 40°C [104°F]), rapid breathing, dry COUGH, and in some cases stabbing pains as lungs expand to inhale. Usually heals within a week, with or without antibiotics.

If either type of pneumonia is suspected, ②, especially if child has difficulty breathing, sucks ribs inwards in effort to breathe, or turns blue around the lips or tongue.

Specific remedies to be given every 5 minutes for up to 10 doses or until help arrives
- Stabbing pains around rib cage, made worse by breathing in, high fever, eyes wide and staring, child also delirious *Belladonna 30c*
- Pain on breathing in, aggravated by slightest movement but alleviated by lying on painful side, child very thirsty at infrequent intervals *Bryonia 30c*
- Symptoms come on suddenly, especially after a fright or exposure to cold wind, child fearful *Aconite 30c*
- Brownish phlegm coughed up, child craves cold drinks but vomits as soon as they become warm in stomach, wants to be cuddled and reassured *Phosphorus 6c*

Rash see FEVER

Retinoblastoma see also TUMOURS OF THE EYE
A malignant tumour of the retina, affecting one or both eyes, most commonly seen in children under age of five; sometimes detectable as a SQUINT, which is why a squint should always be investigated, and in later stages may be visible as a white mass through pupil. Condition often runs in families. Radiotherapy is very effective if tumour is spotted early enough; if not, the affected eye may have to be removed to prevent tumours developing in other parts of the body. See CANCER for homeopathic treatment.

Rheumatic fever
An allergic reaction to streptococcal infections, causing acute inflammation of the joints, RHEUMATIC HEART DISEASE (inflammation of and damage to heart muscles, heart valves, and tissues surrounding heart), and in some cases chorea or St. Vitus' dance

(inflammation of the brain). Acute stage occurs in childhood but effects are long-term. Condition has a hereditary component and is associated with cold, damp weather. Usually onsets 7–28 days after streptococcal SORE THROAT. Symptoms are FEVER, intermittent pain and swelling in joints, and a pink, blotchy rash. If child shows these symptoms, 12. Orthodox treatment is bed rest and penicillin, with some authorities recommending antibiotics to prevent recurrence. Author's view is that EXPERT CONSTITUTIONAL HOMEOPATHIC TREATMENT should be tried after a first attack, with long-term antibiotics as an option if a second attack occurs.

Specific remedies to be given ½-hourly for up to 10 doses while waiting for help
- Painful joints, child restless and frightened *Aconite 30c*
- Child sweats profusely, especially at night, sweat smells unpleasant, copious saliva *Mercurius 6c*
- Slightest movement makes joint pains worse, child irritable, wants to be left alone, very thirsty at long intervals *Bryonia 30c*
- Moderately severe attack, especially if child catches chill after exertion in cold, damp weather *Dulcamara 6c*
- Pains shift from one joint to another, child feels better out of doors but worse after fatty food, tearful *Pulsatilla 6c*

Rickets
Bone deformities such as bow-leggedness caused by lack of Vitamin D and sometimes calcium in diet, or by lack of sunshine (sunlight encourages skin to manufacture Vitamin D). Most at risk are children who are dark-skinned and undernourished. In Britain Vitamin D is usually supplemented in infancy in the form of A, C, and D vitamin drops. If GP diagnoses condition, drops will be prescribed; follow prescribed dosage exactly, as large doses of vitamin D can be harmful.

Ringworm (tinea)
Nothing to do with worms! A fungal infection of the skin, so called because it causes red, scaly patches which heal from the middle outwards. Can affect scalp (hair falls out leaving bald patches), feet (causing ATHLETE'S FOOT), groin, armpits, or trunk. Very contagious, spread by contact in swimming pools and washrooms, and by contact with pets and other animals.

Specific remedies to be given every 4 hours for up to 10 doses
- Infected scalp *Sulphur 6c* then *Sepia 6c* if no improvement
- Infection confined to trunk *Tellurium 6c*

If feet are infected, see remedies for ATHLETE'S FOOT.

Self-help Wash affected areas with soap, wipe dry with surgical spirit, and dab with cod liver oil. If lesions persist, apply anti-fungal ointment (preferably one that does not contain steroids) or selenium-containing shampoo for up to 1 week. Keep child away from school until lesions heal. Destroy all combs, brushes, headgear, etc. which may have been in contact with lesions, and thoroughly wash and dry all clothes. Take pets to homeopathic vet and have them checked for ringworm; destroy all suspect bedding.

Roseola infantum

Virus infection of children aged between six months and three years. Incubation period variable. Symptoms are high FEVER, followed by swollen neck glands and pink rash on trunk, lasting for about a week. Child remains infectious for 5 days after onset of fever.

Specific remedies to be given every 4 hours for up to 10 doses

- High temperature, eyes staring, child delirious, neck glands tender *Belladonna 30c*
- Child tearful, clinging, not thirsty, craves fresh air *Pulsatilla 6c*
- Swollen glands, ear pains on swallowing, symptoms alleviated by cold drinks *Phytolacca 6c*

Rubella (German measles) see also RUBELLA p. 291

A mild but very infectious viral illness, seldom serious in children – ENCEPHALITIS is an extremely rare complication – but very serious during first 3 months of pregnancy. One attack usually confers immunity for life. Incubation is 14–21 days, and infection usually runs its course in 4–5 days. First stage is mild fever; second stage is swollen glands behind ears (when rubbed, glands feel like hard peas); third stage is orange-pink rash which spreads from face to rest of body.

Specific remedies to be given every 4 hours for up to 10 doses once rubella is diagnosed

- Swollen glands, ear pains on swallowing, symptoms alleviated by cold drinks *Phytolacca 6c*
- Onset of rash, child tearful and red-eyed, yellow catarrh *Pulsatilla 6c*

Immunization To minimize risk of rubella in pregnancy, most GPs advise immunization of girls at puberty, if they have not already had the disease. Even if your daughter has had rubella, your GP might be prepared to do a blood test to confirm immunity. Homeopathic immunization, using Rubella 30c nosode (see p. 12 for definition of nosode), can be given as part of preconceptual care if your daughter is unable to have the ordinary immunization but is nevertheless at risk.

Scarlet fever (scarlatina)

Infection caused by streptococcal bacteria, less contagious today thanks to modern hygiene and living standards, decreased virulence of the bacteria, and widespread use of antibiotics. Incubation is 1–6 days. First stage is FEVER, SORE THROAT, and vomiting; second stage is development of scarlet rash, with characteristic inflamed, 'strawberry' tongue. Rash peels, and child recovers within a week. Complications are rare, but include RHEUMATIC FEVER, acute inflammation and pain in joints, and acute NEPHRITIS. Conventional treatment is penicillin.

Specific remedies

- If scarlet fever is suspected *Belladonna 30c* every hour for up to 10 doses; if no improvement, [12]
- As a preventive, if child has been in contact with scarlet fever *Belladonna 30c* once a day for up to 10 days

School phobia

Child dreads going to school. May be due to factors at home or at school, with negative emotions translating themselves into HEADACHE, ABDOMINAL PAIN, NAUSEA AND VOMITING, and FAINTING. Symptoms usually worse on weekday mornings, better at weekends and during vacations. If there is tension in family, child may feel he or she needs to stay at home to prevent something terrible happening. For a child who feels insecure and lacks self-confidence, home is the safest place to be. Problems at school can be very real – difficulty with school work, fear of teachers, teasing, bullying, poor relationships with other children – and should not be ignored. Talk to both child and teachers to find cause. Constitutional homeopathic treatment may improve matters.

Specific remedies to be given once a day in morning, weekdays only, for up to 3 weeks

- Child impulsive, finds it difficult to concentrate, lacks self-confidence, cannot explain why school is so terrifying, worry often accompanied by diarrhoea *Argentum nit. 30c*
- Child tired, exhausted, shaky, dreads performing on stage or in front of class *Gelsemium 30c*
- Child very apprehensive about a new situation, insecure, tends to show off to compensate, craves sweet things *Lycopodium 30c*
- Child hates school toilets, either because they are dirty or because he or she cannot go to toilet with other children nearby *Natrum mur. 30c*
- Child mentally sluggish, apprehensive, lacks initiative, poor physical stamina, clumsy, bad at games, hates being laughed at, very fond of eggs *Calcarea 30c*

Sleep problems see also SLEEP PROBLEMS pp. 121–3

Except when child is ill, disturbed sleep may be due to irregular bedtimes, overtiredness, meals and drinks of tea or coffee too close to bedtime, food ALLERGY, stuffy bedrooms, too few or too many bedclothes, noise, or disruption of the child's regular sleeping pattern by the arrival of a new baby or the start of new school term; if the child gets up to go to the toilet several times a night, he or she may have a urinary tract infection. Often, however, tension and ANXIETY are to blame. Nightmares and night terrors (in which the child wakes screaming and terrified) are usually considered to be anxiety attacks, and can be brought on by a frightening story or an incident on television. At some time or another they are common in most young children. Sleepwalking, which is more common in children between the age of five and ten, occurs because those parts of the brain which control the muscles stay awake.

Need for sleep decreases with age. Newborn babies need about 16 hours, two-year-olds about 12 hours, six-year-olds about 10 hours, and twelve-year-olds about 9 hours. Sleep encourages brain to manufacture growth hormone, which in turn encourages body to manufacture proteins for growth and repair. Sudden friskiness around bedtime is a reliable sign that child is exhausted and needs to switch off. Persistent sleep problems require constitutional treatment.

Specific remedies to be given at bedtime for up to 14 nights; if no improvement, consult your homeopath
- Disturbed sleep due to shock or fright *Aconite 30c*
- Child sleeps with eyes open, moans in sleep, irritable and impossible to please when awake *Chamomilla 30c*
- Sleeplessness due to excitement and nerves, child apprehensive by nature *Gelsemium 30c*
- Child irritable, wakes around 4 am *Nux 30c*
- Child sleeps on stomach, grinds teeth and jerks violently during sleep, wakes in a fright, suffers from worms *Cina 30c*
- Child wakes in an excited state and starts playing with toys *Coffea 30c*
- Child sleeps lightly, jerks in sleep, disturbed sleep triggered off by emotional upset *Ignatia 30c*
- Sleepwalking, especially if child is thin and has a large head *Silicea 30c*
- Child weeps and screams in sleep *Phosphorus 30c*
- Child has night terrors, sleepwalks, has fidgety hands *Kali brom. 30c*
- Child starts and cries out in anxiety during sleep, has head sweats *Calcarea 30c*
- Child sleeps for short periods only, moans during sleep *Antimonium tart. 30c*
- One disturbed night causes bad sleep pattern for several nights afterwards *Cocculus 30c*

Self-help Give hot, milky drinks (not cocoa) or herbal infusions (chamomile, valerian, passionflower, skullcap) at bedtime. Relax child with a warm bath before bed, and avoid late meals.

If child wakes screaming and crying, offer comfort and reassurance but don't ask what is the matter; discuss it in the morning. If the crying continues, put your head round the door every 10 minutes or so just to reassure the child that you are still there, but don't pick him or her up or offer a drink. He or she may cry for an hour or more before going to sleep again, but the next time sleep usually comes more quickly, and the next time more quickly still, until sleep is unbroken right through the night.

If child is crying but asleep, do not wake him or her. If child sleepwalks, gently guide him or her back to bed, and put a gate at top of stairs to prevent accidents.

If child becomes frisky at bedtime, goes to bed tense, and wakes easily in first sleep, try bringing bedtime forward by 15 minutes each night until sleep is continuous; if child then starts waking too early in the morning, move bedtime back by 15 minutes each night until he or she sleeps later.

Always look for the underlying causes, mental or physical, of disturbed sleep, and never punish a child by sending him or her to bed, or bed and bedroom will become tense, uncomfortable places. If sleep problems appear to have an emotional origin, psychotherapy or family therapy should be considered.

Sore throat see SORE THROAT p. 174

Speech difficulties see also STAMMERING
May be due to partial or total DEAFNESS, excitement, or ANXIETY, or may be associated with late development generally. Poor language development is also one of the features of AUTISM.

Until the age of about three months, babies' communications with the outside world are purely expressive – crying expresses hunger, pain, or fear, gurgling, whimpering, and cooing express pleasanter, less distressing emotions. After that their repertoire extends to making sounds which are a reaction to what is going on around them; they begin to babble, experimentally, trying to compare the pitch and rhythm of noises they are making with the sounds they hear and see adults making. Babies the world over make similar noises, regardless of the language their parents speak. Between the age of seven and nine months, distinct syllables emerge and are joined together – 'boo-boo' may not sound very impressive, but it demonstrates an innate grasp of the basic components of language. After that, as every day passes, there is increasing interest in conversations and attempts to chip in with shouts and 'singing'. By the end of the first year certain sounds are being associated with well known objects. During the second year the process of attaching words to objects and actions speeds up; simple noun-verb combinations like 'Mummy do' develop. In the third year vocabulary and syntax broaden to the point where simple questions can be asked. At this age most children can understand and hold simple conversations, and communicate their thoughts and needs.

Partial or total deafness can manifest itself at various stages of speech development: under the age of six months the baby may fail to react to the sounds of voices; at around six months there may be a failure to progress beyond the babbling stage; at the age of one year or more the child may fail to develop words or speak very indistinctly.

Late speech development is not unusual, even when there is no deafness and no sign of late development in other areas; as a parent there are a number of things you can do to help (see self-help measures below).

Where late speech development is associated with late walking, slow growth, physical abnormality or emotional stress, see your GP. In addition to tackling the underlying problem, he or she may recommend speech therapy.

Lisping, STAMMERING, and other pronunciation difficulties are quite common and children usually grow out of them. Try not to make an issue out of them – you'll only make the child more anxious – but if they are severe enough to embarrass the child or cause unintelligibility, then your GP may refer you to a speech therapist.

If nervousness or stress seems to be the cause of speech difficulties, constitutional treatment would be appropriate.

Self-help Whether your child has speech difficulties or not, the following strategies are recommended.

For children under one year: look directly at the child's face when you are talking to him or her; read simple books and point out objects as you say their names; as you dress or undress the child, name each item of clothing; talk about things the child is interested in.

For children over one year: talk naturally about objects which are physically present; always name the objects you are talking about ('Where is your hat?' rather than 'Where is it?'); use your face and hands to convey meaning, even you if have to ham it up a bit; don't bore the child by always correcting mistakes; try hard to understand what the child is saying the first time he or she says it – asking for things to be repeated is very demoralizing.

It would also be worth checking whether the child is exposed to high levels of lead (see toxic metals p. 349) in the atmosphere.

Squint see also SQUINT pp. 156–7

Not usually apparent until child is three months old, often associated with SHORT SIGHT or LONG SIGHT in one eye, which becomes lazy; usually correctable if treated early enough. Squint may be constant or it may come and go; usually the child does not see double, unlike someone who develops a squint in later life. GP will refer child to an opthalmologist to discover the cause; usually the good eye is patched, forcing the child to use the lazy one; if this does not achieve normal coordination, an operation may be necessary. In very rare cases, a squint may be a sign of RETINOBLASTOMA, a malignant tumour of the retina.

Specific remedies to be given 3 times daily for up to 21 days during specialist treatment
• *Gelsemium 6c*
• If Gelsemium does not seem to help *Alumina 6*

If neither of the above remedies is effective, see your homeopath.

Stammering

Repetitive stumbling over consonants at beginnings of words, usually a sign of STRESS in children over five and not improved by trying hard not to stammer. Conventional treatment is speech therapy. Constitutional treatment may help if stammering is part of a larger picture of nervousness, INSECURITY and LACK OF CONFIDENCE.

Specific remedies to be given 3 times daily for up to 14 days
• Child excitable, given to muttering, flailing limb movements *Stramoniuim 6c*
• Child talks too fast and trips over words, making stammering worse *Hyoscyamus 6c*
• General twitching of limbs *Zinc 6c*
• Nervous spasms of face and limbs *Cuprum 6c*
• Nervous tics, stammering and nervousness worse with cold *Agaricus 6c*
• Trembling tongue, too much saliva in mouth *Mercurius 6c*
• Child irritable and over-critical *Nux 6c*

Self-help Reduce amount of copper in child's environment and diet.

Still's disease

An AUTOIMMUNE DISEASE similar to RHEUMATOID ARTHRITIS. Usually onsets between age of two and five, but often disappears at puberty. Symptoms are intermittent, and include FEVER, joint pains, WEIGHT LOSS, loss of appetite (see APPETITE CHANGES), and sometimes ANAEMIA, swollen lymph glands, and eye trouble. If most of the above symptoms are present, 12 . Conventional treatment is by anti-inflammatory drugs, physiotherapy, and splinting affected limb. Constitutional homeopathic treatment is recommended.

Specific remedies to be given 4 times daily for up to 5 days
• Symptoms brought on by cold, damp weather, aggravated by rest and by first movements after rest, alleviated by continued movement *Rhus tox. 6c*
• Symptoms aggravated by slightest movement, soothed by rest and cold applications *Bryonia 30c*
• Skin over affected joints red, swollen, and shiny, stinging pains in joints aggravated by heat or slightest pressure *Apis 30c*

- Symptoms come on after injury *Arnica 30c*
- Symptoms worse in cold, rainy weather, especially if child has become overheated *Dulcamara 6c*
- Pains flit from joint to joint and feel worse for heat, child tearful and clinging *Pulsatilla 6c*

Stomach ache see ABDOMINAL PAIN

Tantrums

Outbursts of angry crying, shouting, and screaming if demands are not instantly met. Tensions within the family, lack of parental affection, inconsistent discipline, and other factors which encourage INSECURITY are usually the reason, but a food ALLERGY is sometimes at the root of the problem. Constitutional homeopathic treatment can help.

Specific remedies to be given once daily for up to 1 week
- Child cross, touchy, rejects all efforts to please, may also have worms and grind teeth in sleep *Cina 30c*
- Child impatient, impossible to please, only placated by being carried around *Chamomilla 30c*
- Child prickly, hyper-critical, touchier than ever after overeating *Nux 30c*
- Child generally dissatisfied with life, very malicious, seems to go into tantrums in spite of himself or herself *Tuberculinum 30c*

Teething

Sore gums, irritability, and stomach upsets during eruption of milk teeth. Babies cut their first teeth around age of six months, and all 20 milk teeth (8 incisors, 4 canines, 8 molars) are usually through by the end of the third year. Homeopathic remedies are extremely effective against the pain and discomfort of teething. The small flaps of skin pushed aside as the molar teeth come through are quite natural; they separate from the gum in due course.

Specific remedies to be given every 30 minutes, or more frequently if pain is severe, for up to 10 doses
- Child irritable, wants to be carried around, makes a fuss when put in cot, one cheek hot and red, the other pale *Chamomilla 30c*
- Child flushed and hot, pupils wide and staring *Belladonna 30c*
- Child thin, with a big head, tends to have sweaty feet and head, dislikes milk *Silicea 6c*
- Child nervous, restless *Actaea 6c*
- Child has mouth ulcers, is startled by sudden noises, dislikes downward motion *Borax 6c*
- Teeth have poor enamel and decay easily and quickly *Kreosotum 6c*
- Sore gums and diarrhoea, or copious salivation *Mercurius 6c*
- Acute pain and high temperature *Aconite 30c*
- Sore gums, child fretful and colicky *Colocynth 6c*

- Teething symptoms accompanied by constipation and ineffectual straining to pass stools *Nux 6c*

Self-help Give *Calc. Phos.* and *Calc. Fluor* (see Tissue Salts p. 388) throughout teething period.

Threadworms

Tiny, white, thread-like worms which infest the rectum, causing itching around anus and sometimes mild, colicky abdominal pain. If child scratches, then sucks fingers or touches food, he or she can be reinfected by mouth. Conventional treatment is by antiworm drugs such as Pripsin and Vermox, but the senna and dyestuffs these contain can cause diarrhoea.

Specific remedies to be taken 3 times daily for up to 14 days; if there is no improvement, see your homeopath
- Itchy bottom, child irritable, picks nose, grinds teeth, is very hungry, dark rings under eyes *Cina 6c*
- Itchy bottom and itchy nose, itchiness worse in evening, child restless in sleep, complains of crawling sensation in rectum after passing stools *Teucrium 6c*
- Standby remedy if above remedies fail *Santoninum 6c*

Self-help Insist that child brushes up his or her personal hygiene. Hands should be washed thoroughly after going to toilet, after touching pets, and always before eating. Fingernails should be cut short and scrubbed occasionally. Pyjamas should be worn in preference to nightdresses to discourage child from scratching, and changed frequently. Pets should be wormed.

Thrombocytopenia see PLATELET DISORDERS

Toilet training problems see also
BEDWETTING, ENCOPRESIS
Before the age of eighteen months most children are simply unable to make the connection between the urge to pass water or stool and the results of doing so. Control of bladder and bowels is something that develops gradually between the age of eighteen months and midway through the fourth year, although accidents can happen up to the age of five or older. Setbacks are quite common after illness or major upsets in routine, such as the arrival of a new baby or tension in the family; if the problem continues for more than a week, see your GP or go to a homeopath for constitutional treatment. Soiling is usually caused by CONSTIPATION, which in turn can be caused by insufficient roughage in the diet or by retention of faeces for emotional reasons; again, if the problem continues for more than a week, consult your GP or homeopath.

Self-help It is important not to hurry or force toilet training. Unlike you, the child has little to gain from putting urine or faeces in a potty rather than in a nappy or on the ground. Try to avoid making the child feel disgusting or guilty about the products of his or her own body. Introduce the potty at around eighteen months, and give it to the child whenever he or she expresses the need to pass water or stool. Once the connection between the potty and the urge to go to the toilet has been established, try to be matter of fact about the results – don't freak out if the child misses or go into rhapsodies if he or she succeeds. Once the potty has been mastered, encourage the child to use a child seat on an adult toilet – a small step may be necessary at first. Until the age of about two and a half, a nappy is necessary at night; if the child has been dry for several nights running, remove the nappy but keep a water-proof sheet on the bed. Occasional bedwetting is quite normal up to the age of about four.

Tonsillitis

Infected tonsils. The tonsils are two small sacs of lymphatic tissue on either side of the root of the tongue whose function is to build up immunity to common infectious organisms and to protect the throat and lungs from infection; they are at their most active in childhood when many infections are encountered for the first time, and reach full size when the child is six or seven. Today tonsils are no longer routinely removed after one or two episodes of acute infection; removal is only considered if infection is chronic or recurs severely many times over a number of years. Recurrent tonsillitis requires constitutional treatment.

Symptoms of tonsillitis include SORE THROAT, FEVER, and feeling generally ill; the tonsils themselves look bright red to begin with, then become covered with a slimy, whitish film. To establish diagnosis in acute situation, 48. Conventional treatment is with antibiotics or paracetamol, and antiseptic gargles. Homeopathy offers the remedies listed below, but if child does not respond within 24 hours call GP again or call your homeopath.

Specific remedies to be given every 2 hours for up to 10 doses during acute attack
- Raw throat, high fever with delirium, staring eyes, tonsils bright red *Belladonna 30c*
- Child says throat hurts but is not thirsty, whole neck region tender and sensitive to slightest pressure, uvula (flap of skin at back of throat) very swollen and shiny *Apis 30c*
- Child chilly, irritable and unreasonable, hates undressing or leaving warmth of bed, says pains in throat feel like splinters or fish hooks, pus from tonsils tastes unpleasant *Hepar sulph. 6c*
- Tonsils dark red, swollen and sore, tongue swollen, glands in neck swollen and tender, breath smells foul, copious saliva *Mercurius 6c*
- Left tonsil most infected and painful, and dark purple in appearance, severe pain on swallowing, pain worse after sleep and worse for warmth, also worse when child drinks but better when he or she eats something, child hates neck-hugging clothes or bedclothes *Lachesis 6c*
- Child very poorly, throat pain extends up to ears, neck glands swollen, tonsils dark red, hot, and swollen, throat feels rough and constricted *Phytolacca 6c*
- Infection starts in right tonsil and moves to left, child has high fever and feels most ill between 4 and 8 am, throat soothed by hot drinks *Lycopodium 6c*

Self-help Give plenty to drink, and apply hot and cold compresses around neck. Boost intake of Vitamin C. Garlic is also good for infected tonsils. Gargle with sage tea.

Toothache see also TOOTHACHE p. 169
Toothache accompanied by fever may be a TOOTH ABSCESS. Call your dentist within 12 hours.

Tooth decay see also CARIES
From the moment they erupt, teeth are vulnerable to decay. Bacteria act on sugars in the mouth to form plaque, an acidic substance which erodes the outer enamel, causing cavities and the familiar pain of TOOTHACHE. For more information on dental problems, see pp. 166–70.

Self-help To minimize tooth decay, oral hygiene should begin as soon as first milk teeth erupt. Restrict sugary foods to twice a week at most. Clean child's teeth after every meal or at least twice a day, using a soft brush, and encourage child to do the same. If you live in a low-fluoride area, give fluoride supplements 5 days out of 7 until age of twelve. Cod liver oil, and other foods containing Vitamins A and D, also help to toughen teeth.

Undescended testicles (cryptorchidism)
The testes, the male reproductive organs, migrate from the abdomen into the scrotum before birth. In pre-term babies the process may not be complete. If, for some reason, the testes become stuck in the inguinal canal (the route by which they descend from abdomen to scrotum) and have not descended by the age of five, surgery may be necessary. While testes are inside the body, they are unable to mature and produce sperm.

Specific remedies to be given twice daily; if no improvement after 2 months, consult your homeopath
- Left testicle descended, but not right *Clematis 30c*
- Neither testicle descended, boy very puny for age *Aurum 30c*

Vulvovaginitis
Redness, soreness and itchiness around vulva (vaginal opening), usually caused by germs in faeces being

transferred to vulva by wiping bottom from back to front rather than from front to back, but sometimes the result of a foreign body in the vagina or an ALLERGY to wool or nylon underwear. May also be associated with BEDWETTING or THREADWORMS. If itchiness is accompanied by smelly discharge from vagina, 48 .

Specific remedies to be given 4 times daily for up to 5 days; if no improvement within 1 week, consult your GP or homeopath
- Intermittent greenish/yellowish, sticky discharge *Hydrastis 6c*
- Vulva burning and itchy, marked constipation *Alumina 6c*
- Smelly discharge, eczema or scaly skin in groin, child suffering from diarrhoea *Sulphur 6c*

Self-help Change child's underwear daily, and give a daily bath without bath salts or bath oils. If allergy suspected, change to cotton underwear. Encourage child to wipe bottom from front to back.

Whooping cough (pertussis)
A highly infectious illness caused by bacteria, serious in very young children and occasionally fatal in babies. Incubation is 1–2 weeks. Child is most infectious during first week of infection, and remains infectious for up to 3 weeks after onset of infection. First stage is runny nose and mild FEVER. Second stage is a COUGH which becomes more and more severe, beginning with a spasm and ending with a characteristic whoop as child fights to regain breath. Coughing may be violent enough to cause cyanosis (blue extremities), NOSE-BLEEDS, burst blood vessels in the eyes, and vomiting, and can last for anything from 2–10 weeks. Complications include PNEUMONIA, leading to permanent lung damage, and also BRAIN DAMAGE due to burst blood vessels in the brain. A second attack may be triggered off within a year of the first if child is prone to COLDS and is in poor health.

If you suspect your child has been in contact with whooping cough or may be developing it, 48 . GP may decide to give an antibiotic, which will kill bacteria before they take hold or at least reduce severity of attack. Give child live yoghurt daily for 5 days after course of antibiotics finishes; this restores beneficial intestinal bacteria destroyed by antibiotic. If child's lips or fingers turn blue during coughing bouts, ②.

Specific remedies to be given after every attack of coughing for up to 2 days; if no improvement, or if unsure which remedy to give, consult your homeopath
- Throat feels dry and tickly, impulse to cough is so violent that child vomits and can scarcely breathe between coughs, clasps stomach in pain when coughing, feels chilly and restless, symptoms worse after midnight *Drosera 6c*
- Hard, dry, hacking cough comes on around 3 am, child very chilly and exhausted, eyelids puffy *Kali carb. 6c*
- Coughing worse at night when child is warm in bed, alleviated by drinking cold water, vomited mucus is transparent and stringy *Coccus 6c*
- Paroxysms of coughing leave child breathless and exhausted, whooping intakes of breath cause lips to turn blue, cramps in toes and fingers (typically, thumbs are tucked into palms), drinks of cold water seem to help *Cuprum 6c*
- Stringy, yellow mucus coughed up *Kali bichrom. 6c*
- Child cries and complains of stomach pains before coughing attack comes on, has bursting feeling in head, cough worse at night and when lying down, better after coughing up mucus, then dry tickling in throat starts again and attack is repeated, with whooping and retching, child red in face, eyes puffy and bulging *Belladonna 6c*
- Child feels sick most of the time, becomes rigid, pale and breathless, then relaxes and vomits, which ends attack *Ipecac. 6c*

Immunization Orthodox immunization is offered as part of 'triple' vaccine (diptheria, tetanus, whooping cough). Adverse reactions are exceedingly rare, despite reports in the popular press. The 'triple' gives 60-80 per cent protection but should not be given if your child has a fever or if any member of your immediate family has a history of fits. There has been no research comparing the efficacy of orthodox and homeopathic immunization, but there is plenty of anecdotal evidence that *Pertussin 30c* nosode (see p. 12 for definition of nosode) prevents the graver complications of whooping cough.

Self-help Do not give cough suppressants. Encourage child to eat little and often, and to sit up and lean forward during bouts of coughing. If child vomits frequently, keep a bowl within easy reach, and wash it out each time child is sick. Keep child away from other children until infectious stage is over.

Wilm's tumour
Malignant tumour of kidney, usually occurring during first three years of life. Signs are swollen stomach, ABDOMINAL PAIN, FEVER, and occasionally BLOOD IN URINE. Conventional treatment is surgery, and drugs or radiation therapy. See CANCER for homeopathic treatment.

SPECIAL PROBLEMS IN ADOLESCENTS

THE hormonal changes that initiate transition from childhood to adulthood begin around the age of 10 or 11 in girls, and a year or so later in boys. This is reflected in the earlier sexual maturity of girls, and in their earlier spurt in weight and height gain (see charts on p. 312). Although the order in which the events of puberty occur is more or less the same in most youngsters, the age at which these events happen varies considerably.

In most boys the first signs of puberty – an increase in testicle size and a darkening of the skin of the scrotum – occur between the age of 11 and 12; six months to a year later pubic hair appears and the penis starts to grow; at the same time the prostate gland and the vesicles in which sperm is stored start to enlarge. The first ejaculation of semen, often during a 'wet dream', usually occurs about a year after the penis starts to grow. At the age of 13 or 14 the larynx begins to enlarge and the voice deepens, unreliably at first. At about the same time hair appears on the upper lip and chin, under the arms, and on the rest of the body. By the age of 17 most boys are sexually mature, though it may take another year for them to reach full height, and another year again before chest and body hair reach full luxuriance.

In girls the first sign of puberty is slight swelling of the breasts; this usually happens between the age of 10 and 11. Pubic hair begins to appear at around the same time, before underarm hair. Most girls have their first period (menarche) between the age of 12½ and 13½, just after their rate of height gain reaches its peak, but menarche at 11 or 14 is not at all uncommon. Menstruation is irregular at first, but usually settles down to a 26–28 day cycle by the age of 16. At the same age height gain levels off.

Adolescence is a time of great emotional and intellectual change too, a time when families need to give the most, and also take the most. A teenager has to negotiate some very tricky conflicts, between dependence and independence, between values held by parents and those held by peers, between wanting to be as free as a bird and having to make commitments. If parents are not prepared to be very open about their own feelings, about their own attitudes to sex, drugs, politics, and the world in general, and about their own experiences of growing up, the conflicts of adolescence can be very painful and very lonely, and are likely to repeat themselves in later life. A balance has to be struck between over-strictness and laissez faire. Laying down the law too heavily is likely to cause humiliation and resentment, but not making any rules is likely to be misconstrued as not caring.

No matter how untidy, loud, rude, hostile, and rebellious adolescents may be in their efforts to achieve a sense of self, what they need most is love and understanding, and their own 'space', physically as well as emotionally. Once they realise and accept that parents also need their own space, the stage is set for healthy transition to adulthood.

Acne

Spotty skin on face, neck, or back caused by the boost which higher hormone levels give to the production of oily sebum and the growth rate of cells in the epidermis; clogged by a mixture of dead cells and sebum, some sebaceous glands become inflamed, forming raised, red spots or pus-filled pimples; squeezing and picking do not improve matters. Condition is often more severe in boys than girls, but skin usually clears in late teens or early twenties. Lasting scars are rare. In some cases foods such as chocolate, cheese, and nuts, and fizzy citrus drinks and junk foods in general seem to aggravate condition; STRESS, steroids, and anti-epilepsy drugs may also play a part. In severe cases GP may prescribe an antiseptic lotion which peels top layer of skin, or antibiotics, hormones, or drugs based on Vitamin A. Homeopathic medicine regards acne as a symptom of fundamental imbalance, so treatment is long-term and constitutional; however, the remedies and self-help measures below may produce some improvement.

Specific remedies to be taken 3 times daily for up to 14 day
- Itchy spots, fidgety feet, restless sleep, unpleasant dreams *Kali brom. 6c*
- Long-standing acne, rough hard skin, condition aggravated by washing, especially if person tends not to feel the cold and is prone to diarrhoea first thing in morning *Sulphur 6c*
- Blind pimples and weeping pustules which form yellow crusts, spots slow to heal *Calcarea sulph. 6c*
- Large spots which look like boils *Hepar sulph. 6c*
- Spots made worse by rich, fatty food, especially if person is fair-haired, cries easily, and dislikes stuffy rooms *Pulsatilla 6c*
- Where pus-filled pimples are main feature *Antimonium tart. 6c*
- Where skin scars easily *Silicea 6c*

Self-help Sunlight, Vitamins A and B₆, and zinc all have a beneficial effect, although zinc may interfere with the absorption of some orthodox drugs given for acne. Avoid refined carbohydrates and iodine (in some cough mixtures, seaweed, etc). The Liver Diet on p. 352, followed for 1 month, should also have a positive effect. Thoroughly wash affected areas twice a day – that will remove excess sebum and dead cells. Do not take vengeance on spots by scrubbing them – damaged,

---

abraded skin easily becomes infected. Mildly antiseptic over-the-counter preparations should be used very sparingly as they can cause sensitization reactions.

Addiction see ADDICTION p. 108, DRUG ADDICTION, ALCOHOLISM

Anorexia see ANOREXIA p. 110

Blushing

Increased blood flow to face, ears, neck, etc. accompanying shame, embarrassment, and other thoughts/emotions which the blusher would prefer to hide; usually a passing phase, often linked with sexual inexperience or insecurity, and with emotional problems generally. Homeopathic constitutional treatment is recommended if blushing is part of a wider picture; if not, the remedies below may help.

Specific remedies to be taken as required for up to 10 doses
- Face normally pale, personality outgoing and rather excitable, fear of thunder and the dark *Phosphorus 6c*
- Where person is fair-haired, timid, cries easily, craves affection, and dislikes hot stuffy rooms *Pulsatilla 6c*
- Blushing causes faintness, especially if person has tendency to become anaemic *Ferrum phos. 6c*

Body odour see also PERSPIRATION PROBLEMS

Sweat glands in groin and under arms begin to broadcast their special odours around age of 15 or 16 in girls and a year or two later in boys. Most adolescent worries about body odour are related to these unfamiliar smells rather than to excessive sweating; STRESS increases sweating, and many girls find they sweat more during their periods. Fresh sweat does not usually smell unpleasant; odour becomes offensive when bacteria breed in stale sweat; daily washing, and alkalinity of soap, discourage bacteria. If sweating is related to stress, constitutional treatment is recommended; otherwise, one of the remedies below may be helpful.

Specific remedies to be taken hourly for up to 10 doses as required
- Sour-smelling perspiration, especially during exercise or sleep, person overweight and feels the cold *Calcarea 6c*
- Cold sweats, worst on feet, person slim and feels the cold, especially cold draughts around head *Silicea 6c*
- Sweat smells unpleasant, person tends to sweat in both hot and cold situations, and may produce a lot of saliva *Mercurius 6c*
- Skin looks dirty, odour persists even after washing *Psorinum 6c*

Delayed puberty

Girls tend to follow their mothers and boys their fathers in the timing of puberty (see p. 336); chronic illness and malnutrition can delay onset; puberty also comes later in children who are very thin or small for their age. If growth spurt has not taken place by age of 15, there may be cause for concern. Constitutional homeopathic treatment may be necessary, but if child is generally healthy one of the remedies below should be tried first; if there is no improvement after 2 months, see your GP or homeopath.

Specific remedies to be given every 12 hours for up to 3 weeks
- Child thin, with a large head, chilly, prone to head sweats, generally timid but can be obstinate at times *Silicea 6c*
- Child flabby and overweight, chilly, prone to sour sweats, mentally and physically sluggish *Calcarea 6c*
- Child mentally and physically immature for age, plagued by sore throats, tonsillitis, and swollen glands, delayed periods *Baryta 6c*

Delayed periods (see also MENSTRUAL PROBLEMS) Periods usually begin between age of 11 and 14, becoming regular at 15 or 16. If first period (menarche) has not occurred by age of 16, GP should be consulted; cause may be ANAEMIA, STRESS, or an imperforate hymen (sheet of tissue completely blocking outflow of blood from vagina). Constitutional homeopathic treatment may be necessary, but the remedies below should be tried first; if there is no improvement after 2 months, see your GP or homeopath.

Specific remedies to be given every 12 hours for up to 3 weeks
- Girl prone to nosebleeds *Bryonia 6c*
- Girl who is timid, often feels chilly, cries easily, suffers from headaches, prefers being in open air, feels sick when she eats rich food *Pulsatilla 6c*
- Lack of periods associated with constipation and anaemia, especially if girl has pear-shaped figure, worries a lot, and hates sympathy *Natrum mur. 6c*
- Sinking feeling in pit of stomach around 11 am, hot flushes, tension headaches, craving for fatty foods *Sulphur 6c*
- Depression, chilliness, weakness, eczema behind ears, mucous discharge from vagina *Graphites 6c*
- Girl overweight, nervous, and worried, complains of unusual fluttering and throbbing of heart, suffers from abdominal pain around 3 pm, sour belching from indigestion, redness and smarting of vulva, face flushed and pale by turns *Kali carb. 6c*

Depression see also DEPRESSION p. 113

Usually due to external factors such as exams, unemployment, breaking up with a girlfriend or boyfriend, or experimenting with drugs or alcohol (see DRUG ADDICTION, ALCOHOLISM); may also be aftermath of a viral illness such as GLANDULAR FEVER. See p. 277 for description of symptoms and treatment.

For explanation of other symbols, see page 107

Exam funk

Extreme ANXIETY about sitting exams, amounting almost to a PHOBIA; feelings of panic and inability to concentrate during exams; may be severe enough to cause stomach upsets, DIARRHOEA, HEADACHE, etc. Often there are problems in the home which make study difficult, or child may feel overwhelmed by parental pressure to achieve high marks. Lack of self-confidence and inability to concentrate may benefit from constitutional homeopathic treatment, but the remedies below are worth trying first.

Specific remedies to be given hourly for up to 10 doses before exams
- Diarrhoea and stomach upsets before exams, the more child tries to control thoughts the less he or she is able to concentrate *Argentum nit. 6c*
- Child almost paralysed with fear at thought of exam, with limbs weak and wobbly, despite conscientious studying *Gelsemium 6c*
- Child very apprehensive, tries to bolster self-confidence by bragging and behaving outrageously, even violently, before exam, settles down once exam starts *Lycopodium 6c*
- Headache brought on by studying, child prone to unpleasantly sweaty feet *Silicea 6c*
- School work tends to cause headaches, child slow in talking and of a rather solitary disposition *Natrum mur. 6c*
- Child emotionally and physically immature for age *Baryta 6c*
- Where emotional problems make it difficult for child to concentrate while studying *Anacardium 6c*

Self-help Start revising in plenty of time. Divide material to be revised into manageable units and do one or two units a day. This will leave some time for leisure activities. Rest immediately before the exam.

Phimosis

Foreskin which is too tight to draw back from head of penis; may not be diagnosed until first erection, which causes considerable pain, although condition is usually diagnosed much earlier; showing child, from age of 3 or so onwards, how to draw back foreskin to wash underneath it may help to prevent problem. Condition may require surgical removal of foreskin (see CIRCUMCISION), but in meantime one of the remedies below might help.

Specific remedies to be given 3 times daily for up to 14 days
- Itching and irritation under foreskin, ejaculation during sleep *Mercurius 6c*
- Painful erections, foreskin swollen, with itchy pimples on it *Jacaranda 6c*

Self-help If foreskin itches, bathe it and head of penis with Hypericum and Calendula solution (5 drops of mother tincture of each to 0.25 litre (½ pint) warm water).

Scoliosis

Sideways curvature of spine, causing asymmetry of ribcage, and in severe cases shortness of breath and recurrent chest infections; abnormality may be present at birth or develop during puberty, perhaps because adolescent growth spurt reveals latent weakness of spinal muscles; curvature tends to worsen rapidly unless diagnosed and treated early. Physiotherapy to strengthen back muscles is first resort; chiropractic and osteopathy are alternative therapies towards same end. If exercise and manipulation do not work, a spinal brace may have to be fitted and worn for a year or so to straighten spine. Condition requires care of an EXPERIENCED HOMEOPATH; a change of diet may be an essential part of treatment.

Shyness

A defence against being thought uninteresting, silly, inexperienced, etc. In reality, most 'shy' people are thoughtful and sensitive – traits which are much more attractive than brashness and loudness – but they reject themselves rather than risk the pain of being rejected by others; the signals that go with shyness – avoidance of eye contact, folded arms, crossed legs, muttered or monosyllabic replies to questions – are also those which tell other people 'I am not interested in you'.

Constitutional homeopathic treatment is recommended if shyness is part of general insecurity and lack of self-confidence. If shyness is only a problem in certain situations, select an appropriate remedy from the list below.

Specific remedies to be taken hourly for up to 10 doses before or during situation which causes apprehension
- Person quiet and sensitive, cries and blushes easily, panics in hot stuffy rooms *Pulsatilla 6c*
- Person timid, inclined to break down in tears, sometimes obstinate, feels the cold, especially cold winds *Silicea 6c*
- Person very pale, highly strung, fearful, desperately in need of affection and reassurance *Phosphorus 6c*
- Great nervousness about new situations, tendency to conceal nervousness by bragging and behaving outrageously or violently *Lycopodium 6c*

Self-help It often helps to admit being shy; that way, other people make a little more effort to break the ice and draw you out. Try to concentrate on the other person, not on yourself. Relax. Watch and listen. Is everyone else consistently brilliant and witty? Of course not. Ask open questions like 'What do you think of . . .' or 'How do you feel about . . .' rather than questions like 'What do you do?' or 'Have you been to see . . .' which invite factual, potentially dialogue-stopping answers.

SPECIAL PROBLEMS OF THE ELDERLY

THE disorders included in this section of the book are particularly associated with the elderly; readers are also referred to the section on nutrition in the elderly on p. 25.

The physical effects of ageing are too well known to need description here; all body systems tend to become less efficient with age, but the rate at which this happens depends greatly on habits of mind and body. It is perfectly possible to be old and healthy, but it is not possible to be old and 21.

The older we get, the more we are obliged to recognize that health is something more than the flawless working of perfect physical parts; it has a great deal to do with being connected with self, family, friends, local community, and society at large in as many positive ways as possible. As the physical fabric develops a creak here and a crack there, these connections become even more precious. Preparation for retirement is not the action of a pessimist or defeatist; the earlier you can imagine and plan a life which is not centred around full-time work the better.

Although orthodox drugs can be life-savers in many conditions which afflict the elderly, their use should be limited to the minimum effective dose. An ageing body is unable to metabolize drugs with the speed and efficiency of a young one, and so side effects are likely to be more marked. In this respect homeopathic remedies have a great advantage; they do not tax the system while trying to assist it.

It is in old age that constitutional weaknesses or imbalances achieve their fullest expression; many layers of disease, affecting many systems and organs, may have accumulated. Where gross pathological changes have occurred, homeopathic treatment is unlikely to send them into reverse, but with good constitutional treatment the quality of an elderly person's life, his or her sense of vitality and well-being, can be greatly improved.

Confusion see also CONFUSION p. 112
Not knowing what day or time of day it is, not recognizing people or surroundings, not remembering events of minutes or hours ago. Usually happens because supply of oxygen or glucose to brain is disrupted.

Confusion is one of the symptoms of HYPOTHERMIA (dangerous loss of body heat, person's abdomen feels cold); this is an emergency, so give First Aid (see p. 101). If confusion comes on gradually after a fall or a head injury, and is accompanied by ABNORMAL SLEEPINESS OR DROWSINESS, NUMBNESS or weakness, or HEADACHE and NAUSEA, cause may be a subdural haemorrhage (see BRAIN HAEMORRHAGE); appropriate action is ②.

Sometimes the symptoms of a subdural haemorrhage are difficult to distinguish from those of SENILE DEMENTIA, although generally speaking the confusion, patchy short-term memory, and personality changes which accompany senile dementia are of slower onset; in some cases, however, these symptoms may be due to vitamin deficiency rather than senility (see nutrition in the elderly p. 25).

Other conditions which may be responsible for confusion are HIGH BLOOD PRESSURE, hypothyroidism (see THYROID PROBLEMS), HYPOGLYCAEMIA (usually from lack of food), or a BRAIN TUMOUR. It should also be remembered that alcohol and drugs have considerable capacity to cause confusion in the elderly, as have infections.

Specific remedy to be taken every hour for up to 10 doses where confusion is acute and of sudden onset; if no improvement within 12 hours, see your GP
- Fever, red face, staring eyes, person upset by slightest jarring *Belladonna 30c*

Specific remedies to be taken every 12 hours for up to 3 weeks where confusion is chronic; if no improvement, see your homeopath
- Confusion due to senile dementia *Baryta 6c*
- Confusion associated with delusions and flights of fancy *Cannabis ind. 6c*

Depression see also DEPRESSION p. 113
Often associated with loneliness, low income, losing friends and relatives, feeling left behind and out of touch, becoming dependent on others, worries about health, fear of DEATH AND DYING... Occasionally symptoms of depression – lethargy, social withdrawal, lack of concentration, forgetfulness, poor sleep, loss of appetite etc. – are mistaken for SENILE DEMENTIA; unlike senile dementia, however, depression is treatable. See DEPRESSION p. 113 and ANXIETY for homeopathic remedies and other forms of treatment.

Dizziness see also DIZZINESS pp. 126–7
Disorders which most often affect balance in old age are PARKINSON'S DISEASE (degeneration of nerve centres responsible for coordinating movement), ARTERIOSCLEROSIS (hardening and narrowing of arteries, especially those which supply brain), OSTEOARTHRITIS (especially in hips and knees), and CERVICAL SPONDYLOSIS (bony growths on neck vertebrae which press on spinal cord and blood vessels to head). Treatment of underlying disorder may alleviate balance problem.

Specific remedies to be taken every 8 hours; if no improvement within 2 weeks, see your GP or homeopath

- Standing up from sitting or lying position causes dizziness, or dizziness which comes on after an injury, dizziness wears off lying down *Arnica 6c*
- Dizziness made worse by movement, with nausea *Theridion 6c*
- Dizziness worse in cold weather, coughing causes seepage of urine *Causticum 6c*
- Poor circulation due to arteriosclerosis, walking out of doors improves circulation, feeling weak and weary and wanting to lie down *Baryta 6c*
- Senile dementia and loss of concentration, dizziness worse between 4 and 8 pm *Lycopodium 6c*
- Poor circulation, dizziness worse in cold weather and when lying on left side *Silicea 6c*

Falls and accidents

The older we get, the more accident-prone we become. Reflexes, eyesight, hearing, and sense of smell are not what they were, balance may be precarious (see conditions which cause DIZZINESS), joints are less supple, bones more brittle, and so on. Women's bones fracture more easily than men's due to thinning of the bones after menopause (see FRACTURES, OSTEOPOROSIS). Skin and blood vessels are also more fragile, leading to easy BRUISING and laceration.

If a fracture is suspected, (999) and give First Aid (see p. 99). If person becomes confused or drowsy, or complains of numbness or nausea, (2), even if there are no cuts, bruises, or broken bones; accident may have caused a subdural haemorrhage (see BRAIN HAEMORRHAGE).

If person is unable to move or call for help after an accident, secondary consequences may be more serious than those of the accident itself; these include HYPOTHERMIA (if person is cold), PNEUMONIA (if accident occurs out of doors), SHOCK (excessive bleeding), and BURNS (if person has fallen against a radiator, for example).

Circulation problems caused by ATHEROSCLEROSIS or ARTERIOSCLEROSIS may mean that injured tissues are slow to heal. Immobility after injury can also weaken bones and muscles, and hasten degenerative changes in joints. In addition, person may lose confidence in ability to get around or succumb to DEPRESSION.

See conditions mentioned above for appropriate homeopathic remedies. However, immediately after a fall give *Arnica 30c* every 15 minutes for up to 6 doses.

Self-help If you have had a bad fall, see your GP as quickly as possible; there are no medals for soldiering on unaided.

The best way to forestall accidents is to keep as physically and mentally active as possible, and pay close attention to nutrition (see p. 25). Your diet should include plenty of Vitamin C and zinc, for example. If you suffer from bouts of weakness or unsteadiness, see your GP; you may have a disorder which is easily cured.

If you live alone, try to get a relative or neighbour to visit you, or at least telephone you, at a set time every day; if you don't answer the door or the 'phone, they will know that something is wrong. Special alarm schemes are available in some areas, but these tend to be expensive; contact your local Social Security office or social services department if you have difficulty finding the money. You may also be eligible for once-only help with the cost of rewiring, installing safe heating, extra lights, guard rails, etc.

To minimize risk of accidents make sure all rugs and floor coverings are secure, keep steps and stairs well lit, and never overload electricity points or place lamps or appliances in places where you are likely to trip over the flex. Wear shoes that fit properly, with laces that are not likely to trip you up, and make sure your slippers have non-slip soles; use a non-slip mat in the bath. If you have to get up during the night, don't blunder around in the dark; have a light beside your bed. If you are unsteady on your feet, use a stick, and make sure steps and stairs have a solid handrail or banisters. Keep everything you need in low cupboards or on shelves which you can reach easily – no climbing up on chairs or stools and overbalancing. If you wear glasses, don't go walking in your reading glasses.

Hypothermia see also First Aid p. 101

Develops when body temperature drops below 35°C (95°F); with age, the body becomes less efficient at monitoring temperature and less able to maintain core temperature when surroundings are cold. Symptoms are apathy, unwillingness to move or speak, CONFUSION, and ABNORMAL SLEEPINESS or DROWSINESS; person's hands and feet feel cold, but surer sign of low body temperature is a cold abdomen. If hypothermia persists, person becomes unconscious; death then follows within a few hours. Once temperature has fallen to 25°C (77°F), odds against recovery are 3 to 1.

Prevention If you have an elderly relative or neighbour who is house-bound or an invalid, and on a low income, visit him or her as often as possible in cold weather. If he or she is not eating properly or not using heating because of the cost, he or she may be eligible for meals on wheels (contact local social services department) or attendance allowance, or help with fuel bills, draught-proofing, extra clothes or blankets, etc. (your local post office or Social Security office will have leaflets). A temperature of less than 20°C (68°F) in a living room or bedroom is too low.

Incontinence of urine see also INCONTINENCE OF URINE p. 235

Not an inevitable part of ageing. In most cases loss of control is secondary to treatable disorders such as urinary tract infections (see CYSTITIS), CONSTIPATION (hard-packed faecal matter in bowel pressing on

---

(999) Emergency – call GP (or dial 999) immediately. (2) Consult your doctor if no improvement within 2 hours

bladder), an enlarged prostate gland (see PROSTATE PROBLEMS), and PRURITIS VULVAE (itchy vulva), or brought on by drugs or prolonged immobility. Loss of bladder or bowel control after a STROKE or SPINAL CORD INJURY can occur at any age; provided damage to brain or spinal cord is not too severe, disability may only be temporary. STRESS INCONTINENCE (momentary loss of control when laughing, coughing, sneezing, lifting, etc. due to weakness of pelvic floor muscles) is primarily a female problem, more typical of the young and middle-aged than of the elderly.

Incontinence is characteristic of later stages of SENILE DEMENTIA; cause is self-neglect and general loss of inhibition rather than any physical disability.

If incontinence cannot be controlled by drugs, GP may advise catheterization (urine continuously drains into a bag through a small tube inserted into bladder); for advice on special underwear, consult your GP or health visitor.

If incontinence is caused by infection, select a remedy from those listed under CYSTITIS or prostatitis (see PROSTATE PROBLEMS; otherwise, choose a remedy from the list below. If there is no improvement within 3 days, see your GP.

Specific remedies to be given 4 times daily for up to 3 days
- Weak, trembly legs, drooping eyelids *Gelsemium 6c*
- Incontinence made worse by coughing or laughing *Causticum 6c*
- Inability to control bladder, with pain in neck of bladder, frequent urge to urinate, urination relieves pain *Ferrum phos. 6c*
- Involuntary dribbles of urine, person very irritable *Nux 6c*

Self-help To minimize amount of urine in bladder at any one time, and to improve bladder control, pass urine at regular, frequent intervals – use a digital watch with a bleeper to remind yourself. Drink sparingly before bedtime, and keep a chamber-pot or commode in the bedroom for emergencies.

Incontinence of faeces
Much less common than incontinence of urine; causes include infections such as GASTROENTERITIS, loss of nervous control after a STROKE or SPINAL CORD INJURY, SENILE DEMENTIA, and even DEPRESSION. In special cases, if underlying cause is not treatable, surgery to tighten anal sphincter muscles may be advised; a small electrical device can also be implanted in rectum to improve sphincter control. Occasionally CONSTIPATION, or rather lack of fibre in diet, is the cause of incontinence; hard mass of faeces blocks bowel and interferes with normal expulsion mechanism, but liquid matter may seep out; regular bowel action can usually be restored with laxatives or enemas. Homeopathic and natural remedies for constipation are described on pp. 223–4.

Self-help Eat a high-fibre diet, even if constipation is not an obvious problem. Involuntary bowel movements most often occur an hour or so after meals.

Senile dementia
Progressive wasting of brain cells or loss of brain function due to hardening of arteries (see ARTERIO-SCLEROSIS); onset is slow, over years rather than months. Short-term memory is affected first – person occasionally forgets what happened hours or minutes ago, and has difficulty following conversations and trains of thought, or making sense of what he or she sees or reads. In early stages, person is well aware of what is happening; even in later stages, confusion may be punctuated by moments of lucidity. With memory and reasoning impaired, person loses interest in activities which were once enjoyable; habitual behaviours which make up 'personality' break down; there is increasing emotional and physical instability, with unpredictable switches between apathy and aggression; social inhibitions, and sometimes sexual inhibitions, also go out of the window.

However, the label of senile dementia should not be too hastily applied. Failing eyesight or hearing, nutritional deficiencies, alcohol, drugs, underactivity of thyroid gland (see THYROID PROBLEMS), a BRAIN TUMOUR, a slow BRAIN HAEMORRHAGE, a STROKE or HEART ATTACK, HYPOTHERMIA, HYPOGLYCAEMIA, urinary tract infections, and DEPRESSION can also produce confused mental states; in many cases, treatment of underlying cause improves intellectual performance.

Homeopathic medicine offers a number of specific remedies for failing mental powers; if the remedy you choose produces no improvement within 1 month, see your homeopath.

Specific remedies to be given every 12 hours for up to 2 weeks
- Person once intellectually sharp and ambitious, now thin and withered, lacking in self-confidence, afraid of being alone, always using wrong words *Lycopodium 30c*
- Degenerative changes in blood vessels, enlarged prostate gland, weakness and tiredness, problems exacerbated by cold *Baryta 30c*
- Partial paralysis, blood vessels supplying brain affected by arteriosclerosis *Aurum iod. 30c*
- Atherosclerosis, craving for salt, person highly strung and very apprehensive *Phosphorus 30c*

Self-help Make sure the diet contains plenty of Vitamins B and C, and also zinc and magnesium.

Skin problems
With age, the skin becomes thinner and loses its elasticity. As part of this process tiny blood vessels in skin may be damaged; as blood seeps out, wine-

coloured blotches form under skin, most commonly on backs of hands, forearms, and lower legs; blotches come and go but never entirely disappear; condition is quite harmless, despite its medical name, *senile purpura*. Like other forms of BRUISING, purpura may be helped by taking extra Vitamin C. Many old people also develop oddly pigmented patches of skin; these are usually nothing to worry about – they may have something to do with faulty fat metabolism or Vitamin E deficiency – but to be on the safe side, read WARTS AND MOLES pp. 144, 148. Itchy skin is also common in old age; in most cases it is due to dryness and can be relieved by using moisturizers; occasionally, however, it is a sign of JAUNDICE (yellowish skin and eye whites, dark urine, pale stools).

Specific remedies to be given 4 times daily for up to 14 days
- Itchy skin made worse by washing and by bed warmth, diarrhoea in morning *Sulphur 6c*
- Dirty-looking skin, especially in cold weather *Psorinum 6c*
- Excessive oily perspiration, made worse by heat and cold *Mercurius 6c*
- Burning sensation in skin, person chilly, restless, and anxious *Arsenicum 6c*

Trigeminal neuralgia see also NEURITIS AND NEURALGIA

Bouts of severe, shooting pain in one side of face, lasting for seconds or minutes, brought on by touch or pressure, chewing, draughts, etc., and caused by damage to trigeminal nerve, although cause of damage is not known; if muscles on affected side of face go into spasm, a facial tic develops; condition is most common in people over 70. If shooting pains occur in conjunction with a sinus, ear, or tooth infection, cause is probably not trigeminal neuralgia but temporary inflammation of trigeminal nerve. If drugs do not prevent neuralgia attacks, GP may recommend an operation to partially destroy trigeminal nerve. However, provided infection has been ruled out, author recommends homeopathic treatment as first resort; if the remedies below produce no improvement within 2 weeks, see your homeopath.

Specific remedies to be taken 4 times daily for up to 14 days
- Intolerable pain in ear, made worse by slightest movement, face flushed, acid indigestion *Verbascum 6c*
- Burning pains which wear off with exercise or exertion, weakness, restlessness *Arsenicum 6c*
- Tearing, stinging pains made worse by cold and damp, relieved by pressure *Colocynth 6c*
- Neuralgia on right side of face *Kalmia 6c*
- Neuralgia on left side of face, tearing pains, twitching muscles, face very pale, noise makes symptoms worse, pressure makes them better *Spigelia 6c*

NOTE TO PART 6

Dosage Doses advised are deliberately on the safe side and may not be high enough to give benefit, but it is recommended that higher dosages should only be taken under the care of a practitioner experienced in nutritional medicine.

Side Effects refer to effects of much larger doses on the whole than those recommended in this book.

PART 6

NUTRITIONAL SUPPLEMENTS AND SPECIAL DIETS

Are supplements necessary?

Supplements should not be needed providing that one is eating a good, well-balanced, wholegrain diet with plenty of raw organically grown vegetables and fruit. There is concern, however, that certain agricultural processes have led to losses of specific nutrients in the food chain. There are also specific times when supplementation may be required, such as when taking certain drugs, oral contraceptive pills, during pregnancy and while lactating, during and after weight loss, and if you are elderly. If you feel that you are generally under par i.e. physically low in energy or mentally lethargic, there is no harm in taking a multi vitamin and mineral supplement for a month. I would recommend that you take one that is not time-released, which contains less than 25 mg of each of the major B vitamins (B1, 5, 6) and has a zinc to copper ratio of not less than 14 to 1.

The quality of supplements

Nutritional supplements are available from one of four sources. Chemists, health food shops, your doctor and specialist mail order companies. Supplements from the chemist are very strictly controlled as to their content but chemist's shops tend not to include such a wide range of vitamins and minerals in their multivitamin preparations as health food shops, and they frequently contain tartrazine and other additives which may upset people who are prone to allergies.

Rules for prescribing supplements

Deficiencies. When you read through the Ailments Section, you may find under certain complaints that there may be a need for certain nutrients, such as vitamin C or zinc. This means that either the ailment is thought to be due to a deficiency of these nutrients or that it responds to increasing their intake in the diet, although you are not necessarily deficient in them.

If you have this complaint, turn to the nutrient section which follows. This will tell you which foods contain the recommended nutrient, and you should increase your intake of those foods for one month. If this does not help, then take a supplement, in the amount equal to, or less than, that which is advised as a maximum for another month. If there is still no improvement, see your GP, a nutritionally trained physician or a dietician. If you do feel better then you may continue taking the supplement, but stop for two days a week. I have deliberately erred on the cautious side when advising dosages of nutrients. However, apart from with fat-soluble vitamins and certain minerals like selenium, it is rare to find side-effects occurring even if you are taking up to 100 times more than the RDA. Any supplement not mentioned below may also be taken, but stop for two days a week after one month, and watch the health press for possible hazards.

RDAS and food labelling

You may have seen Recommended Daily Allowance (RDA) requirements for various nutrients. These are based on whether a nutrient is essential for the body's health, and the amount required to prevent deficiency and disease. RDAs vary considerably from country to country, and although not ideal, RDAs work reasonably well to prevent nutritional disease.

Legally required labels on packets show the chemical analysis of the nutritional and calorific contents of food. Putting nutrition into numerical terms like this makes it easier to match foods to average requirements.

Reading the label

Vitamins are normally measured in: mg (milligrams: one thousandth of a gram); mcg (micrograms: one thousandth of a milligram i.e. one millionth of a gram); IU (International units: a measurement of biological activity rather than weight). There are only three vitamins that are still sometimes measured in international units: Vitamins A, D, and E. These are the conversions: Vitamin A, One IU = 0.3 mcg retinol; Vitamin A (as beta carotene), One IU = 0.1 mcg retinol; Vitamin D, One IU = 0.025 mcg; Vitamin E, One IU = 0.83 mg–1.12 mg depending on the form of Vitamin E used.

EFAs (Essential fatty Acids – Linoleic and Linolenic acids)

Required for integrity of cell walls and the production of potent chemicals such as the prostaglandins.

Found in: Vegetables, grains, wheat, beans, spinach, fish, especially oily fish like mackerel.

Supplements available as: oil filled capsules. These should be taken orally or broken open and the oil rubbed into unbroken skin, on the inner arms or legs, for example. Trade names are Glanolyn, Efamol, Oil of Evening Primrose (containing gammalinoleic acid).

Max EPA contains docosahexaenoic and eko-sapentoeic acid.

RDA: Not given. Maximum dosage – less than 1 gm a day of Efamol. Up to 4 capsules a day of Max EPA.

N.B. Always give supplements of zinc, magnesium, Vitamins C, E and B complex and selenium when taking EFAs.

Avoid Oil of Evening Primrose if you are epileptic and Max EPA if you have a bleeding disorder, except under medical supervision.

Vitamin A

Important for the functioning of the eyes and cell membranes. Too little may lead to night blindness, scaly skin and poor growth. Vitamin A may also be involved in resistance to certain diseases.

Found in: offal, cheese, eggs, butter, margarine, fish oils, green, yellow and orange vegetables, e.g. carrots, cabbage and spinach.

Supplements available as: tablets, oil-filled capsules, bottles of oil e.g. cod liver oil, all of which are taken orally. Maximum dose 15,000 IUs daily unless you are pregnant – see below.

RDA Children – 400–700 mcgs
       Women – 800 mcgs
       Pregnant or lactating women – 1200 mcgs
       Men – 1000 mcgs

Side-effects: If you take a supplement of more than 9000 mcg or 30,000 IU, you may suffer from nausea, vomiting, dizziness, dry, scaling skin, hair loss, fatigue or headaches.

N.B. Do not take more than 10,000 IU or 3000 mcg daily if you are or could become pregnant, as this could harm the foetus.

Vitamin B1 (or thiamine)

Needed for carbohydrate metabolism; deficiency may cause irritability, depression, loss of concentration, fatigue and insomnia. In alcoholics and the elderly, deficiency can cause loss of memory and heart failure.

Found in: Whole cereals, nuts, beans, peas, pulses, yeast, pork, beef, liver, wholemeal bread.

Supplements available as: Capsules or tablets, usually found in combination with other B vitamins.

RDA Children 0.3–0.9 mg
       Women – 0.9 mg
       Pregnant and lactating women 1 mg–1.1 mg
       Men – 1.2 mg
       Maximum dose under 50 mg a day.

Vitamin B2 (riboflavin)

Aids in the metabolism of fats, carbohydrates and proteins. Deficiency can lead to soreness of the lips and tongue, and photophobia (intolerance of bright light).

Found in: liver, offal, milk, cheese, eggs, fish, green vegetables, yeast extract.

Supplements available as pills or tablets usually with other B vitamins.

RDA: Children 0.6–0.8 mg
        Women 1.3 mg
        Lactating and pregnant women 2 mg
        Men 1.8 mg
        Maximum dose 50 mg a day.

Side Effects: Supplements containing B2 may cause urine to become yellow.

N.B. The level of B2 in milk decreases on exposure to light.

Vitamin B3 (niacin, nicotinic acid or nicotanamide)

Involved in general metabolism. Deficiency can lead to irritability, loss of memory and dementia, dermatitis and headache.

Found in: Meat, fish, pulses, wholegrains, offal, nuts.

Supplements available in many forms, usually in combination with other B vitamins.

RDA: Children 5 mg–19 mg
        Women 15 mg
        Pregnant women 18 mg
        Lactating women 21 mg
        Men 18 mg
        Maximum dose, less than 100 mg a day.

Side Effects: High doses may alter liver function tests and can aggravate diabetes and cause depression. These effects wear off after stopping the supplements. It can also cause uncomfortable flushing of the skin, but this usually passes off.

N.B. The B3 in maize corn has to be liberated with alkali or hot ash before it is available to the body.

Vitamin B5 (or pantotenic acid)

Helps with the metabolism of fats, carbohydrates and proteins. Deficiency leads to fatigue, emotional swings and numbness.

Found in: a wide variety of foods. High levels in eggs, wholegrain cereals and meat.

Supplements available in mainly B complex tablets.

RDA 5–10 mg per day
       Maximum dose 100 mg per day.

Vitamin B6 (or pyroxidine)

Also involved in the metabolism of all three main types of nutrients, and of minerals and certain body chemicals called neuro-transmitters. Deficiency leads to irritability, insomnia, dermatitis, and reduced resistance to infection.

Found in: Liver, whole grain cereals, nuts, seeds, bananas, most fruits, green leafy vegetables and avocados.

Supplements available in many forms, usually but not always in combination with other B vitamins.

RDA: (USA) Pregnant women 2.5 mg per day
Lactating mothers: 2.5 mg per day
Adults 1.5–2 mg per day
Maximum dose 50 mg a day.

Side effects: B6 can aggravate a B2 deficiency and very large doses of over 2000 mg a day have been reported to cause nerve damage. Doses of over 100 mg have been reported to produce an increase in dreaming and wakefulness.

Vitamin B12 (or cobalamine)

Necessary for both haemoglobin production and the functioning of the nervous system. Deficiency results in anaemia and lack of co-ordination; it may not always be caused by lack of B12 in the diet, but by inadequate absorption of the vitamin from the intestine.

Found in: Offal, fish, pork, eggs, cheese, yogurt, milk and brewers yeast.

Supplements available in tablets from health food shops and chemists.

RDA: 3–4 mcg
Maximum dose, less than 100 mcg

Folic acid (or folate)

Closely linked to B12 and the workings of the nervous system. Anaemia and mental problems may result from its deficiency. Inadequate intake is especially common in pregnancy and may contribute to the risk of spina bifida.

Found in: Liver, spinach, broccoli tops, asparagus, beets, kidney, cabbage, lettuce, avocados, nuts and wheatgerm.

Supplements available in tablets from health food shops or chemists.

RDA: (USA) Children 45 mcg–300 mcg
Adults 400 mcg
Pregnant women 800 mcg
Lactating women 500 mcg
Maximum dose, less than 400 mcg

Side effects: Avoid if on certain drugs, used to treat epilepsy or if you have an oestrogen-dependent breast tumour. It should not be taken on its own for too long without B12 in case a B12 deficiency is masked and damage results to the central nervous system. Toxicity can result if more than 15 mg per day is taken, causing distension and flatulence, nausea, loss of appetite, sleep disturbances, vivid dreams, malaise and irritability.

Vitamin C (or ascorbic acid)

Has a central role in cell metabolism and helps to prevent infection and repair injury. It also aids absorption of iron. Deficiency results in the bleeding gums and bruised, dry skin of scurvy. Extra vitamin C may be required by the elderly, heavy smokers and drinkers, women taking the contraceptive pill, and those on other medications such as aspirin, antibiotics or steroids.

Found in: most fruit and vegetables – preferably raw; milk, liver and kidney and new potatoes.

Supplements available in powder, soluble tablets, pills. It is probably best to give a natural vitamin C which usually comes from Acerola cherries. Synthetic ones are usually described as ascorbic acid. Natural vitamin C preparations usually also contain bioflavonoids thought to be necessary for its proper functioning. A form of bioflavonoids (oxyrutin) is available on prescription only for varicose veins.

RDA: Children 8 mg–14 mg
Adults 30 mg
Pregnant women and lactating women 50 mg
Maximum dose on or under 500 mg a day.

Side effects: See your GP if you are taking it as a supplement. It may react with drugs such as PAS, salycilates, amphetamines, anti-depressants and Warfarin. Over 50 gms a day there is shown to be an increase in the excretion of calcium, iron and manganese in the urine, with reduced availability of zinc, copper and increased uric acid and oxalic acid excretion. You should avoid vitamin C supplementation if you suffer from glucose-6-dehydrogenase deficiency (an inborn error of metabolism).

N.B. If you suddenly stop supplementation of large doses of vitamin C, it may precipitate scurvy, so gradually cut it down over a period of a few weeks. Suddenly stopping supplementation has also been reported as causing sleeplessness, sore tongue, constipation, diarrhoea, canker sores, pain on passing urine and reduced fertility in women, abortion in large doses (over 6 gm).

Vitamin D (or calciferol)

Needed for the absorption and metabolism of calcium. Its deficiency may lead to rickets or osteomalacia. It can be synthesized by the body when skin is exposed to sunlight. This is the major source for the body.

It is also found in fish liver oils, vegetable and animal oils and in dairy products.

Supplements available in capsules of cod or halibut liver oil, bottled cod liver oil or tablets.

RDA: Children 10 mcg
        Women 2.5 mcg
        Pregnant and lactating women 10 mcg
        Maximum dose 400 units

Side effects: usually caused by taking more than 100,000 units a day – high blood levels of calcium with stone formation in the kidney, joints, blood vessels, heart and lungs; loss of appetite, nausea and vomiting, thirst, increased production of urine, constipation or diarrhoea, pains in the head and weakness. Avoid supplementation if you have sarcoidosis and high blood calcium and are often exposed to sunlight.

Vitamin E (or tocopherol)
Involved in the breakdown of fats. It is especially necessary for women on the contraceptive pill, or those who are pregnant or menopausal.

Found in: vegetable oil, wheat germ, sunflower seed, safflower oil, eggs, butter and wholemeal cereals. (Destroyed by rancid oils and deep-freezing.)

Supplements available as capsules, pills, tablets, oils. It may be found as naturally derived vitamin E – usually expressed as amounts in IUs, or as synthetic vitamin E, usually expressed in mgs. Also available in droplet form for better absorption from specialised manufacturers.

RDA: (USA) Children 3 mg–10 mg
        Women 80 mg
        Pregnant women 10 mg
        Lactating women 11 mg
        Men 10 mg
        Maximum dose 100 units

Side effects: Can interfere with iron absorption so it should be given at different meals. It should not be given to patients on anti-coagulants without medical supervision. Dosages of 300 mg interfere with the immune system, 600 mg causes lowering of the triglyceride and thyroid levels, 900 mgs depression and fatigue, 3,200 mgs diarrhoea, depression, headache, blurred vision, cramps, dizziness, skin rash, irritability of the gastro-intestinal tract, increase in blood pressure, gynaecomastia (swelling of the breasts), vaginal bleeding, hypoglycaemia, stomatitis, chapped lips and reproductive disturbances. Diabetics should be aware of hypoglycaemia attacks if taking large doses of Vitamin E.

Vitamin K
Plays a role in the clotting of blood at the site of a wound. It is especially important in newborn babies.

Found in: spinach, cabbage, lettuce, wheat germ, tomatoes, oil, eggs, liver.

RDA: 30–40 mcg

Supplements: Not recommended because of its toxicity. Injectible, vitamin K is used in hospitals to prevent haemorrhagic disease of the new-born which is particularly common in premature babies, and babies of mothers who are on anti-epileptic drugs. It is now given routinely as the disease can cause permanent brain damage. It also interacts with drugs which stop the blood clotting (anticoagulants).

Calcium
Found in bones, teeth, muscles, nerves and blood; there is more than 1 kg (2¼ lb) in the body. Its absorption in the digestive system is affected by vitamin D, magnesium, bran (which can inhibit absorption), phosphorus, fats, the oestrogen hormones and the parathyroid glands. Deficiency results in osteoporosis (brittle bones). Growing children and older women need a lot of calcium.

Found in: milk (particularly skimmed milk), cheese, wholemeal bread, sesame seeds, soya flour, haricot beans, almonds, parsley, spinach, broccoli, turnip, hard water, herring roe and fish.

Supplements available in soluble and non-soluble tablets.

RDA: Children up to   8 – 300 mg
                          9–14 – 700 mg
                          15–17 – 600 mg
        Adults 300 mg
        Pregnant and lactating women 500 mg
        Maximum dose 1 gm (1000 mgs)

Side effects: It has been suggested by some authorities that milk is not a good source of calcium to rely on, partly because of the commonness of allergic reactions and also because it lacks magnesium, which can lead to a magnesium deficiency, especially in children drinking large quantities. It is usually not toxic in healthy persons. Do not give at the same time of day as magnesium and manganese. Ensure stomach acidity is satisfactory.

Magnesium
Necessary for metabolism of proteins and carbohydrates. There is a long list of deficiency conditions which includes mental problems, heart rhythm disturbances, menstrual problems, high blood pressure and constipation.

Found in: green vegetables, wholegrain cereals and nuts, shrimps, soya beans and hard water.

Supplements available in powders, tablets or in combination with amino acids or B vitamins.

RDA: (USA) Male – 350 mgs
Female – 300 mgs
Pregnant and lactating women –
450mgs
Maximum dose – 200 mgs a day. If
taking calcium as well, you should take
2 parts calcium to 1 part magnesium.

Side effects: Rare.

N.B. Don't take after meals, can cause diarrhoea.

Phosphorus

Found in bones and in all cells, especially those of the nervous system. Deficiency may result in muscle weakness and anaemia.

Found in: foods rich in calcium and protein.

Supplements available are rarely necessary as this mineral is widespread in foods.

RDA: (USA) Adults – 800 mg
Pregnancy and lactation 12 mg

Side effects: None known unless large doses lead to increased requirements of calcium and magnesium.

Iron

Necessary for the formation of the haemoglobin which carries oxygen in red blood cells. Deficiency leads to anaemia.

Found in: Sausage, liver, fish, eggs, pulses, oatmeal, millet, barley, wheat, cane molasses, wholemeal bread, nuts and seeds and green vegetables.

Supplements available in tablets, usually bound to another substance to help absorption and sometimes combined with vitamins or folic acid. Take with vitamin C.

RDA: Children 6–12 mg
Women 12 mg
Pregnant women 13 mg
Lactating women 15 mg
Men 10 mg
Maximum dose – 60 mg of elemental iron daily unless under medical supervision. Avoid supplementing with more than 2 parts iron to 1 part zinc.

Side effects: Siderosis, which is a condition usually developed as a result of taking supplements or cheap wine, causing iron to be deposited in the liver, pancreas, lungs, spleen or heart causing damage, with symptoms of dizziness, weight loss, headache, shortage or breath and fatigue.

N.B. Tannin, e.g. in tea, inhibits absorption of iron, so limit your tea intake.

Zinc

Involved in the absorption and metabolism of vitamins, carbohydrates and phosphorus. It is found especially in the reproductive organs. Deficiency can slow growth and bring on infertility. It is also associated with skin disorders, impaired healing, loss of taste or smell, and white spots on nails.

Found in: oysters, meat, ginger, wholegrains, nuts and seeds, green vegetables, yeast, legumes, milk and eggs.

Supplements available in capsules, soluble tablets, sometimes combined with other substances to aid absorption.

RDA: (USA) Adults – 15 mgs
Pregnant and lactating women – 25 mgs
Maximum dose – less than 25 mgs

Side effects: Over 150 mgs daily for 6 weeks may cause weakening of the immune system and over 200 mgs a day may cause collapse. If on more than 15 mg a day, don't take within 1 hour of food.

N.B. Zinc has been found to alleviate acne in some cases.

Iodine

Essential for the production of the hormone Thyroxine, which is responsible for regulating the metabolic rate, ensuring normal growth and maintaining skin and hair. A deficiency may lead to goitre, a swelling of the thyroid gland which is located in the neck.

Found in: Sea food, seaweed, kelp, lava bread, iodised salt and fish liver oils.

Supplements available in kelp or iodine tablets or solution, capsules of fish oils from chemists, health food shops or on prescription.

RDA: (USA) Males 130 mcg
Females 100 mcg
Pregnant women 125 mcg
Lactating women 150 mcg
Maximum dose – The addition of natural sources of iodine to the diet should be used for supplementation. Use iodine itself only under a doctor's supervision.

Sodium

Involved in the body's fluid balance and nerve and muscle function. Deficiency may lead to cramps, exhaustion, nausea and circulatory problems.

Found in: Salt, meat, fish, yeast extract, bread, butter, vegetables, margarine, biscuits and cheese.

Supplements available in salt.

RDA: (USA) 300 mg
Don't supplement unless dehydrated and then only very carefully

Side effects: May cause high blood pressure or loss of potassium.

Potassium

Plays an important role in water balance and nerve and muscle function. Deficiency symptoms include cramps, fatigue, heart irregularities and headache.

Found in: milk, beef, soya flour, dried fruits, vegetables, cereals. A vegetarian diet has a better sodium and potassium balance than an omnivorous one.

Supplements available in tablets of potassium chloride and other salts, salt substitutes such as ruthmol, also found combined with diuretic tablets.

RDA: (USA) 900 mg

Side effects: Weakness and heart problems. High doses in the elderly can seriously affect kidney function.

N.B. Use salt substitutes containing potassium such as ruthmol, but don't take more than you would if using ordinary salt. Take it with or after food to avoid stomach irritation.

Copper

Found in many enzymes and is essential for healthy blood cells and bones. Anaemia and skeletal defects, raised blood cholesterol and lowered fertility are among the symptoms of deficiency.

Found in: liver, kidney, nuts, shellfish, legumes, stone fruits, yeast, cocoa, wholemeal cereal, water.

Supplements are rarely needed, as copper is found in many foods.

RDA: (USA) 3 mgs

Manganese

Involved in growth, nervous system function, and hormonal, fat and vitamin metabolism. Symptoms of deficiency include cartilage problems, low fertility and birth defects, growth retardation.

Found in: fresh vegetables, nuts, spices, wholegrains, tea.

Supplements available in tablets prepared in conjunction with amino acids and other substances to help absorption.

RDA: (USA) 5 mgs
　　　　　　　Maximum dose – 10 mg

Side effects: irritability, tremor, muscle rigidity.

Fluoride

Contributes to strong bones and teeth and helps to prevent dental decay.

Found in: China tea, sea food, hard water, wheat, carrots, beets, currants, cabbage leaves.

RDA: (USA) 4 mg
　　　　　　　Do not take as a supplement unless painting the teeth or taking fluoride tablets is recommended by dentist. Use fluoride toothpaste. If taking fluoride tablets, stop at weekends after one month's continual use.

Side effects: Mottling of teeth, hardening of bone.

Chromium

Involved with blood-sugar regulation and the hormone insulin (see diabetes). Clouding of the cornea, atherosclerosis and low fertility are symptoms of deficiency.

Found in: blackstrap molasses, honey, brewers' yeast, whole wheat bread, nuts, shellfish, kidney, liver, grape juice, black pepper.

Supplements available in brewers' yeast, solution of chromic chloride.

RDA: (USA) 0.2 mg
　　　　　　Maximum dose – 200 mg

Side effects: very large doses may be cancer forming. Glucose tolerance factor chromium preparations are more active but are yeast derived and people with yeast allergies should avoid them.

Selenium

Necessary for healthy liver, heart and white blood cells. Liver disease, skin problems, cancer and arthritis may indicate deficiency.

Found in: brewers' yeast, sesame seeds, garlic, eggs, fish, shellfish, offal and vegetables.

Supplements available in tablets or solution.

RDA: 0.2 mg
　　　　　Maximum dose less than 0.2 mg

Side effects: Dental decay in children under 12, hair loss, brittle nails, fatigue, skin rash, loss of appetite, sour taste in mouth, possibly congenital malformations.

Silicon

Important for healthy teeth, arteries and growth generally.

Found in: unrefined grains. Used as an additive to stop foods clogging up or foaming.

Do not supplement.

Nickel

May be involved in regularising blood sugar levels and fat metabolism. Congenital defects have been linked to its deficiency.

Found in: most nickel enters the system from environment as nickel is widespread in coins, jewellery, kitchen appliances etc.

RDA: Unknown

Side effects: may cause dermatitis and cancer of the lung.

Toxic or Excess Effects of Vitamins and Minerals

On reading the ailments section you may have found that your ailment may be due to an excess of certain nutrients or toxic vitamins. If it is a mineral or vitamin, check the mineral supplement that you are taking and if it contains this particular nutrient then stop taking it. If it is a toxic metal, then look at the toxic sources and remove them, then get a hair analysis done, and if it is positive see your nutritionist or your GP who may test your blood and advise on which steps to take.

General points about avoiding toxic metals

1. Avoid tobacco smoke at home and at work, exhaust fumes, cooking in unsuitable containers.
2. Eat plenty of fibre and nutrient-rich vegetables and fruit.
3. Don't buy fruit and vegetables from displays on stalls or outside shops where they may have been exposed to leaded exhaust fumes.
4. Correct any nutritional deficiencies you may have by improving your diet.
5. Don't allow young children to suck lead soldiers.

Lead

There are over 10,000 papers on the toxicity of lead. High levels of lead are known to produce potentially fatal results such as anaemia, and other symptoms may include colicky abdominal pains, damage to the peripheral nerves or brain; however, many authorities are now convinced that lower levels than originally thought can cause sub-acute poisoning, leading to still births and congenital abnormalities, learning and behavioural problems, cancer, heart disease and high blood pressure, kidney and metabolic disease immune dysfunction and vague symptoms such as lethargy, depression, muscular aches and pains and frequent infections.

Sources: traffic fumes, unlined copper food pans, dust, polluted water from flaking lead pipes, or lead alloy sealed copper piping, cracked lead-glazed earthenware, lead soldiers, dust and dirt, vegetables grown by the roadside or exposed to traffic fumes, bone meal, dolomite, cigarette ash and tobacco, and occupational exposure.

N.B. Since 1986, no white interior paints have contained lead, nor since 1987 have any coloured interior paints.

Mercury

As with lead, high levels of mercury contamination are known to cause problems, mainly with the nervous system. It is said that hatters suffered from mercury poisoning as a result of the mercury used in the old days in hat production (hence the expression 'mad as a hatter'). However it is now thought that even quite small quantities of mercury may cause problems. Symptoms may include a muscular sclerosis type of degeneration.

Sources: tuna fish, fish from water polluted by effluent, especially from papermaking factories, drinking water, weed killers, dental amalgam, seed wheat and thermometers.

Cadmium

Cadmium displaces zinc from the enzyme system. The effect on the body is mainly centred around the kidney and it may cause high blood pressure.

Sources: cigarette smoke, plumbing alloys, soil, people living in cadmium hotspots near industrial works, also it is widespread in many foods and in rubber tyres, old plaster and carpet backing. It is particularly dangerous to pregnant women and children.

Aluminium

This mainly affects the central nervous system, bone metabolism, liver and kidneys. It may be involved in child hyperactivity and joint problems, and has been incriminated in Alzheimers disease (PRE-SENILE DEMENTIA p. 134).

Sources: aluminium pans – especially when used to cook vegetables or fruit (e.g. rhubarb, apples), pressure cookers, teapots, cake tins, pie tins, roasting pans, baking foil, foil saucers, coffemate, water, antacids, domestic water and water boilers, yogurt pot lids, fruit juice containers, TV dinners in foil, etc. It is released from the soil by acid rain. It is aggravated by a deficiency of magnesium and calcium.

Arsenic

This is found in shellfish, insecticides and animal feed additives, and poison, wall paper and ceramics. Very large doses can be fatal. It is also found in the ground near tin mines, e.g. in Cornwall, and a degree of tolerance can be built up by eating vegetables grown there.

Therapeutic Diets

One of the criticisms thrown at orthodox doctors is that they treat people like they treat cars. In one sense this is true. Like a car, a body will only run properly if it is given the right fuel at the right time. It is clear however that great variations exist and what is a good way of eating for one person may be disastrous for another. I believe that everybody should look at the food they eat and the way they eat it at least once in their lives, preferably when they are in good health. This should be done in the spirit of taking general responsibility for one's own health. Part of which is to find out the most efficient fuel supply for your body and should be part of a total programme including exercise, attention to life style and avoidance of stress etc. If you feel you could do with a cleanout, try a limited fast (see below); this could be followed by a liver diet (p. 352) over one month but remember to substitute permitted for forbidden foods and eat enough quantity and variety of foods. Chew carefully and try to be in a quiet frame of mind at mealtimes.

Allergies
It is not the intention of any of these diets to unmask allergies but several of them may exclude certain foods or complete food groups altogether. If you find when you start the diet that you get a severe reaction, or that when stopping the diet and going back to your usual eating habits, the symptoms which have disappeared whilst you were on the diet come back suddenly, it is possible that you do have an allergic reaction to something you are eating. This may need to be evaluated further by elimination diets. I suggest you read the section on allergies (pp. 271–73) and, if necessary, consult a book which deals more extensively with exclusion diets such as Stephen Davies and Allan Stewart's *Nutritional Medicine* or see a nutritionally qualified physician.

Fasting
Sheldon, a respected naturopath, defined the difference between starvation and fasting like this – as long as hunger is lacking it is fasting, but when hunger returns you are starving. Fasting results in the resting of the digestive tract, mobilisation of the detoxification mechanism and an increase in the activity of the healing powers. It is an excellent introduction to observing the effects that certain foods have on you, and of course the effects of not eating at all. One of these is the release of toxins, previously stored in deposits of fat, into the system. This can mean that the liver, which is responsible for sifting out toxins, becomes overworked. To avoid this, it is advised that you take fruit juices, not just water, when you're fasting, as these can help to stimulate the body's own de-toxification powers, while slowing down the rate of toxin release. You should not go into a fast straight from your usual diet, but have a day or two on raw vegetables and fruit, and similarly when you break the fast, have a couple of days on fruit and vegetables before going on to carbohydrates and then proteins. It is better to start gradually with fasting, so maybe do it for one day the first time, two days the next and so on. Fasting on a regular basis of, say one day a week, is probably better than a long fast once a year. Apart from prevention of certain illnesses, fasting can be helpful in cases of acute febrile illnesses, skin rashes, gastro enteritis, rheumatism, asthma, sinusitis, cholecystitis and colitis. When used as a preventative it is not uncommon to go through a healing crisis somewhere between the third and fourth day, where there is a drop

in blood sugar, loss of appetite, coating of the tongue and acetone on the breath. After this healing crisis there is a gradual return to appetite. The tongue becomes clean and you feel generally better, almost as if you were walking on air.

There are however certain points to remember before starting a fast:

1.   Only do so when you can be sure of being relaxed, and not under pressure – physical or mental.
2.   Accept that you will not be able to smoke during the fasting period as it would make you very light-headed (as well as being a pollutant to the body).
3.   Obtain your doctor's clearance if you are known to have a severe allergy, or are taking a course of prescribed drugs.
4.   If you are seriously ill or very run down you'd do better to wait until you're stronger before fasting.
5.   *Do not fast* if you are hypoglycaemic or dependent on alcohol or drugs.

Notes for people undertaking the diets
On reading through the ailments and diseases section you may be referred to one of the diets from the following pages. These diets should not be undertaken as a punishment but as a challenge to you to find new foods to eat and new ways of cooking. If, however, you are suffering from a severe illness or are on orthodox drugs, it is better to ask your physician if it is all right to start the diet. However, it is very unlikely that any of these diets will lead to problems, provided that a wide enough variety of foods is eaten and that you eat them in sensible quantities. Remember that to get sufficient protein you need to mix grains and pulses in a ratio of 2 : 1, and of that mixture you only need ¾ of the weight of meat that you'd normally eat.

Tips for cooking pulses
Never add salt to pulses while they're boiling as this toughens the skins.

Always boil red kidney beans *vigorously* for 10 minutes at the start of cooking to destroy the natural toxins they contain, and remember to throw away the cooking liquids afterwards.

Pulses and legumes will cook more quickly if you first soak them overnight in plenty of cold water.

The Arthritis Diet
This is an alkaline diet used for the treatment of osteoarthritis and rheumatoid arthritis and other conditions where over-acidity is thought to play a part. Naturopaths believe that arthritis is caused by the accumulation of toxic acids in the joints. These acids are thought to come naturally from the intestine, and from a failure of the body's metabolism to detoxify them when in excess in the diet. Time limit – maximum – of the diet is one month and it then should be relaxed either by introducing forbidden foods one at a time or

by having any of the foods previously not permitted on two occasions during the week.

Opinions on the efficacy of this diet in the treatment of arthritis and other 'acid' conditions vary from ridicule from the orthodox medical profession to claims of miraculous cures from naturopaths. The dietary recommendations given here represent a cross section of these opinions. They should be adhered to until the condition has stabilised. Remember to relax the restrictions after one month; then they can be relaxed further – although certain items should be avoided for life, such as white bread, junk food etc., except on very rare occasions. The dietary advice that follows on these pages should be followed strictly unless otherwise directed by your practitioner. These recommendations are an adjunct to individual homeopathic prescriptions and are designed to give your body the best possible chance to heal itself.

Foods to avoid	*Foods allowed*
A. Red meat (beef, lamb, pork)	A. White fish. Pulses (peas, beans, lentils etc). Chicken – two meals a week only. Egg – two meals of two eggs a week only.
B. Cow's milk, cheese and yogurt	B. Goat's milk, cheese and yogurt. Soya milk.
C. Brown and white wheat flour, bran. (Do not use any produce where wheat starch, edible starch, cereal binder, cereal filler or cereal protein are listed as ingredients.)	C. Oats, brown rice, corn (maize), buckwheat pasta, millet, 100% rye crispbread e.g. *Ryvita*, sugar-free oatcakes, sugar-free muesli e.g. *Waitrose's*.
D. Citrus fruit, fruit covered in wax, such as imported apples.	D. All other fruit. Dried fruit. Tomatoes twice a week only.
E.	E. All vegetables
F. Dry roasted nuts	F. All other nuts especially hazel, almond, cashew and walnut.
G. Sugar and foods containing sugar. Syrup, treacle and honey.	G. Sugar cane molasses, dried fruit, sugar-free jams such as *Nature's Store, Robertsons* and *Whole Earth* products.
H. Coffee, decaffeinated coffee, cocoa, tea, alcohol.	H. Grain coffees (*Caro Extra* for example) herbal teas, *Maté* and *Rooibosch* teas, suitable unsweetened fruit juices, unsalted instant soup, vegetable juices.
I. Salt, pepper, vinegar.	I. *Ruthmol* salt, *Martlett* salt-free salad cream, *Vecon* vegetarian stock cubes.
J. Butter and margarine – use as little as possible	J. Vegetable margarine *(Vitaseig, Vitaquell, Tomor)* vegetable oil.
K. Chocolate	K. Carob

Hay diet

This is a variation of the Arthritis Diet which was developed by Dr Hay, an American physician who cured himself of kidney disease in the early part of the 20th century. It is a food combination diet based on digestive requirements because different dietary constituents need different conditions to be digested.

Along with dietary changes, Dr Hay also advised fresh air, exercise and general life style changes. The basic rules of his diet are, starches and sugar should not be eaten with proteins and acid fruits at the same meal; vegetables, salads and fruits should play a major part in the diet; proteins, starches and fats should be eaten in small quantities and only wholegrain unprocessed starches should be used; and finally at least four to four and a half hours should elapse between meals of different food groups.

It is particularly useful in patients with chronic digestive disorder such as flatulence, constipation, indigestion and obesity, and I would advise you to read *Food Combining for Health* by Doris Grant.

Yeast and Mould Free Diet

This could be called the anti candida diet; it should be combined with low carbohydrate diet and followed for a month but be careful to substitute permitted for forbidden foods, eat proper quantities of food and do not do the diet if you are on drugs without first consulting your GP or nutritionally trained physician. If after a month the symptoms have disappeared but return when you go onto an ordinary diet, you should seek the help of your homeopath or nutritionally trained physician.

For further information read *Candida Albicans* by Leon Chaitow.

Yeasts and fungi are used in many food preparation processes, and can be introduced into foods inadvertently. Brewers' and bakers' yeasts are two strains of the organism: mostly people who react to one will react to the other. Yeast and wheatgerm are the two major sources of B-group vitamins. Persons who react to yeast may also react to mushrooms and truffles. No list can be comprehensive but yeast is certainly found in the following:

Bakery products: All bread, buns, biscuits, cakes etc. except possibly unleavened bread.
Alcoholic beverages: All alcoholic drinks depend on yeasts to produce the alcohol – they are all risky. So is root beer.

Other beverages: Citrus fruit drinks and juices – only home-squeezed are yeast-free. Malted milk, malted drinks.

Cereals: Malted cereals, malted dairy foods for babies, cereals enriched with vitamins.

Condiments: Pickles, salad dressings, mayonnaise, horseradish sauce, tomato sauce, barbecue sauce, French dressing etc. Mustard, ketchup, sauerkraut, olives, chilli peppers, tamari and soy sauce, vinegar.

Dairy products: All cheese including cottage cheese and cheese spreads, buttermilk, milk enriched with vitamins.

Fungi: Mushrooms, mushroom sauce, truffles, etc contain organisms closely related to yeast.

Meat products: Hamburgers, sausages and cooked meats made with bread or breadcrumbs, Marmite, Oxo, Bovril, Vegemite, gravy browning and all similar extracts.

Vitamins: All B-vitamin preparations are likely to be derived from yeast unless otherwise stated, but most manufacturers do make some B-vitamin preparations free of yeast. Some selenium-rich foods.

Mould foods: These foods either belong to the mould family, encourage moulds, or are prepared with them: buttermilk, sour cream, cheese snacks, peanuts, sour milk products, cheese dressings, cream cheese, pistachios, antibiotics. Many dairy products, eggs and meat contain antibiotics in small quantities. Eat sparingly.

Sugar foods: Sugar, sucrose, fructose, maltose, lactose, glycogen, glucose, milk, sweets, chocolate, sweet biscuits, cakes, candies, cookies, puddings, desserts, canned food, packaged food, hamburgers, honey, mannitol, sorbitol, galactose, monosaccharides, polysaccharides, date sugar, turbinado sugar, molasses, maple syrup, most bottle juices, all soft drinks, tonic water, milkshakes, raisins, dried apricots, dates, prunes, dried figs, other dried fruit.

N.B. Shop or restaurant 'beef' or 'hamburgers' may contain added sugar.

Liver diet

This diet has been used to good effect by a naturopath and by a homeopathic doctor in the treatment of a variety of conditions where malfunctions of the liver is suspected. Its purpose is to avoid those foods which the liver finds difficult to process. Time limit: one month. Then have 'forbidden' foods twice weekly.

Foods to avoid	Foods to be eaten in unlimited quantities
A Meat, fowl	A Fish (white preferred, limited tinned fish with oil washed off), Pulses – beans, peas and lentils.
B Eggs	B Tofu – a soya milk product also known as bean curd available from Chinese food shops.
C Refined bread and cereals	C Wholemeal bread, unsweetened whole grain cereals and wholegrains – brown rice, wholewheat pasta.
D Sugar, foods containing sugar, syrup, treacle, honey.	D Molasses, unsweetened jams (refrigerate after opening), Marmite.
E Cow's and goat's milk and products e.g. cheese	E Soya milks
F Tomatoes, citrus fruit, bananas, avocados	F Vegetables, pineapples, grapes, melons. Suitable fruits tinned in natural juice.
G Nuts (except almonds)	G Almonds, sunflower and sesame seeds
H Coffee, cocoa, alcohol, 2 cups of tea only a day	H Grain coffees, herb teas, suitable unsweetened fruit juice, *Rooibosch* and *maté* teas
I Chocolate	I Carob powder
J Fried food	J Food can be sautéed using cold-pressed margarine or oil or vegetable butter.

Restricted foods: Berries (strawberries, raspberries, gooseberries etc) and apricots, peaches, sultanas, raisins and dates can be eaten twice a week in unlimited quantities. Less than one eighth teaspoon salt can be taken daily.

Suggested menu plan

Uncooked breakfast – muesli or breakfast cereal and soya milk or some suitable fruit juice. Wholemeal toast and suitable margarine or spread.

Cooked breakfast – Mushroom on toast or white fish. Porridge and soya milk.

Main meal – white fish/pulse dish/textured vegetable protein. TVP is available from health food shops – two meals weekly only. Wholemeal pasta/brown rice/ potatoes. Fresh vegetables, some uncooked if possible i.e. as a side salad with the meal.

Desserts – suitable fruits, with or without wholemeal pastry or crumble. Desserts based on soya milk. Brown rice puddings with soya milk.

Smaller meals – wholemeal sandwiches with a suitable filling i.e. Marmite, pear/apple spread, tahini spread, lentil or bean spread. Salad. Suitable fresh or stewed fruit. Home-made soup and wholemeal bread.

Blood Sugar Levelling Diet

This is used in the treatment of diabetes and hypoglycaemia (pp. 257–58), with a time limit of one month. After this if the diet has been successful in helping the symptoms you should keep off tea, coffee, sugar and alcohol except for the odd occasion and be careful to keep up your two hourly snacks. You can now have bread and potatoes as often as you like but not as snacks. In other words only have sandwiches or crisps as part of a light meal; and always have them with slow burning foods i.e. lentil soup.

On this diet you may feel slightly worse before you feel better, but that should not last for more than a few days. You may have a headache caused by caffeine withdrawal. If you are on drugs or insulin see your own doctor or a nutritionally qualified physician. Make sure that you substitute permitted for forbidden foods and that you have a wide variety of food and eat the proper amount, chew well and eat in a quiet frame of mind.

Recent research regarding the glycaemic index of food, which gives an indication of the rate at which food is converted into glucose, suggests that the higher the index, the greater the rate of conversion and the less desirable these foods may be for those with a blood sugar problem. These are the foods which are avoided in this diet. There appear to be many differences between very similar foods and their ability to affect the index, and all the previous rules about simple and complex carbohydrates have now been proven to be unreliable. One point, however, which is probably valid is that like anthracite coal, small packages seem to burn slowly whilst large ones seem to burn quickly. When food is in its natural state, wheat for example, it will have a low glycaemic index, but as soon as the package is broken i.e. by grinding it into flour, the glycaemic index rises. For this reason, legumes such as lentils, kidney and soya beans are extremely good for patients who have blood sugar problems. Possible symptoms of reactive hypoglycaemia include confusion, forgetfulness, difficulty in concentration, depression, loss of sense of meaning or purpose in life, anxiety, phobias, suicide, anti-social and asocial behaviour, headaches, dizziness, numbness, staggering, fainting or blackout, twitching of muscles, convulsions, fatigue, bloating, abdominal spasm, muscle and joint pain, backache, colitis and cold sweats. These symptoms often manifest themselves before breakfast, two hours after exercise or emotional stress. They are always of sudden onset.

It is important on this diet to eat little and often. You should eat three meals a day but these should not be large meals. Between each meal you should take a snack – *so that you are eating something every two hours.* Snacks should consist of raw nuts or seeds (such as pumpkin or sunflower), a glass of milk, yogurt, bombay mix or unsweetened oatcakes i.e. Patersons. It is probably easiest to work out a menu for two weeks in advance to ensure that the restrictions on certain foods (see below) are adhered to. If weight is a problem, you may include protein powder or capsules once or twice daily instead of a snack.

Food to avoid completely	*Substitute which can be eaten in unlimited quantities*
A All refined and processed food	A Unsweetened oatcakes, 100% rye crispbread, wholemeal pasta, pulses – all types of beans, peas, lentils etc., brown rice.
B All forms of sugar, honey, all sweets and confectionary, all products containing sugar, glucose, glucose syrup, honey, dextrose, fructose etc.	B Sugar-cane molasses may be used for sweetening in cooking. As a honey substitute, use unsweetened jams such as those made by Robertsons, Nature's Store and Whole Earth.
C Cereals containing sugar	C Unsweetened muesli, porridge, nut butters, e.g. cashew nut butter.
D Cakes and biscuits, pies, puddings, bananas, custard	D Fruit including citrus fruit, fresh or stewed without sugar, yogurt, cottage cheese, raw nuts, seeds, pancakes.
E Tea, coffee, alcohol, soft drinks, hot chocolate, Ovaltine	E Cow's milk, grain coffee e.g. Caro Extra, herb teas, maté and Rooibosch teas, unsweetened fruit juice, vegetable juice.
F Potatoes	F All other vegetables wholemeal pasta, pulses etc.
G Cough syrups, laxatives, medications with caffeine, relish, ketchup, mustard, sauces	G Olive oil, sunflower oil

And no smoking!

Food which may be eaten in limited quantities: Each week you may eat two meals using white fish, two meals using meat, and two meals using eggs (two eggs to each meal), white pasta may be eaten twice a week. 1–2 slices of rye bread may be eaten every day or 1 slice of wholemeal bread. Wholemeal flour may be used for cooking pastry and flans which may be eaten twice a week. Only one eighth teaspoon salt is allowed daily. Butter or margarine in small amounts is permitted on bread etc. Cook with oil. Raisins and other dried fruits are allowed in small quantities twice a week only. Full fat cheese may be eaten twice a week.

Suggested meal pattern
Uncooked breakfast: Grapefruit segments fresh or canned in natural juice. Muesli, rye crispbread, fresh fruit.
Cooked breakfast: Poached or boiled eggs, pancakes,

porridge, unsweetened baked beans, mushrooms or tomatoes on toast.

Lunch or supper: Meat, white fish, cheese or eggs. Vegetable purées can be used to replace gravy or other sauces. Wholemeal pasta, pulse dishes. Vegetables, salads.

Uncooked lunch or evening meal: Salads, bread or toast, rye crispbread, with suitable spread – lentil paste, cottage cheese, unsweetened jam, vegetable pâté etc.

Desserts: Fresh or stewed fruit, baked apples, nuts, yogurt, fruit fools made with stewed fruit and yogurt. Pancakes made with wholemeal flour.

Colon Diet

There are basically two circumstances under which dietary regimes which act specifically on the colon may be employed. The first, and most common, is having a disease actually affecting the colon, such as irritable bowel syndrome or a form of colitis. If you are suffering from a severe form of colitis, such as Chrohn's disease, or if you are on any drugs, then you should not use any of the following diets without asking your GP or nutrionally qualified physician. The most common diet for the colon is a high fibre diet which aims to give more than 30 grams of fibre a day. This is done by a) eating less refined carbohydrate, b) eating plenty of fresh fruit and vegetables, c) eating wholegrain cereals and d) eating larger than usual quantities of pulses and legumes such as peas, lentils, beans etc. Once again, the twice a week rule, page 24 applies.

Then there is the food exclusion diet for the colon. Researchers in Cambridge have found that the five most common food groups to cause irritable bowel syndrome, as measured by levels of prostaglandins in the rectum, are reflected in the colon diet which avoids wheat, corn, dairy products, tea, coffee, citrus fruits. These can either be stopped all at once, or one at a time, then reintroduced to see whether previous symptoms disappear when these foods are excluded, and return when they are included again. If you find that any one food seems to make the irritable bowel worse, then you can cut it down, say to twice a week, but remember to find a substitute. If you find that it is causing problems even when you are having it only twice a week, then you should consult your homeopath or nutritionally qualified physician about it.

Natural Laxatives*

Linseed tea: dissolve 1 dessertspoon of linseeds in 1 pint water. Simmer for 10 minutes, strain and drink 1 cup 10 minutes before food.

Linseed meal: dissolve 1 dessertspoon of linseeds in water and take up to 3 times a day. For best results, allow to soak overnight.

Blackstrap molasses: take 1 dessertspoon 3 times a day.

Colon Cleansing

The other way in which nutrition can be used to help the colon is if it is felt that toxins are being absorbed from the colon and going up in the portal system to the liver where they are causing sluggishness of the liver, leading to such symptoms as headaches, irritability, hangover feelings, general lack of energy and mild depression. There may be also other specific symptoms such as joint pains. The colon plan is best carried out along with the liver diet which should not be attempted by anyone with bowel trouble or who is on drugs without the consent of their GP or nutritionally qualified physician. The ingredients of the colon cleanse are:

1. *Alfalfa tablets:* start with one tablet three times a day after meals, followed by water, and build up to four tablets three times a day.

2. *Acidophilus capsules:* which are a concentrate of a healthy bacteria normally found in the colon: take one capsule a day, building up to one capsule three times a day ten minutes before food. These capsules should be kept in the refrigerator once the package is opened. Each capsule should be around 500 mg, and if you cannot obtain acidophilus capsules, have one carton of live plain yogurt daily.

3. *Psyllium husks:* start with half a teaspoon a day building up to 3 teaspoonfuls a day taken in a small amount of water. Drink two cups of water immediately afterwards. The husks do not dissolve well and you may find it easier to take them in soda water or other aerated drinks as the bubbles appear to help them stay dispersed, thus making them easier to swallow. If you cannot obtain psyllium husks, use linseeds in the same manner, but starting with half a dessertspoon and building up to 3 dessertspoons.

All these products are natural and should not cause problems such as pain, constipation or diarrhoea. Should you feel, however, that they are upsetting you, stop everything and then reintroduce them one by one to find out what is causing the trouble. Discuss the problem with your homeopath or nutritionally qualified physician. The bowel programme can be continued for up to three months providing it is not causing any problems. If you experience a lot of flatulence it may be that the alfalfa is clearing out the toxins faster than the psyllium husks or linseeds can remove them; stop the alfalfa for a few days to see if this helps.

* Reprinted by permission of Dr B. Jensen, D.C.

APPENDIX

60 REMEDY PICTURES

ALL homeopathic remedies have a double personality. On the one hand they are known to *cause* a range of symptoms in perfectly healthy people. On the other hand, by the law of similars, they are known to *alleviate* the same symptoms in people who are unwell. However, remedies which match physical symptoms only may not be enough to provoke a return to health. Ideally, to provoke the greatest healing, a remedy should match the physical symptoms, the mental symptoms, and the constitution of the person concerned.

So if you have selected, from the lists of remedies in PART 5 – Ailments and Diseases or in the General Remedy Finder, a remedy which seems to fit the physical symptoms of the person you wish to treat, look it up in this section of the book and see if it also fits the mental symptoms and general constitution of that person. If it does, it is likely to be very effective. If two or more remedies appear suitable on physical or mental grounds, check which is most suitable on constitutional grounds; again, the remedy which most closely matches the constitutional picture will be the most effective. This is why none of the remedies mentioned in this book is, of itself, homeopathic. For example, *Antimonium tart. 6c* is a homeopathic remedy, homeopathically prepared by successive dilution and succussion, but it will have little effect unless the person it is prescribed for is young, elderly, or very weak.

The following pages describe 60 of the most commonly used homeopathic remedies. Each has a distinct personality, as you will see. Many of them have 'complementary' remedies, remedies whose actions are similar or compatible, and likely to complete a cure once the primary remedy has done its work. Others have 'antidoting' remedies or substances which effectively cancel out their effects. If you need to antidote the effects of a remedy, choose the antidote which best matches your unwelcome symptoms. Still others have 'incompatible' or 'inimical' remedies which, when taken in conjunction with them or in close succession, have the effect of thoroughly confusing the Vital Force. Obviously, antidoting and incompatible remedy combinations should be avoided. One or two of the remedies described are also 'specifics', routinely prescribed for certain ailments whatever the constitution of the patient.

The remedy pictures in this book have been compiled from the writings of Hahnemann himself, and from those of James Tyler Kent, Margaret Tyler, and J. H. Clark. Also woven into them are the author's own observations and notes made during absorbing lectures by Margery Blackie, George Vithoulkas, and Francisco Eizyaga.

Aconite

From *Aconitum napellus*, blue monkshood, blue aconite, wolfsbane. The homeopathic remedy is prepared from the whole fresh plant as it comes into flower and is traditionally used to relieve states of acute or chronic tension just before they manifest as inflammation before they result in unusual discharge.

Constitutional indications Adults who respond well to Aconite are usually full-blooded, strong and healthy-looking. Aconite babies tend to be rosy and chubby.

Mental symptoms alleviated Many aspects of behaviour dictated by fear; fear of dying, even predicting hour of own death; agoraphobia; feeling of haste and hurry; specific or free-floating anxiety, which shows itself in the face; restlessness, tossing and turning in sleep.

Physical symptoms alleviated Eye pain or inflammation caused by injury; congested blood vessels in eye; fever which comes on suddenly, with skin hot, dry and angry-looking; tingling sensation in hands and feet; hollow-sounding, crowing cough; great thirst.

The above symptoms are often brought on by shock, fright, exposure to dry, cold winds, and occasionally by intensely hot weather. They are generally made worse by warm rooms, cigarette smoke, music and lying on the affected side; they also tend to be worse in the evening and at night. Fresh air is usually beneficial.

Remedies which follow well Arnica, Belladonna, Ipecac., Bryonia, Silicea, Sulphur.

Complementary remedy Sulphur.

Antidoting remedies/substances Nux, Coffea; acid fruits, wine, coffee, lemonade.

Allium

From *Allium cepa*, the red onion. The homeopathic remedy is made from the whole fresh plant in July/August. Onion contains an acrid, volatile principle which stimulates the tear glands and the mucous membranes of the upper respiratory tract. At one time is was used to cure worms, earache, and bites from mad dogs.

Constitutional indications None in particular.

Mental symptoms alleviated Fear of pain.

Physical symptoms alleviated Headache centred behind forehead; earache in children; streaming eyes, with bland discharge; streaming nose, with discharge which makes nostrils and upper lip sore; stuffed up nose, with discharge from alternate nostrils; toothache in molar area, shifting from left side to right or from one tooth to another; hoarseness, early stages of laryngitis; coughing which causes splitting, tearing sensation in throat – person clutches throat in alarm; coughing brought on by cold air; neuralgic pains; in babies, abdominal colic.

The above symptoms are aggravated by warm rooms, cold or damp, and the smell of flowers; they also tend to start on the left side and move to the right. Cool rooms and fresh air usually improve things.

Complementary remedies Phosphorus, Thuja, Pulsatilla.

Antidoting remedies Arnica, Chamomilla, Veratrum.

Alumina

The homeopathic remedy is prepared from aluminium oxide. Aluminium, absorbed in significant amounts from cooking utensils, causes mental processes to slow down. Its homeopathic derivative is used to treat sluggishness generally.

Constitutional indications Alumina is most effective with people who are confused or senile; those who respond best are usually thin, with dried-up, greyish skin and dry, sore mucous membranes.

Mental symptoms alleviated Confusion, sense of unreality, of time slowing down; feeling pressured and hurried inside despite outward slowness; apprehension, feeling that something awful is about to happen; feeling as if one is talking, hearing, smelling, and seeing through someone else's mouth, ears, nose, and eyes; deep despair, feeling that everything is dark; suicidal or homicidal thoughts at sight of knives or blood.

Physical symptoms alleviated Dizziness on closing eyes; sensation of cobwebs over face; dry skin which feels as if ants are crawling beneath it; sluggish reactions to nervous stimuli; numbness in legs; feeling of heaviness, possibly followed by paralysis; difficulty swallowing solids, with constricted feeling in throat; craving for fruit and vegetables, and for indigestible items such as pencils, chalk, tea leaves, coffee grounds; aversion to meat and beer; difficulty passing urine – stomach muscles have to work hard to empty bladder; in women, profuse, irritant vaginal discharge; lazy bowels – great straining to pass stools, even when stools are soft and rectum is full, with stomach muscles rather than rectal muscles doing the straining; feeling that there is still something to come even when bowels have been opened.

The above symptoms are not improved by cold air, or by items such as wine, vinegar, pepper, salt or potatoes and other starchy foods; discomfort is usually worst in the morning.

Complementary remedy Bryonia.

Antidoting remedies Ipecac., Chamomilla.

Anacardium

From *Anacardium orientale*, the marking nut tree. The homeopathic remedy is made from cardol, a blackish juice extracted from the pith between the shell and the kernel of the nuts. The juice is used, in India and elsewhere, to mark linen and to etch away moles on the skin.

Constitutional indications Anacardium is highly beneficial to people who have an inferiority complex and are trying hard to prove themselves; they suffer from extreme inner conflict and have, as the saying goes, 'a devil on one shoulder and an angel on the other'. Children who suddenly give up studying for exams, saying they can't remember what they are reading, are candidates for Anacardium.

Mental symptoms alleviated Lack of self-confidence, perhaps masked by callous, cruel or sadistic behaviour; confusion between reality and fantasy; extreme suspicion and mistrust of others; a persecution complex; tendency to swear a lot.

Physical symptoms alleviated Tight 'bandaged' feeling around leg or arm; duodenal ulcers which cause intense discomfort two hours after eating but improve immediately after eating.

The above symptoms are made worse by hot baths, showers, or compresses.

Remedy which follows well Platinum.

Antidoting remedies Coffea, Rhus tox.

Antimonium

The source of this remedy is antimony sulphide. Antimony poisoning causes headaches, coughing and wheezing, loss of libido, painful urination, abdominal pain, skin eruptions and general debility.

Constitutional indications Antimony is most useful in children and in elderly people. Greediness, sentimentality, a great susceptibility to the charms of moonlight, and a propensity for falling madly in love are often encountered among Antimony types. Physically, such people are often fat, despite a chronic loss of appetite, and may suffer from deformed feet or sores around the mouth.

Mental symptoms alleviated In children, an aversion to being looked at or touched; in adults, bursts of lunatic behaviour, wanting to shoot oneself, finding life unbearable.

Physical symptoms alleviated Itchy scalp, falling hair; red, inflamed eyelids; sore nostrils; coughing, made worse by staring into fire; painful corns or calluses on feet; chronic loss of appetite; belching which smells of food just eaten; in old people, alternate bouts of constipation and diarrhoea.

The above symptoms are exacerbated by heat (from the sun or from the fire) and by eating, and specifically by wine, acid beverages, bread, pastry and pork; they also tend to get worse in the evening, at night and in moonlight. Rest is usually beneficial.

Complementary remedy Sulphur.

Antidoting remedy Hepar sulph.

Antimonium tart.

This remedy is made from potassium tartrate of antimony, also known as tartar emetic, which is both an irritant, causing excessive production of phlegm, and a depressant.

Constitutional indications Antimonium tart. is most beneficial to the very old and very young, and to people who are too weak to cough up phlegm.

Mental symptoms alleviated Drowsiness; irritability, especially when disturbed.

Physical symptoms alleviated Headache which feels like a tight band around the head (made worse by coughing); face pale or cyanosed (bluish), and cold to the touch; tongue thickly coated, but red in centre and around edges; wheezing, with a rattling sound in the chest; inability to cough up phlegm; nausea, relieved by vomiting; lack of thirst, or if thirsty a craving for things which are sour or acidic; legs puffy with retained fluid.

All of these symptoms are aggravated by warm rooms, damp cold, movement or lying down, and tend to become worse between 3 and 4 a.m. Milk and sour foods are also aggravating. Cold air and sitting up usually offer relief.

Antidoting remedies Pulsatilla, Sepia.

Apis

From *Apis mellifica*, the honey bee The remedy is prepared from whole bees dissolved in alcohol. Bee stings, as many people know to their cost, cause rapid, watery swellings which smart and burn; anaphylactic reactions can involve the heart and brain.

Constitutional indications None in particular.

Mental symptoms alleviated Depression; irritability; sudden jealousy, suspicion, over-sensitivity.

Physical symptoms alleviated Watery swellings on mouth or eyelids; swelling which spreads to throat and hinders breathing; oedema; fever accompanied by dry skin and a violent headache, with shivering in late afternoon; fever with lack of thirst; any head pain which causes sudden, piercing screams; scanty urination (increased urination indicates that Apis is working well).

The above symptoms tend to start on the right side, then shift to the left; they are aggravated by sleep, touch, pressure, heat and stuffy rooms, and generally get worse in the late afternoon. Fresh air, cold bathing and undressing bring relief.

Complementary remedies Natrum mur. and, if lymph system is involved and glands are swollen, Baryta carb.

Warning: Because of its action on the kidneys, Apis is not recommended in a lower potency than 30c during pregnancy.

Argentum Nit.

The source of this remedy is silver nitrate, once known as Hell Stone or Devil's Stone because of its corrosive and sometimes lethal effect. Chronic silver nitrate poisoning causes the skin to turn permanently blue and damages the kidneys, liver, spleen and aorta. Acute poisoning – not uncommon in the days when silver nitrate was used to cauterize wounds after surgery – causes severe respiratory difficulties.

Constitutional indications Argentum nit. is especially good for people who do jobs which call for quick thinking and a good memory, where the emphasis is on performance. Into this category come actors, singers, business executives, lecturers, students, etc. Most Argentum nit. types are extroverts, but much of their behaviour is motivated by a fear of failure.

Mental symptoms Confusion and loss of mental control under stress, head full of irrational thoughts; feeling that one is only just able to resist dangerous impulses, such as throwing onself in front of a train or leaping from a high window; mental exhaustion; sense of hurry and pressure, of going faster and faster; insecurity, forcing oneself to do things because one is afraid of failing; forming irrational notions about things; fear of crowds, fear of heights, fear of being late for trains, appointments, etc., fear of being crushed by tall buildings; always expecting something unpleasant to happen around the next corner; anxiety when faced with the unusual or unexpected, sometimes accompanied by diarrhoea.

Physical symptoms alleviated Headaches which come on gradually but disappear suddenly, brought on excitement, overwork, travel, sugary foods, etc., and associated with sore, tense neck muscles – pain, usually centred in left temple, wears off in fresh air or if pressure is applied, but becomes more intense if one talks, stoops or moves about; dizziness when looking up at or down from tall buildings; epilepsy; conjunctivitis; stringy mucus in mouth; asthma, relieved by moist air and warmth; warts; sweating brought on by anxiety; palpitations brought on by anxiety, and made worse by lying on left side; craving for salt, sugar and cold food; flatulence, not relieved by belching; vomiting and diarrhoea (greenish stools) brought on by anxiety, worse in hot weather; in babies, diarrhoea during weaning; in women, bearing down sensation in womb, or prolapse of womb.

The above symptoms are not helped by warmth, sugary foods, eating, or emotional problems; they also tend to be worse at night, when there is a moon, and during menstruation. Fresh air and cold usually bring relief.

Antidoting remedy Natrum mur.

Arnica
From *Arnica montana*, leopard's bane or Fallkraut. The homeopathic remedy is made from the whole fresh plant or just the root, or from the dried flowers, and is traditionally used to minimize the immediate effects of shock, falls, bruising, bleeding, and injuries caused by blunt objects. It also helps traumatized tissues to heal.

Constitutional indications Those who derive most benefit from Arnica tend to be rather morose and morbidly imaginative. No matter how ill they feel they are likely to deny that anything is wrong with them and refuse to see a doctor.

Mental symptoms alleviated Wanting to be left alone; hypochondriac tendencies; hopelessness; indifference; restlessness; tossing and turning in bed at night and blaming it on hardness of bed; nightmares about robbers, muddy waters, horrible incidents in the past, etc., from which one wakes mortally afraid and clutching heart; impatience; absentmindedness; inability to concentrate, because one is easily distracted and startled; fear of sudden death.

Physical symptoms alleviated Head feels hot, body cold; concussion; black eyes; eyestrain; cold nose; bad breath; sore gums after dentistry; fever which causes stupor, prostration, even unconsciousness; eczema; boils; broken capillaries internally and on surface of skin, especially after childbirth or injury; sore muscles due to unaccustomed exercise; sprained joints; tennis elbow; in children, whooping cough in which coughing is preceded by crying; aversion to milk and meat; craving for pickles and vinegary foods; foul-smelling stools; faecal incontinence during nightmares.

The above symptoms improve as one starts to move around, then get worse as movement continues. Lying down, with the head lower than the feet, can bring relief. Heat, rest and light pressure generally aggravate matters.

Complementary remedies Aconite, Ipecac.

Antidoting remedy Camphora.

Arsenicum
The source of this remedy is arsenic trioxide, also known as *Arsenicum album*. At one time arsenic was used to treat syphilis, anthrax, yaws and other diseases, and also widely used in manufacturing processes. It causes weakness, loss of appetite, vomiting, heaviness and discomfort in the stomach, diarrhoea, neuritis, a runny nose, skin eruptions, pigmentation of the skin, and eczema.

Constitutional indications Those who benefit most from Arsenicum are deeply insecure and have an almost insatiable need for comfort and consolation. Arsenicum children are highly strung and delicate, with fine skin and hair; although mentally and physically agile, and often precocious, they get pushed around at school. Arsenicum adults have an anxious, frightened appearance and look as if they are wasting away. Because of their fundamental insecurity, any complaints they have tend to recur.

Mental symptoms alleviated Fear of being alone or going out alone, fear of being burgled, fear of the dark, fear of failure, fear of having an incurable illness – all of which sap the intellect and will; feeling that one is about to die unless the doctor is called; restlessness due to anxiety; thoughts of suicide; great fastidiousness and orderliness in one's dress and habits; irritability; seeing evil omens everywhere and refusing to be reassured; religious mania; possessiveness; hoarding and miserliness; not wanting to meet friends and acquaintances for fear of having offended them; great sensitivity to touch, smell and cold; night terrors; waking at the slightest noise, especially between midnight and 2 a.m., and getting up and walking about; feeling sleepy but unable to get to sleep.

Physical symptoms alleviated Headaches at 3-weekly intervals, accompanied by dizziness and vomiting, aggravated by pressure and the smell of food or cigarette smoke, but relieved by movement and by cold applications if applied early enough – pain burns and throbs, starting at bridge of nose and extending over entire head, which feels extremely tender; stinging, watering eyes; sneezing, with catarrh which stings and burns, soothed by sniffing warm water up nose; red, swollen lower lip, soothed by hot applications; dry, cracked lips, or pale, bleeding lips; intensely sore mouth ulcers, with a red, glazed-looking tongue; asthma brought on by anxiety, with severe breathlessness between midnight and 2 a.m. which obliges one to sit up to breathe, often improved by warmth and sniffing warm water up nose; early stages of heart failure, with fluid retention, especially around ankles; tendency to bleed easily; veins which feel as if ice-cold or boiling water were flowing through them; rough, scaly, cracked skin; lack of perspiration, or profuse perspiration; vomiting, with vomit which stings; wanting frequent sips of water; wanting to eat only fatty or sour foods; diarrhoea, often accompanied by vomiting, brought on by cold winds or overindulgence in ripe fruit, vegetables, iced foods or alcohol – stools are watery, scant, frequent and foul-smelling, and cause soreness around the anus and burning pains in rectum; dehydration and collapse due to diarrhoea, especially in children.

The above symptoms are often helped by warmth, hot drinks, and an extra pillow when lying down. The sight or smell of food, cold food or cold drinks, and cold dry winds tend to exacerbate them; discomfort is usually worst on the right side and between midnight and 2 a.m.

Complementary remedies Rhus tox., Carbo veg., Phosphorus, Thuja, Scale.

Antidoting remedies Opium, Camphor, China, Hepar sulph., Nux.

Baryta carb.
The source of this remedy is barium carbonate which, in large amounts, causes nausea, vomiting, convulsions, and diarrhoea.

Constitutional indications Baryta carb. is most effective in the very young and the very old. Children who benefit from it are mentally and physically slow, very skinny for their age, and pot-bellied; they also tend to have wrinkled skin and a vacant expression on their face. Elderly people who respond well tend to be obese. Both groups may also suffer from hormone problems.

Mental symptoms alleviated Extreme shyness; fear of people and situations; lack of concentration; forgetfulness; immature behaviour.

Physical problems alleviated Headaches which improve in open air but get worse in hot sun or in front of fire; swollen tonsils, with swollen lymph glands in neck and abdomen; cough which gets worse in evening but wears off after midnight, relieved by lying on stomach; muscle aches after eating or sleeping; sebaceous cysts; fatty tumours or warts; sore feet due to excessive perspiration and use of foot antiperspirants/deodorants; atherosclerosis, with degeneration of walls of arteries; high blood pressure; aneurysms; palpitations, made worse by exertion; griping pains in stomach, relieved by lying on stomach.

The above symptoms are intensified by cold, damp, rinsing in cold water, hot meals, excitement, raising the arms, dwelling on aches and pains, and by the presence of strangers; they also tend to get worse when lying on the left side. Cold food and being left alone generally improve matters.

Complementary remedies Dulcamara, Psorinum, Silicea.

Incompatible/inimical remedy Calcarea carb.

Belladonna
From *Atropa belladonna*, deadly nightshade. The homeopathic remedy is made from the whole fresh plant, which is highly poisonous, containing the alkaloids atropine, hyoscamine, and scopolamine. The symptoms of deadly nightshade poisoning are giddiness, confusion, increasingly excited, incoherent or violent behaviour, a dry mouth and throat, flushed face, wide staring pupils, and difficulty speaking and swallowing. A high fever develops, sometimes accompanied by convulsions. Drowsiness and coma ensue, and eventually death.

Constitutional indications The kind of person who responds most markedly to Belladonna is sturdily built, apparently in rude health, and vigorous in mind and body.

Mental symptoms alleviated Restlessness; wild, incoherent, excited behaviour; maniacal laughter; racing imagination; hallucinations; jumpiness and fear when approached; feeling dazed and stupid; horrible dreams; feeling sleepy but not able to sleep.

Physical syymptoms alleviated Unusual sensitivity to light, noise, touch, pressure, motion, jarring, pain; fits; throbbing headaches which feel as if all the blood in the body has gone to the head (made worse by sun, cold, shock, menstruation, movement, stooping, eye movements); hot, flushed face, with pale mouth and lips; earache, especially on right side (made worse by getting head wet or cold); dilated, staring pupils, and intolerance of light; bright red tongue, sometimes raw around edges but coated in middle; in infants, teething pains; spasms of dry, tickly coughing made worse by talking; sore throat, tender to the touch, and throat pains which cause head and neck to jerk; sudden contraction of throat on swallowing; thirst for lemon juice, not alleviated by drinking it; inflammation of the kidneys; jerking and twitching in sleep; burning, dry, flushed and throbbing skin, with cold hands and feet

Many of the symptoms above are made worse by jarring, motion, light, noise, pressure, sun, having the hair cut and lying down. They also tend to be worse on the right side and at night from 11 p.m. onwards. They are often relieved by standing, sitting upright, staying in the warm and applying warmth to the affected parts.

Specific use Scarlet fever.

Complementary remedy Calcarea carb.

Antidoting remedies/substances Camphora, Coffea, Opium, Aconite; acetic acid (in fruit, lemon juice, vinegar), tea, coffee.

Bryonia

From *Bryonia alba* (also known as *B. dioica*), white, red or common bryony. The homeopathic remedy is made from the whole fresh plant. Because it affects fibrous tissues, serous membranes (membranes which secrete fluids), ligaments around joints, the broad part of tendons, and the coating of nerves, all of which can become inflamed and painful with rheumatism, Bryonia is frequently prescribed for rheumatism sufferers, especially if fever is present as well.

Constitutional indications The kind of person who responds to Bryonia is often of rather plodding intelligence, rubicund and well-fleshed, with a dark complexion and dark hair; he or she often gets stitching pains, and is easily angered or irritated.

Mental symptoms alleviated Feeling tired, languid, reluctant to move or speak when spoken to; feeling dull and stupid in the head, as if the head is about to fly to bits, but irritable with it; delusions about being away from home, or wanting to go home, when already at home; wanting something but not knowing what, wanting things impossible to get, or refusing things once they are offered; fear of death, of

not regaining health; hopelessness; job or financial worries, especially after a dispute with someone in authority; worry dreams, often about money or job.

Physical symptoms alleviated Bursting headaches, made worse by slightest movement, also by too much food or alcohol, hot drinks, colds and coughing, but relieved by firm pressure and cold; heavy eyelids and stabbing pains in the eyes; dry, sore, itchy lips; foul, coated tongue; dry, constricted throat; extreme thirst at long intervals; vomiting after rich fatty foods and hot drinks; craving for meat and unusual foods; stomach feels as if there is a stone in it – the sensation is made worse by pressure; stools which are large, hard, crumbly, black or burnt-looking; in women, breasts which are hard and inflamed, as if there is an abscess brewing, made worse by slightest movement; chest pains severe enough to make one clutch chest and head when coughing; pains around rib cage, made worse by coughing, drinking and warm rooms, and worse at night; cold hands and feet; in rheumatism sufferers, joints which are hot, swollen and painful, and made worse by cold draughts and slightest movement; profuse, sour-smelling sweat.

Many of the symptoms above are made worse by excitement, bright light, noise, touch, movement, and eating. They are also worse in the mornings, around 9 p.m. (when delirium and fever tend to reach a peak), and around 3 a.m. Cold, dry winds and draughts should be avoided. Cool air and firm, cool pressure on affected parts generally bring relief.

Complementary remedies Natrum mur., Natrum sulph. and, to a lesser extent, Alumina.

Antidoting remedies Aconite, Chamomilla, Nux.

Calcarea

The source of this remedy is calcium carbonate derived from oyster shells. Calcium is essential for healthy bones and for the proper functioning of nerves and muscles.

Constitutional indications Adults who respond well to Calcarea are usually fair, flabby and overweight, and have a cold, clammy handshake. Children who respond well tend to be tubby and clumsy, with a chalky pale complexion, coarse skin and coarse, curly hair; they are also prone to head sweats at night. Calcarea types are among the few mortals who actually feel better when they are constipated.

Mental symptoms alleviated Depression; emotional fragility; fear of making a fool of oneself, fear of the dark, fear of losing one's mind; inability to apply oneself after emotional upsets; mania for work, followed by sudden laziness and preoccupation with oneself and one's ailments; passivity, reluctance to answer questions; resentment; preoccupation with trivia, fiddling with small objects, doodling; feeling sorry for oneself and weeping from self-pity; going over and over details of illness/ailments until others feel like hitting one on the head; poor memory, forgetting what one has just been reading; tendency towards intense religiosity – reading Bible all day, for example; cruelty to people and animals, but shedding tears when relating incidents of cruelty; difficulty getting to sleep, then waking and worrying about what might go wrong; night terrors.

Physical symptoms alleviated Head sweats at night; head which feels cold and damp; in babies, a large head and fontanelles which are slow to close; headaches centred on · right temple, brought on by extreme heat or cold, or by becoming overheated; headaches caused by missing breakfast; dizziness; acute eye infections, with redness of white of eyes, especially in right eye; cataract; persistent, unpleasant-smelling discharge from ears; nasal polyps; swollen tonsils and adenoids; late or complicated teething; swollen neck glands; perspiration on chest; coarse skin with large pores; sweaty eczema; chilblains; copious perspiration, with bland or offensive odour; scoliosis or crookedness of the spine; in infants, late walking and unsteadiness on legs due to overweight; hanging feet out of bed at night because soles are burning hot; poor co-ordination, clumsiness; hearty appetite, with craving for eggs, pickles and acid foods, sweet things, and raw potatoes; in children, wanting to eat soap and other indigestible items such as soil and chalk; aversion to coffee, meat and milk (milk tends to aggravate other symptoms); strong-smelling urine; gallstones; piles; feeling better when constipated, worse when bowel movements are soft or loose; in women, early or abnormally heavy periods.

The above symptoms are exacerbated by draughts, cold, cold damp winds, and exertion, and are felt most intensely between 2 and 3 a.m. They wear off in the morning, improve with constipation, and are generally relieved by lying on the affected side.

Complementary remedies Rhus tox., Belladonna, Lycopodium, Phosphorus, Silicea, Platinum.

Antidoting remedies Camphora, Ipecac., Nitric ac., Nux.

Incompatible/inimical remedies Bryonia, Sulphur.

Calcarea phos.
The homeopathic remedy is prepared from calcium phosphate, also used as a Tissue Salt (see p. 35).

Constitutional indications Calcarea phos. suits people who are discontented, uncertain what they want; such people are usually thin (thinner than Calcarea types) and have dark hair, long legs, and a sagging abdomen; as babies they may have been late in walking. Late-developing adolescents with muddy skin also respond well to Calcarea phos.

Mental symptoms alleviated Nervousness, restlessness, fidgeting; dislike of routine; need for stimulation; difficulty getting up in the morning.

Physical symptoms alleviated In babies, delayed closure of fontanelles; headaches in children of school age; numbness or crawling sensations in hands and feet; sweaty scalp; delayed or complicated teething, with rapid tooth decay; painful bones and joints; growing pains; fractures which are slow to heal; craving for bacon rinds and strong-tasting foods; poor digestion, with stomach ache after meals, proneness to vomiting, and upsets after eating ice cream; splattery, greenish stools.

The above symptoms are usually aggravated by damp, cold, changeable weather, melting snow, exertion, lifting things and worrying; grief, bad news, sexual excesses and disappointments in love also have a negative effect. Summer and warm dry weather often produce dramatic improvement.

Complementary remedies Ruta, Hepar sulph.

Cantharis
The source of this remedy is *Cantharis* (or *Lytta*) *vesicatoria*, a species of beetle misleadingly called Spanish fly, which contains a rapid-acting irritant called cantharidin. In traditional medicine Spanish fly was used to cause blistering, increase fluid loss, treat baldness, procure abortion and provoke sexual desire. Patients who took it experienced burning pains in the throat and stomach, difficulty swallowing, nausea, vomiting, diarrhoea and a frantic urge to pass water; the unlucky ones went into convulsions, even into a coma.

Constitutional indications Cantharis should be the remedy of first resort for individuals who look as if they are suffering intensely.

Mental symptoms Paroxysms of rage, made worse by looking at shiny objects or touching throat while drinking; excessive desire for sex, amounting to a frantic itch for intercourse; extreme anxiety; screaming; being insolent, querulous, irritable, even violent; losing consciousness.

Physical symptoms alleviated Seeing things in shades of yellow; burning sensation in throat; urgent thirst, with reluctance to drink because drinking causes spasms of breathlessness; no appetite for food; burning sensation in stomach; loathing for tobacco; pleurisy, accompanied by sweating and palpitations; erysipelas; burns and scalds relieved by cold applications; insect bites with a blackish centre; redness and infection which spreads within 4 hours; swelling and suppurating rashes on hands; ice-cold hands with finger nails which feel red hot; burning sensation on soles of feet at night; severe cystitis, with scalding inflammation which worsens rapidly and cannot be ignored; burning pains in abdomen which feel as if intestinal lining has been stripped raw; severe distention of abdomen; diarrhoea which burns and scalds.

The above symptoms are exacerbated by touch, movement, coffee and cold water, and tend to get worse in the afternoon. However, they respond to warmth and gentle massage, and can be soothed by belching and passing wind; they are least troublesome at night and in the morning.

Complementary remedies Belladonna, Mercurius, Phosphorus, Sepia, Sulphur.

Antidoting remedies Aconite, Pulsatilla, Camphora.

Carbo veg.
The source of this homeopathic remedy is vegetable charcoal, made from beech, birch or poplar wood. Its main action is the removal of excess mucus from the digestive system. In the pre-pharmaceutical era vegetable charcoal was used to absorb gases and check fermentation.

Constitutional indications Carbo veg. is most beneficial to people who complain of not having felt really well since a particular illness or accident. Mental sluggishness is one of the first symptoms they mention.

Mental symptoms alleviated Slow thought processes and lack of mental energy; patchy, unreliable memory; preferring daylight to darkness; fear of the supernatural; lack of interest in news and current affairs; fixed ideas.

Physical symptoms alleviated Headaches in the morning, especially after overeating – head feels hot and heavy; fainting easily; dizziness and nausea; face which is purplish or has a greenish pallor; red-tipped nose; bitter, salty taste in mouth; cold breath and tongue; hoarseness; spasmodic cough, with gagging, choking and vomiting of mucus; bronchitis, especially in elderly people who smoke; clumsiness, poor co-ordination; cold, bluish hands and feet; cold, clammy skin; wanting to be fanned because body feels burning hot inside although skin is cold; internal or external bleeding; poor venous circulation, or varicose veins which bleed; gangrene; cold, puffy legs; aversion to meat and milk; craving for salty or acid foods, sweet things and coffee;

digestive problems, no matter what kinds of food are eaten; most foods, but particularly fats, cause wind; burning sensation in stomach, heartburn, sour belching and regurgitation of food; indigestion made worse by overeating, eating rich foods, or eating too late in evening.

The above symptoms are generally relieved by cold, fresh air and belching. Fatty foods, milk, coffee and wine only exacerbate discomfort, which is most marked in warm, wet weather, in the evening and when lying down.

Complementary remedies Kali carb., Phosphorus, Pulsatilla.

Antidoting remedies Nux, Camphora, Arsenicum, Ambra.

Causticum
This remedy, made from quicklime (calcium oxide) and potassium bisulphate, was invented by Samuel Hahnemann himself. It is especially good for conditions which involve local paralysis, burning sensations, rawness, soreness or skin eruptions which have been suppressed by steroids, etc.

Constitutional indications Those who derive most benefit from Causticum tend to be dark-haired, dark-eyed, sallow-skinned, weak and rather rigid in their thinking. Children who respond well to Causticum are often very excitable and outgoing, thoroughly involved in everything going on around them and deeply concerned about injustice.

Mental symptoms alleviated Pessimism, depression, anxiety; intellectual laziness; sudden tears and floods of emotion; intense sympathy with people or animals in pain or trouble; lack of self-reliance; irritability; wanting to criticize everything; suspicion and distrust which mask timidity and nervousness; in children, not wanting to go to bed at night.

Physical symptoms alleviated Dizziness when bending forwards or sideways, as if there were an empty space between brain and skull; Bell's palsy; rushing and roaring in ears; hearing echo of own voice; colds which go to the ears; drooping eyelids, dimmed vision, momentary sight loss; soreness inside nose and thick yellow catarrh; post-nasal drip, relieved by cold drinks; dry, tickly cough; hoarseness, especially in morning; scraped feeling in throat, with painless loss of voice; paralysis of vocal cords; rheumatism, with muscular stiffness due to contracted tendons; stiff neck after sitting in a draught; deformed joints, with sharp, tearing pains in them; warts on face or fingers; scars or healed injury sites which become sore again; in women, early periods with scanty flow which stops at night or when lying down; stress incontinence; cystitis, with delayed urination despite intense urging.

The above symptoms are often worse on the right side, but respond to damp and warmth. Cold dry winds, sweet foods, coffee, grief and fright have a deleterious effect.

Complementary remedies Carbo veg., Petroselinum.

Incompatible/inimical remedies Phosphorus, Coffea.

Chamomilla

From *Matricaria chamomilla*, German chamomile. The homeopathic remedy is made from the whole fresh plant. In herbal form, chamomile is used to treat nervous complaints and womb problems.

Constitutional indications Individuals who respond best to Chamomilla have a very low pain threshold and are often bad-tempered and complaining. Complaints often begin with the words 'I can't bear. . .'

Mental symptoms alleviated Inner turmoil; rudeness; spitefulness; being bad-tempered with everyone and everything, including oneself; being impossible to please, rather like a child who is quiet when carried but screams when put down; slightest pain or discomfort at night makes one jump out of bed and walk about.

Physical symptoms alleviated Slightest pain causes sweating and fainting; numb feeling in head; convulsions brought on by anger; throbbing sensation in one half of head, relieved by bending head back; one cheek red, the other pale; severe earache, with congested, blocked feeling in affected ear; tinnitus; teething, especially if accompanied by fever and greenish diarrhoea; toothache which responds to cold rinsing but flares up with hot drinks and also at night; yellow, coated tongue; heartburn; dry, hacking cough; coughing in sleep, and also when angry; feeling sleepy but unable to get to sleep; drowsiness in morning; anxiety dreams which cause one to start out of sleep and get angry; moaning and crying in sleep; skin which feels very hot; sticking feet out of bed at night to cool them; in women, heavy periods accompanied by severe labour-like pains; abdominal pain which causes legs to be drawn up; tearing pains in general; diarrhoea, with thin, slimy, pale green stools; stools which are hot and smell of rotten eggs.

The above symptoms are almost always made worse by bad temper, and also by heat, cold winds, fresh air and belching; they also tend to be worse at night, from 9 p.m. onwards. Warm wet weather and fasting often improve matters; children feel better if they are carried.

Complementary remedies Belladonna, Magnesia phos.

Antidoting remedies Camphora, Nux, Pulsatilla.

Chelidonium

From *Chelidonium majus*, the greater celandine. The homeopathic remedy is prepared from the whole plant when it is in flower, or from the root only. Its main action is on the liver.

Constitutional indications Chelidonium has an affinity with thin, fair, lethargic people.

Mental symptoms alleviated Depression; anxiety; pessimism and despondency; mental sluggishness, unwillingness to make any effort; tendency to brood; weepiness.

Physical symptoms alleviated Headaches accompanied by great heaviness, lethargy and drowsiness; lead-in-the-head feeling; hangovers which prevent one sitting up or standing up; cataracts; drowsiness during the day; coated tongue, with teeth marks on it; asthma which comes on at night; pain around lower angle of right shoulder blade; upset stomach, with nausea and vomiting; craving for cheese and hot drinks (sometimes aversion to cheese); liverishness, with dizziness and vomiting; distention of upper abdomen.

The above symptoms are generally made worse by movement, heat, touch and changes in the weather; they also tend to affect the right side, and are especially marked early in the morning and around 4 a.m. and 4 p.m. Milk, hot drinks, eating and firm pressure usually bring relief.

Complementary remedies Lycopodium, Bryonia.

Antidoting remedy Chamomilla.

China

From *Cinchona calisaya*, an evergreen shrub from South America. The homeopathic remedy is made from the dried bark, also known as Peruvian bark, which yields quinine, used to treat malaria and also to cause abortion. Quinine causes contractions of the bronchi, spleen and uterus, irritation of the stomach, cochlea, and retina, loss of protein in the urine, and heat, fever and sweating. Its homeopathic derivative is very beneficial after debilitating illness or excessive loss of body fluids.

Constitutional indications Individuals of an artistic or poetic nature usually respond well to China.

Mental symptoms alleviated Apathy, indifference; inability to concentrate; emotional fragility, jumpiness, edginess; nervous exhaustion; outbursts of anger despite mild nature; inability to express feelings face to face; building castles in the air, playing the hero in dreams; reliving day's events in dreams.

Physical symptoms alleviated Headaches which wear off by pressing painful area but intensify if hair is combed; neuralgia; dizziness; convulsions; haemorrhages and nosebleeds; tinnitus; weak, jumpy muscles; fever, with alternate bouts of sweating and shivering, refusing to drink during sweats but wanting to drink during chills; profuse sweating; flushing and shivering generally, in absence of fever; sallow, yellowish complexion; skin which is very sensitive to touch; swollen ankles; belching which does not relieve indigestion; sensation of food being stuck behind breastbone; aversion to butter and fatty foods; craving for alcohol; gastroenteritis; gall bladder problems; uncomfortable flatulence, made worse by movement; blood in urine; swollen liver and spleen; frothy, yellow, chopped-egg stools.

The above symptoms are not improved by food, cold, draughts, movement or touching affected areas; they also tend to be worse at night and in the autumn. Sleep, warmth and firm pressure are usually helpful.

Complementary remedies Ferrum, Calcarea phos.

Antidoting remedies Arnica, Arsenicum, Ipecac.

Colocynth
From *Citrullus colocynthus*, the bitter apple or bitter cucumber. The homeopathic derivative is most commonly used to relieve anger and destructive effects of anger, and severe abdominal pain. It is made from the pulp of the fruit, which contains colocynthin, a substance which acts on the bowels, causing great pain and painful straining when stools are passed; the stools themselves become very watery.

Constitutional indications Colocynth is best suited to people who are fair-haired and fair-skinned.

Mental symptoms alleviated Anger and indignation; extreme irritability, made worse by questioning; embarrassment caused by offensive remarks.

Physical symptoms alleviated Dizziness when standing with head to left; headaches which improve by applying warmth or pressure; trigeminal neuralgia; stomach pain, with nausea and vomiting; shooting, nervy pains in kidney area or around ovaries; sciatica; gout; rheumatism; agonising abdominal pain, alleviated by lying on side with knees drawn up to chin; spasmodic abdominal pain with diarrhoea, relieved by passing wind.

All of the symptoms above are aggravated by anger and

indignation, and also by eating, drinking and damp cold; they also tend to be worst around 4 p.m. Firm pressure, warmth, sleep, coffee and passing wind usually produce improvement.

Antidoting remedies Coffea, Staphysagria, Chamomilla.

Dioscorea
From *Dioscorea villosa*, the wild yam The homeopathic remedy is made from the fresh root, which contains a substance called dioscorene, highly irritant to the nerves supplying the bowels.

Constitutional indications None in particular.

Mental symptoms alleviated Calling things by the wrong name.

Physical symptoms alleviated Pain in centre of chest and down both arms, accompanied by breathlessness; sinking feeling in stomach; general discomfort in upper abdomen; belching, especially after drinking tea; pain in liver area (right upper abdomen), radiating to right nipple; constant abdominal pain, punctuated by spasms of acute pain which radiate to other parts of the body, even to fingers and toes.

All the symptoms above tend to get worse in the evening and at night, and are not helped by doubling up or lying down. Standing up, stretching, walking about out of doors and applying pressure usually improve matters.

Antidoting remedies Chamomilla, Camphora.

Dulcamara
From *Solanum dulcamara*, woody nightshade or bittersweet. This plant contains an alkaloid called solanin, which paralyses the vagus nerve and causes the heart to pump faster. The homeopathic remedy is prepared from the stems and leaves of the plant just before it comes into flower, and is traditionally used to treat conditions brought on by changes from warm to cold, or from warm to damp and cold.

Constitutional indications None in particular.

Mental symptoms alleviated None in particular.

Physical symptoms alleviated Paralysis or weakness made worse by cold and damp; sore, itchy, bleeding or encrusted eruptions on face or scalp; ringworm; large, smooth, fleshy or flat warts; urticaria; catarrh which gets worse in warm rooms; hoarseness; coughing up large amounts of phlegm; coughing made worse by lying down; pain around navel; yellow or greenish diarrhoea; difficulty opening bowels or urinating after catching a chill.

Most of the symptoms above improve with warmth and movement. Immobility, damp cold, getting wet and cooling down rapidly after sweating profusely tend to make them worse.

Complementary remedy Baryta carb.

Antidoting remedies Camphora, Cuprum.

Incompatible/inimical remedies Belladonna, Lachesis.

Euphrasia

From *Euphrasia officinalis* (also known as *E. sticta*), common eyebright. The homeopathic remedy is made from the whole fresh plant, traditionally used as a cure for eye ailments. The poet Milton wrote that the Archangel 'Purged with Euphrasy and Rue the visual nerve, for he had much to see'.

Constitutional indications None in particular.

Mental symptoms alleviated None in particular.

Physical symptoms alleviated Bursting headaches; profuse, stinging discharge from eyes; watering eyes; conjunctivitis; intolerance of bright light; dimmed vision; sticky mucus or little blisters on cornea; hot, red cheeks; bland, watery catarrh; early stages of measles; in women, short, painful periods in which flow lasts for only an hour a day, or cessation of periods accompanied by eye problems; in men, prostatitis; constipation.

The above symptoms are generally aggravated by warmth, south winds, bright light and being indoors; they also tend to be worse in the evening. Coffee and darkened rooms often bring relief.

Antidoting remedies Camphora, Pulsatilla.

Ferrum phos.

The homeopathic remedy is prepared from iron phosphate, one of the Tissue Salts (see p. 35). It is most beneficial in the first stages of inflammation, when extra blood flows to affected areas.

Constitutional indications People who respond best to Ferrum phos. are often rather pale, anaemic and complaining, and prone to sudden, fiery congestion of the face.

Mental symptoms alleviated None in particular.

Physical symptoms alleviated Headaches which improve by bathing forehead in cold water; pale face which flushes easily; head colds which begin with nosebleeds; earache; hoarseness, laryngitis; dry, hacking cough with pain in chest; rheumatic joints, with raised temperature and shooting pains which intensify on starting to move but wear off with gentle exercise; fevers which onset slowly, especially if face is pale with red spots on cheeks, if pulse is weak and rapid, and if chill comes on around 1 p.m.; haemorrhages, especially if blood is bright red; aversion to meat and milk; craving for stimulants; sour belching, and vomiting of undigested food; in women, periods at 3-weekly intervals, with heavy, dragging pain in uterus and pain around apex of head, or dryness of vagina; stress incontinence, with wetting at night; early stages of dysentery, with blood in stools.

The above symptoms are generally made worse by jarring touching, moving, lying on right side, being too hot, being exposed to the sun, and by not perspiring as one should or suppressing perspiration with anti-perspirants; they also tend to be more marked between 4 and 6 a.m. Cold applications and gentle exercise usually bring relief.

Complementary remedies Kali mur., Kali phos., Calcarea phos.

Gelsemium

From *Gelsemium sempervirens*, yellow jasmine. The homeopathic remedy is prepared from the root of the fresh plant which contains an alkaloid which interferes with nervous control of breathing and movement, causing paralysis, trembling and inflammation.

Constitutional indications Individuals of limited intelligence, who are dull and heavy-looking and have a bluish tinge to their skin, often respond well to Gelsemium. The remedy is also beneficial for heavy smokers.

Mental symptoms alleviated Fears and phobias accompanied by trembling and the need to pass urine; fears often centred around falling, throwing oneself from a great height, going to the dentist, having surgery, heart suddenly stopping if one does not move; dullness and drowsiness; inability to sleep because of excitement; nervousness and a sense of inadequacy.

Physical symptoms alleviated Heavy head which feels as if there is a tight band around it; headaches which wear off after urinating, vomiting or sleeping but which intensify with bright light and movement; dizziness, faintness; scalp which feels sore; face which looks flushed, heavy, hot and sweaty; earache; heavy, drooping eyelids; visual disturbances or double vision; burning pain in right eye; summer colds with mild fever, sneezing and watery catarrh; nasty taste in mouth; numb, trembling tongue with a thick yellow coating; sore throat with red tonsils, with earache and difficulty swallowing, often associated with anxiety and made worse by hot drinks; dry cough; heavy, tired, aching, trembling limbs, accompanied by pain in neck; twitch or tremor of single muscles, which feel cold and tingly; flu-like chills up and down back, with intermittent waves of heat; lack of thirst; in women, painful periods or pain in uterus unconnected with periods.

The above symptoms are generally worse early in the day and at bedtime; sun, heat, damp, fog, tobacco, impending thunder, excitement, emotional stress, apprehension, worrying about symptoms, and worrying about performing in public tend to make them worse. Open air, exercise, passing urine, taking stimulants or alcohol, applying local heat and bending forward all produce improvement.

Antidoting remedies Coffea, China, Digitalis.

Glonoinum

The source of this remedy is the explosive liquid nitroglycerine. The active principle in nitroglycerine is nitrous oxide or 'laughing gas' which causes blood vessels to dilate, lowering blood pressure.

Constitutional indications Glonoinum is most effective in women who have high blood pressure, especially if they are flushed and overweight.

Mental symptoms alleviated Confusion; loss of sense of place or direction.

Physical symptoms alleviated Bursting sensation in head and neck; dizziness; headaches, especially if caused by extremes of heat or cold, jolting or jarring, strong emotions, or cessation of periods; in women, hot flushes during menopause.

The above symptoms tend to be made worse by heat, exertion, noise, sunlight and bright lights, wine, stimulants, tight or heavy clothing and lying too close to the floor. Cold air and cold applications, firm pressure, bending the head back, and lying with head higher than hips all seem to relieve symptoms.

Antidoting remedy Aconite.

Graphites

The homeopathic remedy is made from plumbago or black lead, a mixture of carbon, iron and silica. At one time black lead was used to treat cold sores.

Constitutional indications Elderly women who are overweight, constipated, chilly and rather melancholy respond well to Graphites. So do coarse-featured, dark-haired individuals with earthy complexions. The Graphites type often does hard manual work in the open air or drives heavy goods vehicles.

Mental symptoms alleviated Indecisiveness, timidity, unresponsiveness to external events; poor short-term memory; awareness that mind is not fully alert and in control causes anxiety; occasional depression; easily startled; tendency to become maudlin and weepy when listening to music.

Physical symptoms alleviated Hair loss; numbness and cramps in hands and feet; intolerance of bright light; deafness which improves with background noise; weepy eczema behind ears; face which feels as if there is a cobweb over it; periodically feeling very hot and sweaty, usually followed by a nosebleed; swollen glands; rough, dry, cracked skin; keloids; cold sores; tendency for slightest cut or abrasion to turn septic; skin lesions which exude thick honey-coloured pus; hardening of old scars; duodenal ulcers, soothed by hot food and by lying down, or duodenal ulcers which alternate with skin complaints; aversion to sweets, fish and salty foods; in women, late periods accompanied by constipation, infrequent or scanty periods, enlarged ovaries or hardening of the breasts; constipation, with large, knotty stools passed with a lot of straining.

The above symptoms tend to wear off in the dark or after sleep, but are aggravated by cold, sweet foods, seafood and suppression of skin eruptions with steroids, etc. Discomfort is often worse during periods and usually located on the left side.

Complementary remedies Hepar sulph, Lycopodium.

Antidoting remedies Nux, Aconite, Arsenicum, China.

Hamamelis

From *Macrophylla dioica* (also known as *M. virginica*), witch hazel. The homeopathic remedy, made from the bark of the twigs and roots which contain a substance which causes veins to haemorrhage, is traditionally used to improve venous circulation and alleviate bruising and soreness.

Constitutional indications None in particular.

Mental symptoms alleviated Depression and withdrawal – wanting to be left alone and not talked to; wanting others to show due respect; restlessness; irritability; grandiose ideas.

Physical symptoms alleviated Headaches, often relieved by nosebleeds, open air, reading, thinking or talking; eyes which are painful and bloodshot; injuries which cause soreness and bruising; tender, rheumatic joints; tickly cough, with blood-flecked phlegm; varicose veins; phlebitis; venous bleeding which is slow to stop; epididymitis; urethritis; in women, inflammation of uterus or ovaries, ovulation pain or heavy menstrual bleeding, with very sore abdomen.

The symptoms above are often made worse by warm damp air, pressure and movement.

Complementary remedy Ferrum.

Antidoting remedy Arnica.

Hepar sulph.

The source of this remedy is calcium sulphide, obtained by heating together the calcareous inner layer of oyster shells with flowers of sulphur. At one time this preparation was used to antidote the effects of the many forms of physic containing mercury.

Constitutional indications Hepar sulph. is best suited to individuals who are overweight, flabby, pale, sluggish and rather depressed; such people tend to look as if they have been through a lot, and gratefully sink into the nearest chair.

Mental symptoms alleviated Irritability with self and others which hides anxiety; great sensitivity to touch, pain, cold dry air, noise, disturbance of any kind; tendency to be hasty, impulsive and to want change for change's sake; taking unreasonable likes and dislikes to people; taking offence easily; outward calm conceals restlessness; feeling hard done by and telling others how everything in the past has gone wrong.

Physical symptoms alleviated Slightest pain causes fainting; sinusitis, with sinus areas very tender, made worse by bending forward but relieved by warmth; corneal ulcers; conjunctivitis; cold sores or ulcers at corner of lips; colds which start with an itchy throat; fish-bone-in-throat sensation; sore throat which causes ear pain when swallowing; hoarseness or loss of voice; choking or intense pain on swallowing, relieved by wrapping something warm around neck; tonsillitis, with swollen glands in neck; dry, hoarse cough brought on by exposure to cold; hollow, crowing cough with loose, rattling phlegm in chest, with retching and vomiting, worse at night; exhausting cough worse between 6 p.m. and midnight; influenza, with sneezing, fever, sweating and craving for warmth despite high temperature; abcesses or boils, with sour-smelling sweat; constant thirst for sips of fluid (children may not be thirsty at all); craving for fats, condiments and sour, vinegary foods; aversion to alcohol; diarrhoea, made worse by eating ripe, juicy fruit, vegetables, and iced foods.

The above symptoms are generally aggravated by cold air and draughts, undressing and touching affected parts, and are generally most intense in the morning and when lying on the affected side. Eating a meal, staying in the warm, applying compresses and wrapping the head up all improve matters.

Remedies which follow well Calcarea, Calcarea sulph.

Complementary remedy Calendula.

Antidoting remedies Belladonna, Chamomilla, Silicea, Kali iod.

Hyoscyamus

From *Hyoscyamus niger*, henbane. The homeopathic remedy is made from the whole fresh plant and mainly affects the nervous system.

Constitutional indications Hyoscyamus is most effective in the senile and elderly, and in individuals who mutter to themselves or hold conversations with people who are absent or dead. The Hyoscyamus type tends to live in a world of his or her own.

Mental symptoms alleviated Incoherent, excited behaviour not due to infection or fever; obsessional behaviour; fearfulness, jealousy, suspicion; tendency to talk and act obscenely.

Physical symptoms alleviated Involuntary jerking of head, arms and hands; cough relieved by sitting up but worse lying down; twitching in every muscle, with awkward, angular movements; extremely sensitive skin; desire to undress and throw bedclothes off; frequent urge to pass water, though flow is infrequent and scanty; frequent urge to open bowels, with small, infrequent stools.

The above symptoms are generally improved by stooping, but are more troublesome at night, and not improved by eating or lying down.

Antidoting remedies Belladonna, Camphora.

Hypericum

From *Hypericum perforatum*, St John's wort. The homeopathic remedy is made from the whole fresh plant and is mainly used to treat nerve injuries, its principle action being on the central nervous system.

Constitutional indications None in particular.

Mental symptoms alleviated Drowsiness; depression.

Physical symptoms alleviated Concussion; neuralgia; heavy, icy cold sensation in head; head which feels elongated, as if lifted up high into the air; eye injuries; discomfort after going to dentist; toothache, with pulling or tearing pains; coated tongue with a clean tip; severe shooting pains which travel in an upward direction; back pain which travels up or down spine; puncture wounds caused by nails, splinters or bites; crushed fingers or toes; thirst; a craving for wine or hot drinks; nausea; in women, late periods, accompanied by headaches; diarrhoea, with loose yellowish stools, made worse by overheating; painful, bleeding piles; nervy pains in rectum.

The above symptoms are often relieved by tilting the head back, but tend to get worse in cold, damp or foggy conditions and in warm stuffy rooms; being touched or exposing any part of the body is usually detrimental.

Antidoting remedies Arsenicum, Chamomilla.

Ignatia

From *Ignatia amara,* also known as *Strychnos ignatia,* St Ignatius' bean. The homeopathic remedy is made from the seed pods, which contain the powerful poison strychnine. Strychnine acts on the central nervous system.

Constitutional indications Ignatia is most effective in children who are bright, precocious and highly strung, and in adults who are alert, nervous, rather pale, given to sighing and yawning, and wear a rather strained expression on their face, often with frequent blinking or a facial tic. Ignatia types are very fragile emotionally, inclined to be perverse and unpredictable. Women who respond well to Ignatia are often artistic.

Mental symptoms alleviated Rapid changes of mood; apprehension, fear of going out alone, fear of being seen to take initiative; suddenly bursting into tears; tendency to be self-pitying, self-blaming and hysterical; easily shocked, easily knocked off emotional perch by grief, love, worry; mild depression; little capacity for anger or violence; sensitivity to noise, especially when studying; inability to work; wanting to be socially responsible and well thought of.

Physical symptoms alleviated Headaches which feel as if a nail is being driven into side of head, made more intense by lying on painful side; nervous headaches in children, relieved by heat but made worse by coffee; fainting in confined spaces; beads of sweat on forehead and upper lip which disappear when eating; sour taste in mouth; hiccups, or spasmodic, irritating cough; febrile convulsions; feeling very thirsty with a chill; red face which is chilly to the touch; inflammation, relieved by firm pressure; extreme sensitivity to pain; pain concentrated in small areas; choking; tickly cough; sore throat which improves on eating solids; feeling as if there is a hard lump in the throat; craving for unusual foods when ill; craving for sour or acidic foods; upper abdominal pain, nausea and vomiting, alleviated by eating; in women, painful spasms of uterus during periods; constipation due to emotional factors; piles; rectal spasms, or prolapse of rectum which causes sharp upward-shooting pains.

The above symptoms are often relieved by eating, urinating, firm pressure, walking as well as resting, lying on the painful side and by external heat. Fear, anxiety, fresh air, cold, being overdressed, coffee, brandy, tobacco and strong odours are generally irritants; symptoms also tend to be worse in the morning and after meals.

Complementary remedy Natrum mur.

Antidoting remedies Pulsatilla, Cocculus, Chamomilla.

Incompatible/inimical remedies Coffea, Tabacum, Nux.

Ipecac.

From *Cephaelis* (or *Psychotria*) *ipecacuanha,* ipecacuanha. The homeopathic remedy is made from the dried root, whose active principle, emetine, is used in orthodox medicine as an emetic and expectorant. In herbal medicine, ipecacuanha is used to treat dermatitis.

Constitutional indications None in particular.

Mental symptoms alleviated Anxiety; fear of death; contempt for everything around one; moroseness.

Physical symptoms alleviated Fainting; nosebleeds; feeling chilly most of the time; suffocation or difficulty breathing; desire to cough and vomit simultaneously; constant nausea, not relieved by vomiting; asthma, gasping for air; pale, cold, sweaty skin; back pain; profuse bleeding or haemorrhaging, with loss of bright red blood; blood slow to clot; weak pulse; lack of thirst.

The above symptoms tend to come and go, but are usually worse in winter, aggravated by moving about as well as lying down, and can be brought on by embarrassment or stress.

Complementary remedies Cuprum, Arnica.

Antidoting remedies Arsenicum, China, Tabacum.

Kali carb.

The source of this remedy is potassium carbonate.

Constitutional indications Those who benefit most from Kali carb. tend to be sallow-skinned, physically weak, flabby and flat-footed; they are often depressed, dogmatic, inclined to see issues as black or white and have a strong sense of duty; bookkeeping, translating, the law and police work tend to attract the Kali carb. type.

Mental symptoms alleviated Feeling scared stiff, unhappy, irritable, worried about one's future; sense of failure; forgetfulness; nervousness; feeling overwhelmed when alone; sensation of bed sinking into floor as one falls asleep.

Physical symptoms alleviated Headaches behind temples; dizziness brought on by yawning or cold wind; excessive puffiness between eyebrows and upper eyelids; eyes stuck together in morning; stuffed-up nose, worse in warm rooms; watery, yellowish catarrh which causes choking or vomiting; cheesy taste in mouth; throat feels as if there is a lump in it, with a stinging pain on swallowing; backache, especially before periods; stitch-like pains, cutting pains, burning pains, with painful areas clammy or sweaty; asthma which worsens around 3 a.m., obliging one to sit up; chest pain unrelated to inhaling or exhaling, aggravated by pressure and lying on right side but relieved by leaning forwards; dry, hoarse cough and loss of voice; stomach often affected by shocks and emotional upsets; craving for sweet, starchy, or acid foods, and sour drinks; heavy weight in pit of stomach; nausea followed by sour, watery vomiting; choking on food; bloated abdomen, with griping pains; abdomen distended and full of wind, discomfort relieved by bending over or leaning back but increased by drinking ice cold water; in women, premenstrual weakness and depression, or period pains which feel like labour pains.

The above symptoms are often helped by warmth, moisture and movement, and tend to wear off during the day; they are aggravated by hot drinks, coffee, cold surroundings, changes in the weather, pressure, touch, rest and lying on the affected side, and come on most strongly after sexual intercourse and between 2 and 4 a.m.

Complementary remedy Carbo veg.

Antidoting remedy Coffea.

Lachesis

From *Lachesis trigonocephalus*, the bushmaster or surucucu snake of South America. The homeopathic remedy is made from the venom which, depending on the size of the victim, inhibits nerve impulses within the heart and causes death very swiftly, or interferes with blood clotting and speeds up the rate at which red blood cells are destroyed, which causes slow death from jaundice, infection or blood loss.

Constitutional indications Lachesis is especially effective in people who are tremulous, rather bloated in appearance and in need of relief from nervous over-stimulation; many such people also have red hair and freckles.

Mental symptoms alleviated Talkativeness, nervousness, restlessness, irritability; tendency to be suspicious and distrustful, sometimes obsessively so; occasional depression; jealousy over petty things; unsociability, especially first thing in morning.

Physical symptoms alleviated Headaches, often made worse by periods, bright light, hot sun; throbbing or bursting headaches aggravated by stooping and by movement generally; *petit mal* epilepsy; fainting; horror of putting things in ears; puffy, purplish face; habit of putting tongue out and flicking it over lips; ropy, foul-tasting saliva; trembling tongue which is dry, red, brown or black and fissured; left-sided sore throat, with pain in left ear when swallowing; throat which feels swollen and constricted, worse for hot drinks, hot applications and tight things around neck, but better for eating hot food; back of throat looks dark purple and inflamed; waking up choking, with swollen neck glands; pneumonia, accompanied by general weakness, a weak heart and fever; hot sweats and shivering, relieved by eating but aggravated by sleep; skin ulcers and wounds which have a bluish margin to them; boils which are red and angry-looking but painless; swollen, engorged veins which make skin look bluish; rapid, weak, irregular pulse; throbbing sensations in various parts of the body, often accompanied by headache; palpitations and fainting; angina and difficulty breathing; swollen glands generally; great thirst; increased appetite; stomach pains with vomiting, made worse by tight clothing; craving for oysters, coffee, and alcohol; appendicitis; anal spasm and bleeding piles; in women, spasmodic, congestive period pains, relieved by flow of blood, premenstrual syndrome, or menopausal hot flushes.

The above symptoms are not improved by touch, hot or warm baths, hot drinks, closing eyes, or going to sleep; they also tend to be worse in the spring and more noticeable on the left side. They do improve, however, when there is some sort of discharge.

Complementary remedies Crotalus, Lycopodium, Hepar sulph.

Antidoting remedies/substances Arsenicum, Mercurius; alcohol, salt.

Ledum

From *Ledum palustre*, marsh tea or wild rosemary. The homeopathic remedy is made from the whole fresh or dried plant and is traditionally used to heal puncture wounds and soothe pains which ascend from the lower part of the body.

Constitutional indications None in particular.

Mental symptoms alleviated Anxiety; timidity; moroseness, wanting to be left alone; hatred for fellow human beings; impatience, working oneself into a state of extreme anger.

Physical symptoms alleviated Black eyes; stiff joints which loosen up when bathed in cold water; cold, puffy, purplish skin, especially in cold weather.

The above symptoms are not helped by touch or warmth, and tend to get worse at night. Cold applications are usually beneficial.

Lycopodium

From *Lycopodium clavatum*, wolf's claw club moss. The homeopathic remedy is made from the powdery spores, which have the property of floating on water and flaring up when sprinkled on a naked flame.

Constitutional indications The Lycopodium type usually has a handshake which is so firm that it hurts, and a haughty, unfriendly air; other characteristics are leanness, a stooping posture and an unhealthily sallow skin, often with many lines and wrinkles. Such people tend to gravitate towards politics, teaching, the law and the priesthood.

Mental symptoms alleviated Anxiety, nervousness, insecurity, impatience; cowardice – physical, moral or social; dread of being left on one's own; tendency to be secretive; inability to sleep at night because brain goes over and over day's events; mental fatigue, despite braininess; slow to get into gear in mornings; tightness with money; great sensitivity to noise or smells; hypochondria; memory difficulties; aversion to new challenges; ambition; in children, preferring to bury nose in a book rather than play with other children; talking and laughing in sleep, night terrors, tendency to wake around 4 a.m., sense of apprehension on waking in morning.

Physical symptoms alleviated Neuralgia-type headaches, alleviated by open air but aggravated by pressure or indigestion; haemorrhaging of blood vessels in eye; early degeneration of retina; chronic catarrh; nostrils which flare on inhaling; mouth which feels dry and swollen; right-sided sore throat, made worse by cold drinks; tracheitis; right-sided pneumonia; obstinate, dry, tickly cough; scalding pain between shoulder blades; slow recovery after flu, or post-viral syndrome; hands and feet hot and dry, or right foot much hotter than left; psoriasis on palms of hands; aneurysms; throbbing sensation in arteries; thyrotoxicosis; craving for sweet foods; aversion to onions; in children, aversion to breakfast due to hatred of school; ravenous hunger, followed by discomfort after a few mouthfuls; getting indigestion if one has to wait for food; often feeling and being sick; in men, increased libido accompanied by inability to achieve or sustain erection, or enlarged prostate; reddish urine with sandy sediment in it; distended abdomen, full of wind; lazy bowels, constipation or spasm of anal sphincter making it impossible to pass stools despite straining; constipation in infants; bleeding piles.

The above symptoms are often relieved by sympathy, movement, undressing, cold surroundings, or a hot meal or a hot drink in the evening; symptoms also tend to wear off after midnight. Stuffy rooms, tight clothing and overeating usually aggravate matters; symptoms are often worse on the right side and cause most discomfort between 4 and 8 p.m.

Complementary remedies Calcarea, Sulphur.

Antidoting remedies Camphora, Pulsatilla, Causticum.

Magnesia phos.

The homeopathic remedy is made from magnesium phosphate, one of the Tissue Salts (see p. 35). It has an anti-spasmodic effect.

Constitutional indications Magnesia phos. is most beneficial to people who are thin, dark, nervous, tired, and exhausted.

Mental symptoms alleviated Inability to think clearly; moaning and complaining.

Physical symptoms alleviated Headaches made worse by mental exertion; dizziness brought on by movement; tendency to fall forward when eyes are closed; involuntary, jerky movements of face, hands and arms; in teenage girls, a red, flushed face; neuralgia in right eye or right ear, made worse by washing in cold water; toothache which improves with heat; ulcers on gums, accompanied by swollen neck glands; teething trouble; hiccups; retching; weak or twitching muscles; cramping, nerve pains which improve with warmth and pressure but worsen with cold and strenuous exercise; writer's cramp; belching which does not relieve stomach discomfort; craving for cold drinks; abdominal pain and wind, relieved by warmth and pressure; bloated, distended abdomen, relieved by loosening clothing, walking about or passing wind; period pains, relieved by heat, or early periods, with dark, stringy discharge; constipation.

The above symptoms are almost always relieved by warmth, pressure and bending double; they tend to be worse on the right side and at night, and can be exacerbated by touch, undressing and cold.

Antidoting remedies Belladonna, Gelsemium, Lachesis.

Mercurius

The source of this remedy is black oxide of mercury. Mercury, liberally used in many medicinal preparations at one time, cannot be efficiently eliminated by the body and results in chronic or acute poisoning.

Constitutional indications The Mercurius type is usually light-haired, with slow speech and slow, rather drugged reactions.

Mental symptoms alleviated Feeling dull, slow, muddle-headed; not knowing what to say; nervousness, timidity, suspicion, mistrust, anxiety, restlessness, irritability; sense of haste and hurry; talking very rapidly; poor comprehension and poor memory; lack of willpower; finding that time passes very slowly; weariness and disenchantment with life.

Physical symptoms alleviated Neuralgia; loss of sensation in any part of body; congestive, vice-like headaches; burning pain over left temple; tight band of pain over nose and above eyes; encrusted lesions on scalp, with smelly discharge; profuse discharge of pus from ears, with earache which is made worse by warmth of bed; chronic conjunctivitis, with margins of eyelids red, swollen and stuck together; eyes which sting and water profusely, with a severe ache behind eyeballs, made worse by glare of fire; acrid, watery catarrh; sneezing which makes nose feel raw and scalded, especially in sunshine; open sores on nostrils, aggravated by damp; slimy saliva which stains pillow during sleep; swollen gums; numb or sore gums; trembling tongue, or swollen tongue with teeth marks on it; foul breath; metallic taste in mouth; loose teeth in infected, reddened gums; swollen, raw, dark red throat, or ulcers which constrict throat and make swallowing painful; throat pain accompanied by hot sweats; smarting jaw, worse on right side; cough which produces yellow phlegm, often worse at right and in warm rooms; paroxysms of coughing made worse by warm or damp conditions, smoking and lying on right side; weak, trembling muscles; aching joints; breaking out in hot, drenching sweats, which chill skin as they evaporate; profuse, oily sweats which seem to make other symptoms worse, especially at night; blisters or pus-filled eruptions on skin; open sores; ulcers which itch and sting, especially in bed; low blood pressure; swollen glands; craving for cold drinks or stimulants; stomach upsets, especially after eating sweets and solids; in men, increased production of smegma, with head of penis sensitive and sore; in women, profuse vaginal discharge; alternate bouts of constipation and diarrhoea; chronic dysentery, with raw, sore anus; greenish stools with blood in them; painful urging to pass stools; cutting pains in abdomen; excessive production of urine with protein in it.

The above symptoms tend to improve with rest and wrapping up well. Changes in temperature, heat and cold, being warm in bed, dampness and perspiration are generally aggravating; symptoms also tend to right-sided and worse at night.

Complementary remedy Badiaga, Sulphur.

Antidoting remedies Hepar sulph., Aurum, Mezereum.

Incompatible/inimical remedy Silicea.

Natrum mur.

The source of this remedy is common salt, sodium chloride.

Constitutional indications Natrum mur. is of most benefit to people of squarish build who tend walk on their heels; they may be sandy- or dark-haired, but often have greasy skin and a cracked lower lip; although they appear deliberate and self-assured, they can be inward-looking and vulnerable. Skinny children with hard, nodular lymph glands also respond well to Natrum mur.

Mental symptoms alleviated Impatience, clumsiness, touchiness; getting worked up over trivial things; screaming with rage; crying with laughter; often feeling depressed or down in the dumps, especially in morning; anxiety; difficulty expressing true feelings; feeling wounded or humiliated; relieving feelings by locking oneself away and crying; fear of the dark and of thunder; remaining dry-eyed when bereaved; poor sense of humour; sentimentality; brooding over injustice; politeness which hides hardness and ruthlessness; being easy to get on with socially but very difficult to live with – pretending not to want attention, then resentful at not getting it or nasty if one does; expecting others to take an interest in one's problems, and being resentful if they don't.

Physical symptoms alleviated Blinding migraines with zig-zag lines in front of eyes, often brought on by eyestrain, sunlight, travel, crowded public places, emotional trauma, or exercise; migraine headaches which cause sweating; headaches in teenage girls; bursting headaches, or headaches which feel as if inside of head is being attacked by a battery of hammers, often worse between 10 and 11 a.m.; headaches which start at back of head, then radiate all over; left-sided headaches, especially when head is down, alleviated by fresh air; waking up feeling more dead than alive; sensitive scalp; protruding eyes; hot sweaty hands; numb hands; warts on palms of hands; greasy skin; goitre; palpitations and faintness, made worse by lying down; raised blood pressure; anaemia; disorders of the spleen; backache which improves with firm pressure; transparent catarrh; boils in nose; painful spots under nose; nose swollen on one side; cold sores and a higher than normal temperature; cracked lower lip; lips and tongue which feel numb; geographical tongue; hairy tongue; mouth ulcers; increased appetite, or very small appetite; craving for salty foods, fresh milk and beer; aversion to fat, meat, coffee and sour wine; aversion to salt; indigestion, made worse by tobacco; indigestion which is cured by fasting or eating very little; duodenal ulcers which suddenly start to bleed; in women, dry or sore vagina, vaginismus, watery vaginal discharge, amenorrhea caused by stress, shock or grief, irregular periods, feeling unwell just before and just after periods, swollen ankles before periods; bedwetting; constipation, with dry hard stools; an anal fissure which bleeds.

The above symptoms are generally relieved by fresh air, fasting, cold baths, and a firm bed; they tend to worsen around 10 a.m. and in extremely cold or thundery weather, and are not improved by mental or physical exertion, talking, writing, jarring, noise, music, warmth, bright light, hot sun, draughts, seaside air or sympathy.

Complementary remedies Apis, Sepia, Thuja.

Antidoting remedies Arsenicum, Phosphorus.

Natrum sulph.

The source of this remedy is Glauber's salts or sodium sulphate, a constituent of many spa waters and also used as a Tissue Salt (see p. 35).

Constitutional indications Natrum sulph. is especially indicated for people who are pale, tired, ill-looking, and who are sensitive and have been hurt many times.

Mental symptoms alleviated Gloominess and taciturnity; bad temper; emotional turmoil and confusion, often made worse by talking or being spoken to; feeling torn between desire to live and desire to die; suicidal feelings; timidity; anxiety; dreams of running water.

Physical symptoms alleviated Bursting, vice-like headaches at back of head and behind forehead; headaches centred on crown of head; headaches brought on by head injuries; dry mouth, with cracked and blistered lips, ulcers on tongue and palate as if from eating strong spices; copious thin saliva; reluctance to eat; asthma made worse by cold and damp; greenish phlegm; difficulty breathing, especially between 4 and 5 a.m. or on fourth or fifth day of a cold – breathing is not eased by pressure on chest or by warm or wet applications; cough which produces loose phlegm and disturbs sleep, relieved by lying on left side but aggravated by pressure; suddenly sitting up in bed in order to cough up phlegm; pain in left side of chest; empty feeling in chest, with loose phlegm; rheumatic aches and pains on left side; compressed feeling in elbows, especially in damp or stormy weather; tenderness or sharp, stitch-like pains in liver area, aggravated by tight clothing and hot sun; abdomen which rumbles with painful wind, and inability to pass wind; abdominal cramps; bowel movements which oblige one to get out of bed around 5 a.m.; urine scanty and stinging.

The above symptoms are generally relieved by keeping dry and changing position frequently. Damp, cold or wet conditions, sea air, listening to music and lying on left side usually exacerbate symptoms, which tend to be worse in the morning.

Complementary remedies Arsenicum, Thuja.

Nux

From *Nux vomica*, the poison nut tree. The homeopathic remedy is made from the dried, ripe seeds, which contain strychnine, a powerful poison which acts on the central nervous system; in small doses strychnine makes perceptions more vivid and increases production of saliva; in larger doses it causes tetany or muscular spasm, and death from respiratory failure.

Constitutional indications Several physical types respond well to Nux, although self-reliance, efficiency and a liking for hard work tend to be common characteristics, which explains why many *Nux* types are managers, supervisors, or entrepreneurs. Some *Nux* types are well-groomed, hearty, and full of life, others slouch as if they have been up all night; many are thin, prematurely bald, suffer from indigestion and irascibility, and aspire to the finer things of life; complexion may be dry, lined and sallow, with rings under the eyes.

Mental symptoms alleviated Fanatical precision and tidiness; irritability; using anger and violence to dominate others; setting high standards which drive others to distraction; craving respect and admiration; pompous, extravagant talk, never expressing worries or doubts; anxiety, hopelessness, weariness; anger and frustration when things go badly; concern for health of others, but not for own; impulsiveness.

Physical symptoms alleviated Hangovers from too much alcohol; waking up with a thick head, or a head which feels very fragile, or a headache which feels like a nail being driven in above the eyes; 24-hour flu, with shivering and stiff, aching muscles; insomnia, made worse by overwork or abuse of alcohol or narcotics; tickly nose which causes sneezing; sneezing which stops out of doors; blocked nose at night, runny nose during the day; nose which feels hot and sore; uncomfortably dry mouth and thickly coated tongue; difficulty swallowing (food goes down then gets stuck); racking cough, with retching; tickly cough, with pain in larynx; backache relieved by sitting up or turning over in bed; when ill, craving fatty foods and finding bread, meat, coffee and tobacco repugnant; occasional cravings for sour foods; a liking for spirits; being very fussy about freshness of food; liking pungent, spicy foods; indigestion and vomiting; in women, early periods which are prolonged and heavy, irregular periods, tendency to faint just before periods, or periods accompanied by urge to pass water and stools; constipation; diarrhoea after eating juicy fruit, vegetables or rice; abdominal cramps, soothed by heat but aggravated by pressure; colicky pains which cause nausea but wear off when bowels are opened; piles which make rectal contractions painful and ineffectual.

The above symptoms are generally relieved by warmth, sleep, firm pressure and washing or wet applications; they also tend to abate in the evening and when the person is left alone. Cold, wind, dryness, noise, spices, stimulants, narcotics, eating, getting angry and being touched tend to make symptoms worse; symptoms are also worse in winter and between 3 and 4 a.m.

Antidoting remedies Coffea, Ignatia, Cocculus.

Incompatible/inimical remedy Zinc.

Opium

From *Papaver sominiferum*, the opium poppy. The homeopathic remedy is made from the dried milky juice which exudes from the green seed capsules. Heroin, morphine and many other drugs are derivatives of opium, which has a vitality-lowering effect.

Constitutional indications None in particular.

Mental symptoms alleviated Apathy, lack of enthusiasm; not complaining when complaint is justified; over-excitement; fright and after-effects of fright.

Physical symptoms alleviated Strokes; delirium tremens; sneezing; irregular breathing; sweaty or clammy skin.

The above symptoms tend to be aggravated by warmth and get markedly worse during and after sleep; they improve in cold surroundings, especially if one keeps moving.

Antidoting remedies/substances Ipecac, Nux, Passiflora; black coffee.

Phosphoric ac.

This remedy is made from phosphoric acid, whose chief action is on the nervous system. Too much phosphoric acid can cause gastroenteritis.

Constitutional indications Phosphoric ac. has most affinity with children or young people who are growing fast and becoming thin and gangly. It is also indicated in people whose constitution, originally strong, has been undermined by a particularly virulent illness, by excessive loss of body fluids, or by grief or depression. Most Phosphoric ac. types have a mild, yielding temperament.

Mental symptoms alleviated Apathy; indifference to people and surroundings; difficulty understanding what is going on.

Physical symptoms alleviated Headaches which are made worse by noise, especially music; during acute illness, drowsiness or semi-consciousness; weak chest; coughing; profuse, painless diarrhoea which makes one feel better rather than worse.

The above symptoms are not improved by noise, music, strong odours, bad news, cold draughts, wind, snowy air, or by sitting, standing or being touched. They do respond, however, to walking, fresh air, and sleep, even a short nap.

Antidoting remedy Coffea.

Phosphorus

This remedy is made from amorphous phosphorus.

Constitutional indications Phosphorus is most appropriate in thin children who are tall for their age, delicate and desperate for reassurance; if they appear to stare, it is often because they are scared. Adults who respond best to Phosphorus are usually well-proportioned and have a fine skin which blushes easily, but may be dark or fair, with a coppery tinge to the hair; they are intelligent, gregarious and sometimes artistic, but their passions tend to be shortlived and regretted afterwards; they are drawn towards selling, politics and humanitarian endeavours.

Mental symptoms alleviated Nervous tension, especially from overwork; loathing exams and homework; bottling things up, reluctance to talk about problems; indifference to family and friends when ill; wanting to be in the limelight; fear of dark, thunder, being alone, dying; tendency to see catastrophe around every corner; great sensitivity to atmosphere.

Physical symptoms alleviated Headaches which are made worse by heat but wear off after eating or bathing forehead in cold water; dry skin; extremities often feel very hot; poor circulation in fingers, although plunging hands into hot water causes nausea; red, smarting eyes, made worse by bright light and cold air; print appears red and lights have green haloes around them; hearing echoes of own voice; difficulty picking out human voice from other sounds; beads of perspiration on forehead or upper lip, especially in moments of mental or physical stress; heart noticeably affected by emotion, causing palpitations, faintness or a feeling of suffocation; small, weak pulse; profound anaemia; fever, with alternate bouts of sweating and shivering; nosebleeds, brought on by blowing nose; chronic catarrh; dry mouth and stiff tongue with brownish centre; bleeding gums; sensitive larynx, hoarseness, losing voice; dry, tickly cough made worse by talking, laughing and cold air, possibly causing retching and vomiting; rust-coloured phlegm; pneumonia, made worse by lying on bad side or on back; tight feeling in chest or under breastbone, especially after a chill; acute asthma or bronchitis; laboured breathing; respiratory symptoms which improve in a warm atmosphere but worsen lying down or after eating; hiccups; burning pains in region of spine; numbness or loss of co-ordination; cramps; cold knees, especially at night; craving for salty food, meat, ice cream and cold drinks; aversion to sweet things; heartburn, soothed by eating; sensation of pressure in stomach; nausea; peptic ulcer, signalled by mouth filling with saliva; bleeding from lining of stomach, especially in pregnancy; sexual problems which are vividly felt but not resolved; in women, excessive desire for sex.

The above symptoms are generally improved by sleep, friction, fresh air, lying on right side, drinking and being touched. Physical or mental exertion, hot meals and hot drinks, and lying on painful side make matters worse; symptoms are also more marked between sunset and midnight, and in thundery or changeable weather.

Complementary remedies Arsenicum, Allium, Lycopodium, Silicea.

Antidoting remedies Nux.

Incompatible/inimical remedy Causticum.

Phytolacca

From *Phytolacca decandra*, poke root. The homeopathic remedy is made from the fresh leaves or the ripe berries, or in winter from the fresh root. The active principle on which the remedy depends affects the nervous system, the throat, the digestive system and fibrous tissues throughout the body, including the tissue which sheath bones.

Constitutional indications None in particular.

Mental symptoms alleviated Indifference to people and things; expecting to die.

Physical symptoms alleviated Shooting pains which feel like electric shocks; dizziness on standing up from sitting position; pain in eyeballs which seems to improve in open air; desire to clench teeth and gums together; swollen, painful throat which makes swallowing difficult, aggravated by hot drinks, with pain in root of tongue and up eustachian tube into ear – on inspection back of throat looks dry, dark red and congested; stiff neck which hurts if moved and gets worse at night (if Bryonia or Rhus tox. fail); hip pain, relieved by rubbing; nausea relieved by vomiting; in women, breasts which feel stony-hard and painful, but less painful with pressure, or lumpy breasts with

discharge from nipples and pain extending backwards from nipple.

The above symptoms tend to be exacerbated by cold, cold damp rooms, bed warmth, movement and menstruation; they are often worse at night and on the right side of the body.

Antidoting remedies Belladonna, Mezereum.

Incompatible/inimical remedy Mercurius.

Pulsatilla

From *Pulsatilla nigricans*, the pasque flower. The homeopathic remedy is made from the whole plant when it is in flower.

Constitutional indications Children who are small, fair, fine-boned, bright and cheerful, but also shy and sensitive and blush easily respond well to Pulsatilla. So do slightly plumper, darker, more languid children who crave affection but find it difficult to give. Adults who are shy, gentle, fair-skinned or fair-haired, and rather plump also benefit from Pulsatilla. The Pulsatilla type is easily led, easily moulded and rather changeable.

Mental symptoms alleviated Depression; tendency to yield and give way to others; preference for a sheltered life; sympathy with people or animals in distress, sometimes to the point of tears; self-consciousness; longing for attention and affection; obliging others by laughing at their jokes and antics; always wanting someone else in room; fear of death and insanity; little obstinacy or determination; rare anger.

Physical symptoms alleviated Headaches centred above eyes, alleviated by firm pressure, aggravated by indigestion, and worse in evening; fainting, especially in hot stuffy rooms; corneal ulcers, styes or conjunctivitis; fever, with lack of thirst; blocked up nose at night, runny nose during day; yellowish, bland catarrh, better in open air and worse in warm; loss of smell; acute sinusitis; nosebleeds; white, coated tongue and bad taste in mouth; dry mouth and lack of thirst; toothache; pricking sensation in gums, relieved by cold air but aggravated by warmth; dry throat; a loose cough, with greenish phlegm in morning; low back-ache, not improved by movement; flitting joint pains which wear off with exercise and cold applications but get worse with heat; sleeping with hands above head; disturbed sleep due to rich food or overheated bedroom (moderate excercise before bed gives a sound night's sleep); mild anaemia; palpitations; varicose veins; stomach which is tight and tense in morning, and easily upset by rich or fatty food, especially pork; sensation of pressure under breastbone after meals; craving for sweet things; rumbling, gurgling stomach;

in women, thick, creamy, smarting discharge from vagina, late periods, or cessation of periods, especially after shock, acute infection or illness; in both sexes, increased desire for sex; bedwetting; bowels loose, with no two stools alike.

The above symptoms are often relieved by crying, raising the hands above the head, gentle exercise, fresh air and cold drinks or cold applications; sympathy also has a positive effect. Sun, heat, changes in temperature, rich or fatty foods and lying on painful side usually intensify symptoms, which are worse in the evening and at night.

Complementary remedies Coffea, Nux, Chamomilla.

Rhus tox.

From *Rhus toxicodendron*, poison ivy, a North American species. The homeopathic remedy is made from the fresh leaves, which are very poisonous if touched, although some people are immune to them. Traditionally Rhus tox. is used to relieve stiffness, whether physical, mental or emotional.

Constitutional indications None in particular, beyond a lack of flexibility in mind and body.

Mental symptoms alleviated Bursting into tears for no particular reason; restlessness, nervousness and irritability; depression or thoughts of suicide; deriving little enjoyment from senses; great mistrust of, and fear of being poisoned by, drugs and other remedies; dreaming of strenuous physical exercise.

Physical symptoms alleviated Dizzy feeling, as if brain were loose inside head, made worse by walking or standing up; head feels heavy, as if hung over; high temperature, accompanied by delirium and confusion, brought down by sweating; fever brought on by a chill; eczema, in which skin is red, swollen and blistered, and burns and itches; patches of red skin, with clear demarcation line between red areas and unaffected areas; eyes swollen, brimming with painful tears; eyelids stuck together; sensitive scalp; violent throbbing sensation in nose, which is blocked in evening; dry, fissured tongue, brownish with red tip; jaws which make a cracking sound when chewing; teeth which feel loose or too long; bitter taste in mouth; swollen throat; irritating cough, which wears off when talking or singing; stiff, painful muscles which seize up with rest but loosen up with exercise and heat; stiffness in lower back; numbness in arms and legs; stitching pains made worse by cold and damp; craving for cold drinks; nausea and vomiting; drowsiness after eating; in women, early periods, which are heavy and prolonged, or burning pains in vagina, made worse by heat; bedwetting; passing large quantities of urine; frothy, smelly diarrhoea, without abdominal pain; abdominal pain relieved by lying prone.

The above symptoms are generally improved by keeping on the move or changing position frequently, and staying warm and dry. They tend to be aggravated by rest, starting to move after rest, taking clothes off, cold winds and thundery weather; they also intensify at night.

Complementary remedies Bryonia, Calcarea carb., Phytolacca.

Antidoting remedies Anacardium, Croton.

Incompatible/inimical remedies Mezereum, Graphites, Apis.

Ruta

From *Ruta graveolens*, rue, also known as herb-of-grace and herb-of-repentance. The homeopathic remedy is made from the whole fresh plant before it comes into flower. Herbals refer to rue as 'an antidote to all dangerous poisons' and as a defence against witches! In homeopathy Ruta has virtue against restlessness and bruising.

Constitutional indications None in particular.

Mental symptoms alleviated Anxiety; quarrelsomeness, always contradicting people; depression, dissatisfaction with self and others.

Physical symptoms alleviated Headaches due to eyestrain, often brought on by reading fine print and made worse by alcohol; eyes which look red and feel hot; infection of tooth sockets after extraction; weak chest and difficulty breathing, with localized pain over breastbone; tendon injuries and bruised bones; sciatica, often worse at night when lying down; deep aching in the bones; painful bruises; prolapse of rectum, made worse by stooping and crouching; constipation, with large stools which are difficult to pass, alternating with loose stools full of blood and frothy mucus; tearing or stitching pains in rectum.

The symptoms above are generally improved by movement but made worse by cold, damp, rest, and lying down.

Complementary remedy Calcarea phos.

Antidoting remedy Camphora.

Sepia

The source of this remedy is cuttlefish ink. Sepia is used in conditions characterized by stasis, a state of stoppage in which nervous and hormonal impulses seem to be cancelling each other out.

Constitutional indications Those who respond best to Sepia tend to be tall, lean and narrow-hipped, with soft facial features, dark hair, brown eyes shadows under the eyes, and a sallow complexion (sometimes with a yellow-brown saddle across the nose and cheeks). Although they look tired and low-spirited, they perk up with exercise. Women going through the menopause also respond well to Sepia.

Mental symptoms alleviated Indifference, even to loved ones; irritability and snappiness with family and friends, making one difficult to live with, but cordiality with strangers; inability to conceal thoughts, coupled with wish to hide away physically; selfishness, bottled up anger, despair, fear that something dreadful is about to happen; crying when talking about symptoms or illness; physical and mental torpor, despite ability to be the life and soul of the party; being overwhelmed by life and resentful of one's lot; tendency to be greedy and opinionated; tendency to play the martyr.

Physical symptoms alleviated Headaches accompanied by nausea, especially in evening (often relieved by vomiting or wrapping head, but made worse by stuffy rooms, jarring, noise, tobacco, crowded places and menstruation); dizziness which feels like a ball rolling around in the head; baldness; extreme sensitivity to odours; constant catarrh, which tastes salty; throat which is sensitive to the slightest pressure; pale lips, coated tongue and sour taste in mouth; milk and fatty foods cause indigestion, especially in evening; smell of cooking causes nausea; craving for spicy, pungent foods and for wine and vinegar; aching back and sides, relieved by exercise and pressure but made worse by standing; unbearably itchy skin, with patches of brown-yellow discolouration; vitiligo; smelly foot sweats; low blood pressure; palpitations; flushing hot and cold by turns; congested veins; bedwetting in first stage of sleep; in men, sexual problems or exhaustion after sex; flatulence and tenderness in abdomen, relieved by lying on right side; in women, upsets in menstrual cycle, hot flushes during menopause, sagging or prolapsed womb, pain during intercourse, aversion to sex and to being touched.

The above symptoms tend to wear off after food, sleep, exercise or hot applications, and in thundery weather. They are generally made worse by cold, tobacco, mental fatigue and exertion in hot, damp conditions, and are most marked in the early morning, in the evening, in the build-up to a storm and on the left side.

Remedy which follows well Guaiacum.

Complementary remedies Natrum mur., Phosphorus, Nux.

Inimical remedies Lachesis, Pulsatilla.

Silicea

The source of this remedy is flint, which is primarily silica or silicon dioxide, one of the Tissue Salts (see p. 35). Silica is essential for growth and bone development, is present in connective tissue, and helps to keep cartilage flexible and skin permeable.

Constitutional indication Silicea is of most benefit to children who are puny and lacking in stamina, especially if they have a rather large, sweaty head, delicate skin, sandy hair, blue eyes and small hands and feet. Such children tend to be very lively and friendly, angels if managed properly but devils if they are not. Intellectual adults also benefit from it.

Mental symptoms alleviated Feeling pushed around and taking frustration out on subordinates; self doubts, lack of confidence and assertiveness, fear of failure; overworking or being over-conscientious to point of exhaustion; obstinacy and tenacity balanced by sense of fun, ready wit, gentleness and flashes of courage; occasional spitefulness, especially over small things; disturbed sleep when under stress.

Physical symptoms alleviated Right-sided migraines, worse around midday but relieved by pressure; headaches which are relieved by urination but made worse by mental or physical exertion (pain starts at back of head and extends over one eye); tinnitus; glue ear; sore lower eyelids; chronic catarrh, with cracked skin at side of nose; stuttering; aversion to meat, and to hot foods because they cause sweating; thirst; profuse perspiration, with very smelly feet; unhealthy-looking skin, with spots or pimples; fingers which go dead and icy cold in winter; poor nails with hard skin around them, which tends to split; lack of push when passing stools, so stools slip back inside rectum.

The symptoms above are generally aggravated by lying on the left side, getting pins and needles, undressing, washing and bathing and sudden cessation or suppression of sweat. They also tend to be worse in the morning, in damp or draughty conditions, in cold windy weather, and when the moon is new. Matters often improve in the summer, and in wet or damp conditions; the head needs to be wrapped up well.

Complementary remedies Thuja, Sanicula, Pulsatilla, Fluoric ac.

Incompatible/inimical remedy Mercurius.

Spongia

This remedy is prepared from the common sponge, toasted. The active constituents of sponge are iodine and bromine, which in excessive amounts irritate and inflame the larynx, trachea, thyroid gland, heart and testicles.

Constitutional indications Spongia is most effective in people who are light-haired, blue-eyed, lean and rather dried-up looking. It is especially good if tuberculosis or chest complaints run in the family.

Mental symptoms alleviated Anxiety, apprehension, fear of dying.

Physical symptoms alleviated General feeling of heaviness and exhaustion, with rushes of blood to chest, neck and face; colds which begin with a tickly throat, which is very sensitive to touch; congested feeling in larynx; hoarseness, with sore, burning sensation in larynx; enlarged thyroid gland; dry mucous membranes; dry, sibilant cough which sounds like a saw grating through a plank of wood, made worse by sweating and cold drinks; croup, with marked wheezing during intakes of breath, although chest is clear on examination; waking from sleep feeling as if one is suffocating; palpitations, especially around midnight and during menstruation.

The above symptoms cause most discomfort when talking, swallowing, moving about, lying with the head lower than the feet and touching affected areas; they also tend to be worst around midnight. Warm food, warm drinks and sitting up usually produce some improvement.

Complementary remedies Aconite, Hepar sulph.

Antidoting remedy Camphora.

Staphysagria

From *Delphinium staphysagria*, stavesacre or palmated larkspur. The homeopathic remedy is made from the seeds, which contain a substance used to kill head lice.

Constitutional indications Those who benefit most from Staphysagria tend to suppress their emotions, especially when they are in love. Though mild and gentle on the surface, there is often great emotional turmoil underneath.

Mental symptoms alleviated Bottled up anger, which tends to make other symptoms worse; impatience, spitefulness; a tendency to dwell on old insults; easily wounded by words; melancholy.

Physical symptoms alleviated Stupefying headache (the 'head-full-of-lead' feeling), made worse by yawning or by excessive sexual activity; styes or lumps on eyelids; bursting pain in eyeballs; itching above and behind ears; toothaches which are aggravated by biting, chewing or touching affected tooth, especially during menstruation; cuts and surgical incisions; eczema; ravenous appetite, even when stomach is full; nausea after abdominal operations; craving for tobacco;

urogenital problems, especially after first intercourse – cystitis, painful stretching of vagina.

The symptoms above generally improve with warmth, or after breakfast or a good night's sleep. Anger, indignation, self-denial, grief, sexual excess and being touched, especially on affected parts, tend to make symptoms worse; smoking and dehydration are also aggravating.

Complementary remedies Causticum, Colocynth.

Antidoting remedies Camphora.

Incompatible/inimical remedy Ranunculus.

Sulphur

This remedy is made from flowers of sulphur. Medicinally, sulphur is a purgative and increases the production of urea (from the breakdown of protein) in the liver. It is also a constituent of albumin and epithelial tissue. At one time sulphur was extensively used to treat rheumatism.

Constitutional indications Sulphur is most beneficial to people who have small, red-rimmed eyes and long lashes, a rather dirty-looking complexion, a lean body and stooping shoulders. It may also be appropriate for small, scrawny individuals, or for those who are ruddy-faced and full-bodied. The Sulphur type also tends to be egotistical, a would-be intellectual, a dabbler in philosophy.

Mental symptoms alleviated Shiftless, lazy, couldn't-care-less attitude; lack of energy and willpower; tendency to live by wits rather than hard work; liking to get one's own way; tendency towards melancholy, self-pity, hypochondria; finding crude talk or behaviour distasteful; always professing readiness to help others; daydreaming; dabbling in too many projects at a time and tending to lose heart; suddenly becoming awkward, indecisive and having difficulty understanding what is going on; tendency to wake around 3 a.m.

Physical symptoms alleviated Headaches which are made worse by fresh air but wear off in warm rooms; hair which is glossy but falls out; dry, scaly skin and scalp; skin which looks dirty even though clean; occasional sweating; palms of hands and soles of feet burning hot (bedclothes may be thrown off at night to cool feet); patches of itchy red skin made worse by warmth, washing or scratching; conjunctivitis or red eyes; chronic greenish catarrh; sensitivity to bad smells; coughing which often ends with sneezing; sore, burning lips; suddenly becoming hot and flushed in the face; giddiness and flushing, especially on getting out of bed in morning; suffocating feeling, especially at night; oppressive, burning sensation in chest, with shooting pains in back, made worse by deep breathing or lying on back; tendency to regurgitate food; irregular meals and ravenous appetite for all the wrong things (fat, salt, sugar, spicy foods, spirits), especially around 11 a.m. and 11 p.m.; acid stomach and vomiting; sinking feeling in stomach, worse around 11 a.m.; frequent thirst; hypoglycaemia; low back pain, spreading to groin; stiff joints which make a cracking noise; muscle cramps, made worse by bathing; chronic diarrhoea, worse around 5 a.m., and inflammation around anus; anal fissures.

The above symptoms are generally improved by fresh air, staying warm and dry, or lying on the right side. Immobility, prolonged standing, too many clothes, damp cold, washing, being too warm in bed and drinking alcohol often aggravate matters; symptoms also tend to be worse in the morning and at night, exhibiting a 12-hour cycle.

Complementary remedies Aconite, Aloe, Nux, Psorinum.

Antidoting remedies Camphora, Chamomilla, China, Mercurius, Rhus tox., Sepia, Thuja.

Tarentula
This source of this remedy is *Lycosa tarentula*, a large black spider found in Southern Europe. Its bite was reputed to cause tarantism or dancing mania. The homeopathic remedy is made from the whole live spider and is traditionally used to relieve conditions in which frantic, tormented behaviour is the chief characteristic.

Constitutional indications None in particular.

Mental symptoms alleviated Sudden mood changes; laughter and gaiety which suddenly turn to spitefulness and destructiveness; incredibly quick, foxy reactions; extreme restlessness, wanting everything immediately, never waiting in queues; constant need to busy oneself.

Physical symptoms alleviated Inability to keep still; restless legs, made worse by walking; dizziness; numbness; in women, pruritis vulvae.

The above symptoms are made worse by noise, walking, being touched and seeing other people in trouble. Bright colours, music and open air usually make things better.

Antidoting remedy Lachesis

Thuja
From *Thuja occidentalis, arbor vitae* or tree of life The homeopathic remedy is made from the fresh green twigs, which contain a substance which affects the concentration of salt, water and electrolytes in the body. Thuja is most appropriate where areas of pain are small and localized.

Constitutional indications Thuja is most beneficial in people who have a greasy skin and take little interest in their appearance, especially if they are also unattractive, deceitful and manipulative. Small, fine-boned children who are slightly backward or have difficulty expressing themselves also respond well to Thuja.

Mental symptoms alleviated Paranoia (feeling that one is under someone else's influence or always in their presence); reluctance to talk; being very sensitive, easily wounded, often moved to tears by music; conscientiousness; physical activity makes thoughts and emotions less intense; restless sleep, especially on moonlit nights, talking in sleep, dreaming of dead people or of falling.

Physical symptoms alleviated Headaches brought on by overtiredness, overexcitement or stress; chronic greenish-yellow catarrh; clean red tongue; tooth decay; inflamed and swollen gums; asthma; inflamed and swollen joints; brittle bones; warts which weep or bleed; greasy or pale, waxy skin, with exposed areas inclined to sweat; perspiration which smells offensive and stains clothes yellow; left side of body feels cold; fair hair which extends down spine; lack of appetite early in the day; indigestion caused by drinking tea; urinary infections; in women, vaginal and uterine infections, scanty or early periods, severe period pains centred over left ovary, or miscarriages; soft, pale, greasy stools, and grumbling, gurgling bowels.

The symptoms above are generally aggravated by damp cold, vaccination, sunlight and bright lights, bed warmth, fatty foods and coffee; they also tend to be worse on the left side, at night and at the beginning of the day or just after breakfast, and when the moon is waxing. Drawing up the limbs or lying on the affected side often improves matters.

Complementary remedies Sabina, Arsenicum, Natrum sulph., Silicea.

Antidoting remedies Mercurius, Camphora.

Urtica
From *Urtica urens*, the small stinging nettle. The homeopathic remedy is made from the fresh plant when it is in flower. As the old rhyme says, *a propos* of nettles: 'Cut them in June, come back again soon. Cut them in July and you cut them down truly.' Urtica is traditionally used to alleviate conditions accompanied by burning or scalding sensations.

Constitutional indications Urtica is especially helpful to people who suffer from gout or high uric acid levels.

Mental symptoms alleviated None in particular.

Physical symptoms alleviated Rheumatic pain; neuritis and neuralgia; itchy or blotchy skin, or skin which is hot and blistered; in women, lack of breast milk, or pruritis vulvae.

The symptoms above are generally made worse by touch, cold damp air, water, and snow.

Antidoting substance Dock leaves.

Veratrum

From *Veratrum album*, white hellebore. The homeopathic remedy is made from the roots just before the plant comes into flower, and is traditionally used in cases of collapse, where there is profuse cold sweating.

Constitutional indications None in particular.

Mental symptoms alleviated Excitement, excessive enthusiasm; being overcritical; tendency to brood in silence, but hating to be left alone; melancholy, fear of dying.

Physical symptoms alleviated Extremely cold, sweaty skin, perhaps with a bluish tinge; weak, rapid pulse; violent reactions to pain; muscles which feel weak or paralysed; cramps in calves; extreme thirst; heavy vomiting; cramping pains in abdomen, accompanied by violent diarrhoea.

The above symptoms are often relieved by warmth and by walking, but aggravated by damp cold, drinking, opening bowels, or becoming frightened; they are often worse at night.

Antidoting remedies Camphora, Aconite, China, Staphysagria.

USEFUL ADDRESSES

Many of the organizations listed below have regional or local branches whose addresses and telephone numbers can be obtained from your local library or Citizens Advice Bureau. They will also be listed in your local Yellow Pages telephone directory, usually under 'Charitable & benevolent organisations', or 'Disabled – amenities and information', or 'Social service & welfare organisations'. The Samaritans and Alcoholics Anonymous are always listed in the local information section at the front of residential and business telephone directories.

Where no telephone number is given, please write. If you are requesting leaflets or printed information, do send a stamped, addressed envelope.

SPECIFIC DISORDERS

For more information about national organizations concerned with various diseases and handicaps contact:

The Patients Association, Room 33, 18 Charing Cross Road, London WC2H 0HR, tel 071-240 0671 and ask for their booklet *Self-Help and the Patient*, price £2.95 (post free).

AAA (Action Against Allergy), 43 The Downs, London SW20 8HG, tel 081-947 5082

National Ankylosing Spondylitis Society, 6 Grosvenor Crescent, London SW1X 7ER, tel 071-235 9585

Anorexic Aid, *(support and information for anorexics and their families),* The Priory Centre, 11 Priory Road, High Wycombe, Bucks. HP13 6SL, tel 0494 21431

Arthritic Association, 122 Three Bridges Road, Crawley, West Sussex RH10 1JP, tel 0293 22041

Arthritis Care (formerly British Rheumatism and Arthritis Association), 6 Grosvenor Crescent, London SW1X 7ER, tel 071-235 0902/5

Asthma Society and Friends of Asthma Research Council, 300 Upper Street, London N1 2XX, tel 071-226 2260

Back Pain Association, 31-33 Park Road, Teddington, Middlesex TW11 0AB, tel 081-977 5474/5

Royal National Institute for the Blind (RNIB), 224 Great Portland Street, London W1N 6AA, tel 071-388 1266

Cancer Contact, *(group for sufferers and ex-sufferers interested in exploring 'gentle treatment' of cancer),* Organiser: 6 Meadows, Hassocks, W. Sussex BN6 8EH, tel 07918 4754

Cancer Help Centre, Grove House, Cornwallis Grove, Clifton, Bristol BA8 4PG, tel 0272 743216

International Cerebral Palsy Society, 5A Netherhall Gardens, London NW3 5RN, tel 071-794 9761

Chest, Heart and Stroke Association, Tavistock House North, Tavistock Square, London WC1H 9JE, tel 071-387 3012/3/4

Coeliac Society of the United Kingdom, P.O. Box 181, London NW2 2QY, tel 081-459 2440

National Association for Colitis and Crohn's Disease (NACC), 98a London Road, St Albans, Herts. AL1 1NX

Coronary Prevention Group, 60 Great Ormond Street, London WC1N 3HR, tel 071-833 3687

Royal National Institute for the Deaf (RNID), 105 Gower Street, London WC1E 6AH, tel 071-387 8033

Depressives Associated, P.O. Box 5, Castletown, Portland, Dorset DT5 1BQ

British Diabetic Association, 10 Queen Anne Street, London W1M 0BD, tel 071-323 1531

British Dyslexia Association, Church Lane, Peppard, Oxfordshire RG9 5JN, tel 049 17699

National Eczema Society, Tavistock House North, Tavistock Square, London WC1H 9SR, tel 071-388 4097

Endometriosis Society, 65 Holmdene Avenue, Herne Hill, London SE24 9LD, tel 071-737 4764

British Epilepsy Association, 40 Hanover Square, Leeds LS3 1BE, tel 0532 439 393

Friedreich's Ataxia Group, Burleigh Lodge, Knowle Lane, Cranleigh, Surrey GU6 8RD, tel 0483 272741

Guillain Barre Syndrome Support Group, Foxley, Holdingham, Sleaford, Lincs. NG34 8NR, tel 0529 304615

Haemophilia Society, P.O. Box 9, 16 Trinity Street, London SE1 1DE, tel 071-407 1010

Headway – National Head Injuries Association, 200 Mansfield Road, Nottingham NG1 3HX, tel 0602 622383

Herpes Association, 41 North Road, London N7 9DP, tel 071-609 9061

British Kidney Patient Association (BKPA), Bordon, Hampshire, GU35 9JZ, tel 04203 2021/2

Lupus Group, *(support for sufferers from systemic lupus erythematosus)*, 6 Grosvenor Crescent, London SW1X 7ER, tel 071-235 0902/5

MENCAP (Royal Society for Mentally Handicapped Children and Adults), MENCAP National Centre, 123 Golden Lane, London EC1Y 0RT, tel 071-253 9433

British Migraine Association, 178a High Road, Byfleet, Weybridge, Surrey KT14 7ED, tel 0932 52468

Migraine Trust, 45 Great Ormond Street, London WC1N 3HD, tel 071-278 2676

Motor Neurone Disease Association, 61 Derngate, Northampton NN1 1VE, tel 0604 22269/250505

Action for Research into Multiple Sclerosis (ARMS), 4a Chapel Hill , Stansted, Essex CM24 8AG, tel 0279 815553 or 081-568 2255 (counselling service)

Multiple Sclerosis Society of Great Britain and Northern Ireland, 25 Effie Road, London SW6 1EE, tel 071-736 6267

Muscular Dystrophy Group of Great Britain and Northern Ireland, Nattrass House, 35 Macaulay Road, Clapham, London SW4 0QP, tel 071-720 8055

Myalgic Encephalomyelitis Association, P.O. Box 8, Stanford-le-Hope, Essex SS17 8EX, tel 0375 642466

National Association for the Relief of Paget's Disease, 413 Middleton Road, Manchester M24 4QZ, tel 061 643 1998

Intractable Pain Society of Great Britain and Ireland, Pain Relief Clinic, Basingstoke District Hospital, Aldermaston Road, Basingstoke, Hants. RG24 9NA, tel 0256 473202

Parkinson's Disease Society, 36 Portland Place, London W1N 3DG, tel 071-323 1174

National Society for Phenylketonuria (PKU) and Allied Disorders, Worth Cottage, Lower Scholes, Pickels Hill, Keighley, West Yorkshire BD22 0RR, tel 0535 44865

Phobics Society, 4 Cheltenham Road, Chorlton-cum-Hardy, Manchester M21 1QN, tel 061 881 1937

National Association for Premenstrual Syndrome, 25 Market Street, Guildford, Surrey GU1 4LB, tel 0483 572715 or 0483 572806 (daytime helpline)

Premenstrual Advisory Service, P.O. Box 268, Hove, Sussex, tel 0273 771366

Psoriasis Association, 7 Milton Street, Northampton NN2 7JG, tel 0604 711129

Raynaud's Association Trust, 40 Bladon Crescent, Alsager, Cheshire ST7 2BG, tel 09363 5167

Schizophrenia Association of Great Britain, International Schizophrenia Centre, Bryn Hyfryd, The Crescent, Bangor, Gwynedd LL57 2AG, tel 0248 354042

National Association for Sickle Cell Anaemia Research (OSCAR), 200A High Road, Wood Green, London N22 4HH, tel 081-889 4844/3300

Spastics Society, 12 Park Crescent, London W1N 4EQ, tel 071-636 5020

Spinal Injuries Association, Yeoman House, 76 St James's Lane, London N10 3DF, tel 081-444 2121

UK Thalassaemia Society, 107 Nightingale Lane, London N8 7QY, tel 081-348 0437

British Tinnitus Association, c/o Royal National Institute for the Deaf, 105 Gower Street, London WC1E 6AH, tel 071-387 8033

CHILDREN AND PARENTS

National Autistic Society, 276 Willesden Lane, London NW2 5RB, tel 081-451 1114

Research Group 'Fund' for Autists, 49 Orchard Avenue, Shirley, Croydon, Surrey CR0 7NE, tel 081-777 0095

Children's Cancer Help Centre, 14 Kingsway, Petts Wood, Orpington, Kent BR5 1PR, tel 0689 35455

National Childbirth Trust, *(preparation for birth and parenthood)*, 9 Queensborough Terrace, London W2 3TB, tel 071-221 3833

Foundation for the Study of Infant Deaths, Cot Death Research and Support, 15 Belgrave Square, London SW1X 8PS, tel 071-235 1721/0965

CRY-SIS, *(support group for parents of babies who cry excessively)*, BM-CRY-SIS, London WC1N 3XX, tel 071-404 0501

Cystic Fibrosis Trust, Alexandra House, 5 Blyth Riad, Bromley, Kent BR1 3RS, tel 081-464 7211

National Deaf Children's Society, 45 Hereford Road, London W2 5AH, tel 071-229 9272/4

Down's Syndrome Association, 1st Floor, 12-13 Clapham Common South Side, London SW4 7AA, tel 071-720 0008

Foresight (Association for the Promotion of Preconceptual Care), The Old Vicarage, Church Lane, Witley, Godalming, Surrey GU8 5PN, tel 042879 4500

Hyperactive Children's Support Group, 59 Meadowside, Angmering, Nr. Littlehampton, West Sussex BN16 4BW, tel 0903 725182

La Leche League of Great Britain, *(breastfeeding advice and information)*, BM 3424, London WC1V 6XX, tel 071-242 1278

Association for Improvements in the Maternity Services (AIMS), 163 Liverpool Road, London N1 0RF, tel 071-278 5628

National Council for One-Parent Families, 255 Kentish Town Road, London NW5 2AB, tel 071-267 1361

National Society for the Prevention of Cruelty to Children (NSPCC), 67 Saffron Hill, London EC1N 8RS, tel 071-242 1626

Association of Child Psychologists, Burg House, New End Square, London NW3 1LT, tel 071-794 8881

Association for Spina Bifida and Hydrocephalus, 22 Upper Woburn Place, London WC1H 0EP, tel 071-388 1382

Association of Parents of Vaccine Damaged Children, 2 Church Street, Shipton-on-Stour, Warwickshire CV36 4AP, tel 0608 61595

ADDICTION

Action on Smoking and Health (ASH), 27 Mortimer Street, London W1N 7RH, tel 071-637 9843

Al-Anon Family Groups UK and Eire, *(support for relatives and friends of alcoholics)*, 305 Gray's Inn Road, London WC1X 8QF, tel 071-833 3471

Alcoholics Anonymous, P.O. Box 514, 11 Redcliffe Gardens, London SW10 9BQ, tel 071-352 9779

Families Anonymous, *(support for families and friends of drug abusers)*, 88 Caledonian Road, London N7 9DN, tel 071-278 8805

Gamblers Anonymous, 17/23 Blantyre Street, London SW10 0DT, tel 071-352 3060 (24-hour service)

Narcotics Anonymous, *(support for those wishing to come off drugs)*, P.O. Box 246, London SW10 0DP, tel 071-351 6794/6066/6067

Release, *(advice and referral for those with drug-related problems)*, 347a Upper Street, London N1 0PD, tel 071-837 5602 (office hours) or 071-603 8654 (24-hour emergency service)

SCODA (Standing Committee on Drug Abuse), 1-4 Hatton Place, Hatton Garden, London EC1N 8ND, tel 071-430 2341

TRANX (Tranquillizer Recovery and New Existence), *(support for those wishing to come off medically* *prescribed minor tranquilizers)*, 17 Peel Road, Harrow, Middlesex HA3 7QX, tel 081-427 2065

The DHSS publishes various leaflets designed to help drug abusers and their families. These should be available from your local Health Authority (see local Yellow Pages telephone directory under 'Health Authorities & services') or you can obtain them direct by writing to:

DHSS Leaflets Unit, *(drug misuse)*, Dept. DM, P.O. Box 21, Stanmore, Middlesex HA7 1AY

DHSS Leaflets Unit, *(solvent abuse)*, Department M50S 13–39 Standard Road, London NW10 6DF

OTHER PROBLEMS

Albany Trust, *(counselling for sexual and relationship problems)*, 24 Chester Square, London SW1W 9HS, tel 071-730 5871

Body Positive, *(support and advice for people who are HIV positive)*, BM AIDS, London WC1N 3XX, tel 071-833 2971

Brook Advisory Centres, *(national network for young people, offering birth control advice, confidential pregnancy testing, and abortion counselling)*, 153a East Street, London SE17 2SD, tel 071-708 1234

National Association of Citizens' Advice Bureaux, Myddelton House, 115-123 Pentonville Road, London N1 9LZ, tel 071-833 2181

Counsel and Care for the Elderly, *(advice and information for elderly people)*, 131 Middlesex Street, London E1 7JF, tel 071-621 1624

Cruse, The National Organisation for the Widowed and their Children, *(support for the bereaved)*, Cruse House, 126 Sheen Road, Richmond, Surrey TW9 1UR, tel 081-940 4818/9047

Disabled Living Foundation, 380-384 Harrow Road, London W9 2HU, tel 071-289 6111

Family Planning Association, *(advice and information on all aspects of sexuality, birth control, and sexual problems)*, 27-35 Mortimer Street, London W1N 7RJ, tel 071-636 7866

Terence Higgins Trust, *(help and support for AIDS sufferers and for those who are HIV positive)*, BM AIDS, London WC1N 3XX, tel 071-833 2971

Medic-Alert Foundation, *(Medic-Alert emblem warns police, ambulance and medical services that wearer has a*

hidden medical condition that may affect emergency care), 11-13 Clifton Terrace, London N4 3JP, tel 071-263 8596

British Pregnancy Advisory Service, *(advice on birth control and pregnancy, pregnancy testing, abortion counselling)*, Austy Manor, Wootten Wawen, Solihull, West Midlands B95 6BX, tel 056 42 3225

Rape Crisis Centre, *(counselling, and medical and legal help, for victims of rape or sexual assault – women only)*, P.O. Box 69, London WC1X 9NJ, tel 071-278 3956 or 071-837 1600 (24-hour emergency service)

RELATE (formerly National Marriage Guidance Council), Herbert Gray College, Little Church Street, Rugby CV21 3AP, tel 0788 73241

Health and Safety Executive, *(advice and information on safety in the workplace)*, Baynard's House, 1-13 Chepstow Place, London W2 4TF, tel 071-229 3456

Samaritans, *(help for the suicidal or despairing – telephones at local branches are staffed 24 hours a day, 7 days a week; see local information section at front of local residential or business telephone directory for telephone number)*, 17 Uxbridge Road, Slough SL1 1SN, tel 75 32713 (administrative enquiries only)

Sanity, *(research into nutritional and biochemical factors in mental illness)*, 63 Cole Park Road, Twickenham, Middlesex TW1 1HT

SPOD – Association to aid the Sexual and Personal Relationships of People with a Disability, 286 Camden Road, London N7 0BJ, tel 071-607 8851

Vegan Society, 33-35 George Street, Oxford, Oxon OX1 2AY, tel 0865 722166

Vegetarian Society, Parkdale, Dunham Road, Altrincham, Cheshire WA14 4QG, tel 061 928 0793

Weight Watchers, 11-12 Fairacres, Dedworth Road, Windsor, Berkshire SL4 4UY, tel 07535 856751

Women's Health Concern, Flat 17, Earls Terrace, London W8 6LP, tel 071-602 6669

CLINICS

Marigold Treatment Centre, *(homeopathic chiropody clinic)*, 134 Montrose Avenue, Edgeware, Middlesex HA8 0DR, tel 081-959 5421

Midlands Asthma and Allergy Research Clinic, 12 Vernon Street, Derby DE1 1ST, tel 0332 362461

Anthroposophical Medical Treatment Centre, Park Attwood Therapeutic Centre, Trimpley, Bewdley, Worcestershire DY12 1RE, tel 02997 444

Wholistic Research Company, (*evaluates and markets equipment designed to make home environment healthier*), Bright Haven, Robins Lane, Lolworth, Cambridge CB3 8HH, tel 0954 81074

COMPLEMENTARY MEDICINE

Information about acupuncture, chiropractic, homeopathy, medical herbalism, naturopathy, and osteopathy can be obtained from:

Council for Complementary and Alternative Medicine (CCAM), Suite 1, 19a Cavendish Square, London W1M 9AD, tel 071-409 1440

Information about other complementary and alternative therapies, in addition to those mentioned above, can be obtained from:

Institute for Complementary Medicine (ICM), 21 Portland Place, London W1N 3AF, tel 071-636 9543

Postal enquiries, enclosing a large stamped, self-addressed envelope, would be appreciated. Both CCAM and ICM keep lists of skilled practitioners and also monitor training standards and qualifications.

Information can also be obtained from the organizations listed below, although it should be emphasized that for reasons of space this list is not comprehensive. By including some organizations and not others no recommendation or criticism is intended. Where no telephone number is given, postal contact is preferred.

British Acupuncture Association and Register, 34 Alderney Street, London SW1V 4EV, tel 071-834 1012

College of Traditional Chinese Acupuncture, Tao House, Queensway, Leamington Spa, Warwickshire CV32 5EZ, tel 0926 39347

Council for Acupuncture, Suite 1, 19a Cavendish Square, London W1M 9AD, tel 071-409 1440

Medical Acupuncture Society, 15 Devonshire Place, London W1N 1PB, tel 071-935 7575

Traditional Acupuncture Society, 1 The Ridgeway, Stratford-on-Avon, Warwickshire CV37 9JI, tel 0789 298798

International Register of Oriental Medicine (UK), Green Hedges House, Green Hedges Avenue, East Grinstead, East Sussex RH19 1DZ, tel 0342 313106/7

Register of Traditional Chinese Medicine, 7A Thorndean Street, London SW18 4HE, tel 081-947 1879

Society of Teachers of the Alexander Technique, 10 London House, 266 Fulham Road, London SW10 9EL, tel 071-351 0828

Alternative Sitting, P.O. Box 19, Chipping Norton, Oxfordshire OX7 6NY, tel 060871 8875

Association of Tisserand Aromatherapists, P.O. Box 746, Brighton, East Sussex BN1 3BN, tel 0273 204214 or 0865 56262

International Federation of Aromatherapists, 46 Dalkeith Road, London SE21 8LS

British Association for Autogenic Training and Therapy, 101 Harley Street, London W1N 1DF, tel 071-935 1811

Bates Association of Eyesight Training, 128 Merton Road, London SW18 5SP. Send an SAE for more information

Candida Albicans Advice Group, P.O. Box 89, East Grinstead, West Sussex RH19 1YY

British Chiropractic Association, 5 First Avenue, Chelmsford, Essex CM1 1RX, tel 0245 358487

National Federation of Spiritual Healers, Old Manor Farm Studio, Church Street, Sunbury-on-Thames, Middlesex TW16 6RG, tel 0932 783164

National Institute of Medical Herbalists, 41 Hatherley Road, Winchester, Hampshire SO22 6RR, tel 0962 68776

British Society of Medical and Dental Hypnosis, 42 Links Road, P.O. Box 6, Ashstead, Surrey KT21 2HT, tel 03722 73522

European Society of Medical Hypnosis, 3 Troy Road, Morely, Leeds LS27 8JJ, tel 0532 533494

Association of Hypnotists and Psychotherapists, 25 Market Square, Nelson, Lancs BB9 7LP, tel 02822 699378

UK College of Hypnotherapy and Counselling, 10 Alexander Street, London W2 5NT, tel 071-727 2006 and 071-221 1796

British Register of Iridologists, 6 Gold Street, Saffron Walden, Essex CB10 1EJ, tel 0799 26138

National Council and Register of Iridologists, 80 Portland Road, Bournemouth, Dorset BH9 1NQ, tel 0202 529793

Northern Institute of Massage, 100 Waterloo Road, Blackpool, Lancs FY4 1AW, tel 0253 403548

West London School of Therapeutic Massage, 41 St Luke's Road, London W11 1DD, tel 071-229 4672

British Naturopathic and Osteopathic Association, 6 Netherhall Gardens, London NW3 5RR, tel 071-435 8728

British Society for Nutritional Medicine, P. O. Box 3AP, London W1A 3AP, tel 071-637 1561

Institute for Optimum Nutrition, 5 Jerdon Place, London SW6 1BE, tel 071-385 7984

British Dental Society for Clinical Nutrition, Flat 1, Welbeck House, 62 Welbeck Street, London W1M 7HB, tel 071-486 3127

Centre for Nutritional Studies, 21 Upton Close, Henley-on-Thames, Oxon RG9 1BT, tel 0491 572435

Nutritional Eye Health Centre, Sanctuary House, Oulton Road, Oulton, Norfolk NR32 4QZ, tel 0502 83294

General Council and Register of Osteopaths, 1-4 Suffolk Street, London SW1Y 4HG, tel 071-839 2060

British Osteopathic Association, 8-10 Euston Place, London NW1 6QH, tel 071-262 5250

College of Osteopaths, 110 Thorkhill Road, Thames Ditton, Surrey KT7 0UW, tel 081-398 3308

Chartered Society of Physiotherapy, 14 Bedford Row, London WC1R 4ED, tel 071-242 1941

London and Counties Society of Physiologists, 100 Waterloo Road, Blackpool, Lancs. FY4 1AW, tel 0253 403548

British Association for Counselling, *(information about counselling services for personal relationship and psychosexual problems)*, 37a Sheep Street, Rugby CV21 3BC, tel 0788 78328

British Association of Psychotherapists, 12 Hendon Lane, London N3 3PR, tel 081-346 1747

Institute for Group Analysis, 1 Daleham Gardens, London NW3 5BY, tel 071-431 2693

Institute of Psychoanalysis, 63-65 New Cavendish Street, London W1M 7RD, tel 071-580 4952

Society of Analytical Psychology, 1 Daleham Gardens, London NW3 5BY, tel 071-435 7696

London Centre for Psychotherapy, *(counselling and individual or group psychotherapy at moderate fees)*, 274 Upper Street, London N1 2UA, tel 071-359 7371

Association of Reflexologists, 37 Standale Grove, Ruislip, Middlesex HA4 7UA , tel 0895 635621

British Reflexology Association, 12 Pond Road, London SE3 9JL, tel 081-852 60602

International Institute of Reflexology, 28 Hollyfield Avenue, Friern Barnet, London N11 3BY, tel 081-368 0865

College of Reflexology, 9 Mead Road, Shenley, Radlett, Herts WD7 9DA, tel 09276 7192

Shiatsu Society, 19 Langside Park, Kilbarchan, Renfrewshire PA10 2EP, tel 05057 4657

Yoga for Health Foundation, Ickwell Bury, Ickwell Green, Nr. Biggleswade, Beds. SG18 9EF, tel 0767 27271

British Wheel of Yoga, 80 Leckhampton Road, Cheltenham, Glos. GL53 0BN

HOMEOPATHY
If you are looking for a homeopathic practitioner in your area, or want to know where the nearest homeopathic pharmacy is, the following organizations will be pleased to help you.

Homoeopathic Development Foundation, 19A Cavendish Square, London W1M 9AD, tel 071-629 3205

The Faculty of Homoeopathy, The Royal London Homoeopathic Hospital, Great Ormond Street, London WC1N 3HR, tel 071-837 3091 ext. 85 or 72

The British Homoeopathic Association, 27a Devonshire Street, London WC1N 1RJ, tel 071-935 2163

The Hahnemann Society, Hahnemann House, 2 Powis Place, Great Ormond Street, London WC1 3HT, tel 071-837 3297/278 7900

Society of Homoeopaths, *(has register of non-medically qualified homeopaths)*, 2 Artizan Road, Northampton NN1 4HU, tel 0604 21400

Homeopaths who are GPs and working as family doctors within the National Health Service can refer patients to consultants in the following NHS homeopathic hospitals:

Bristol Homoeopathic Hospital, Cotham Road, Cotham, Bristol BS6 6JU, tel 0272 731231

Glasgow Homoeopathic Hospital, 100 Great Western Road, Glasgow G12 0RN, tel 041 339 0382

Department of Homoeopathic Medicine, Mossley Hill Hospital, Park Avenue, Liverpool L18 8BU, tel 051 724 2335

The Royal London Homoeopathic Hospital, Great Ormond Street, London WC1N 3HR, tel 071-837 8833 (071-837 7821 for appointments)

Tunbridge Wells Homoeopathic Hospital, Church Road, Tunbridge Wells, Kent TN1 1JU, tel 0892 42977

Most chemists and healthfood shops stock a limited range of homeopathic remedies. For the full range of remedies, however, one has to go to a specialized pharmacy or direct to the manufacturer. All products can be supplied by post.

Ainsworths, 38 New Cavendish Street, London W1M 7LH, tel 071-935 5330

Buxton and Grant, 176 Whiteladies Road, Bristol BS8 2XU, tel 0272 735025

Galen Pharmacy, 1 South Terrace, South Street, Dorchester, Dorset DT1 1DE, tel 0305 63996

Goulds, 14 Crowndale Road, London NW1 1TT, tel 071-388 4752 or 071-387 1888

Nelson's Pharmacies Ltd, 73 Duke Street, London W1M 6BY, tel 071-629 3118

A Nelson & Co., *(licensed manufacturer)*, 5 Endeavour Way, London SW19 9UH, tel 081-946 8527

Weleda (UK) Ltd, *(licensed manufacturer)*, Heanor Road, Ilkeston, Derbyshire DE7 8DR, tel 0602 303151

Phials, storage boxes, unmedicated tablets and other homeopathic supplies can be obtained by post from:

The Homeopathic Supply Company, 4 Nelson Road, Sherringham, Norfolk NR26 8BU, tel 0263 824683

Biochemic Tissue Salts and Combination Remedies can generally be obtained from homeopathic pharmacies, healthfood shops, and from some chemists, or direct from:

New Era Laboratories Ltd, Marfleet, Hull HU9 5NJ, tel 0482 75234

Bach Flower Remedies are stocked by homeopathic pharmacies and some healthfood shops, or can be bought from:

Bach Flower Remedies Ltd, Mount Vernon, Sotwell, Wallingford, Oxon OX10 0PZ, tel 0491 39489

BIBLIOGRAPHY

HOMEOPATHY

Bannerjee, P. N. *Chronic Diseases: Cause and Cure* Homoeopathy Prachar Karjalaya, Calcutta, 1931

Boericke, W. *Materia Medica with Repertory* Boericke and Tafel, Philadelphia, 1927

Borland, D. M. *Children's Types* British Homoeopathic Association, 1940

Borland, D. M. *Digestive Drugs* British Homoeopathic Association, 1940

Borland, D. M. *Pneumonias* British Homoeopathic Association

Bradford, T. L. *The Life and Letters of Samuel Hahnemann* Royal Publishing House, Calcutta, 1970

Campbell, A. *The Two Faces of Homoeopathy* Robert Hale, 1984

Clark, J. H. *Dictionary of Materia Medica* 3 vols., Homoeopathic Publishing Company, London 1925

Clark, J. H. *Clinical Repertory* Homoeopathic Publishing Company, London, 1904

Clark, J. H. *The Prescriber* Homoeopathic Publishing Company, London, 8th edition, 1952

Clark, J. H. *Indigestion* James Epps, 7th edition, 1912

Gibson, D. H. *First Aid Homoeopathy in Accidents and Ailments* British Homoeopathic Association, 9th edition, 1982

Haehl, R. *Samuel Hahnemann: His Life and Work* 2 vols., Homoeopathic Publishing Company, London, 1922

Hahnemann, Samuel *The Chronic Diseases* 2 vols., translated by L. H. Tafel from 2nd enlarged German edition of 1835, Winger and Company, Calcutta

Hobhouse, R. W. *The Life of Samuel Hahnemann* World Homoeopathic Links, New Delhi, 1984

Hughes, R. *The Manual of Pharmaco-Dynamics* Leith and Ross, 1899

Jahr, G. H. G. *Diseases of Females* Bhatta-Charrya and Company, Calcutta, 1939

Jouanny, J. *Essentials of Homoeopathic Therapeutics* Laboratoire Boiron, Lyon, 1985

Kent, J. T. *Materia Medica* Sinha Roy, Calcutta, 2nd edition, 1970

Kent, J. T. *Lectures on Homoeopathic Philosophy* Erhart and Carl, Chicago, 4th edition, 1937

Kent, J. T. *Final General Repertory* eds. Chand, D. H. and Schmidt, P. Natural Homoeopathic Pharmacy, New Delhi, 2nd edition, 1982

Lessell, C. B. *Homoeopathy for Physicians* Thorsons, 1983

Nash, E. D. *Leaders in Homoeopathic Therapeutics* Boericke and Tafel, Philadelphia, 1946

Neatby, E. A. and Stoneham, T. G. *A Manual of Homoeopathic Therapeutics* Staple Press, 1948

Ostrum, H. I. *Leucorrhea* Set, Dey and Company, Calcutta, 1937

Panos, Maesimund B. and Heimlich, Jane *Homeopathic Medicine at Home* Corgi, 1980

Pratt, N. *Homoeopathic Prescribing* Beaconsfield Publishers, 1980

Roberts, A. H. *The Principles and Art of Cure by Homoeopathy* Homoeopathic Publishing Company, London, 1936

Royal, G. *Diseases of the Brain and Nerves* Boericke and Tafel, Philadelphia, 1928

Sharma, C. *A Manual of Homoeopathy and Natural Medicine* Turnstone Press, 1975

Smith, Trevor *Homoeopathic Medicine* Thorsens, 1982

Smith, Trevor *Homoeopathic Treatment of Emotional Illness* Thorsens, 1983

Smith, Trevor *A Woman's Guide to Homoeopathic Medicine* Thorsons, 1984

Stevenson, J. H. *Helping Yourself with Homoeopathic Remedies* Thorsons, 1976

Tyler, Margaret L. *Homoeopathic Drug Pictures* Health Science Press, 1952

Tyler, Margaret L. and Weir, Sir John *Acute Conditions, Injuries, etc.* British Homoeopathic Association

Wheeler, C. E. *The Principles and Practice of Homoeopathy* Heinemann, 1940

Yingling, W. A. *The Accoucheur's Emergency Manual* Set, Dey and Company, Calcutta, 1936

GENERAL MEDICINE

Baily and Love's: A Short Practice of Surgery revised by Rains, A. J. and Capper, W. M. H. K. Lewis, 14th edition, 1968

Barker, J. E. *Chronic Constipation* John Murray, 1927

Barnes, B. O. and Galton, L. *Hypothyroidism* Thomas Crowell Company, New York, 1976

Benenson, A. S. *The Control of Communicable Diseases in Man* American Public Health Association, Washington, 1975

Bradford, R. W. and Culbert, M. L. *The Metabolic Management of Cancer* Robert Bradford Foundation, California, 1979

Bradford, R. W. and Culbert, M. L. *International Protocols for Individualized Integrated Metabolic Programs and Cancer Management* Robert Bradford Foundation, California, 1981

Cheraskin, E., Ringsdorf, W. M. and Clark, J. W. *Diet and Disease* Keats Health Science, Connecticut, 1977

Crouch, J. E. and McClintick, J. R. *Human Anatomy and Physiology* John Wiley and Sons, New York, 1976

Davidson's Principles of Medicine ed. McLeod, John, Churchill Livingstone, 12th edition, 1977

Davidson, Sir S., Passmore, R., Brock, J. E. and Trusswell, A. S. *Human Nutrition and Dietetics* Churchill Livingstone, 7th edition, 1979

Dorland's Illustrated Medical Dictionary W. R. Saunders, Philadelphia, 26th edition, 1981

Draper, I. T. *Lecture Notes on Neurology* Blackwell, 2nd edition, 1968

Ellison, W. B. and Mitchell, R. G. *Diseases in Infancy and Childhood* E. and S. Churchill, Edinburgh, 1968

Foxen, E. H. M. *Lecture Notes on Diseases of the Ear, Nose and Throat* Blackwell, 2nd edition, 1968

Fredericks, C. *Psycho-Nutrition* Grosset & Dunlap, New York, 1976

Freed, D. L. J. *The Health Hazards of Milk* Bailliere Tindall, 1984

Fry, L. *Dermatology: An Illustrated Guide* Update Publications, 1973

Gerson, M. *Cancer Therapy* Totality Books, California, 3rd edition, 1977

Glaister, J. *Medical Jurisprudence and Toxicology* Churchill Livingtone, 6th edition, 1930

Herxheimer, A. *Side Effects of Drugs* vol. 7, Excerpta Medica, Amsterdam, 1972

Hutchison, J. H. *Practical Paediatric Problems* 4th edition, Lloyd-Luke, 1975

Jensen, B. *Nature has the Remedy* Unity Press, California, 1978

Lawrence, D. R. and Bennett, P. N. *Clinical Pharmacology* Churchill Livingstone, 5th edition, 1980

Ledermann, E. K. *Natural Therapy* Watson & Co., 1953

Lindlahr, H. *Practice of Natural Therapeutics* vol. 2, ed. Proby, J. C. P., C. W. Daniel Company, 1981

McCance and Widdowson *The Composition of Foods* Paul, A. A. and Southgate D. A. T., HMSO, London, 1978

McLeod, J. *Clinical Examination* Churchill Livingstone, 1967

Pfeiffer, C. *Mental and Elemental Nutrients* Keats Publishing Company, Connecticut, 1975

Roe, D. A. *Drug-Induced Nutritional Deficiencies* AVI Publishing Company, Connecticut, 1976

Schauss, A. *Diet, Crime and Delinquency* Parker House, California, 1981

Schroeder, H. *The Poisons Around Us* Keats Publishing Company, Connecticut, 1974

Tomlinson, H. *Aluminium Utensils* L. N. Fowler & Co., 1967

Tredgold, R. F. and Wolff, B. K. *UCH Notes of Psychiatry* Gerald Duckworth, 1970

Walter, J. W. and Israel, M. S. *General Pathology* Churchill Livingstone, 2nd edition, 1965

Warin, J. F., Ironside, A. G. and Mandal, B. K. *Lecture Notes on Infectious Diseases* Blackwell, 3rd edition, 1980

Williams, R. J. and Kalita, D. W. eds. *The Physician's Handbook on Orthomolecular Medicine* Keats Publishing Company, Connecticut, 1977

Williams, P. L. and Warwick, R., eds. *Gray's Anatomy* Churchill Livingstone, 1980

JOURNALS AND PERIODICALS

Doctor
British Journal of Holistic Medicine
British Homoeopathic Journal
Homoeopathy
Homoeopathy Today
Journal of Alternative and Complementary Medicine
Mimm's Magazine
Update
communications from the British Homoeopathy Research Group

Books for further reading

NUTRITION

Ash, Janet and Robert, Dulcie *Happiness is Junk-free Food* Thorsons, 1986

Ballantine, R. *Diet and Nutrition* Himalayan National Institute, Pennsylvania 1978

Budd, M. L. *Low Blood Sugar* Thorsons, 1984

Colgan, M. *Your Personal Vitamin Profile* Blond & Briggs, 1983

Davies, S. and Stewart, A. *Nutritional Medicine* Pan Books, 1987

Elliot, Rose *Vegetarian Mother and Baby Book* Fontana, 1984

Grant, Doris *Food Combining for Health* Thorsons, 1984

Hall, R. H. *Food for Nought* Vintage Books, New York, 1976

Hanssen, M. *E for Additives* Thorsons, 1984

Hasslam, David *Eat It Up: A Parent's Guide to Problems* Macdonald, 1986

Marks, J. *A Guide to the Vitamins* Medical and Technical Publishing, 1975

Marshall, Janette *Shopping for Health* Penguin, 1987

Null, G. *The New Vegetarian* William Morrow & Co., New York, 1978

Pleshette, J. *Health on Your Plate* Hamlyn, 1983

Reuben, D. *The Save Your Life Diet* Ballantine, New York, 1981

Shute, Wilfrid *The Vitamin E Book* Keats Publishing Company, Connecticut, 1975

Stanway, A. *Trace Elements* Vandyke Books, 1983

Tatchell, J. *You and Your Food* Usborne, 1985

Templeton, Louise *The Right Food for Your Kids* Century, 1984

Weaver, Gillian *Feeding Time: How to Cope with Your Child's Eating Problems* Columbus, 1985

GENERAL HEALTH

BMA Family Doctor Home Adviser ed. Smith, T., Dorling Kindersley, 1986

Davidson, J. *Subtle Energy* C. W. Daniel Company, 1986

Davis, Adele *Let's Get Well* Unwin, 1966

Dawood, R. *Traveller's Health* Oxford University Press, 1986

Gardner, A. W. and Roylance, P. J. *New Essential First Aid* Pan Books, 1980

Jensen, B. *Tissue Cleansing through Bowel Management* Bernard Jensen, California, 1980

Leach, P. *Baby and Child* revised edition, Penguin, 1989

The Macmillan Guide to Family Health ed. Smith T., Macmillan, 1982

Physical Fitness: The 11-minute Plan for Men Penguin 1987

Physical Fitness: The 12-minute Plan for Women Penguin 1987

West, R. *The Family Guide to Children's Ailments* Hamlyn, 1983

Ziff, S. *The Toxic Time Bomb* Thorsons, 1984

SPECIFIC PROBLEMS

Chaitow, L. *Candida Albicans* Thorsons, 1985

Chaitow, L. *Vaccination and Immunization* C. W. Daniel Company, 1987

Chaitow, L. and Martin, S. *A World Without AIDS* Thorson, 1988

Cutland, L. *Kick Heroin* Sky Books, 1985

Davidson, J. *Subtle Energy* C. W. Daniel Company, 1986

Davidson, J. *Radiation: what it is, what it does to you, and what we can do about it* C. W. Daniel Company, 1986

Ditzler, James and Ditzler, Joyce *Coming Off Drugs* Papermac, 1986

Grant, E. *The Bitter Pill* Elm Tree Books, 1985

Kilmartin, Angela *Understanding Cystitis* Heinemann, 1973

Kilmartin, Angela *Victims of Thrush and Cystitis* Arrow Books, 1986

Randolph, T. G and Moss, R. W. *Allergies* Turnstone Press, 1981

Woodward, B. *Wired* Faber and Faber, 1984

HOMEOPATHY AND OTHER THERAPIES

Bach, Edward *Heal Thyself* C. W. Daniel Company, 1931, reprinted 1978

Bach, Edward *The Twelve Healers and Other Remedies* C. W. Daniel Company, 1933, reprinted 1973

Blackie, Margery G. *The Patient Not the Cure: The Challenge of Homeopathy* Macdonald & Jane's, 1976

Blackie, Margery G. *Classical Homoeopathy* Beaconsfield Publishers, 1986

Chancellor, P. M. *Handbook of the Bach Flower Remedies* C. W. Daniel Company, 1971, reprinted 1977

Coulter, C. *Portraits of Homeopathic Medicines* (2 vols) North Atlantic Books, Berkeley, 1986

Coulter, H. *Divided Legacy* (3 vols) North Atlantic Books, Berkeley, 1986

Gilbert, P. *A Doctor's Guide to Helping Yourself with Biochemic Tissue Salts* Thorsons, 1984

Hahnemann, Samuel *The Organon of Medicine* tr. Kunli, J., Naude A., and Pendleton, P., Gollancz, 1986

Inglis, B. and West, R. *Alternative Health Guide* Michael Joseph, 1983

Newman-Turner, R. *Naturopathic Medicine* Thorsons, 1984

Tisserand, R. *The Art of Aromatherapy* C. W. Daniel Company, 1977

Ullman, D. *Homeopathy: Medicine for the 21st Century* Thorsons, Wellingborough, 1989

Vithoulkas, George *The Science of Homoeopathy* Grove Press, New York, 1980

Vlamis, G. *Flowers to the Rescue* Thorsons, 1986

INDEX

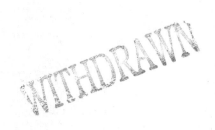